Clinical Gastroenterology

Series Editor
George Y. Wu, Div of Gastroenterology-Hepatology, Univ of Connecticut
School of Medicine, Farmington, CT, USA

Clinical Gastroenterology is a series of concise monographs on diseases commonly encountered in the clinical practice of Internal Medicine and Gastroenterology. Particular emphasis is placed on areas in which knowledge is advancing rapidly. Each volume is concise, concentrating on "clinical pearls," and new advances in diagnostic and therapeutic technology.

Volumes in the series include practical information of companies or laboratories that perform specialized testing, relative costs of diagnostic and therapeutic options. An emphasis is placed on illustrations, especially diagrams and diagnostic/therapeutic algorithms to permit rapid acquisition of practical information that is not readily available in the major texts. Additional unique features include summaries of key points, recommendations, and indications for requesting GI subspecialty consultation.

The series is of great value to Gastroenterologists and Hepatologists interested in the latest practical developments in the field as well as Internists who have particular interests or large numbers of patients with particular diseases in the field of Gastroenterology-Hepatology.

Marko Banić • Damir Erceg
Editors

Drug Interactions in Gastroenterology

A Clinical Guide

Springer

Editors
Marko Banić
Division for IBD and Clinical Nutrition,
Department of Gastroenterology,
Hepatology and Clinical Nutrition
Dubrava University Hospital
Zagreb, Croatia

Damir Erceg
Srebrnjak Children's Hospital
Zagreb, Croatia

ISSN 2197-7399 ISSN 2197-7704 (electronic)
Clinical Gastroenterology
ISBN 978-3-031-69802-6 ISBN 978-3-031-69800-2 (eBook)
https://doi.org/10.1007/978-3-031-69800-2

This Humana imprint is published by the registered company Springer Nature Switzerland AG
The registered company address is: Gewerbestrasse 11, 6330 Cham, Switzerland

Dedicated to all the health professionals who fought COVID-19 pandemic and to those who during that struggle succumbed.

Preface

The nature of digestive diseases represents the reflection of modern civilization and society, characterized by prolonged life expectancy, comorbidity, comedication, and the need for a multidisciplinary approach in patients' management. During the past several years, we have witnessed the evolution of concepts in the treatment of complex digestive diseases, which have significantly improved disease outcomes and patients' quality of life. However, the therapeutic decisions in these patients are often complicated by the need for combined and sequential drug use, taking into account the patients' comorbidities. The discussions with other gastroenterologists, clinical pharmacologists, abdominal surgeons, and microbiologists during numerous occasions in conferences and medical rounds inspired the editors to work on the idea of this book as a clinical guide in dealing with drug interactions in gastroenterology.

Altogether, this book brings 32 chapters, organized into 5 parts. Part I consists of four chapters revealing the journey from substance to drug and highlighting legal and regulatory aspects, the preclinical and clinical research cycle of drug discovery, and the importance of considering drug–drug interactions in clinical medicine. The five chapters in Part II deal with the basic pharmacology of GI drugs, including antisecretory and motility agents, anti-inflammatory and antimicrobial drugs, and mucosal protective agents. Part III is dedicated to the paradigm of distinction between adverse drug reactions and drug interactions and to understanding the basic mechanisms, enzymes, and transporters involved in different types of drug interactions. In this part of the book, the chapters discuss how to avoid drug interactions and also deal with the pharmacogenomics of drug used in gastroenterology and the interactions of these drugs with herbs and food. Part IV discusses comorbidity and the influence of various conditions and diseases on drug interactions, such as cardiorespiratory, renal, and hepatic conditions, immune-mediated diseases, and nervous system disorders. In this part of the book, a very important chapter reveals the impact of the functional status of the gastrointestinal mucosa on oral drug absorption.

The efforts of the authors of chapters in Part V of the book focus on presenting and explaining the clinical aspects of comorbidity in patients with digestive diseases, highlighting the most significant drug interactions in the treatment of acid-related disorders, intestinal inflammation, liver and pancreatobiliary disorders, and functional gastrointestinal disorders.

The authors and editors hope that this book, representing a clinical guide, will drive the attention of potential readers to the importance of recognizing the most common drug interactions in gastroenterology. The content of this clinical guide is aimed at helping health professionals avoid these harmful events and offer patients better disease outcomes.

In general, we believe that our endeavour has the potential to expand the knowledge of medical students and various healthcare professionals while also enhancing the theoretical and practical skills of specialists in different biomedical fields who are involved in treating patients with digestive diseases.

Zagreb, Croatia — Marko Banić
Zagreb, Croatia — Damir Erceg

Acknowledgements

It was not an easy task to conduct the editorial work on this book, *Drug Interactions in Gastroenterology: A Clinical Guide*. We would like to express our gratitude to the people who supported the idea and helped us finalize the project.

The editors would like to extend their special thanks to Professor emeritus George Y. Wu, the editor of the Springer Clinical Gastroenterology Book Series, who supported the general idea of this book.

We started the project with Sheik Mohideen K and finalized it with the help of Ameena Qobrtaj, Maria Christi, Margaret Moore, Paige Rpperger, and Sinchu Mohan. The editors would also like to extend their gratitude to all the members of the Springer Nature editorial team who worked on this book, for their patience, understanding, and dedication.

The time required to carry out and finalize the project somehow encroached upon our family life, and we would like to thank our spouses, Ruža and Sanja, and our children, Luka, Mihael, and Ivan, for their love and support.

The editors would also like to extend their gratitude to all the contributors who did a great job.

Marko Banić
Damir Erceg

Contents

Contributors

Aurora Antolović Amidžić Department of Pharmacology, Faculty of Medicine, J.J. Strossmayer University of Osijek, Osijek, Croatia

Department of Pharmacy, University Hospital Center Osijek, Osijek, Croatia

Roberto Antolović Catholic University of Croatia, Zagreb, Croatia

Žarko Babić Department of Interventional Gastroenterology, Dubrava University Hospital, Zagreb, Croatia

Lidija Bach-Rojecky Faculty of Pharmacy and Biochemistry, University of Zagreb, Zagreb, Croatia

Vesna Bačić Vrca Department of Clinical Pharmacy, Dubrava University Hospital, Zagreb, Croatia

Marko Banić Division for IBD and Clinical Nutrition, Department of Gastroenterology, Hepatology and Clinical Nutrition, Dubrava University Hospital, Zagreb, Croatia

School of Medicine, University of Zagreb, Zagreb, Croatia

School of Medicine, University of Rijeka, Rijeka, Croatia

Ines Baotić Zabok General Hospital and the Croatian Veterans Hospital, Zabok, Croatia

Silvio Bašić Department of Neurology, Dubrava University Hospital, Zagreb, Croatia

Department of Neurology and Neurosurgery, Faculty of Dental Medicine and Health, J. J. Strossmayer University of Osijek, Osijek, Croatia

Milenko Bevanda Division of Gastroenterology and Hepatology, Department of Internal Medicine, University Hospital Mostar, Mostar, Bosnia and Herzegovina

School of Medicine, University of Mostar, Mostar, Bosnia and Herzegovina

Ines Bilić Ćurčić Department of Pharmacology, Faculty of Medicine, J. J. Strossmayer University of Osijek, Osijek, Croatia

Department of Endocrinology, University Hospital Center Osijek, Osijek, Croatia

Alen Bišćanin Department of Gastroenterology and Hepatology, Sestre Milosrdnice University Hospital Center, Zagreb, Croatia

Kristina Bojanić Department of Biophysics and Radiology, Faculty of Dental Medicine and Health Osijek, J. J. Strossmayer University of Osijek, Osijek, Croatia

Department of Biophysics and Radiology, Faculty of Medicine, J. J. Strossmayer University of Osijek, Osijek, Croatia

Department of Radiology, University Hospital Center Osijek, Osijek, Croatia

Tomislav Bokun Department of Gastroenterology, Hepatology and Clinical Nutrition, Dubrava University Hospital, Zagreb, Croatia

Faculty of Pharmacy and Biochemistry, University of Zagreb, Zagreb, Croatia

School of Medicine, University of Zagreb, Zagreb, Croatia

Marko Luka Bošković Dr. Ivan Barbot Neuropscyhiatric Hospital, Popovača, Croatia

Marko Brinar School of Medicine, University of Zagreb, Zagreb, Croatia

Division of Gastroenterology and Hepatology, Department of Internal Medicine, University Hospital Center Zagreb, Zagreb, Croatia

Camelia Bucsa Pharmacovigilance Research Center, Iuliu Hatieganu University of Medicine and Pharmacy, Cluj-Napoca, Cluj, Romania

Petra Ćaćić Department of Gastroenterology and Hepatology, Sestre Milosrdnice University Hospital Center, Zagreb, Croatia

Rok Čivljak Dr. Fran Mihaljević, University Hospital for Infectious Diseases, Zagreb, Croatia

School of Medicine, University of Zagreb, Zagreb, Croatia

Agostino Di Ciaula Clinica Medica “A. Murri”, AOUC Policlinico, Bari, Italy

Viktor Domislović Department of Gastroenterology and Hepatology, University Hospital Center Zagreb, Zagreb, Croatia

Dan Dumitrascu Department of Internal Medicine, Iuliu Hatieganu University of Medicine and Pharmacy, Cluj-Napoca, Romania

Ivan Durlen Department of Nephrology and Dialysis, Dubrava University Hospital, Zagreb, Croatia

Kristina Duspara Department of Pharmacology, Faculty of Medicine, J. J. Strossmayer University of Osijek, Osijek, Croatia

Department of Pharmacology and Biochemistry, Faculty of Dental Medicine and Health Osijek, J. J. Strossmayer University of Osijek, Osijek, Croatia

Public Health Institution, Tuzla, Bosnia and Herzegovina

Damir Erceg Srebrnjak Children's Hospital, Zagreb, Croatia

School of Medicine, Catholic University of Croatia, Zagreb, Croatia

Department of Pharmacology and Biochemistry, Faculty of Dental Medicine and Health Osijek, J. J. Strossmayer University of Osijek, Osijek, Croatia

Department of Pharmacology, Faculty of Medicine, J. J. Strossmayer University of Osijek, Osijek, Croatia

Hrvoje Falak Division of Cardiovascular Diseases, Department of Internal Medicine, Dubrava University Hospital, Zagreb, Croatia

Andreea Farcas Pharmacovigilance Research Center, Iuliu Hatieganu University of Medicine and Pharmacy, Cluj-Napoca, Cluj, Romania

Tajana Filipec Kanižaj Department of Gastroenterology, Merkur University Hospital, Zagreb, Croatia

Romana Gjergja Juraški Srebrnjak Children's Hospital, Zagreb, Croatia

Faculty of Medicine, J.J. Strossmayer University of Osijek, Osijek, Croatia

Ivica Grgurević School of Medicine, University of Zagreb, Zagreb, Croatia

Department of Gastroenterology, Hepatology and Clinical Nutrition, University Hospital Dubrava, Zagreb, Croatia

Faculty of Pharmacy and Biochemistry, University of Zagreb, Zagreb, Croatia

Danijela Grizelj Division of Cardiovascular Diseases, Department of Internal Medicine, Dubrava University Hospital, Zagreb, Croatia

Ivica Horvatić School of Medicine, University of Zagreb, Zagreb, Croatia

Faculty of Pharmacy and Biochemistry, University of Zagreb, Zagreb, Croatia

Department of Nephrology and Dialysis, Dubrava University Hospital, Zagreb, Croatia

Dubravko Jelić Selvita d.o.o, Zagreb, Croatia

Lucija Virović Jukić Department of Gastroenterology and Hepatology, Sestre Milosrdnice University Hospital Center, Zagreb, Croatia

School of Medicine, University of Zagreb, Zagreb, Croatia

Duško Kardum University North, Varaždin, Croatia

Department of Gastroenterology, Merkur University Hospital, Zagreb, Croatia

Faculty of Medicine, J.J. Strossmayer University of Osijek, Osijek, Croatia

Tomislav Kizivat Clinical Institute of Nuclear Medicine and Radiation Protection, University Hospital Center Osijek, Osijek, Croatia

Department for Nuclear Medicine and Oncology, Faculty of Medicine, J. J. Strossmayer University of Osijek, Osijek, Croatia

Sanja Klobučar Department of Endocrinology, Diabetes and Metabolic Diseases, University Hospital Center Rijeka, Rijeka, Croatia

Mia Knobloch Department of Gastroenterology and Hepatology, Sveti Duh University Hospital, Zagreb, Croatia

Željko Krznarić School of Medicine, University of Zagreb, Zagreb, Croatia

Division of Gastroenterology and Hepatology, Department of Internal Medicine, University Hospital Center Zagreb, Zagreb, Croatia

Milan Kujundžić Department of Gastroenterology, Hepatology and Clinical Nutrition, Dubrava University Hospital, Zagreb, Croatia

Lucija Kuna Department of Pharmacology and Biochemistry, Faculty of Dental Medicine and Health, J. J. Strossmayer University of Osijek, Osijek, Croatia

Robert Likić School of Medicine, University of Zagreb, Zagreb, Croatia

Division for Clinical Pharmacology and Therapeutics, Department of Internal Medicine, University Hospital Center Zagreb, Zagreb, Croatia

Marina Madunić Zabok General Hospital and the Croatian Veterans Hospital, Zabok, Croatia

Ivana Mareković Department for Clinical and Molecular Microbiology, University Clinical Hospital Center Zagreb, Zagreb, Croatia

Ivana Marinović Department of Endocrinology, Dubrava University Hospital, Zagreb, Croatia

Ivana Marković Department of Neurology, Dubrava University Hospital, Zagreb, Croatia

Department of Neurology and Neurosurgery, Faculty of Dental Medicine and Health, J. J. Strossmayer University of Osijek, Osijek, Croatia

Darko Marković Selvita d.o.o, Zagreb, Croatia

Marija Martinović Vuk Vrhovac University Clinic for Diabetes, Endocrinology and Metabolic Diseases, Merkur University Hospital, Zagreb, Croatia

Marinko Marušić Department of Gastroenterology and Hepatology, Sveti Duh University Hospital, Zagreb, Croatia

Faculty of Medicine, J. J. Strossmayer University of Osijek, Osijek, Croatia

Faculty of Health Studies, University of Rijeka, Rijeka, Croatia

Srećko Marušić Department of Endocrinology, Dubrava University Hospital, Zagreb, Croatia

School of Medicine, University of Zagreb, Zagreb, Croatia

Mladen Merćep Department of Translational Research, Mediterranean Institute of Life Sciences-MedILS, Split, Croatia

Department of Biotechnology, University of Rijeka, Rijeka, Croatia

Ivana Mikolašević Department of Gastroenterology, University Hospital Center Rijeka, Rijeka, Croatia

School of Medicine, University of Rijeka, Rijeka, Croatia

Marina Mudrovčić Pharmacies Baričević, Zagreb, Croatia

Vjera Ninčević Department of Pharmacology, Faculty of Medicine, J. J. Strossmayer University of Osijek, Osijek, Croatia

Department of Pharmacology and Biochemistry, Faculty of Dental Medicine and Health, J. J. Strossmayer University of Osijek, Osijek, Croatia

Doris Ogresta Department of Gastroenterology and Hepatology, Sestre Milosrdnice University Hospital Center, Zagreb, Croatia

Tea Omanović Kolarić Department of Pharmacology and Biochemistry, Faculty of Dental Medicine and Health, J. J. Strossmayer University of Osijek, Osijek, Croatia

Department of Pharmacology, Faculty of Medicine, J. J. Strossmayer University of Osijek, Osijek, Croatia

Matej Paić Department of Gastroenterology and Hepatology, Sveti Duh University Hospital, Zagreb, Croatia

Eva Pavić Department of Nutrition and Dietetics, University Hospital Center Zagreb, Zagreb, Croatia

Marta Perović Mihanović Dr. Fran Mihaljević, University Hospital for Infectious Diseases, Zagreb, Croatia

Gabrijela Perše Department for Clinical and Molecular Microbiology, University Clinical Hospital Center Zagreb, Zagreb, Croatia

Sanja Pleško Department for Clinical and Molecular Microbiology, University Clinical Hospital Center Zagreb, Zagreb, Croatia

Piero Portincasa Clinica Medica "A. Murri", Department of Precision and Regenerative Medicine and Ionian Area (DiMePre-J), University of Bari Medical School, Bari, Italy

Dragan Primorac St. Catherine Specialty Hospital, Zagreb, Croatia

School of Medicine, University of Split, Split, Croatia

Eberly College of Science, State College, Penn State University, University Park, PA, USA

The Henry C. Lee College of Criminal Justice and Forensic Sciences, University of New Haven, West Haven, CT, USA

Faculty of Medicine, J. J. Strossmayer University of Osijek, Osijek, Croatia

School of Medicine, University of Rijeka, Rijeka, Croatia

Faculty of Dental Medicine and Health, J. J. Strossmayer University of Osijek, Osijek, Croatia

Medical School REGIOMED, Coburg, Germany

Matea Radačić Aumiler Division for Clinical Pharmacology and Therapeutics, Department of Internal Medicine, University Hospital Center Zagreb, Zagreb, Croatia

Department of Biotechnology, University of Rijeka, Rijeka, Croatia

School of Medicine, Catholic University of Croatia, Zagreb, Croatia

Nikola Raguž-Lučić Department of Pharmacology, Faculty of Medicine, J. J. Strossmayer University of Osijek, Osijek, Croatia

Department of Pharmacology and Biochemistry, Faculty of Dental Medicine and Health Osijek, J. J. Strossmayer University of Osijek, Osijek, Croatia

Dario Rahelić Vuk Vrhovac University Clinic for Diabetes, Endocrinology and Metabolic Diseases, Merkur University Hospital, Zagreb, Croatia

School of Medicine, Catholic University of Croatia, Zagreb, Croatia

Faculty of Medicine, J. J. Strossmayer University of Osijek, Osijek, Croatia

Valentina Rahelić Department of Nutrition and Dietetics, University Hospital Center Zagreb, Zagreb, Croatia

Hrvoje Roguljić Department of Internal Medicine, University Hospital Center Osijek, Osijek, Croatia

Department of Pharmacology, Faculty of Medicine, J. J. Strossmayer University of Osijek, Osijek, Croatia

Lucija Romić Vuk Vrhovac University Clinic for Diabetes, Endocrinology and Metabolic Diseases, Merkur University Hospital, Zagreb, Croatia

Ivana Samardžić Department of Clinical Pharmacy, Dubrava University Hospital, Zagreb, Croatia

Department of Endocrinology, Dubrava University Hospital, Zagreb, Croatia

Velimir Šimičević Servier Pharma d.o.o, Zagreb, Croatia

Martina Smolić Department of Pharmacology, Faculty of Medicine, J. J. Strossmayer University of Osijek, Osijek, Croatia

Department of Pharmacology and Biochemistry, Faculty of Dental Medicine and Health Osijek, J. J. Strossmayer University of Osijek, Osijek, Croatia

Robert Smolić Department of Pathophysiology, Faculty of Medicine, J. J. Strossmayer University of Osijek, Osijek, Croatia

Department of Pharmacology and Biochemistry, Faculty of Dental Medicine and Health, J. J. Strossmayer University of Osijek, Osijek, Croatia

Ana Maria Soldo Department of Gastroenterology and Hepatology, Sveti Duh University Hospital, Zagreb, Croatia

Sabina Steiner Srdarević Department of Pharmacology and Biochemistry, Faculty of Dental Medicine and Health Osijek, J. J. Strossmayer University of Osijek, Osijek, Croatia

Zrinka Todorić Department for Clinical and Molecular Microbiology, University Clinical Hospital Center Zagreb, Zagreb, Croatia

Nikolina Tolj Zabok General Hospital and the Croatian Veterans Hospital, Zabok, Croatia

University of Dubrovnik, Dubrovnik, Croatia

Rosana Troskot Perić Department of Gastroenterology and Hepatology, Sveti Duh University Hospital, Zagreb, Croatia

Faculty of Health Studies, University of Rijeka, Rijeka, Croatia

Zabok General Hospital and the Croatian Veterans Hospital, Zabok, Croatia

Mirjana Turkalj Srebrnjak Children's Hospital, Zagreb, Croatia

Faculty of Medicine, J. J. Strossmayer University of Osijek, Osijek, Croatia

Catholic University of Croatia, Zagreb, Croatia

Mario Udovičić Division of Cardiovascular Diseases, Department of Internal Medicine, Dubrava University Hospital, Zagreb, Croatia

Marija Urek Division of Gastroenterology, Hepatology and Clinical Nutrition, Department of Internal Medicine, Dubrava University Hospital, Zagreb, Croatia

School of Medicine, University of Zagreb, Zagreb, Croatia

Aleksandar Včev Department of Pathophysiology and Physiology with Immunology, Faculty of Dental Medicine and Health, J. J. Strossmayer University of Osijek, Osijek, Croatia

Department of Internal Medicine, University Hospital Center Osijek, Osijek, Croatia

Sonja Vukadin Department of Pharmacology and Biochemistry, Faculty of Dental Medicine and Health, J. J. Strossmayer University of Osijek, Osijek, Croatia

Department of Pharmacology, Faculty of Medicine, J. J. Strossmayer University of Osijek, Osijek, Croatia

David Q.-H. Wang Department of Medicine and Genetics, Division of Gastroenterology and Liver Diseases, Marion Bessin Liver Research Center, Einstein-Mount Sinai Diabetes Research Center, Albert Einstein College of Medicine, Bronx, NY, USA

Marko Zelenika Department of Gastroenterology, Hepatology and Clinical Nutrition, Dubrava University Hospital, Zagreb, Croatia

School of Medicine, University of Zagreb, Zagreb, Croatia

Part I

Drug Journey: From Substance to Drug

Regulatory and Legal Aspects of the Drug Lifecycle

1

Velimir Šimičević

Introduction

The European Medicines Agency (EMA) defines a drug/medicinal product as a substance, or combination of substances that are intended to treat, prevent, or diagnose a disease, or to restore, correct, or modify physiological functions by exerting a pharmacological, immunological, or metabolic action [1]. The process to discover, develop, obtain, and maintain regulatory approval for a new drug to be launched onto the market requires an immense amount of time (on average 10 years), effort, and investment (on average 2.8 billion USD, including post-approval research and development costs) [2]. The entire process is highly controlled, and the pharmaceutical industry is considered to be one of the most highly regulated industries in the world with strict restrictions on patenting, testing, marketing and safety of the products supplied. Countries possess their own regulatory authority, which is responsible for enforcing the rules and regulations and issue the guidelines to regulate drug development process, licensing, registration, manufacturing, marketing, labeling, and the product life cycle of pharmaceutical products.

Some of these authorities include:

- The EMA (European Union)—European Medicines Agency (https://www.ema.europa.eu/)
- The FDA (USA)—Food and Drug Administration (www.fda.gov/)
- The PMDA (Japan)—Pharmaceuticals and Medical Devices Agency (https://www.pmda.go.jp/)

V. Šimičević (✉)
Servier Pharma d.o.o, Zagreb, Croatia
e-mail: velimir.simicevic@servier.com

M. Banić, D. Erceg (eds.), *Drug Interactions in Gastroenterology*, Clinical Gastroenterology, https://doi.org/10.1007/978-3-031-69800-2_1

- The MHRA (United Kingdom)—Medicines and Healthcare products Regulatory Agency (https://www.gov.uk/government/organisations/medicines-and-healthcare-products-regulatory-agency/)
- The HC (Canada)—Health Canada (https://www.canada.ca/)
- The TGA (Australia)—Therapeutic Goods Administration (https://tga.gov.au/)

It is the role and responsibility of governments and their regulatory authorities to bring forth and enforce legislative acts and regulations. Regulations are based on the legal acts and define processes to a greater degree. Regulations lead to the creation of guidelines which are then used by regulatory authorities to clarify requirements and provide advice. Guidelines are usually specific to a therapeutic area or technical discipline. It is the responsibility of the pharmaceutical industry to conduct the processes of drug discovery, non-clinical and clinical development as well as post-authorization activities in strict adherence to these acts and regulations, thus preparing documentation which will be used to obtain and maintain the authorization of a drug on the respective market.

Other than national authorities, certain international organizations are also involved in the development and maintenance of safe and efficacious drugs. These organizations include:

- WHO—World Health Organization (www.who.int/)
- ICH—International Council on Harmonization (https://www.ich.org/)[1]
- PIC/S—Pharmaceutical Inspection Co-operation Scheme (https://pic-scheme.org/)
- ISO—International Organization for Standardization (https://www.iso.org/)

They are tasked with the responsibility of developing and promoting high and harmonized standards as well as guidance documents to ensure the quality, safety, and efficiency of products, services, and systems.

The following text will show how the development and maintenance of a drug is impacted by various legislative acts, regulations and guidance documents.

Drug Discovery and Development

Drug Discovery

Drug discovery is the process of identifying potential new medicines. It involves a wide range of various scientific disciplines, including biology, chemistry, and

[1]The International Council on Harmonisation (ICH) was created in April 1990 at a meeting in Brussels. ICH had the initial objective of coordinating the regulatory activities of the European, Japanese and United States regulatory bodies in consultation with the pharmaceutical trade associations from these regions, to discuss and agree the scientific aspects arising from product registration.

pharmacology (see also Chap. 2). Thousands of candidates are identified and screened. On average, only one to two of every 10,000 substances synthesized in laboratories will successfully pass all stages of development required to become a marketable drug [3]. Regulatory authorities have minimal oversight into this phase of the drug development process, yet do provide certain requirements and clear documentation to achieve milestones.

Non-clinical Data

Once a lead compound has been identified, preclinical studies are initiated (see also Chap. 2). Their objective is to determine the pharmacology (efficacy and mode of action, pharmacodynamics) and safety pharmacology (identification of undesirable pharmacodynamic properties that may have relevance to its human safety and investigation of its mechanism) of the compound, its pharmacokinetic and toxicokinetic properties (absorption, distribution, metabolism, and excretion), toxicology (single and repeat-dose toxicity, genotoxicity, carcinogenicity, reproductive/developmental and juvenile toxicity, local tolerance, and immunotoxicity) and environmental risk assessment. These studies are conducted in animal models through model systems in vitro, in vivo or ex vivo. Their primary goal is to predict drug behavior in humans and identify potential risks that may allow for the transition from animal studies to human clinical trials, as well as being used to support regulatory filings. In order to expedite non-clinical requirements for global regulatory submissions, the ICH created a list of guidance documents regarding non-clinical investigations.[2] However, in addition to the ICH, regulatory authorities, such as the EMA (European Union), have also published specific guidelines determining the requirements for non-clinical investigations.

The majority of preclinical studies are conducted in line with Good Laboratory Practice (GLP). GLP is a set of principles intended to assure the quality and integrity of non-clinical laboratory studies that are intended to support research or marketing authorizations for products regulated by government agencies. They define technical matters such as laboratory methods, documentation, data handling, instrument calibration, and much more that are connected with the actual conduct of testing at the non-clinical level. The regulations in the United States can be found in 21 CFR Part 58.1 [4] and, for the European Union, through the Organization for Economic Co-operation and Development (OECD) [5].

Once an adequate amount of preclinical data is gathered and analyzed, the decision to proceed toward clinical trials is taken based on the fact if the collected data in preclinical studies has shown that the drug is safe enough to be administered in human subjects.

In the United States, the applicant must first submit an investigational new drug (IND) application to the FDA (discussed in a later chapter of this book) which is a

[2]The entire set of guidance documents (including non-clinical investigations) may be accessed at https://www.ich.org/page/ich-guidelines.

mandatory requirement to allow clinical investigations on drugs that do not possess a valid approval. Additionally, an IND application also allows the shipment of unapproved drug across state lines in the United States, as only marketed drugs are allowed to be shipped from state to state. In this sense, the IND also has a temporary legal function [6].

In other countries, such as in the European Union, the step to obtain such approval prior to the initiation of clinical trials is not mandatory; however, applicants may contact regulatory authorities in order to request scientific advice that should guide them in conducting the appropriate studies, so that no major objections are likely to be raised during the evaluation of the data [7].

Clinical Data

Clinical research represents the bridge between the basic, non-clinical investigations performed in the laboratory and patients (see also Chap. 3). Setting up clinical studies is a lengthy process, as there are many documents to prepare (e.g. protocols and case report forms (CRFs)), study facilities to be assessed (e.g. study sites, Contract Research Organizations (CROs), and clinical laboratories), regulatory review to be considered and negotiations and agreements with study sites (e.g. contracts, finances, confidentiality, indemnity, and insurance) to be undertaken as well as the manufacturing of the medicinal product to be used in clinical trials (also referred to as the Investigated Medicinal Product—IMP). Similar to GLP governing the conduct of preclinical investigations, clinical studies are conducted in line with Good Clinical Practice (GCP). GCP can be defined as a standard for the design, conduct, performance, monitoring, auditing, recording, analyses, and reporting of clinical trials that provides assurance that the data and reported results are credible and accurate, and that the rights, integrity, and confidentiality of trial subjects have been protected [8].

The various phases of clinical research will be discussed in other chapters of this book and will not be described in detail here. However, they all have a common denominator and that is human subject safety. Therefore all subjects enrolled in clinical trials are closely monitored and the trials themselves are supervised by appropriate regulatory authorities as well as by the Sponsor of the trial itself. All trials that involve a therapeutic intervention with an IMP must be approved by an Independent Ethical Committee (EC) or Institutional Review Board (IRB) prior to approval of the clinical trial itself, and this must be documented in compliance with international guidelines and the local regulations of the country in which the research is conducted [9]. The EC or IRB assesses the informed consent process, benefits and risks and how volunteers will be selected in the process.

Informed consent was first formulated under international law through the Declaration of Helsinki, in response to the atrocities of the Second World War and its principles are still under continuous review and discussion [10] due to the evolving nature of the involved IMPS as well as the nature of the trials themselves.

Furthermore, to ensure that trial subjects are not placed at risk and that the results of clinical trials are unaffected by inadequate safety, quality, or efficacy arising from unsatisfactory manufacturing, procedures for the manufacturing, packaging, labeling, shipping, accounting, reconciling and disposing of IMPs must comply with relevant Good Manufacturing Practice (GMP) requirements. GMP can be defined as a system for ensuring that products are consistently produced and controlled according to quality standards. It is designed to minimize the risks involved in any pharmaceutical production that cannot be eliminated through testing the final product and has been incorporated into local legislation [11, 12].

Submission of Marketing Applications

Once all of the steps in drug development are accomplished and all information and results, including investigations from the preclinical studies as well as the results of all conducted clinical trials, are available, the Common Technical Document (CTD) is prepared [13]. The CTD is a submission dossier that has been designed to provide a common format between Europe, the United States, and Japan for the documentation included in an application for the registration of a human pharmaceutical product, and its structure is detailed in the ICH M4 guidelines [14]. The CTD dossier is divided into five main modules:

Module 1: Administrative information and prescribing information
Module 2: Overviews and summaries of Modules 3–5
Module 3: Quality (pharmaceutical documentation)
Module 4: Non-clinical reports (pharmacology/toxicology)
Module 5: Clinical study reports (clinical trials)

Module 1 is not strictly included in the CTD since it contains documents that are specific to each region, e.g. application forms or the proposed label. The content and format of this module is specific to individual Regulatory Authorities. Unlike Module 1, Modules 2–5, are common to all the regions. The document may also be submitted in electronic form (eCTD).

The (e)CTD provides an accurate format to transfer the obtained product information to the regulatory authority for assessment. In the United States, this is the Food and Drug Administration; in the United Kingdom, the MHRA; in Japan, the PMDA, etc. In the European Union, applicants have the option to submit the application for the marketing authorization of a new drug by three different procedures:

1. **Centralized Procedure (CP)**: There is a single application, a single evaluation and a single authorization issued throughout the European Union. The procedure is mandatory for specific types of medicines: products obtained by means of biotechnology and other high-technology methods, products intended for the treatment of HIV, cancer, diabetes or neurodegenerative diseases and autoimmune diseases, as well as products for orphan medicinal products intended for

the treatment of rare diseases (the prevalence of the condition in the EU must not be more than 5 in 10,000). EMA's Committee for Medicinal Products for Human Use (CHMP) carries out the scientific assessment of the application and give a recommendation on whether the medicine should be marketed or not. However, under EU law, the EMA has no authority to actually permit marketing in the different EU countries. The European Commission is the authorizing body for all centrally authorized products, which takes a legally binding decision based on EMA's recommendation. This decision is issued within 67 days of receipt of EMA's recommendation [15]. Once approved, the product has the same tradename in all EU Member States, and the product information[3] is identical in all Member States.

2. **Decentralized Procedure (DCP)**: The procedure for authorizing medicines in more than one European Union Member State in parallel. It can be used for medicines that do not need to be authorized via the centralized procedure and *have not already been authorized* in any Member State. Briefly, the applicant decides in which countries of the EU the product will be marketed and decides which country will be the Reference Member State (RMS).[4] The application is then submitted to the RMS and the remaining countries in which the product will be marketed (Concerned Member States, CMS). The RMS and CMS validate the submission after which the RMS reviews the application and issues a preliminary assessment report (PAR) to the CMS. The CMS in turn then give their comments and these comments, along with the PAR are sent to the applicant who must respond to any questions or issues. Once the applicant has responded, the RMS issues the Draft Assessment Report to the CMS and Applicant and the CMS then approves the Assessment Report. Following this step, the RMS issues the Marketing Authorization (MA) for its country and each CMS initiates the national phase of the approval in which it approves the product information in the local language. Once approved, the product may the same or different tradename in each of the EU Member States where the product is approved, but the product information is identical in all the CMS [16].
3. **National Procedure (NP)**: A procedure through which authorization of a new product is granted in only *one* European Union Member State. If the applicant wishes to register in another EU Member State, the submission automatically triggers a DCP.

[3]The Product Information consists of the approved Summary of Product Characteristics (SmPC), the labelling and the Patient Information Leaflet (PIL).

[4]The European Union Member State that leads the review of an application in a decentralized procedure.

Post-authorization Activities

After granting a marketing authorization, the marketing authorization holder is obliged, according to applicable laws and regulations, to report to regulatory authorities all variations/post-approval changes to the previously authorized documentation throughout the drug's life cycle. Variations/post-approval changes may be administrative variations (i.e. change of the manufacturer's address, change to the product's tradename), change in the documentation on quality (i.e. change in the manufacturing procedure, quality control methods), change in safety information resulting through new post-authorization studies (i.e. inclusion of new adverse effects in the patient information leaflet or results of clinical data in special population groups such as elderly or hepatically/renally impaired patients) and changes in indications (adding or omitting certain indications). The marketing authorization holder is required to follow the newest scientific and technological advances in the field of development, testing and regulations of drugs and implement them through variations of the medicinal product that is on the market [17, 18].

Particular emphasis must be placed on the change to safety information. As pointed out earlier in the text, the main principle of the drug development process is human safety. As clinical trials have their limitations in this process (in the sense of small number of treated patients compared to the target population, lack of concomitant diseases and/or medication, long-term treatment data are limited, etc.) [19], it is the responsibility and obligation of the marketing authorization holder to continuously collect data regarding the safety of the use of the approved drug. This process falls under the scope of pharmacovigilance, and the data collected is submitted to regulatory authorities in line with the ICH guideline E2C (R2) on periodic benefit-risk evaluation report (PBRER) that has been transferred into local national legislation of various countries [20].

The main focus of the PBRER is the evaluation of relevant new safety information from the available data sources, placed within the context of any pertinent efficacy/effectiveness information that may have become available since the date of the first marketing approval in any country in the world. All pertinent new safety and efficacy/effectiveness information discovered during the reporting interval should be discussed in the appropriate sections of the PBRER. The need for the submission of a PBRER and the frequency of report submission to regulatory authorities are subject to national or regional regulatory requirements and usually depend on such factors as approval dates, the length of time the product has been on the market, and the extent of knowledge of the benefit-risk profile of the product. The PBRER format and content are intended to apply to periodic reports that cover reporting periods of 6 months or longer. Once a drug has been marketed for several years, national or regional regulation may allow the frequency of submission to be extended to longer time intervals, e.g., greater than 1 year for products considered to have an established and acceptable profile or considered to be low risk, however, more frequent PBRERs may continue to be required in other regions [20].

Patents/Data Exclusivity

As stated earlier the process to discover, develop, obtain and maintain regulatory approval for a new drug to be launched onto the market requires an immense amount of time, effort and investment. The manner in which a pharmaceutical company is able to recoup the development costs and to earn profit to invest in the development of future drugs is through the obtaining of patents. Pharmaceutical companies will patent any molecule that shows promise early in the development process [21]. Patents prevent other companies from copying it for 20 years and cover many aspects of the intellectual property of a drug, including the active substance, manufacturing, formulations, and, in some cases, its use. Once a patent has expired, other companies may bring copies of the drug onto the market.

Other than patents, another important intellectual property right is data exclusivity as the pharmaceutical sector is heavily regulated, with significant costs associated with both developing a new medicinal product and generating the data required to get a product to market, protecting that data is important. Data exclusivity is a form of product exclusivity right for medicinal products. The rationale for granting data exclusivity is to compensate the innovator company for the investment it has put in to developing the new medicinal product and to generate the data required to obtain a marketing authorization. An innovator company enjoys a period of data exclusivity during which their preclinical and clinical trials data may not be referenced in the regulatory filings of another company for the same drug substance. Unlike patents which last for 20 years, data exclusivity may vary. For example, in the United States, data exclusivity for a new chemical entity is for 5 years, for an orphan drug 8 years and 12 years for a biologic drug [22] while in the European Union data exclusivity for a new molecule may be upto 11 years (8 years of data exclusivity, followed by 2 years of market exclusivity at which time a generic may be approved by a regulatory authority but may not be placed on the market which may be prolonged by an additional year if a significant new indication for the relevant medicinal product is granted) [23].

Generic Drugs

Although this chapter mainly dealt with the legal and regulatory aspects of the full drug development process that includes preclinical and clinical investigations, it should also be mentioned that the development of generic drugs bears the same legal scrutiny.

Generic drug development uses a different approach and strategy compared to that used to develop an innovator drug product. However, the key factor is that the generic drug manufacturer must meet the same standards with regards to GMP and GCP (in bioequivalency studies) when conducting its development as well as its obligations in the post-authorization period with regards to the quality and safety of the product.

References

1. Medicinal Product. https://www.ema.europa.eu/en/glossary/medicinal-product. Accessed 23 Apr 2022.
2. DiMasi JA, Grabowski HG, Hansen RW. Innovation in the pharmaceutical industry: new estimates of R&D costs. J Health Econ. 2016;47:20–33. https://doi.org/10.1016/j.jhealeco.2016.01.012.
3. The Pharmaceutical Industry in Figures 2021. https://www.efpia.eu/media/602709/the-pharmaceutical-industry-in-figures-2021.pdf. Accessed 23 Apr 2022.
4. CFR—Code of Federal Regulations Title 21 Part 58—Good laboratory practice for nonclinical laboratory studies. https://www.govinfo.gov/app/details/CFR-2011-title21-vol1/CFR-2011-title21-vol1-part58. Accessed 23 Apr 2022.
5. OECD series on principles of good laboratory practice and compliance monitoring. https://www.oecd-ilibrary.org/environment/oecd-series-on-principles-of-good-laboratory-practice-and-compliance-monitoring_2077785x. Accessed 23 Apr 2022.
6. Food and Drug Administration. Investigational new drug (IND) application. https://www.fda.gov/drugs/types-applications/investigational-new-drug-ind-application. Accessed 26 Apr 2022.
7. European Medicines Agency. Scientific advice and protocol assistance. https://www.ema.europa.eu/en/human-regulatory/research-development/scientific-advice-protocol-assistance. Accessed 26 Apr 2022.
8. ICH guideline E6 (R2) Good Clinical Practice (GCP). https://www.ich.org/page/efficacy-guidelines. Accessed 23 Apr 2022.
9. Bohaychuk W, Ball G. Good clinical practices. In: Edwards LD, Fletcher AJ, Fox AW, Stonier PD, editors. Principles and practices of pharmaceutical medicine. 2nd ed. Wiley; 2007.
10. Gupta UC. Informed consent in clinical research: revisiting few concepts and areas. Perspect Clin Res. 2013;4:26–32. https://doi.org/10.4103/2229-3485.106373.
11. EudraLex the rules governing medicinal products in the European Union Volume 4 EU GMP Annex 13: Investigational medicinal products. https://www.gmp-compliance.org/files/guidemgr/2009_06_annex13.pdf. Accessed 23 Apr 2022.
12. FDA Guidance for Industry: guideline for the preparation of investigational new drug products (human and animal). 1991. https://www.fda.gov/regulatory-information/search-fda-guidance-documents. Accessed 23 Apr 2022.
13. Jordan D. An overview of the Common Technical Document (CTD) regulatory dossier. Med Writing. 2014;23(2):101–5.
14. ICH M4 Guideline: Organisation of the common technical document for the registration of pharmaceuticals for human use (R3). https://www.ich.org/page/ctd. Accessed 23 Apr 2022.
15. European Medicines Agency. Authorisation of medicines—centralised authorisation procedure. https://www.ema.europa.eu/en/about-us/what-we-do/authorisation-medicines. Accessed 24 Apr 2022.
16. CMDH. Decentralised procedure member states' standard operating procedure. https://www.hma.eu/human-medicines/cmdh/procedural-guidance/application-for-ma/dcp.html. Accessed 24 Apr 2022.
17. European Medicines Agency. Post-authorisation. https://www.ema.europa.eu/en/human-regulatory/post-authorisation. Accessed 24 Apr 2022.
18. U.S. Department of Health and Human Services Food and Drug Administration Center for Drug Evaluation and Research (CDER). Changes to an approved NDA or ANDA. 2004. https://www.fda.gov/files/drugs/published/Changes-to-an-Approved-NDA-or-ANDA.pdf. Accessed 24 Apr 2022.
19. Beaulieu-Jones BK, Finlayson SG, Yuan W, Altman RB, Kohane IS, Prasad V, Yu KH. Examining the use of real-world evidence in the regulatory process. Clin Pharmacol Ther. 2020;107(4):843–52. https://doi.org/10.1002/cpt.1658. Epub 2019 Nov 14.

20. ICH guideline E2C (R2) on periodic benefit-risk evaluation report (PBRER). https://www.ich.org/page/efficacy-guidelines. Accessed 24 Apr 2022.
21. Lopez G. Patents. In: Edwards LD, Fletcher AJ, Fox AW, Stonier PD, editors. Principles and practices of pharmaceutical medicine. 2nd ed. Wiley; 2007.
22. FDA frequently asked questions on patents and exclusivity. https://www.fda.gov/drugs/development-approval-process-drugs/frequently-asked-questions-patents-and-exclusivity. Accessed 24 Apr 2022.
23. European Medicines Agency. Data exclusivity/Generics/Biosimilars: regulatory and procedural guidance. https://www.ema.europa.eu/en/human-regulatory/marketing-authorisation/guidance-documents/data-exclusivity-generics-biosimilars-regulatory-procedural-guidance. Accessed 24 Apr 2022.

Preclinical Research in Drug Discovery 2

Roberto Antolović, Dubravko Jelić, and Darko Marković

Drug Journey: From Substance to Drug

Preclinical pharmacology and toxicology are essential elements of the drug discovery and development process and are critical in enabling the translation of findings from the laboratory and the clinic. The drug discovery process is complex and involves numerous iterative steps designed to optimise the pharmacological and drug-like properties of a candidate molecule, a New Chemical Entity (NCE), and minimise the potential for side effects and toxicities [1]. The drug discovery and development process of creation of the new drug is long (usually takes 10–15 years on average) and expensive (on average 2.8 billion USD), but highly important process, which can be divided into three main pharmaceutical phases, drug discovery, drug development and drug commercialisation (see also Chap. 1).

Drug discovery research process usually starts with a new original idea about a biologically relevant drug target, which needs to be validated first for its druggability during discovery phases of target validation. Another option is phenotypic-based drug discovery, where deconvolution of possible target(s) is done in later stage of drug discovery process. After completion of this initial phase, new compounds are profiled during hit finding (HF), hit-to-lead (H2L), lead optimisation (LO) and candidate selection (CS) phases. Target validation, discovery, and translational phases hopefully ends up with the clinical trials, such as the first time in human (FTiH), and

R. Antolović (✉)
Catholic University of Croatia, Zagreb, Croatia
e-mail: roberto.antolovic@unicath.hr

D. Jelić · D. Marković
Selvita d.o.o, Zagreb, Croatia
e-mail: dubravko.jelic@selvita.com; darko.markovic@selvita.com

M. Banić, D. Erceg (eds.), *Drug Interactions in Gastroenterology*, Clinical Gastroenterology, https://doi.org/10.1007/978-3-031-69800-2_2

I–III (IV) clinical studies on human subjects, all up to the product marketing (Fig. 2.1).

Such a discovery and development process is long and complicated and is usually associated with a very low chance of success. There are, of course, positive examples and many success stories, where compounds will reach patients and help cure their diseases, which often represents unmet medical needs. Especially important parameter in drug discovery process is integration. Integrated project teams are usually the driving forces of this process. They usually consist chemistry teams, which work together on particular chemical scaffolds and new synthesis methodologies in medicinal chemistry, directed to the generation of new chemical entities. Medicinal chemists usually work together with drug modelling experts (or apply in silico tools) in planning their chemistry tasks. Additionally, integrated research project teams also include a number of biology/pharmacology and DMPK (drug metabolism and pharmacokinetics) experts (both in vitro and in vivo) who are involved in the daily/weekly/monthly testing of the newly synthesised compounds and building of structure-activity relationship (SAR) knowledge. All this enable efficient and fast synthesis/pharmacology optimisation turnover cycles, with creation of higher chances for better lead identification and selection of optimal candidates.

In general, drug discovery research phase is a long-term process, which usually takes many years of hard work within numerous scientific groups and disciplines (Fig. 2.2).

This chapter will focus on the main principles and research activities in the process of preclinical drug discovery and development, starting from different approaches to define a new chemical entity, which may have the pharmacophoretic properties and potential to modify selected target with optimal activity, high specificity and required safety profile.

In the preclinical drug discovery process, few different but overlapping activities are essential for effective hit discovery, lead optimisation, ADME, translational and

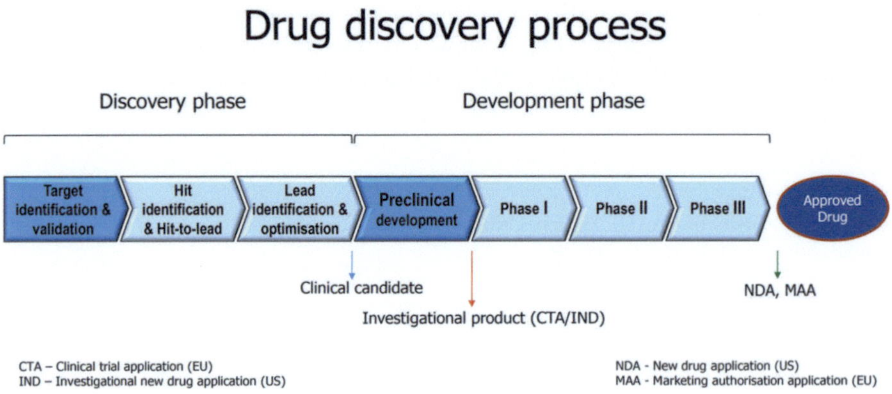

Fig. 2.1 Drug discovery process

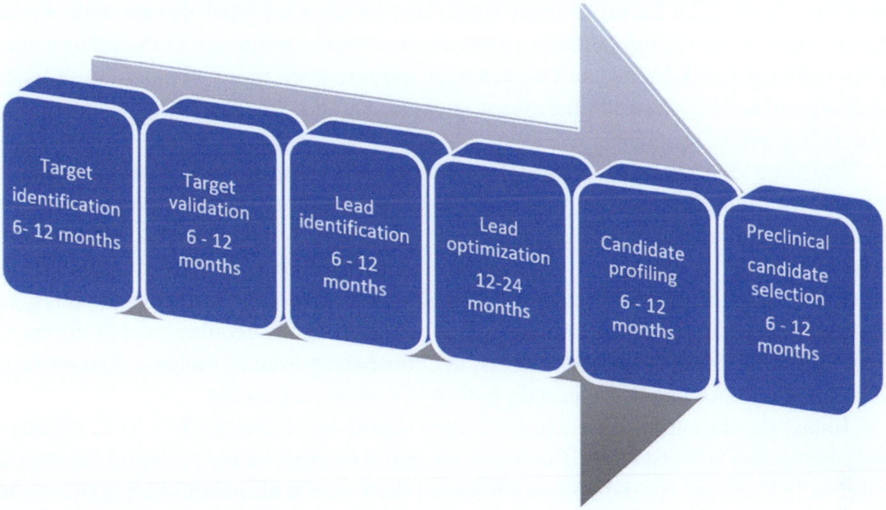

Fig. 2.2 Duration of the major steps in the preclinical drug development

safety profiling, as well as candidate selection in the modern pharmaceutical industry. These activities include:

- Target identification and validation
- Bioassay and in vitro screening development to measure the biological activity (High-Throughput and High-Content Screening)
- Identification of Hits and optimisation of Leads
- Absorption, distribution, metabolism and excretion (ADME) studies
- Ex vivo and translational medicine studies
- In vivo experimental models and Safety Pharmacology
- Preclinical candidate final selection

Target Identification and Validation

A biological target is a broad term which can be applied to a range of biological entities, which may include, e.g., membrane proteins as receptors or cytosolic proteins like enzymes, hormones, genes, RNA, etc. Targets usually play a significant role in the homeostatic misbalance characteristic for particular disease states [2]. A drug should modulate the activity of the therapeutic target or, in other words, the target has to be 'druggable'. At the same time, the modulation of the target under physiological conditions, or in other diseases, should have a minor impact. Today is very well known that certain target classes are more amenable to small molecule drug discovery, for example, G-protein-coupled receptors (GPCRs), whereas larger molecules as antibodies or recombinant proteins are good at blocking protein/protein interactions. Genetic targets are genes or gene products that, in specific diseases, have been found to carry mutations or have a higher disease risk. Good target identification and validation enables increased confidence in the relationship between target and disease and allows us to explore even more whether target modulation will lead to desired pharmacological effect and can also clarify mechanism-based side effects [3].

The drug discovery process is faced today with the identification of growing number of biological targets, which are directly or indirectly connected to a certain disease caused by change of physiological into the pathophysiological process and development of the disease. Understanding of the principles and essential processes in the cell signalling within and between the cells as well as knowing the possible biochemical changes in the signalling pathways on his molecular level is the basic approach which will allow the scientist to choose the potential biological target suitable for the treatment of the certain pathophysiological process.

Today, the data mining of available data stored and ready for use from different data banks has led to a significant increase in the number of the potential biological targets. In this context, data mining refers to the use of a bioinformatics approach to not only help in identifying but also selecting and prioritising potential disease targets [4]. It is estimated that 4479 (22%) of the 20,300 protein-coding genes annotated in Ensemble version 73 are drugged or druggable [5]. The data which are available in commercially available or the data banks of big pharma companies come from a variety of sources including scientific publications and patent information, gene expression data, proteomics, phosphoproteomics, glycomics data, transgenic phenotyping and compound profiling data. Identification approaches also include examining mRNA/protein levels to determine whether they are expressed in disease and if they are correlated with disease exacerbation or progression. Target validation studies apply genetic knockdown, knockout, or if available, the use of well-defined and characterised specific inhibitors or modulators of the certain target or antibodies against the target in question. In vitro cell-based mechanistic studies are used to reveal target characteristics and the pathways connected to the targets. The discovery of small interfering RNA (siRNA) facilitated the use of high-throughput reverse genetic screens whereby specific genes are downregulated and the phenotype is assessed [6]. Similarly, large-scale transfection screens are utilised in order to identify genes responsible for transforming phenotype [7]. All of these in vitro methods directly establish causality to the modification of the target. Another powerful approach is to look for genetic associations; for example, is there a link between a genetic polymorphism and the risk of disease or disease progression, or is the polymorphism functional. An alternative approach is to use phenotypic screening to identify disease-relevant targets as a phage-display antibody library to isolate human monoclonal antibodies (mAbs) that bind to the surface of tumour cells [8].

The most straightforward approach towards assessing protein druggability is a biochemical or cell-based screen of a large compound collection [9]. In this way, the vast number of different types of small molecule hits can be identified and recognised and to achieve that goal, the compound collection must be chemically diverse and large, usually comprising more than 100,000 or even more than one million compounds [10]. Conventional screening depends on a library of drug-like compounds, which is all selected to be consistent with Lipinski's rule of 5 [11].

Bioassay Development to Measure the Biological Activity

The field of bioassay development had evolved considerably since technological advances in basic sciences at the end of the nineteenth and the beginning of the twentieth century improved traditional medicine and serendipitous findings, especially during the early 1990s, when the parallel and combinatorial chemistry, as well as high-throughput biological screening revolution, began. The concept of using a "high-throughput" paradigm for both chemistry and biology within drug discovery has advanced considerably in the last few decades. With advances in automatisation and miniaturisation of biological screening techniques, biological testing is no longer the 'bottleneck' of research and development process [12]. With this development, the productivity of biological screening increased, while the price decreased, which made the high-throughput 'paradigm' available to the broad scientific community. The number of druggable therapeutic targets, types of biological assays, and number of detection methods have greatly increased [13].

High-throughput screening (HTS) is an automatised method for faster and simpler identification of bioactive compounds from different compound collections, using parallel testing in 96 (or more)-well microtitre plates. It involves the use of robotics, data processing, automation, liquid handling devices (including nano pipetting units) and sensitive multifunctional and multiplex detectors for specific assay readouts, which significantly facilitates target-based or phenotypic-based drug discovery (Fig. 2.3).

Microtitre plates (or multiwell plates), with differing numbers of wells (96, 384, 1536, 3456, etc.), as well as various types of (multichannel) pipettes, are among the essential screening tools (Fig. 2.4).

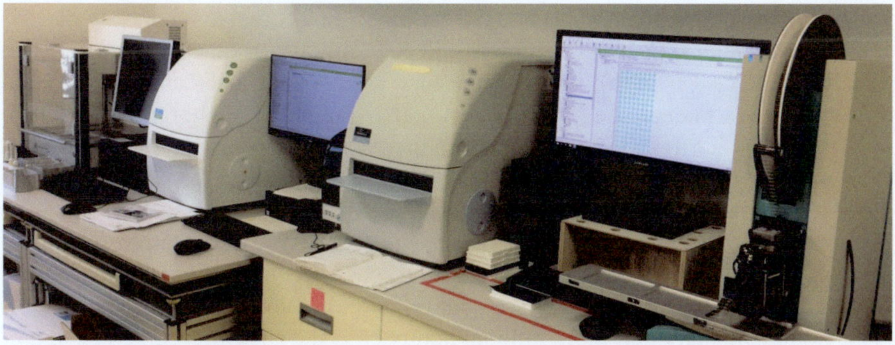

Fig. 2.3 Examples of automated liquid handling devices and multifunctional readers used in biological screening (from left to right): Brand Liquid Handling Station (BrandTech Scientific), EnVision 2105 (Perkin Elmer), EnVision 2104 (Perkin Elmer), Mosquito (SPT labtech). (Picture is taken in Selvita d.o.o. in Zagreb)

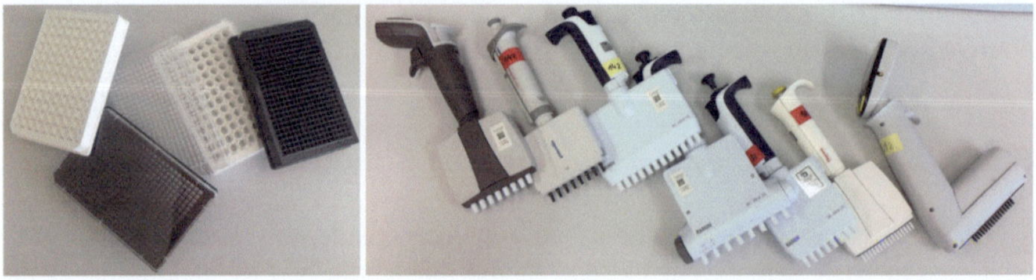

Fig. 2.4 Microtitre plates of various formats (left) and various types of (multichannel) pipettes (right) used for bioassay development and screening

Automation allows the scientist to gain important biological data quickly and precisely, with a high level of reproducibility, following pre-defined activity limits and assay robustness and performance quality control (QC) parameters (Z' as ratio of the means and standard deviations of positive and negative controls, Signal/Background as ratio of maximum to background signal within the assay, and Hill Slope as the highest absolute value of the sigmoidal curve slope). Many logarithmic (dose) response curves follow the familiar symmetrical sigmoidal shape. The main goal of fitting the dose-response curve in many situations is to determine the best-fit value of the XC_{50} value, which is the concentration of tested compound that provokes a response halfway between the top and bottom plateaus of the readout signal (inflection point, or 50% inhibition). If these plateaus are not well defined, the XC_{50} will be very uncertain. The XC_{50} parameter for activity uses the Michaelis-Menten equation, which describes, for example, enzyme activity as a function of substrate concentration [14]. Inhibitory (antagonism) equations fit the IC_{50} ('I' for inhibition), while the stimulation (agonism) equations fit the EC_{50} ('E' for effective). QC criteria parameters are usually checked for every XC_{50} curve.

By using high-quality software for data analysis and management, HTS permits the faster and easier performance of millions of biochemical, genetic or pharmacological tests in vitro. With the objective to improve success rates and cycle times for the discovery of new hits and leads, HTS has become a cornerstone of drug discovery [15]. Although HTS is very efficient and powerful, it consumes a lot of time and materials (i.e. cost is high), but with the increased size of a screening library the efficiency tends to decrease [16]. However, after the initial euphoria and the huge investments which resulted in the fast automatisation and miniaturisation ('ultra HTS' paradigm), a new rational approach to HTS has replaced the ultra HTS paradigm within most drug discovery research sites worldwide. Whereas the emphasis previously had been on a steady increase in capacity ('quantitative increase') through automatisation and miniaturisation, recent years have shown a steady shift towards higher content and quality ('quality increase') for biological test systems [17]. Complementary and more rational approach is the structure-guided design of a ligand with appropriate drug-like properties. This process is also known as Structure-Based Drug Design (SBDD) and exploits structures of the receptor protein or ligand alone, or (if available) the structure of a protein-ligand complex [18].

Within SBDD, large chemical libraries are computationally screened to search for compounds that are complementary to the target. Despite the now essential role of HTS in modern drug discovery, its major drawback is that, apart from the target, the process often has little relevance to the actual pathophysiology of the disease. Thus, a series of elaborate cell biology and animal models are required to prove that a compound is of biological and functional relevance [19].

High-content screening (HCS) is another paradigm complementary with HTS, which combines the efficiency of high-throughput techniques with the capability of cellular imaging to collect quantitative data from complex biological systems [20]. HCS includes any method used to analyse whole cells (live or fixed) or components of cells with a simultaneous readout of several parameters. Automated image-based screening permits the identification of small compounds, which alter cellular phenotypes, and is of interest for the discovery of new pharmaceuticals and new cell biological tools for modifying cell function [21]. High-content screening technology is mainly based on combining automated digital microscopy and flow cytometry, together with IT-systems for the analysis and storage of the data [22], which enabled high-throughput high-content readouts in microtitre plate formats.

In selection and the set-up of a biological screening assay, important factors are sensitivity, precision, time, cost, robustness, simplicity, and the possibilities for automatisation and miniaturisation. After target identification, development and optimisation of the assay is the next step before HTS campaign, performed on the relevant compound collection. Screening process ends up with a discovery of number of hits and potential lead-like structures. Both the quality and the quantity of these lead-like classes are primary drivers for the discovery of the best-in-class medicines. This makes lead generation one of the crucial steps in the drug discovery process [23].

Identification of Hits and Optimisation of Leads

A Hit is a molecule with known structure, which in primary screening has exhibited robust activity with clearly expressed dose-response dependence. The average proportion of hits from an HTS campaign is 1–3% (or more, in case of specific assay or more focused compound library). If the number of hits is too high or too low, this can be a signal that the evaluated target is not druggable, or that the assay is not specific enough, or not sufficiently developed or optimised correctly.

A Lead is the best representative of the structural series of compounds with an overall biological potential that is good enough to advance the group into an integrated new drug discovery research programme.

A Candidate is a member of a lead series of compounds, which has been selected for further (pre)clinical testing. It must fulfil all target product profile (TPP) criteria of activity and safety. This is the final selected compound, which is then profiled as a possible new drug.

In general, when compounds are identified from HTS, they are not always suitable for the initiation of further medicinal chemistry exploration. After the primary screening campaign, a detailed evaluation of the hit molecules obtained is needed where activity has to be demonstrated in secondary screening and a functional test (e.g. cellular or phenotypic assay), or/and in the orthogonal binding assay (e.g. biophysical proof of direct binding). Potential pharmacophores are recognised, an overview of structural similarity with other compounds in the compound collections is generated, testing of different structural analogues of the selected structure is performed, and, in the end, synthesis of new analogues of the hit structure is initiated. For hits from HTS, as a next step in hit evaluation, selectivity, chemical tractability, binding mechanism, pharmacokinetic properties and patentability are usually viewed as more significant than the actual potency of the confirmed hits [23]. This is the start of the lead generation process, whereby numerous structure-activity relationship (SAR) medicinal chemistry cycles are followed within the research project, with iterative improvements of the initial early lead molecule. Further proof of the stoichiometric interaction of the compound with the cellular target is obtained with value-added affinity/interaction biophysical methods, such as NMR, X-ray co-crystallisation, calorimetry or SPR [23].

Selection of the right testing strategy within in vitro biological screening represents one of the most important aspects of the drug discovery process. Apart from the intrinsic biochemical and kinetic challenges in identifying an appropriate modulator for a target, the range of meaningful assays and ligand-identification technologies (HTS, natural products testing, literature, combinatorial chemistry, ligand design, chemogenomics, etc.) can also significantly influence the chances for success [24]. By using biochemical, biophysical, cell-based assays (2D or 3D cultures), organoids, and disease-relevant ex vivo assays on animal/human tissues, usual pharmacological readouts within hit/lead identification and optimisation phases are enzymatic activity (affinity) and competitivity, selectivity towards the same or other target families (e.g. kinases), or binding kinetics (on/off-rate). In various phenotypic or translational assays, different cellular processes are measured, from cell signalling, cell cycle, proliferation, apoptosis and cytotoxicity, to receptor internalisation, gene reporting or other relevant cellular/functional assays. Biochemical assays (end point, or kinetic) are valuable tools, despite the fact that this type of analysis is not performed in its true biological context. Cell-based assays are also widely used, as they have the potential to provide more information about intracellular molecular targets than biochemical or biophysical assays. The right combination of particular assays with the use of appropriate readout technology, such as absorbance, fluorescence, luminescence, radioactivity or electrophysiology, makes the selected assay applicable to any type of in vitro biology (high-throughput) screening [25, 26].

Primary or secondary screening assays can be homogeneous (in solution, 'one-pot assay') or heterogeneous (on a solid phase, with multiple washing steps before reading the plate) [27].

Cell-based assays offer more information on the target and its interactions with cellular cofactors, specific cellular pathways, and on cytotoxicity, membrane permeability, metabolism and stability of the test compounds under physiological conditions. However, besides all the above-mentioned advantages, challenges still exist. To select and make a good, biochemical, biophysical, cell-based assay, or disease-relevant translational assay, it is necessary to implement knowledge and experience by the scientists which understands drug discovery process, in order to improve chances for overall success.

Hit discovery and lead generation are, therefore, far more than just the identification of active compounds—they are the multidisciplinary processes by which the most promising lead candidates are selected from a rigorously assessed molecular series [24].

ADME Studies

Understanding drug metabolism and pharmacokinetics (DMPK) has improved success rates of drug discovery and development in the last two decades and is now routinely incorporated into early drug discovery [28]. As shown in Fig. 2.5, absorption, distribution, metabolism and excretion (ADME) studies are important for each stage of the drug discovery and development. In fact, the ADME parameters obtained from in vitro and in vivo models, which aid in the prediction of drug behaviours inpatients, are important for the decision to advance, hold or terminate a drug candidate [29].

The high-throughput screening in drug discovery for absorption, distribution, metabolism and excretion (ADME) properties has become the norm in the industry. The ADME strategies for drug discovery and development will vary based on the clinical goals of a programme. Consequently, the therapeutic area, the severity and rarity of the disease, the duration of drug treatment, and the ADME properties of

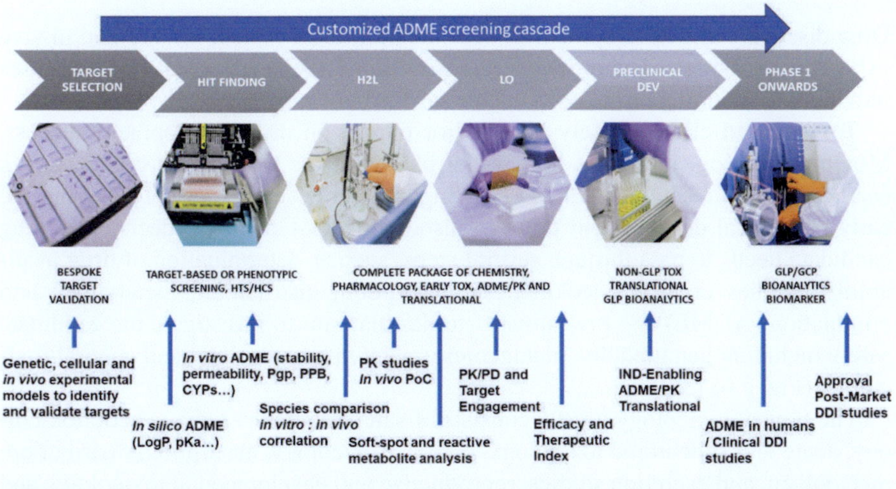

Fig. 2.5 Typical metabolism, ADME and Drug-Drug Interaction (DDI) model systems used in various stages of drug discovery and development. *ADME* absorption, distribution, metabolism and elimination, *PPB* plasma protein binding, *CYP* cytochrome P450, *PoC* proof of concept, *PK/PD* pharmacokinetics/pharmacodynamics, *GLP* good laboratory practice, *IND* investigational new drug

competitive products are factors that should be considered in developing an adequate ADME profile during lead optimisation and candidate selection. The primary goal is to provide a competitive product based on efficacy and adequate safety, avoiding PK-based failures in the clinic. We believe that drug target potency and selectivity should be the principal objective for the drug design strategy prior to lead optimisation; optimal activity and selectivity are the most important early goals for the chemistry of drug design. Thus, moving the classes of molecules with the greatest selectivity in pharmacological properties to lead optimisation is a critical first step in the design strategy for new drugs. The emphasis on structure-pharmacological activity by medicinal chemists prior to lead optimisation provides a more efficient means for compound optimisation than optimising pharmacological and ADME properties in parallel. The appropriate strategy for ADME assays needs to be carefully designed to be performed at hit-to-lead (H2L), early lead optimisation (Early LO) and late lead optimisation (Late LO) stages, which delineates the types of studies that should be performed and the deliverables at each stage. Late LO stage is then followed by the Development Candidate (DC) selection. The optimising of the ADME properties of a drug candidate is a complicated process. Utilisation of high-throughput technologies to eliminate compounds with poor ADME properties at HTS stage has been fruitful in speeding up the candidate selection from a vast number of compounds, but it carries the potential of throwing away potent chemical leads. The toxicity and efficacy have now become the prime candidates for attrition [30].

In Vivo Experimental Models and Safety Pharmacology

Drug discovery and development involve the utilisation of both in vitro and in vivo experimental models. The ultimate goal is to translate the animal model responses into an understanding of the risks vs. effects for human subjects.

Toxicity and clinical safety have major impact on drug development success. Moving toxicological studies into earlier phases of the R&D chain prevents drug candidates with a safety risk from entering clinical development [31]. During the early preclinical development process, also known as Go/No-Go decision, a drug candidate needs to pass through several steps, such as determination of drug availability (studies on pharmacokinetics), absorption, distribution, metabolism and elimination (ADME) and preliminary studies that aim to investigate the candidate safety including genotoxicity, mutagenicity, safety pharmacology and general toxicology (Fig. 2.6) [32].

The typical toxicology profile consists of safety pharmacology, genetic toxicology, acute and subchronic toxicology, chronic toxicology, absorption, distribution, metabolism, and excretion studies, reproductive and developmental toxicology, and an evaluation of carcinogenic potential (Fig. 2.7) [33].

Preclinical toxicology testing of pharmaceutical agents is a very important component of the drug development process. The intrinsic property of an agent adversely affects an organism or the degree to which a substance is able to damage an exposed

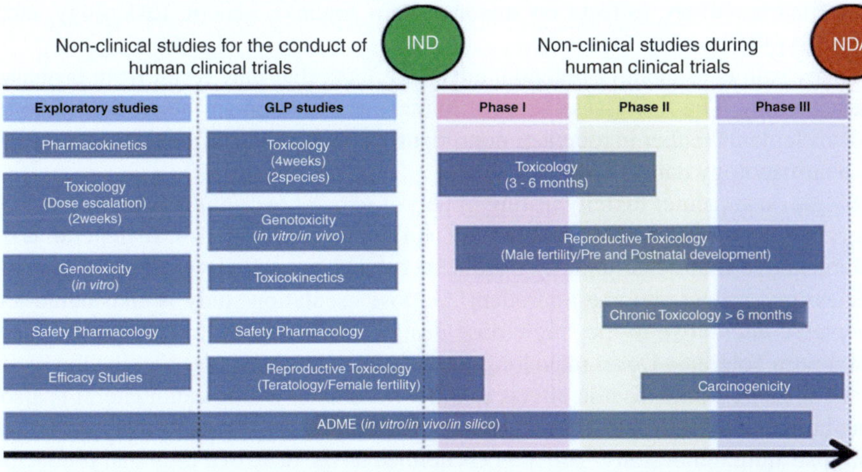

Fig. 2.6 Steps of non-clinical studies in drug development process. *GLP* good laboratory practice, *IND* investigational new drug, *NDA* new drug application, *ADME* absorption, distribution, metabolism and elimination

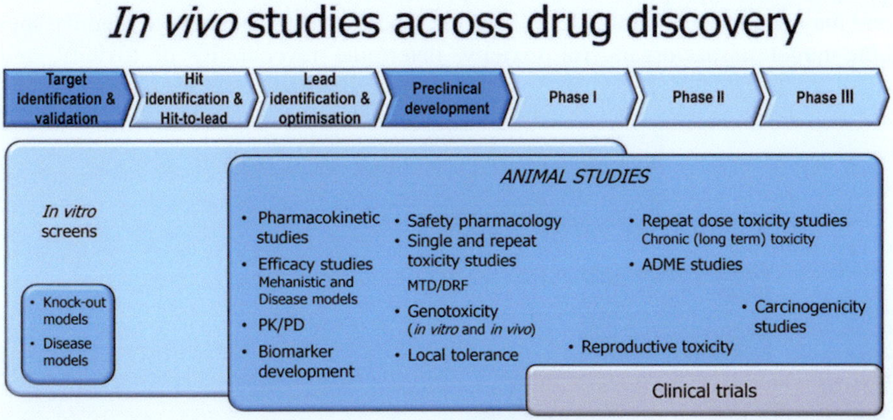

Fig. 2.7 In vivo studies across drug discovery. *PK/PD* pharmacokinetics/pharmacodynamics, *MTD* maximum tolerated dose, *DRF* dose-range finding, *ADME* absorption, distribution, metabolism and elimination

organism. ICH M3 (R2) "Non-clinical safety studies for the conduct of human clinical trials for pharmaceuticals" recommend international standards for, and promote harmonisation of, the non-clinical safety studies recommended to support human clinical trials of a given scope and duration as well as marketing authorisation for pharmaceuticals. Therefore, it requires non-clinical safety studies to be performed on candidate drugs. These studies evaluate general toxicology (in vivo experiments), safety pharmacology (effects on major system organs), genetic toxicology, etc. (Fig. 2.8) [34].

A key role is to identify potential adverse effects that may result from primary pharmacology. The risk assessment for humans is based on an integration of both in vivo elements (either in rodent or nonrodent species) and in vitro (such as secondary pharmacology data).

Single dose (acute) toxicity testing as part of general toxicology is carried out to determine the effect of a single dose on a particular animal species. In general, it is recommended that acute toxicity testing be carried out with two different animal species (one rodent and one nonrodent). A dose escalation study is considered an acceptable alternative to the single-dose design. The rationale for using the MTD (Maximum Tolerated Dose) main long-term studies is to maximise the likelihood of detecting any chronic disease effects or other hazards of a drug candidate. It is also more humane to determine the MTD before conducting any PK or ADME studies to minimise animal morbidity. The MTD is defined as the dose of a drug that produces an acceptable level of toxicity or the highest dose of a drug that does not cause unacceptable side effects. The NOAEL (No-Observed-Adverse-Effect Level) is the highest level of exposure to the drug at which there are no biologically significant increases in the severity or frequency of adverse effects between the treated animal group and the appropriate control group; some effects are not considered adverse, and may be produced at this level [35, 36]. These studies also help to identify specific target tissues/organs for toxicity, determine reversibility of toxicity, and

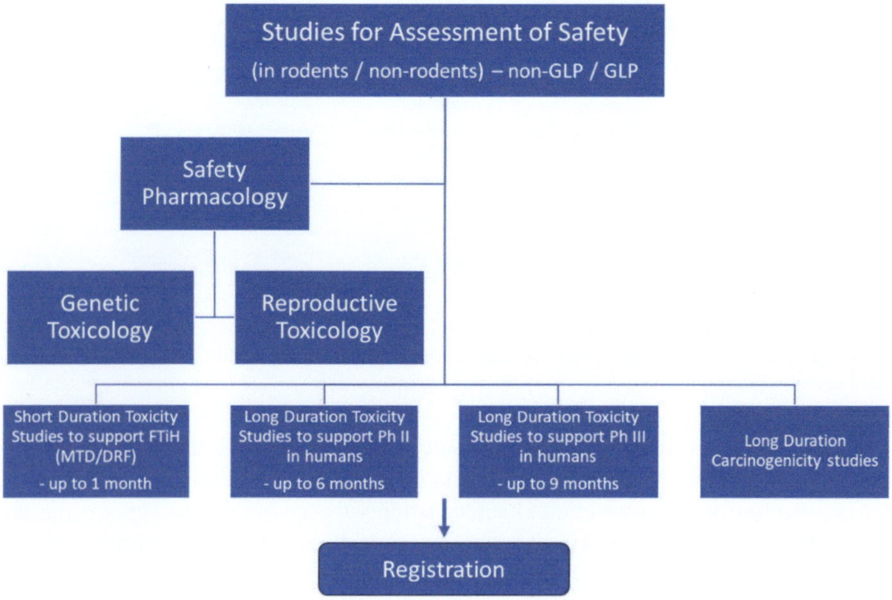

Fig. 2.8 Cascade of general toxicology studies for potential new medicine. *GLP* good laboratory practice, *FTiH* first time in human, *MTD* maximum tolerated dose, *DRF* dose-range finding

identify dosage parameters for repeated-dose toxicity tests. Maximum Tolerated Dose (MTD) studies are used to set the doses for short and long-term toxicology studies in animals and to determine safe starting doses for first-in-man clinical trials.

The primary goal of repeated-dose toxicity studies is to characterise the toxicological profile of the test compound following repeated administration (CPMP/SWP/1042/99 Guideline on repeated-dose toxicity). Repeated-dose toxicity studies are conducted in two mammalian species (one rodent (rats, mice and hamsters) and one nonrodent (dogs, non-human primates, and minipigs)), and their design takes into account the pharmacological relevance, treatment duration, therapeutic indication and scope of the proposed clinical trial they are to support.

All procedures should conform to standards of laboratory animal care. Study design: Healthy young adult animals are randomly assigned to the control and treatment groups. During the study period, animals are monitored for mortality, clinical signs, body weights, and feed consumption daily or periodically. Blood and urine samples are collected at the end of the treatment period (and the end of the recovery period) for clinical pathology analysis. Upon completion of the treatment, animals are euthanised and subjected to a necropsy. Major organs are weighed, and tissue samples are collected for histopathological examination at the end of the treatment period (and end of the recovery period). In general, following the first dose on Day 1 and the last dose, blood samples are collected from each animal in the toxicokinetic group at multiple time points within 24 h for plasma concentration analysis of the test chemical and possible metabolites. The ophthalmological examination can be performed, the same as another testing (local tolerance) during repeated-dose toxicity studies. The study design in nonrodents species are quite similar to that in rodents, except those electrocardiograms (ECG) are usually conducted in nonrodent species (animals are individually housed) to evaluate potential cardiovascular effect of the test compound.

The duration of repeat-dose studies can be short (e.g., daily dosing for up to 14 days), subchronic (up to 3 months), or chronic (longer than 3 months and usually up to 2 years) [37].

Genetic toxicology studies are conducted to assess the potential for induction of genetic mutations or chromosomal damage. Genetic toxicity testing is required for all classes of chemicals and drugs, but its conduct can differ from compound to compound to account for regulatory requirements and choice and design of assays. Figure 2.9 shows some of the most common testing methods for the assessment of genotoxic substances [38].

In conclusion, genetic toxicology needs to answer questions coming from two major directions: hazard and risk identification and high-throughput testing. Safety Pharmacology (SP) (Fig. 2.10) is an essential part of the drug development process that aims to identify and predict adverse effects prior to clinical trials. SP studies are described in the International Conference on Harmonisation (ICH) S7A and S7B guidelines. The aim of Safety Pharmacology is to characterise the pharmacodynamic/pharmacokinetic (PK/PD) relationship of a drug's adverse effects using continuously evolving methodology. The key issues for Safety Pharmacology are detection of an adverse effect liability, projection of the data into safety margin

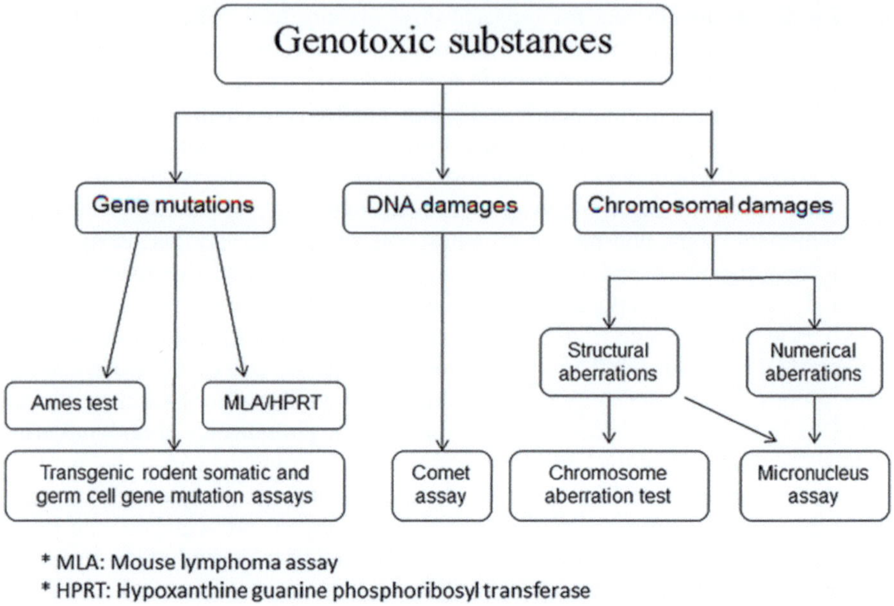

Fig. 2.9 A battery of most common testing methods for the assessment of genotoxic substances

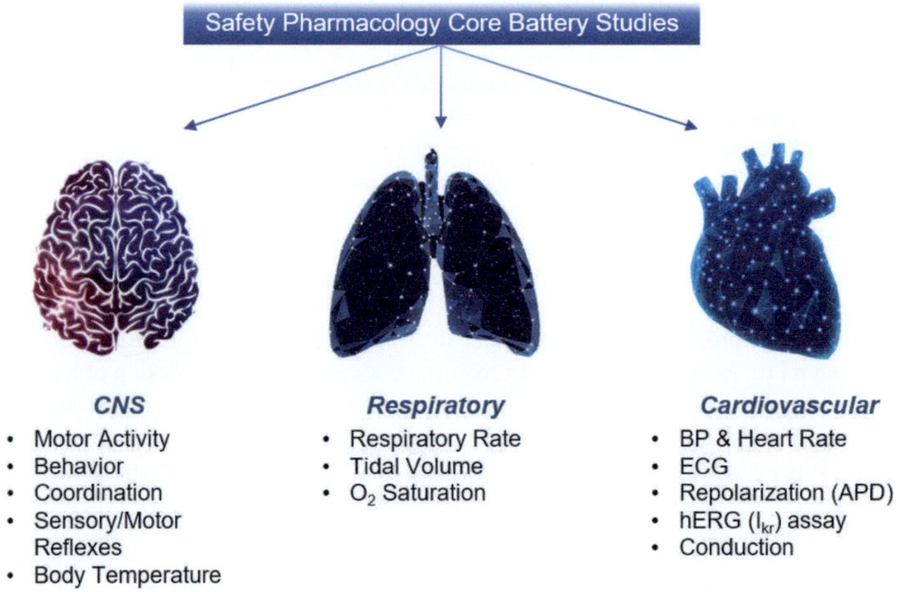

Fig. 2.10 Safety pharmacology core battery studies [38]

calculation and finally clinical safety monitoring [39]. The typical core battery of safety pharmacology studies includes: Central nervous system studies: Irwin test, Cardiovascular system studies: In conscious or anaesthetised animals, hERG and Purkinje studies (in vitro) and Respiratory system studies: whole body plethysmography.

Importantly, the results of the exploratory drug safety studies will be used by the sponsor to judge the potential risks associated with the continued pursuit of a potential development candidate. In many ways, preclinical toxicological investigations in discovery serve the important objective of identifying the most promising candidates to progress into development and onto registration [40].

Preclinical Candidate Final Selection: Final Remarks

Many drugs do not reach the clinical phase of development, mainly for two reasons. The first one is that they do not work in biological systems as expected, which means the activity or specificity of the new chemical entity or both are not good enough, and the second obstacle why the potential drug does not reach the clinical phase might be the safety profile. In that case, the molecule has good activity and target specificity but does not have an expected adequate safety profile. In other words, if a new molecule should reach clinical development as a clinical candidate, that molecule must have completed drug-like properties. It must have appropriate activity and affinity for the therapeutic target and has to be target-specific, which may increase the safety profile of the molecule. On the other hand, one of the critical steps in the preclinical drug development process is a careful and realistic selection of the biologically relevant therapeutic target (target identification), followed by proper target validation, which has to show that modification of the target will lead to the desired pharmacological effect. In order to follow all regulatory and FDA guidelines concerning the pre-requisite safety and efficacy profile of all new drugs on the market, drug discovery research scientists must carefully balance between medicinal chemistry, computational and in silico techniques and tools, phys-chem, in vitro biological, pharmacological, ADME-Tox and in vivo drug screening and profiling methodologies, ending with the safety and bioethical requirements for better and more efficient drug discovery and development. Quite different from many other industries, within drug discovery, a single pharmaceutical product, in this case, a defined compound or biomolecule, makes the difference between failure and great success.

References

1. Williams MM. Preclinical pharmacology and toxicology—contributions to the translational interface. In: Reference module in biomedical sciences. Wiley; 2014.
2. Sams-Dodd F. Drug Discov Today. 2005;10:139–47.
3. Hughes JP, et al. Br J Pharmacol. 2011;162:1239–49.

4. Yang Y, Adelstein SJ, Kassis AI. Drug Discov Today. 2009;14:147–54.
5. Finan C, et al. The druggable genome and support for target identification and validation in drug discovery. Sci Transl Med. 2017;9(383):eaag1166.
6. Xin H, Bernal, et al. J Biomol Screen. 2004;9:286–93.
7. Wan D, et al. Proc Natl Acad Sci USA. 2004;101:15724–9.
8. Kurosawa G, et al. Proc Natl Acad Sci USA. 2008;105:7287–92.
9. Hajduk PJ, et al. Drug Discov Today. 2005;10:1675–82.
10. Surade S, Blundell TL. Chem Biol. 2012;19:42–50.
11. Lipinski CA, et al. Adv Drug Deliv Rev. 2001;46:3–26.
12. Dove A. Nat Biotechnol. 1999;17:859–63.
13. Macarrón R. Drug Discov Today. 2006;11:277–9.
14. Marangoni AG. Enzyme kinetics—a modern approach. Hoboken: Wiley-Interscience; 2003.
15. Kenny BA, et al. Prog Drug Res. 1998;51:245–69.
16. Egner U, Hillig RC. Expert Opin Drug Discov. 2008;3:391–401.
17. Mayr LM, Bojanic D. Curr Opin Pharmacol. 2009;9:580–8.
18. Kalyaanamoorthy S, Chen YP. Drug Discov Today. 2011;16:831–9.
19. Henriksen K, Christiansen C, Karsdal MA. Drug Discov Today. 2011;16:967–75.
20. Zanella F, Lorens JB, Link W. Trends Biotechnol. 2010;28:237–45.
21. Mattiazzi Usaj M, et al. High-content screening for quantitative cell biology. Trend Cell Biol. 2016;26(8):598–611.
22. Eglen RM. Drug Discov World. 2009:25–31.
23. Keserü GM, Makara GM. Drug Discov Today. 2006;11:741–8.
24. Bleicher KH, et al. Nat Rev Drug Discov. 2003;2:369–78.
25. Eglen RM, et al. Curr Chem Genomics. 2008;1:2–10.
26. Fan F, Wood KV. Assay Drug Dev Technol. 2007;5:127–36.
27. Hagan AK, Zuchner T. Anal Bioanal Chem. 2011;400:2847–64.
28. Alavijeh MS, Palmer AM. IDrugs. 2004;7:755–63.
29. Zhang D, et al. Acta Pharm Sin B. 2012;2(6):549–61.
30. Suresh K, et al. Curr Top Med Chem. 2005;5:1033–8.
31. Hornberg JJ, et al. Exploratory toxicology as an integrated part of drug discovery. Part I: Why and how. Drug Discov Today. 2014;19(8):1131–6.
32. Andrade EL, et al. Braz J Med Biol Res. 2016;49(12):e5646.
33. Dorato MA, Buckley LA. Curr Protoc Pharmacol. 2006;10:Unit10.3.
34. Robinson S et al. NC3Rs, Guidance on dose level selection for regulatory general toxicology; 2009.
35. ECETOC. Recognition of, and differentiation between, adverse and non-adverse effects in toxicology studies. Technical Report 85; 2002.
36. Faustman EM, Omenn GS. Risk assessment. In: Klaassen CD, editor. Cassarett and Doull's toxicology the basic science of poisons. 6th ed. New York: McGraw-Hill; 2001. p. 92.
37. Wallace Hayes A, et al. Loomis's essentials of toxicology. 5th ed. Academic; 2019.
38. Ren N, et al. JTransl Med. 2017;15:110.
39. Pugsley MK, et al. Principles of safety pharmacology. Br J Pharmacol. 2008;154(7):1382–99.
40. Bass AS, et al. J Pharmacol Toxicol Methods. 2009;60(1):69–78.

Clinical Research and Regulatory Review 3

Matea Radačić Aumiler and Ines Baotić

Clinical Research: Clinical Trials Phases I–IV

Clinical trials are a crucial aspect in the development of new drugs (see also Chap. 1). Clinical trial is a research study that should be conducted according to the highest ethical principles, safety, and well-being of the subjects to be protected (for details, please see section "Regulatory Review"). The objective of clinical trials is to evaluate the safety and efficacy of the *Investigational New Drug* (IND) or an intervention. After preclinical evaluation of IND has been sufficiently addressed, a pharmaceutical company (IND sponsor) files an *IND Application* to the regulatory to proceed with evaluation of IND in clinical setting (Fig. 3.1).

Each individual involved in the clinical study team should have appropriate education, experience, and training for the respective tasks in compliance with the regulatory requirements. Moreover, there is a confidentiality agreement that is applied to all the documents, IND and subject data obtained in the clinical trial. Clinical study team and conduct of clinical trial in the delegated institution (investigational site) is the responsibility of the individual leading the team—principal investigator (PI). To conduct a study as PI, the physician needs to gain a lot of experience as a co-investigator or subinvestigator, knowing regulations and *the International Conference of Harmonization Good Clinical Practice* (ICH GCP) guidelines pertaining to the ethical conduct through the duration of the trial, how to obtain informed consent, recruit

M. Radačić Aumiler
Division for Clinical Pharmacology and Therapeutics, Department of Internal Medicine, University Hospital Center Zagreb, Zagreb, Croatia

Department of Biotechnology, University of Rijeka, Rijeka, Croatia

School of Medicine, Catholic University of Croatia, Zagreb, Croatia

I. Baotić (✉)
Zabok General Hospital and the Croatian Veterans Hospital, Zabok, Croatia
e-mail: inesbaotic@gmail.com

M. Banić, D. Erceg (eds.), *Drug Interactions in Gastroenterology*, Clinical Gastroenterology, https://doi.org/10.1007/978-3-031-69800-2_3

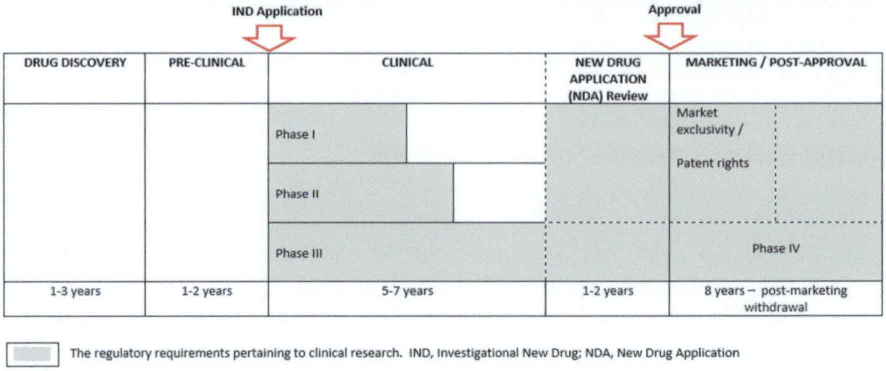

Fig. 3.1 Drug development process

patients and to acquire hands-on diagnostic tests and procedures that are part of on-site visits specified in the study protocol. The progress to PI role requires knowing all applicable laws and regulations, the responsibilities of PI as well as the responsibilities of each and every individual in the clinical study team. Furthermore, the PI role requires the review of study documents ahead of the beginning of a clinical trial, budget negotiations, signing consent to perform the trial at the institution and all necessary documents for the Central or Institutional Review Board approval, and preparing reports on a clinical trial with evaluation of screening and recruitment process, drop-out rate and serious adverse events with a final report after the trial has ended.

Apart from physicians in the team, an important role is the clinical trial coordinator (CTC). The CTC is professional and manages the clinical trial at the investigational site. Although the management is the responsibility of PI, there are more than a few managing tasks that are forwarded to CRC including storage and archiving of clinical trial documents after the end of the trial. Also, an important role is to have a study nurse who is educated and dedicated to working with subjects included in the trial. The study nurse is crucial for educating subjects (on dietary requirements, IND application, blood glucose measurements, explaining the subject's different questioners and helping the subjects to fill those), IND accountability, and as the study nurse is usually the first contact for the subjects they study nurse should ensure the patients are well supported throughout the trial.

There are number of certifications offered that enable thorough education of each individual involved in the clinical study team, additionally showing experience, dedication, and commitment to the position.

Well-conducted clinical trials in phase I, phase II, and phase III with carefully designed study protocols should provide sufficient data for *New Drug Application* (NDA) [1, 2].

Essential documents of any clinical trial are the investigator brochure, study protocol, informed consent, and subject records with medical data.

The investigator's brochure is a document that PI needs to review ahead of the clinical trial beginning at the investigational site and appraise if all the necessary preclinical and clinical (if applicable) data are obtained for the clinical trial of the appropriate phase to be conducted.

The study protocol is an essential document that contains general information on the clinical trial, as well as background information and clinical trial objectives. The protocol defines the design of the clinical trial, duration of the trial, subject criteria for enrollment and exclusion, the data on treatment (IND/control, concomitant drugs, and rescue therapy), all the physical examinations and diagnostic tests, and statistical analysis of the data that would be performed [3].

According to the ICH GCP standards, all patients need to be informed in writing about all relevant aspects of the trial as well as about potential risks/benefits of the IND and procedures ahead of being enrolled in the clinical trial. Therefore, for the patient to be enrolled, the voluntarily informed consent (IC) needs to be signed and dated before any other action taken [3]. After IC agreement has been obtained from the patient (legal representative), the patient becomes clinical trial subject. The subject can withdraw the IC at any time during the trial without stating the reason, and the withdrawal of IC should not interfere with the quality of patients' further medical treatment and care.

The subjects' medical records could be on paper or as e-charts. The medical records usually follow the visits (on investigational site or telephone or electronic) set by study protocol. Either paper or e-charts should contain: the information on patients inclusion/exclusion criteria, general information about age, gender, the type of the disease, the stage of the disease, previous treatment history, other medical conditions, etc. Furthermore, these records should contain all results of the performed physical examinations and diagnostic tests with all reported (serious) adverse events and adverse drug reactions. The medical records in clinical trials are also called "the source data" of the subject and, according to the ICH GCP, it should be stored for 15 years after the end of the trial.

Clinical trials are stratified into phases based on the objectives of the trial. However, the clinical phases are not distinct, consecutive periods but rather markers of milestones in drug development process.

Phase I: In phase I trials the IND is for the first time applied to human subjects ("first in men" studies). Phase I mainly evaluates the safety of an IND and therefore usually includes a small number of healthy volunteers [1]; except for phase I trials of anticipated cancer treatment(s), that are usually carried out in subjects who already have the disease. Investigational objectives in phase I are pharmacokinetics (PK), pharmacodynamics (PD), and toxicity [1].

The PK/PD study evaluates absorption (A), distribution (D), metabolism (M), excretion (E) of IND, and basic efficacy of the IND. If just PK is evaluated those are ADME studies. In phase I, safety is the main target, although as the phase I trials are of short duration with a short exposition of subjects to IND, only adverse drug reactions of acute toxicity could be observed. In this phase, usually 10–30 subjects are involved, and if data is obtained and evaluated to support further investment in safety and more elaborate efficacy testing, the IND goes to phase II [4].

Phase II: Investigational objectives in phase II trials are determining dose-response relationship and finding the most appropriate dose ("dose-finding" studies);

however, for some INDs "dose-finding" may already be evaluated in phase I. Also, further investigating the safety of IND is a continuous objective, as is evaluating the efficacy of IND in subjects with targeted pathology. Much bigger subject groups than in phase I are usually required for phase II trials to be finalized. If an IND has a better safety/efficacy profile than placebo and is equal to or better than the "golden standard" treatment (control) for the targeted disease in primary efficacy or "pivotal" trials, the clinical research and evaluation of the IND is forwarded to phase III clinical trial. Sometimes, there is a differentiation between phase IIA and phase IIB; IIA evaluates the efficacy and safety of IND in subjects with the targeted disease (for instance, diabetes mellitus type II), while IIB trials evaluate the IND in subjects with the disease and its complications (for instance, diabetes mellitus type II with diabetic nephropathy) [4].

Phase III: An IND presenting favorable safety/efficacy profile, in smaller groups of subjects, is further introduced in phase III, in which the initial safety and efficacy data need to be confirmed ("confirmatory" trials) [1]. The confirmatory trials include hundreds or even thousands of subjects, from different investigational centers in different countries ("multicenter" trials). Phase III trials compare IND to the "golden standard" or standard-of-care (SOC) drug [4]. These trials are of longer duration and assess adverse drug reactions in chronic exposure and compare efficacy and safety of IND vs. control. The clinical trial may be terminated ahead of end-of-trial defined by study protocol if the adverse drug reactions are too severe or if IND group has much better efficacy data compared to control [4].

After all necessary IND data from preclinical and clinical trials have been gathered and analyzed the IND sponsor (pharmaceutical industry) submits the NDA for commercialization of the new drug to *the U.S. Food and Drug Administration* (FDA) and/or analog to NDA, the application for marketing authorization to *the European Medicines Agency* (EMA) or outside United States and EU to the appropriate regulatory authority.

Phase IV: Phase IV trials are conducted after NDA approval has been obtained for IND [1]. Since phase IV clinical trials are performed after the drug has been approved and placed on the market, phase IV is also named "post-marketing" trials. For certain marketed drugs phase IV is obligatory regulatory requirement as a part of follow-up measures (FUM) focused on evaluating the long-term safety of these medicinal products in a larger population and "real life" setting. Phase IV trials may also be a part of sponsor (pharmaceutical industry) strategy to better commercialize the new drug as well as to obtain more precise safety profile in certain patient groups (geriatric population, patients with different comorbidities and higher number of concomitant drugs) that were not included in clinical trials after the IND application [1]. The "real-life" setting of phase IV ensures not just a higher number of patients of different age and different comorbidities are exposed to new drug but overall a longer exposure that is crucial for detection of rare adverse events that could not be seen during phase I–III [5, 6]. Furthermore, the potential of the new drug to be effective in certain initially not investigated indications may be detected that may extend the drug being approved in this add-on indications. However, the drug to be approved for the add-on indication requires the drug to be translated back into further preclinical and clinical research for evaluation of safety and efficacy in particular add-on indication [5, 7].

From all the above, the conclusion is that although clinical trials phase I–III are rigorous due to the relatively short duration of trials with narrow definition of subject population quite limited in number, they still do not provide full efficacy nor safety profile of an IND at the time of drug approval. Therefore, the phase IV is necessity to better define the profile of a drug on market [5].

As clinical trials are clinical research studies in which at the time-point defined in the study protocol, intervention (IND/control treatment) is applied, all trials regardless of phase are interventional. Furthermore, as subjects are followed forward through trial duration and data are systematically collected in the process, all clinical trials within the drug development are prospective. Key features of the design of clinical trials phase II and III are randomization, blinding, and the use of control group. Randomization meaning, each subject is put into the active or control treatment group ("trial arms"), by chance (Fig. 3.2). Active treatment group receives IND and control group receives a SOC drug or placebo. If randomization is successful, the two groups should be the same in respect of both measured confounders and unmeasured ones [8]. So, the ideal situation would be to have just the difference between groups in regard of intervention. Although randomization cannot ensure between-treatment balance with respect to all subjects characteristics, it ensures the expectation of balance [1]. Apart from randomization, blinding is another main tool for controlling bias in clinical trials.

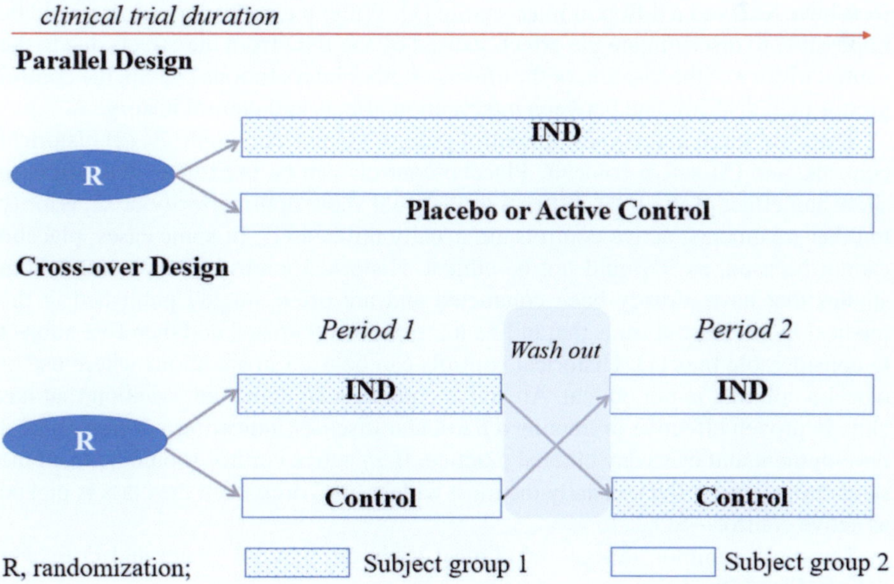

Fig. 3.2 Clinical trial design—parallel and cross over

Blinding is keeping study subjects, investigators, or assessors unaware of the assigned intervention. The purpose of blinding is that their knowledge would not affect their behavior, which can be subtle, unnoticeable, and unintentional and it is less likely they would have biased psychological or physical responses to the intervention [1].

Clinical trials can be "single-blind" indicating blinding of subjects for assigned treatment. "Double-blind" indicating neither the subjects nor the clinical study team know who has received the IND or comparator drug. "Triple-blind" indicating subjects, investigators, and the sponsor are blinded. Trials with no blinding are called "open-label" [4]. As mentioned before, in phase III clinical trials, usually two active interventions are compared. These interventions may have different treatment schedules, may be administered via different routes, or look, taste, or smell different, so a typical way to blind such a study is the "double-dummy" approach that utilizes two placebos, one for each intervention, which is often easier than trying to make the two interventions look like each other. Subjects are then randomized to receive one active treatment and one placebo [1].

A placebo is defined as an inert pill, injection, or other sham intervention that masks as an active intervention, and as it has no activity for the disease treated, it is often called the "sugar pill" and it serves to maintain blinding of treatment assignment. It is used as a control to account for the natural history of disease and for psychological effects [1]. Although placebo has no activity for the disease treated, it can nevertheless provide treatment effects, especially when the endpoint is subjective [1].

Another key feature in clinical trial design is the selection of a control group. The control group ensures data on subjects in "placebo treatment" scenario, or if subjects have received a different intervention [1]. Without a control group, it would be impossible to discriminate the effects caused by the IND from the effects due to the natural history of the disease, or the effects of other interventions [1]. So, the control groups help discriminate between intervention effects and natural history.

There are three main types of control groups: (1) placebo-controls, (2) historical controls, and (3) active controls. Placebo-controls can be used when the aim is to show any effect of the IND. When a trial should show noninferiority or superiority to other treatments, active controls are usually utilized [1]. In some cases, placebo cannot be used, as it would not be ethical. Historical controls are obtained from studies that have already been conducted and are often already published in the medical literature, but trials that utilize it are non-randomized and therefore subject to considerable bias [1]. Historical controls can be used in situations where use of placebo-controls is not ethical. An active control is an active intervention that has already proven effective in treating a particular disease (indication), during clinical development and everyday clinical practice. If an active control should be from the same drug class as IND; usually the most widely used drug from the class is picked as active control—SOC.

The most common designs of clinical trials are parallel group and crossover design (Fig. 3.2).

In parallel group design each subject is randomly assigned to only one treatment, i.e., groups ("trial arms") are assigned to different treatment. In crossover design, each subject receives two or more treatment options, in some periods of time, during the clinical trial. In contrast to a parallel design where patients are randomized to a treatment and remain on that treatment through the whole trial, in crossover design, each subject receives one treatment during the defined time period and afterward crossover to a second treatment for a defined time period. During the course of the crossover trial, those two time periods that subject is on treatment are usually separated by a period called the washout period that ensures the concentration of initial drug the subject was receiving is untraceable—"washed out" from the body. Crossover design can be implemented only for chronic, stable diseases.

The selection of endpoints is of outmost importance in clinical trial design. The selection of the primary endpoint is made to address the primary objective of the trial [1]. The primary endpoint should be clinically relevant, interpretable, sensitive to the effects of intervention, practical, and possible to measure [1]. Endpoints can be objective or subjective. Objective endpoints can be measured, in contrast, subjective endpoints are more susceptible to individual interpretation and subject to bias. Sometimes significant time is needed to observe a definitive endpoint (e.g., death), thus surrogate endpoints can be established, in order to remain predictive of a clinical event and still allow for saving in time.

Regulatory Review

The regulatory review is continuous process through the drug development ensuring applicable laws and regulations with local (institutional) policies and practices are followed (see also Chap. 1). Depending on the drug market region, centralized (CRB) or institutional review boards (IRB) with appointed regulatory bodies are dedicated to regulatory review of clinical trials. The submission of the required clinical trial documents to the CRBs/IRBs and regulatory bodies is the responsibility of the IND sponsor or PI. While, for the NDA review, IND sponsors' application to the FDA, EMA, or appropriate body is required.

Centralized review boards or IRBs, evaluate and follow each clinical trial from the submission up to the end of the trail in particular institution (at the investigational site). The basics of the regulatory review at that point is evaluating if IND sponsor of clinical trial and investigational team are following all applicable laws, regulations, and guidelines. Both, clinical trials phase I–III (pre-marketing) and trials phase IV (post-marketing) are regulated by a set of *the International Conference on Harmonization of Technical Requirements for Registration of Pharmaceuticals for Human Use* (ICH) guidelines [9, 10].

The ICH guidelines are internationally accepted documents summarizing standards for designing, conducting, recording, monitoring, and reporting clinical trials. Based on the topic, the ICH guidelines are divided into four main categories: quality, efficacy, safety, and multidisciplinary, and labeled accordingly as Q for quality, E for efficacy, S for safety, and M for multidisciplinary [10]. Although the safety of human subjects is global highlights ICH guidelines, there are some ICH guidelines that need to be additionally emphasized the one to obtain better overview of the thoroughness of the regulatory approach:

ICH E1 *Clinical Safety for Drugs used in Long-term Treatment* [11]
ICH E2A-E2F *Pharmacovigilance* [12]
ICH E6(R3) *Good Clinical Practice (ICH GCP) in the Final Concept Paper* [13]
ICH E14 *Clinical Evaluation of QT* [14]
ICH S1–S12 *Safety Guidelines* (generally drug development preclinical research guidelines set to detect potential risks ahead of investigational products entering into the clinical phase, except for ICH S7A *Safety Pharmacology Studies for Human Pharmaceuticals*) [15]
ICH M12 *Drug Interaction Studies* (new harmonized guideline under development for assessing drug-drug interactions during investigational product development in clinical phase) [16]

ICH guidelines as well as applicable laws are concordant with ethical principles stated in World Medical Association's *Declaration of Helsinki* that regulate and provide guidance for physicians and other participants in medical research involving human subjects. In year 1964 Declaration of Helsinki was initially developed, however there have been several revisions of Declaration since, last being in 2000. The two ethical principles need to be emphasized: "in the medical research on human subjects, considerations related to the well-being of the human subject should take precedence over the interests of science and society" [17, 18] and "the subjects must be volunteers and informed participants in the research project" [18].

In the EU main documents regulating clinical trials are *the Directive 2001/20/EC* and the *Regulation No 536/2014 of the European Parliament and of the Council* of 16 Apr 2014 on clinical trials on medicinal products for human use [19], and regarding the book topic on drug interactions *the EMA Guideline on the investigation of drug interactions*, 2012 [20]. With each EU Member state incorporating afore mentioned Directive and Regulation in its own drug development regulatory frame. While, in the USA the key documents are *Code of Federal Regulation Title 21 (CFR Title 21)* [21] and *Draft Guidance for Clinical Drug Interaction Studies—Study Design, Data Analysis, and Clinical Implications* [22]. In Japan key applicable documents regulating clinical trials are: *the Ministry of Health and Welfare (MHW) Ordinance No. 28* dated March 27, 1997 partially revised several times, last revision by *Ministry of Health, Labor and Welfare (MHLW) Ordinance No. 9* dated Jan 22, 2016 [23]; and related to the drug interactions, *Guideline on drug interaction for drug development and appropriate provision of information*, 2018 [24]. An overview of development process of the new Japanese guideline for investigating drug interactions with an impact on further drug interaction evaluation within regulatory activities was elaborated in the publication by Ishiguro and colleagues [25].

In order to ensure the appropriate level of transparency in the clinical trials, the regulatory frame in EU, United States, and Japan also set the information and documents that are relevant to be submitted to official database of clinical trials (EU database and clinicaltrials.gov) that are publicly accessible. Also, regulated clinical trial data should not be published in order to protect privacy of subjects/participants and the interests of the pharmaceutical industry.

The NDA review greatly differs from region to region. The main difference in the NDA review process among the members of the ICH is that the United States and Japan have centralized NDA review while in the EU there are four different NDA review procedures: centralized, decentralized, mutual-recognition, and national procedure [26].

The centralized NDA review for marketing of the medicinal product incorporates single U.S. FDA assessment or single EMA or single MHLW assessment with marketing authorization, which is valid thought the United States, EU, and Japan, respectively. In the EU regulatory system for INDs (containing new active substance), centralized NDA review is compulsory if indicated for the treatment of cancer, diabetes, neurodegenerative diseases, autoimmune and other immune dysfunctions, viral diseases such as human immunodeficiency virus (HIV) or acquired immune deficiency syndrome (AIDS) [26]. The centralized review is also compulsory for INDs derived from biotechnology processes, advanced-therapy medicines, orphan medicines and veterinary medicines for use as growth or yield enhancers [26]. For other medicines centralized procedure is optional [26].

Decentralized NDA review is followed when marketing authorization is requested in more than one EU Member state if the medicinal product has not yet been authorized in any EU Member state [27].

And, if medicinal product is already authorized for marketing in one EU Member state by national procedure, pharmaceutical companies can additionally apply for marketing authorization to be recognized in (any) other EU Member states, which is called the drug approval process by mutual-recognition procedure (MRP) [27].

Drug discovery and development process is usually of extensive duration. The time required for an IND to be approved and commercialized is approximately 10 years. However, most of INDs never make it through; as of 5000 researched compounds, just 1 IND is approved. Clinical research formatted in clinical trials, evaluating safety/efficacy profile of IND, is paramount of drug development. And the established set of regulations and guidelines pertaining to clinical research ensures an IND has acceptable quality, safety, and efficacy at the time of the approval, and also ensures further follow-up and evaluation of the drug being on the market.

References

1. Evans SR. Fundamentals of clinical trial design. J Exp Stroke Transl Med. 2010;3(1):19–27. Epub 2010/01/01.
2. Kelly WK, Halabi S. Oncology clinical trials: successful design, conduct and analysis. 2nd ed. Springer; 2018.
3. ClinicalTrials.gov. Bethesda: U.S. National Library of Medicine. 2019 [cited 1 Feb 2020]. https://clinicaltrials.gov/ct2/about-studies/learn.
4. Friedman L, Furberg CD, DeMets D, Reboussin DM, Granger CB. Fundamentals of clinical trials. 5th ed. Springer; 2015.

5. Suvarna V. Phase IV of drug development. Perspect Clin Res. 2010;1(2):57–60. Epub 2010/04/01.
6. Zhang X, Zhang Y, Ye X, Guo X, Zhang T, He J. Overview of phase IV clinical trials for postmarket drug safety surveillance: a status report from the ClinicalTrials.gov registry. BMJ Open. 2016;6(11):e010643. Epub 2016/11/25.
7. Glasser SP, Salas M, Delzell E. Importance and challenges of studying marketed drugs: what is a phase IV study? Common clinical research designs, registries, and self-reporting systems. J Clin Pharmacol. 2007;47(9):1074–86. Epub 2007/09/04.
8. Thiese MS. Observational and interventional study design types; an overview. Biochem Med. 2014;24(2):199–210. Epub 2014/06/28.
9. Lindstrom-Gommers L, Mullin T. International Conference on Harmonization: recent reforms as a driver of global regulatory harmonization and innovation in medical products. Clin Pharmacol Therap. 2019;105(4):926–31. Epub 2018/11/15.
10. ICH. [cited 18 Feb 2020]. https://www.ich.org/page/ich-guidelines.
11. ICH. E1 Guideline the extent of population exposure to assess clinical safety for drugs intended for long-term treatment of non-life-threatening conditions. 1994 [cited 18 Feb 2020]. https://database.ich.org/sites/default/files/E1_Guideline.pdf.
12. ICH. E2A-E2F guidelines pharmacovigilance. 1994 [cited 18 Feb 2020]. https://www.ich.org/page/efficacy-guidelines.
13. ICH. E6(R3) Guideline for good clinical practice. In: Final concept paper. 2019 [cited 18 Feb 2020]. https://database.ich.org/sites/default/files/E6-R3_FinalConceptPaper_2019_1117.pdf.
14. ICH. E14 guideline the clinical evaluation of QT/QTC interval prolongation and proarrhythmic potential for nonantiarrhythmic drugs. 2005 [cited 18 Feb 2020]. https://database.ich.org/sites/default/files/E14_Guideline.pdf.
15. ICH. S7A safety pharmacology studies for human pharmaceuticals. In: Safety guidelines. 2000 [cited 18 Feb 2020]. https://www.ich.org/page/safety-guidelines.
16. ICH. M12 drug interaction studies. In: Final concept paper. 2019 [cited 18 Feb 2020]. https://database.ich.org/sites/default/files/M12_FinalConceptPaper_2019_1117.pdf.
17. Anthony RJYL, Coll RK, Dillon J, Chiu M, Fakudze C, et al. Research ethics boards and the gold standard(s) in literacy and science education research. In: Hand BSM, Yore LD, editors. Quality research in literacy and science education. London: Springer Science+Business Media B.V; 2009.
18. Association WM. Declaration of Helsinki. Bull World Health Organization. 2001 [cited 18 Feb 2020]. https://www.who.int/bulletin/archives/79(4)373.pdf.
19. EC. Regulation (EU) No 536/2014 of the European Parliament and of the Council. Official J Eur Union. 2014 [cited 18 Feb 2020]. https://ec.europa.eu/health/sites/health/files/files/eudralex/vol-1/reg_2014_536/reg_2014_536_en.pdf.
20. EMA. Guideline on the investigation of drug interactions. 2012 [cited 18 Feb 2020]. https://www.ema.europa.eu/en/documents/scientific-guideline/guideline-investigation-drug-interactions_en.pdf.
21. FDA US. CFR—Code of Federal Regulations Title 21. 2019 [cited 18 Feb 2020]. https://www.accessdata.fda.gov/scripts/cdrh/cfdocs/cfcfr/cfrsearch.cfm.
22. FDA. Clinical drug interaction studies—study design, data analysis, and clinical implications guidance for industry. 2017 [cited 18 Feb 2020]. https://www.fda.gov/files/drugs/published/Clinical-Drug-Interaction-Studies-%E2%80%94-Study-Design%2D%2DData-Analysis%2D%2Dand-Clinical-Implications-Guidance-for-Industry.pdf.
23. JPMA. Pharmaceutical Laws and Regulations. 2019 [cited 18 Feb 2020]. http://www.jpma.or.jp/english/parj/pdf/2019e_ch02.pdf.
24. PMDA. Guideline on drug interaction for drug development and appropriate provision of information. 2018 [cited 18 Feb 2020]. https://www.pmda.go.jp/files/000228122.pdf.
25. Ishiguro A, Sato R, Nagai N. Development of a new Japanese guideline on drug interaction for drug development and appropriate provision of information. Drug Metab Pharmacokinet. 2020;35(1):12–7. Epub 2020/01/07.

26. EMA. Authorisation of medicines. 2019 [cited 18 Feb 2020]. https://www.ema.europa.eu/en/about-us/what-we-do/authorisation-medicines.
27. CMDh. Best practise guide for decentralised and mutual recognition procedures. 2018 [cited 18 Feb 2020]. https://www.hma.eu/fileadmin/dateien/Human_Medicines/CMD_h_/procedural_guidance/Application_for_MA/CMDh_068_1996_Rev11_05_2018_clean.pdf.

DDI and Drug Development 4

Damir Erceg and Aurora Antolović Amidžić

Introduction

Drug discovery and development are a very complex processes involving various scientific fields (see also Chaps. 1, 2, and 3). Medicinal chemistry, drug metabolism, biochemistry, formulation, pharmacokinetics, toxicology, and pharmacology are deeply involved in preclinical research. Drug metabolism plays a crucial role in the examination of pharmaco-toxicological effects in study subjects. The ideal drug includes the following characteristics: high aqueous solubility (needed for i.v. dosing), good oral availability (suitable for oral dosing), adequate elimination half-life for dosing interval, balanced clearance among hepatic metabolism, biliary and renal secretion, multiple enzymes including in metabolism, low potential for enzymes and transporters inhibition or induction, good comparability between plasma metabolite profiles in human subjects and species used in toxicological studies [1, 2]. Improvement of safety and PK/PD of new potential drugs together with minimizing bioactivation and low potential DDIs are the main targets. Drug

D. Erceg (✉)
Srebrnjak, Children's Hospital, Zagreb, Croatia

School of Medicine, Catholic University of Croatia, Zagreb, Croatia

Department of Pharmacology and Biochemistry, Faculty of Dental Medicine and Health Osijek, J. J. Strossmayer University of Osijek, Osijek, Croatia

Department of Pharmacology, Faculty of Medicine, J. J. Strossmayer University of Osijek, Osijek, Croatia
e-mail: damir.erceg@unicath.hr; derceg@bolnica-srebrnjak.hr

A. Antolović Amidžić
Department of Pharmacology, Faculty of Medicine, J. J. Strossmayer University of Osijek, Osijek, Croatia

Department of Pharmacy, University Hospital Center Osijek, Osijek, Croatia
e-mail: antolovic.aurora@kbo.hr

M. Banić, D. Erceg (eds.), *Drug Interactions in Gastroenterology*, Clinical Gastroenterology, https://doi.org/10.1007/978-3-031-69800-2_4

metabolism is a sensitive discipline, critical in the phase of drug development, with significant contribution in discovering new chemical entities and bringing them to patients for treating diseases with existing non-adequate therapy [1]. A significant DDI appears when therapeutic failure or toxic effects of the drug are challenged by concomitant application with another medication. The drug-drug interactions (DDIs) are one of the leading cause of ADRs making their evaluation one of the most important parts of contemporary drug development due to safety reasons. The profiling of DDIs and identification of safety risks help us to identify suitable candidates in the discovery phase and enable further reasonable DDI assessment during the process of drug development [3]. The aim of drug development is an integration of knowledge acquired during preclinical and clinical DDI studies in an optimal manner, taking into consideration safety risks after drug approval. The involvement in significant clinical DDIs is a direct consequence of a series of drug withdrawals from the US market in the period from 1998 to 2003 [4]. The first case was related to the drug used for treating angina and hypertension, calcium channel blocker mibefradil. Mibefradil is a strong inhibitor of cytochrome P450 3A (CYP3A) and the efflux transporter P-glycoprotein (P-gp) produced risky and in some cases a fatal interaction with the calcium channel blocker felodipine, sensitive substrates of CYP3A. According to that, the prescribing information for mibefradil was revised, and concomitant use with 26 different drugs was contraindicated. This action was not fruitful, and the manufacturer decided to withdraw the drug from the market in June 1998 due to unfavorable risk-benefit risk and the complexity of prescribing drug information safely and available better therapeutic options without serious DDI risk. This is an illustrative case for PK (metabolic inhibition by a new molecular entity). Other cases of drug withdrawal were related to cisapride, a prokinetic agent for the treatment of gastrointestinal reflux (GER) as well as two antihistaminics, astemizole and terfenadine. All drugs played an important role in the depolarization of and were metabolized and cleared exclusively via CYP 3A4. Their concentration was significantly increased due to the coadministration of inhibitors of this enzyme. Coadministrations with commonly used medications such as antibiotics or grapefruit juice are an increased risk for torsade points (fatal arrhythmia). Also, other non-CYP enzymes can be significantly affected by DDI. An example of a serious DDI involving inhibition of a non-CYP enzyme that has resulted in fatal outcomes is the case of interactions between the antiviral drug sorivudine and the cytotoxic anticancer agent 5-fluorouracil (5-FU) or 5-FU prodrugs that are metabolized by the enzyme dihydropyrimidine dehydrogenase (DPD) [5]. Another example of clinically significant DDIs resulting from inhibition on non-CYP enzymes is the interaction between the xanthine oxidase (XO) inhibitor allopurinol and 6-mercaptopurine (6-MP) or its imidazolyl derivative, azathioprine [6]. Inhibition of XO-mediated metabolism of 6-MP by allopurinol has been shown to result in a fivefold increase in systemic exposure of orally administered 6-MP, necessitating a reduction in the dose of 6-MP or azathioprine in patients requiring coadministration with allopurinol. The interaction between azathioprine and allopurinol can be fatal. As we can see, risk assessment and management of DDI is important for clinical practice, pharma research, and drug regulation. In clinical practice, DDI is important in polypharmacy, oncology, HIV treatment, and in the older population [7]. But last, not least, the identification of clinically important interactions with food (e.g., grapefruit juice) and herbal products described in other chapters is also a serious issue due to perception as innocuous substances without risk (see also Chaps. 14 and 15).

DDIs are usually classified into the following categories:

- Pharmacokinetic (PK) interactions including absorption, distribution, metabolism, or excretion (ADME)—when one drug changes PK parameters from the other.
- Pharmacodynamic (PD) interactions—when one drug could change the effect of the other drug, without affecting its PK.

DDIs examinations may be challenged by retrospective population studies, case reports, or in vitro analyses if the drug is on the market. If the drug is in later stages of clinical development or already on the market, DDIs studies may be triggered by retrospective analyses of population data, case reports, or additional in vitro data. When the drug enters clinical development, this evaluation is typically based on in vitro, animal, and in silico data, but the evaluation is rapidly strengthened by accumulating clinical data. Consequently, the drug of interest can be evaluated either as a substrate (victim drug) or as an inhibitor or inducer (perpetrator drug) of drug-metabolizing enzymes or transporters.

The risk assessment and management of DDIs has an important role in pharmaceutical development, drug regulation, and medical practice generally. These facts emphasize the significance of DDIs and magnified their importance as a public health issue [1, 8]. The scientific advances over the last two decades, resulting in critical enablers that now permit a rational approach to drug interaction risk assessment and clinical pharmacological evaluation. The scientific advances in the last decades facilitate a rational approach for DDI evaluation and risk assessment.

These facilitators are:

- In vitro technology is necessary to examine drug metabolism and DDIs (multiplication of human metabolizing enzymes and transporters, availability of different necessary biological and substances).
- Progress in "in vitro"-"in vivo extrapolation" (IVIVE) as well as in simulation and modeling due to better prediction and optimization DDI s clinical studies.

The drug response and fate of the drug in an organism are essential for the assessment of therapeutic interval as a critical point for the estimation of DDIs and future prescribing instructions [1].

Enzymes and Transporters

The main roles in pharmacokinetics (PK) are reserved for enzymes and transporters (see more in Chap. 12). They are equally important in the activation and fate of drugs in the body. Drugs change their pharmacological activity through metabolic transformations divided into Phase I and II reactions. The metabolic enzymes have the main role in Phase I biotransformation processes such as oxidation, reduction, or hydrolysis, followed by Phase II reactions, that mostly involve covalently binding compounds such as glucuronic acid, glutathione, or sulfate. The examples of Phase II enzymes are uridine diphosphoglucuronosyl transferases (UGTs) and glutathione-*S*-transferases (GSTs). Their products, more polar metabolites are excreted from the body by efflux transporters. There are two main groups of drug transporters: the solute carrier (SLC) and ATP-binding cassette (ABC). Generally, ABC transporters play a vital role in drug disposition (efflux drugs from the liver and kidney), while SLC's primary function is drug influx. DDI, based on metabolism is due to induction or inhibition of metabolic enzymes (mainly CYP 450s or UGT). Some of the drugs with narrow therapeutic windows such as cyclosporine are substrates of both CYP3A4 enzyme and MDR1 transporter [9].

Enzymes

There are 57 families of cytochrome P450. Families 5–51 are responsible for the metabolism and biosynthesis of physiological compounds while families 1–4 are responsible for the metabolism of xenobiotics (general chemicals, natural products, and drugs) [10, 11]. Mainly, the drug metabolism is carried out by the CYP1, 2, and 3 families and occurs in the liver (Fig. 4.1), where the highest concentration of CYP450 is observed. The significance of extrahepatic metabolism in tissues like the

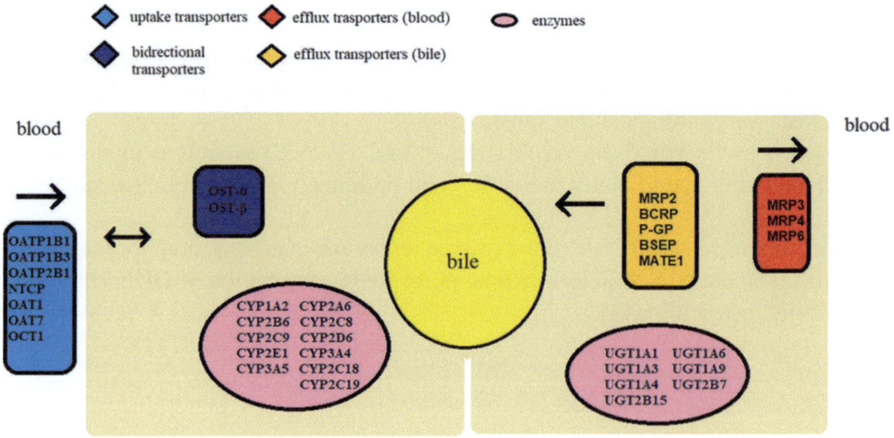

Fig. 4.1 Liver

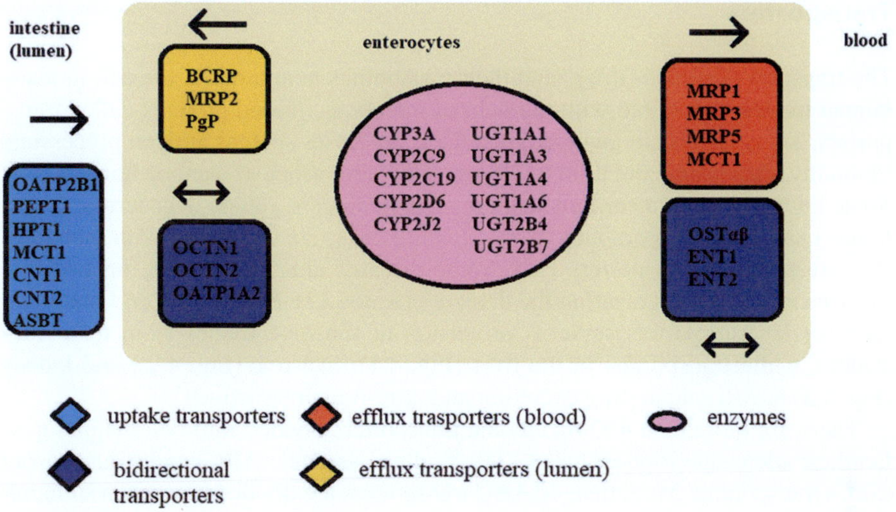

Fig. 4.2 Intestine

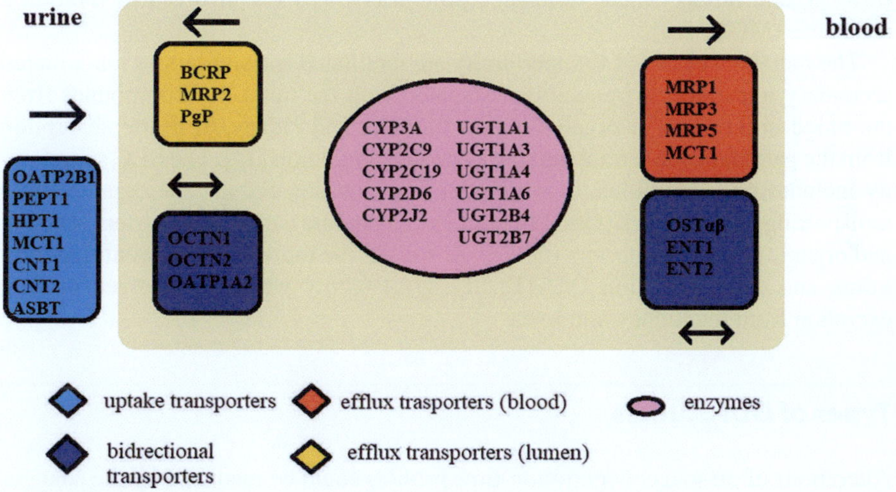

Fig. 4.3 Kidney

intestine (Fig. 4.2), kidney (Fig. 4.3), or lung, however, is also recognized. Only a dozen enzymes belonging to three families (CYP 1, 2, and 3) are involved in the biotransformation of many drugs in clinical use. The five isozymes of cytochromes P450 (1A2, 2C9, 2C19, 2D6, and 3A4) are responsible for more than three-fourths of reactions regarding drug metabolism. The expression of each CYP can be influenced by various factors and can lead to different characteristics such as poor, normal, intermediate, rapid, and ultrarapid metabolizers.

Transporters

The transport of various drugs and their metabolites in and out of the cell in many human tissues is possible with the help of membrane-bound proteins called transporters. Transporters are involved in cellular processes such as antigen processing, immunity, cholesterol and lipid transport, and maintenance of osmotic homeostasis. Some human genetic disorders including cystic fibrosis, retinal degeneration, cholesterol and bile transport, and neurological diseases are connected with mutations in corresponding transporters [12]. Some diseases alter transporter function and expression, in turn aggravating the disease process. The blood-brain and maternal-fetal barrier transporters serve as protection of sensitive tissues from toxic substances, while transporters in the liver (Fig. 4.1), intestine (Fig. 4.2), and kidney (Fig. 4.3) have a role in drug excretion and drug-drug interactions.

There are more than 400 membrane transporters divided into two major superfamilies: adenosine triphosphate (ATP) binding cassettes (ABC) and solute carrier (SLC) transporters. More than 40 ABC transporters are divided into seven subfamilies: White/ABCG, multidrug resistance-associated proteins (MRP)/ABCC, MDR/ABCB, OABP/ABCE, GCN20/ABCF, ABC1/ABCA, ALD/ABCD. ABC transporters such as P-glycoprotein (P-GP), multidrug resistance-associated proteins (MRPs), and breast cancer resistance protein (BCRP) are involved in multidrug resistance (MDR) [13].

The members of the SLC superfamily are facilitated transporters or ion-coupled secondary transporters, frequently associated with the uptake of compounds from the blood into tissues or organs such as the liver and kidney, or in the absorption from the gastrointestinal tract into the systemic circulation [14]. The SLC superfamily includes 65 subfamilies, of which the most investigated are the organic anion transporting polypeptides (OATPs, SLCO), the organic cation transporters (OCTs), and organic anion transporters (OATs), as well as the more recently identified multidrug and toxin extrusion (MATE, SLC47A) family which is involved in drug excretion from the kidney and liver.

Types of DDI Studies

Alterations of plasma concentration-time profiles could be mediated by the changes in different pharmacokinetic processes (absorption, distribution, metabolic, and elimination). The main role in biotransformation and fate of new molecular entity in human body is reserved for enzymes and transporters. In the case of concomitant medications, one drug (victim) can be changed by another drug (perpetrator). The preclinical and clinical development are the parts of the drug development process. Many various factors, such as the mechanism of DDIs, dosing regimen, and exposure-related safety, have an influence on drug development. According to that, the regulatory agencies issued different documents that serve as general guides during drug development. Drugs can be divided into different categories as substrate,

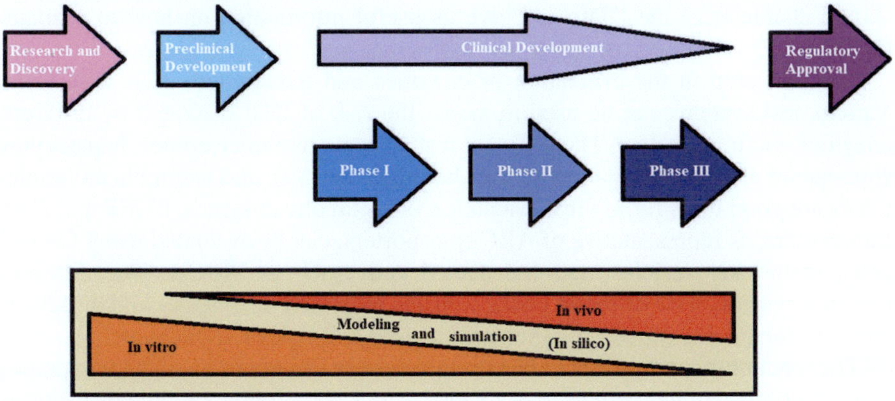

Fig. 4.4 DDI drug development

inducers, and inhibitors. Generally, DDI studies should be performed during preclinical and clinical drug development (Fig. 4.4).

In Vitro Studies

In vitro evaluation of the new drug concerning DDIs involve the following:

- Assessment of the role of enzymes and transporters in the development of new drug.
- Characterizing the relationship between a drug and enzymes/transporters.
- Informing the likelihood of clinical DDIs as well as the need for clinical studies.

DDI may arise from either an investigational drug affecting other medications as well as from other medications affecting the investigational drug. In vitro experiments should be conducted to assess which enzyme is included in drug metabolism, often focusing on CYP enzymes. For example, if a drug is metabolized by one CYP enzyme in vitro and anticipated drug concentration is increased in humans, concomitant medication may lead to higher concentrations and consequently to toxic effects. Also, the concentration level of the drug can be decreased in the case of concomitant medication with an inducer of CYP enzyme, and the result can be that it is an ineffective drug. Furthermore, drug transporters that deliver drugs to and from the enzymes are also important to evaluate due to the possibility of the drug's unexpected systemic exposure. Drug transporter studies provide data on a drug's substrate potential and likelihood of inhibiting the transporter involved in a drug excretion. The results of these studies, in addition to PK data, help us predict the possibility of DDIs. Generally, in vitro evaluation of metabolic enzymes and transporters has to be performed before conducting clinical studies. The clinical studies should characterize the DDIs and give us useful information on how to mitigate the DDIs.

The first step in the evaluation of enzymes and transporters is in vitro tests. Various test systems can be used to assess the risk of DDI mediated by different enzymes and transporters. The different test systems like microsomes, hepatocytes supernatant after centrifugation of liver homogenate (S9), and recombinant human CYPs are good tools for in vitro evaluation of metabolic enzymes. BCRP and P-gp transporters, as representative of ABC transporters, can be evaluated using Caco-2 cells, membrane vesicles, and transfected cells such as MDCK. The different research systems have different characteristics with their advantages and disadvantages, so the choice depends on the specific drug and type of application.

The reaction-phenotyping studies try to determine enzymes involved in metabolism. Inhibition studies help us to evaluate a drug's perpetrator potential by examining enzymes such as CYP P 450 or UGT. The increased plasma level of the victim drug can result in drug toxicity due to reduced metabolism. On the contrary, induction studies can measure the potential to up-regulated metabolizing enzymes and result in reduced efficacy. If NCE is not a CYP substrate, other enzymes are involved in Phase I reactions such as alcohol/aldehyde dehydrogenase (ADH), flavin monooxygenase (FMO), monoamine oxidase (MAO), and xanthine oxidase (XO) should be examined. Enzymes involved in Phase II reactions (conjugation reactions) have a lower incidence of adverse DDIs and less attention in DDI evaluations. In the case of unknown metabolism or if metabolism contributes $\geq 25\%$ of the drug's excretion, in vivo studies with appropriate inhibitors/inducers are necessary, starting with strong inducers/inhibitors. If a positive reaction is noted, a weaker probe should be evaluated using a proper modeling system or clinical study. In vitro results determine a need for further in vivo studies according to DDI guidelines' decision trees. In vitro tools like a nuclear receptor assay or the adenocarcinoma cell line LS 180, which expresses P-gp, investigate the role of the investigational drug as an inducer of transporters. The induction potential in some cases depends on in vivo studies due to a lack of validation in vitro methods.

In vitro science has advanced over the last two decades based on a new model and novel technology. Different cell lines that are transfected with enzymes or transporter proteins (including double transfections), bio-generation of an increasing range of enzymes using mammalian cell or bacterial vectors cryopreserved hepatocytes that will attach for culture and human liver microsomes pooled from many donor livers. All that, together with high-pressure liquid chromatography (HPLC) and fast-scanning MS/MS instrumentation, is ever pushing the limits of detection to far lower levels.

The above-mentioned factors, in conjunction with powerful in silico modeling, now allow scientists to make more accurate predictions about certain kinds of DDIs in vivo and to try and control these by appropriate labeling. As a result, the kinds of interactions that caused high-profile drug withdrawals during the late 1990s (e.g., terfenadine as a victim drug and mibefradil as a perpetrator drug) can now be largely predicted in the laboratory from in vitro data, and it is unlikely that this type of drug withdrawal (based upon inhibition of CYP450 enzymes) will happen again. The regulatory guidance now available in this area provides a solid framework when considering the in vitro information required to assess the DDI potential of a new chemical entity.

Clinical Studies

The human pharmacokinetic data in addition to in vitro studies, are the basis for clinical DDI studies. The investigational drug (or major metabolite) may be a substrate, inhibitor, or inducer for various enzymes or transporters. The guidance includes different decision trees and appropriate methods and models. The key considerations for in vitro studies include a selection of convenient and validated methods and a rational choice of substrate/interacting drug.

There are different types of DDI clinical studies during drug development programs: stand-alone and nested studies [15]. They serve to determine the presence and magnitude of DDI. The stand-alone studies can be divided into index studies and concomitant studies. The index studies assessed the worst-case scenario, while concomitant studies examined DDI in real life after drug approval. The choice of drugs in concomitant studies depends on their frequency of concomitant use and the potential of DDI.

Index Studies

The basis of DDI evaluation is index studies that use perpetrators (inducers or inhibitors) or victims (substrates) with well-known PK and DDI characteristics. The index perpetrators change the function of enzymes and transporters predictably, and they are safe for human use. The index substrate contributes to a specific elimination pathway and has defined interactions with an index inhibitor. According to that, drugs can be further classified on strong or moderate perpetrators or sensitive or moderate sensitive substrates. Typical inhibitors or inducers study evaluate DDI under the "worst-case scenario." For drugs that are evaluated as victims of a DDI, the worst case is the concomitant administration of a strong index inhibitor or inducer of the drug's major metabolic pathway(s), while in drugs evaluated as perpetrators of DDIs, the worst case is the administration of the investigated drug with a sensitive index substrate, ideally at the highest dose level and most frequent dosing schedule of the investigated drug. The drug that increases the AUC of a sensitive index substrate by more than fivefold is designated as a strong inhibitor for that pathway. The moderate inhibitor increases the AUC two- to fivefold. The regulatory agencies maintain a list of recommended index inhibitors or inducers (perpetrators) and substrates (victims) [16].

In Silico Studies

In silico studies extrapolate in vitro data to clinically relevant DDIs. There are three different categories of model-based methods mentioned in regulatory guidances basic (static), mechanistic static, and dynamic models. The use of all models, but especially PBPK, are increasing in the past few years. PBPK are mathematical techniques for predicting ADME processes of investigational drugs in the animal or human body. The pharma companies use them more and more to reduce the number of unnecessary clinical studies. Some publications describe the use of PBPK in DDI drug development and regulatory review [17, 18].

The regulatory agencies have issued guidance documents as a helpful tool for DDI assessment. The history of development regulatory documents is shown in Fig. 4.2.

DDIs Regulatory Guidelines

Drug-drug interactions (DDI) can reduce the therapeutic effect or increase the toxicity of drugs. Also, DDIs were the major cause of drug withdrawal from the market. These facts, together with polypharmacy, have encouraged the main drug regulators such as PMDA (Pharmaceutical Manufacturing Drug Agency), FDA (Food and Drug Administration), and EMA (European Medical Agency) to help developers in the planning and evaluating DDIs. The results were published guidelines with regular updates as a result of the growth of scientific knowledge as well as technical improvement. Many considerations determine the type and design of the studies necessary to perform during drug preclinical and clinical drug development.

The prediction of potential DDIs could be based on the result of preclinical and clinical evaluations as well as recommended probe substrates and specific inhibitors/inducers of drug-metabolizing enzymes and transporters. Compared to earlier versions, new guidance documents contained much more extensive recommendations on in vitro and in vivo studies. Figure 4.5 gives us a short historical review in this field. Sudsakorn et al. recently compared in a review article all existing guidelines issued by EMA, PMDA, and FDA [19].

Europe

Cole et al., in their article EMA, described the development of regulatory DDIs documents in the EU [20]. The committee for Medicinal Products for Human Use (CHMP) prepared and published "Note for Guidance on the Investigation of Drug Interactions" in 1998 after reaching a consensus [21]. This guideline reflected a harmonized EU approach. In 2010, a revision of this guideline was carried out and it came into effect in January 2013 [22]. This guideline is the current one in use in Europe, but in 2017 the EMA announced the intention to revise the guideline [23]. In the meantime, several clarification answers on the guideline were published in

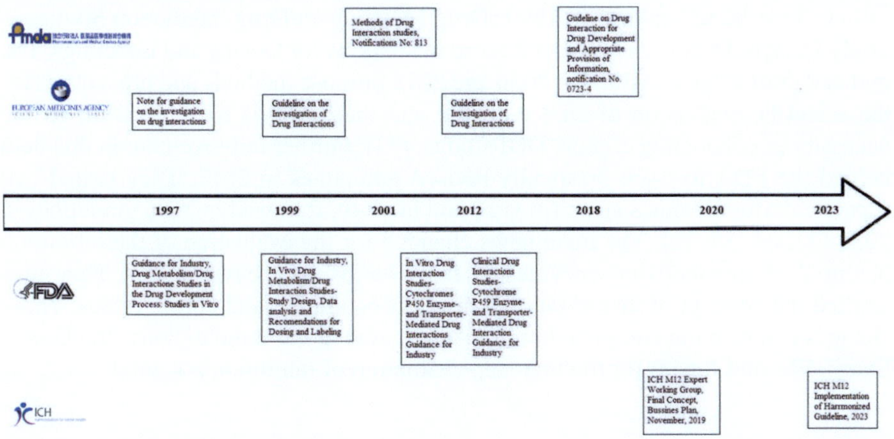

Fig. 4.5 History of DDI guidelines

October 2014 [24]. Also, the PBPK guideline published in 2018 contained information relevant to an assessment of drug interactions [25].

Japan

In Japan, the regulatory document notified by the Ministry of Health, Labour and Welfare (MHLW) in June 2001 was referenced to investigate drug interactions during drug development and review drug interactions during the regulatory approval review [26]. Over the time's Japanese regulatory document was revised as well as documents of other regulators [27, 28]. The Japanese guideline revisions were undertaken by a research group that consisted of academics affiliated with relevant academic societies, personnel engaged in preclinical and clinical development at pharmaceutical companies, and regulators of regulatory authorities. Until the notification of the new Japanese guideline in 2018, a final draft of the guideline was published, and public consultations occurred twice around the time of the final draft publication [29, 30]. Responses to major comments obtained during the public consultation or guideline descriptions requiring appropriate commentary with relevant referenced literature are included in a document on questions and answers that were published along with the new Japanese guideline. Ishiguro et al. presented the highlights of the new Japanese guideline and address the background underlying investigations in a review article [31].

The United States

The first draft of DDI guidelines was published by FDA in 1997 (Drug Metabolism/ Drug Interaction Studies in the Drug Development Process: Studies In Vitro), followed by the second one in 1999 (Drug Metabolism/Drug Interaction Studies—Study Design, Data Analysis, and Recommendations for Dosing and Labeling). The updated draft versions issued in 2006 and 2012 propose methods and procedures for the scientific evaluation of DDI potential and their criteria for a decision on the necessity of conducting clinical DDI studies [32]. Further improvement in this field helped the FDA to issue drastically revised guidelines in 2017. They issued two separate draft guidelines again (in vitro and in vivo), followed by final guidelines in 2020 [33, 34, 35, 36]. The main news changed for the evaluation of the inhibition potential of metabolizing enzymes in the liver using a basic model. They also applied the concept of investigational drug concentration and cutoff values. These changes result in the complete harmonization among the three regions (the United States, EU, and Japan) for the first-step evaluation of inhibition potential.

ICH

The regulatory agencies use a risk-based strategy to assess DDIs in clinical trials because it is impractical to evaluate each DDI during drug development. However, there are some discrepancies in the approach used by agencies. Thus, lack of harmonization contributes to a burden that meets the pharmaceutical industry during product development and may increase drug development costs and delay patient access to new therapeutic products. A harmonized guideline will lead to a consistent approach in designing, conducting, and interpreting DDI studies during the development of a therapeutic product. A consistent approach will reduce uncertainty for the pharmaceutical industry to meet the requirements of multiple regulatory agencies and lead to more efficient utilization of resources. Eventually, this will help reduce the cost and bring treatments faster to the global market for patients who need the therapies. Recently an ICH (International Conference of Harmonisation) initiative on drug interactions has been announced, and this is likely to influence any future revision of guidance [37]. It is anticipated that a Step 2b Guideline will be completed by 4Q of 2021 and that Step 4 will be reached by 2Q of 2023, with implementation to follow in 2023. This guideline will replace regional guidelines.

Conclusion

Evaluation of the DDI potential of a new drug is a very sensitive part of the drug development process, crucial for drug safety. The understanding of the mechanism and prediction of DDI is based on preclinical, in vitro, in silico data but clinical data remain as a central place in the evaluation of DDI risk. It is not possible to predict all permutations of different drug combinations during drug development. In silico models together with mechanistically focused clinical studies help us to better understanding DIIS and its clinical relevance. The drug in the drug development process can be investigated either as a perpetrator or victim of metabolizing enzymes or transporters. There is no standard and optimal schedule to examine DDIs, but the design of each study has to be grounded carefully, based on the availability of in vitro and clinical data to ensure the usefulness of the study and protect the subject's safety [38].

References

1. Zhang Z, Tang W. Drug metabolism in drug discovery and development. Acta Pharm Sin B. 2018;8(5):721–32. https://doi.org/10.1016/j.apsb.2018.04.003.
2. FDA Clinical Pharmacology and Biopharmaceutics Review(s). https://www.accessdata.fda.gov/drugsatfda_docs/nda/2017/208082Orig1s000ClinPharmR.pdf. Accessed 3 Mar 2021.
3. Lyubimov AV, Venkatakrishnan K. DDI risk assessment and evaluation in pharmaceutical development: interfacing drug metabolism and clinical pharmacology. In: Lyubimov AV, editor. Encyclopedia of drug metabolism and interactions. Wiley; 2012. https://doi.org/10.1002/9780470921920.edm118.
4. Huang SM, Lesko LJ. Drug-drug, drug-dietary supplement, and drug-citrus fruit and other food interactions: what have we learned. J Clin Pharmacol. 2004;44(6):559–69.
5. Diasio RB. Sorivudine and 5-fluorouracil: a clinically significant drug-drug interaction due to inhibition of dihydropyrimidine dehydrogenase. Br J Clin Pharmacol. 1998;46(1):1–4.
6. Zimm S, Collins JM, O'Neill D, et al. Inhibition of first-pass metabolism in cancer chemotherapy: interaction of 6-mercaptopurine and allopurinol. Clin Pharmacol Ther. 1983;34(6):810–7.
7. Qato DM, Alexander GC, Conti RM, et al. Use of prescription and over-the-counter medications and dietary supplements among older adults in the United States. JAMA. 2008;300(24):2867–78.
8. U.S. Department of Health and Human Services, Food and Drug Administration, Center for Drug Evaluation and Research (CDER). Draft guidance/guidance for industry. Drug interaction studies: study design, data analysis, implications for dosing, and labeling recommendations. Silver Spring, MD: FDA; 2012. http://www.fda.gov/downloads/Drugs/GuidanceComplianceRegulatoryInformation/Guidances/UCM292362.pdf. Accessed 3 Mar 2021.
9. Hu YF, Qiu W, Liu ZQ, Zhu LJ, et al. Effects of genetic polymorphisms of CYP3A4, CYP3A5 and MDR1 on cyclosporine pharmacokinetics after renal transplantation. Clin Exp Pharmacol Physiol. 2006;33(11):1093–8. https://doi.org/10.1111/j.1440-1681.2006.04492.x.
10. Rendic SP, Guengerich FP. Human family 1–4 cytochrome P450 enzymes involved in the metabolic activation of xenobiotic and physiological chemicals: an update. Arch Toxicol. 2021;95(2):395–472. https://doi.org/10.1007/s00204-020-02971-4.
11. Rendic SP, Peter Guengerich F. Human cytochrome P450 enzymes 5–51 as targets of drugs and natural and environmental compounds: mechanisms, induction, and inhibition—toxic effects and benefits. Drug Metab Rev. 2018;50(3):256–342. https://doi.org/10.1080/03602532.2018.1483401.
12. Liu X. ABC family transporters. In: Liu X, Pan G, editors. Drug transporters in drug disposition, effects and toxicity, Advances in experimental medicine and biology, vol. 1141. Singapore: Springer; 2019. https://doi.org/10.1007/978-981-13-7647-4_2.
13. Schinkel AH, Jonker JW. Mammalian drug efflux transporters of the ATP binding cassette (ABC) family: an overview. Adv Drug Deliv Rev. 2012;64:138–53.
14. Pizzagalli MD, Bensimon A, Superti-Furga G. A guide to plasma membrane solute carrier proteins. FEBS J. 2021;288(9):2784–835. https://doi.org/10.1111/febs.15531.
15. Rekić D, Reynolds KS, Zhao P, et al. Clinical drug-drug interaction evaluations to inform drug use and enable drug access. J Pharm Sci. 2017;106(9):2214–8. https://doi.org/10.1016/j.xphs.2017.04.016.

16. US Department of Health and Human Services, Food and Drug Administration, Center for Drug Evaluation and Research (CDER). Drug development and drug interactions: table of substrates, inhibitors and inducers. Available at: http://www.fda.gov/Drugs/DevelopmentApprovalProcess/DevelopmentResources/DrugInteractionsLabeling/ucm093664.htm. Accessed 9 Dec 2020.
17. Jamei M. Recent advances in development and application of physiologically-based pharmacokinetic (PBPK) models: a transition from academic curiosity to regulatory acceptance. Curr Pharmacol Rep. 2016;2:161–9.
18. Yoshida K, Budha N, Jin JY. Impact of physiologically based pharmacokinetic models on regulatory reviews and product labels: frequent utilization in the field of oncology. Clin Pharmacol Ther. 2017;101(5):597–602. https://doi.org/10.1002/cpt.622.
19. Sudsakorn S, Bahadduri P, Fretland J, Lu C. FDA drug-drug interaction guidance: a comparison analysis and action plan by pharmaceutical industrial scientists. Curr Drug Metab. 2020;21(6):403–26. https://doi.org/10.2174/1389200221666200620210522. Accessed 29 Jun 2021.
20. Cole S, Kerwash E, Andersson A. A summary of the current drug interaction guidance from the European Medicines Agency and considerations of future updates. Drug Metab Pharmacokinet. 2020;35(1):2–11. https://doi.org/10.1016/j.dmpk.2019.11.005.
21. Note for guidance on the investigation of drug interactions. Committee for human medicinal products (CHMP) of the European Medicines agency (EMA). 1998. https://www.ema.europa.eu/en/documents/scientific-guideline/note-guidance-investigation-drug-interactions_en.pdf. Accessed 29 Jan 2021.
22. Guideline on the investigation of drug interactions. Committee for Human Medicinal Products (CHMP) of the European Medicines Agency (EMA). Doc. Ref. CPMP/EWP/560/95/Rev.1 corr.2**. 2012. https://www.ema.europa.eu/en/documents/scientific-guideline/guideline-investigation-drug-interactions_en.pdf.
23. Concept paper on a revision of the Guideline on the investigation of drug interactions. Committee for Human Medicinal Products (CHMP) of the European Medicines Agency (EMA). Doc. Ref. EMEA/CHMP/694687/2016. 2017. https://www.ema.europa.eu/en/documents/scientific-guideline/conceptpaper-revision-guideline-investigation-drug-interactions_en.pdf.
24. Clinical pharmacology and pharmacokinetics: questions and answers. Drug interactions. https://www.ema.europa.eu/en/human-regulatory/research-development/scientific-guidelines/clinicalpharmacology-pharmacokinetics/clinical-pharmacology-pharmacokineticsquestions-answers#2.-drug-interactions-section. Accessed 16 Jul 2019.
25. Guideline on the reporting of physiologically based pharmacokinetic (PBPK) modelling and simulation. Committee for Human Medicinal Products (CHMP) of the European Medicines Agency (EMA). Doc. Ref. EMA/CHMP/458101/2016. 2018. https://www.ema.europa.eu/en/documents/scientific-guideline/guideline-reporting-physiologically-based-pharmacokinetic-pbpk-modellingsimulation_en.pdf.
26. Ministry of Labor and Welfare. Methods of drug interaction studies, notification No. 813, evaluation and licensing division. Japan: Pharmaceuticals Medical Safety Bureau; 2001.
27. European Medicines Agency. Guideline on the investigation of drug interactions, draft, CPMP/EWP/560/95/Rev.1. Committee for Human Medical Products, EU; 2010. https://www.ema.europa.eu/en/documents/scientific-guideline/draft-guideline-investigation-drug-interactions_en.pdf. Accessed 14 Aug 2019.
28. Food and Drug Administration. Guidance for industry, drug interaction studies: study design, data analysis, implications for dosing, and labeling recommendations, DRAFT. Center for Drug Evaluation and Research, U.S. Department of Health and Human Services; 2012.
29. Ministry of Labor and Welfare. Guideline on drug interaction for drug development and appropriate provision of information (final draft), office communication. Japan: Pharmaceutical Evaluation Division, Pharmaceuticals Safety and Environmental Health Bureau; 2014.
30. Ministry of Labor and Welfare. Guideline on drug interaction for drug development and appropriate provision of information, notification No. 0723-4. Japan: Pharmaceutical Evaluation Division, Pharmaceuticals Safety and Environmental Health Bureau; 2018. https://www.pmda.go.jp/files/000228122.pdf. Accessed 14 Aug 2019.

31. Ishiguro A, Sato R, Nagai N. Development of a new Japanese guideline on drug interaction for drug development and appropriate provision of information. Drug Metab Pharmacokinet. 2020;35(1):12–7. https://doi.org/10.1016/j.dmpk.2019.11.009.
32. Yu J, Ritchie TK, Mulgaonkar A, Ragueneau-Majlessi I. Drug disposition and drug-drug interaction data in 2013 FDA new drug applications: a systematic review. Drug Metab Dispos. 2014;42(12):1991–2001. https://doi.org/10.1124/dmd.114.060392.
33. U.S. Food and Drug Administration, FDA Center for Drug Evaluation and Research. Guidance for industry; in vitro metabolism- and transporter-mediated drug-drug interaction studies. Guidance for Industry, Draft Guidance. 2017. https://www.fda.gov/files/drugs/published/In-Vitro-Metabolism%2D%2Dand Transporter-Mediated-Drug-Drug-Interaction-Studies-Guidance for-Industry.pdf.
34. U.S. Food and Drug Administration, FDA Center for Drug Evaluation and Research. Guidance for industry; clinical drug interactions studies—study design, data analysis, and clinical implications. Guidance for Industry, Draft Guidance. 2017. https://www.fda.gov/files/drugs/published/Clinical-Drug-Interaction Studies%2D%2DStudy-Design%2D%2DData-Analysis%2D%2Dand-ClinicalImplications-Guidance-for-Industry.pdf.
35. U.S. Food and Drug Administration, FDA Center for Drug Evaluation and Research. Guidance for industry; clinical drug interaction studies—cytochrome P450 enzyme and transporter mediated drug interactions. 2020. https://www.fda.gov/media/134581/download.
36. U.S. Food and Drug Administration, FDA Center for Drug Evaluation and Research. Guidance for industry; in vitro drug interaction studies—cytochrome P450 enzyme and transporter mediated drug interactions. 2020. https://www.fda.gov/media/134582/download.
37. ICH Assembly Minutes. Charlotte, NC. https://www.ich.org/fileadmin/Public_Web_Site/Meetings/Ass_MC_Meetings_Reports/ICH37Charlotte_Assembly_Minutes_Final_2019_0108.pdf. Accessed 14–15 Nov 2018.
38. Tornio A, Filppula AM, Niemi M, Backman JT. Clinical studies on drug-drug interactions involving metabolism and transport: methodology, pitfalls, and interpretation. Clin Pharmacol Ther. 2019;105(6):1345–61. https://doi.org/10.1002/cpt.1435.

Part II

Basic Pharmacology of GI Drugs

Antisecretory Drugs

5

Robert Smolić, Sonja Vukadin, and Lucija Kuna

Introduction

Antisecretory drugs are used for acid-related gastrointestinal disorders (see also Chap. 27). H2RAs were introduced into practice first, but nowadays PPIs are more used due to their greater potency and relatively good safety profile.

H2 Receptor Antagonists (H2RAs)

H2 receptor blockers or H2 receptor antagonists (H2RAs) represent landmark in the treatment of gastrointestinal disease [1]. Ranitidine, cimetidine, nizatidine and famotidine belong to the most widely used drugs in medicine which are available by prescription and over the counter (OCT); Famotidine, ranitidine, and cimetidine are all available either OTC or by prescription, depending on the dose, while nizatidine is available by prescription only. However, proton pump inhibitors (PPI) are valuable as substitutions for H2RAs in everyday practice [2, 3].

R. Smolić (✉)
Department of Pathophysiology, Faculty of Medicine, J.J. Strossmayer University of Osijek, Osijek, Croatia

Department of Pharmacology and Biochemistry, Faculty of Dental Medicine and Health, J.J. Strossmayer University of Osijek, Osijek, Croatia
e-mail: robert.smolic@mefos.hr; robert.smolic@fdmz.hr

S. Vukadin · L. Kuna
Department of Pharmacology and Biochemistry, Faculty of Dental Medicine and Health, J.J. Strossmayer University of Osijek, Osijek, Croatia
e-mail: lucija.kuna@fdmz.hr

M. Banić, D. Erceg (eds.), *Drug Interactions in Gastroenterology*, Clinical Gastroenterology, https://doi.org/10.1007/978-3-031-69800-2_5

Indications

H2RAs are used to suppress gastric acid secretion in disorders such as:

1. Gastric or duodenal ulcers
2. Gastric hypersecretion
3. Moderate heartburn or indigestion
4. Off-label they may be used for stress ulcer prophylaxis, gastritis, gastrointestinal hemorrhage esophagitis and urticaria

It is important to emphasize that overall effectiveness of H2RAs highly depends on the intensity of dosage regimen, severity of gastric disease and therapy duration. They suppress 24-h gastric acid release by approximately 70%, which makes them less potent than PPIs. H2-RAs inhibit basal gastric secretion, hence, their efficiency has significant role in suppressing nocturnal acid secretion. It is mainly the level of nocturnal acidity that impacts duodenal ulcer healing, therefore, evening dosing of H2RAs antagonists is appropriate therapy in most cases [1, 4].

Mechanism of Action

H2RAs decrease gastric acid production by reversibly binding to histamine H2 receptors on basolateral membrane of gastric parietal cell, thereby inhibiting the effect of histamine [1]. Physiologically, histamine released from enterochromaffin-like (ECL) cells binds to H2 receptor and triggers a cascade that enhances the intracellular cyclic adenosine monophosphate (cAMP). Consequently, cAMP activates the hydrogenpotassium pump that exchanges intracellular hydrogen ions with potassium ions from the gastric lumen. Given H2RAs are competitive inhibitors of histamine at H2-receptors, they cause reduction of acid secretion [5, 6]. Both gastrin and acetylcholine stimulate ECL cells to release histamine; therefore, their effect on parietal cells is also decreased when the H2 receptors are blocked by H2RAs [7]. Figure 5.1 shows mechanism of action of H2RAs.

Pharmacokinetics

H2RAs are well absorbed after oral administration and their mean bioavailability is 50–70% [8]. There are different oral preparations of H2RAs available on market today, such as powder for suspension, syrup, capsule, oral solution, and chewable tablet. The onset of action is about 1 h and duration of action ranges between 4 and 10 h, making them valuable for the on-demand therapy of occasional symptoms. All H2RAs have equivalent effectiviness in reducing gastric acid secretion [9]. Their therapeutic concentration is reached quickly after intravenous dosing and maintained for 4–5 h for cimetidine, 6–8 h for ranitidine, and 10–12 h for famotidine. Unlike PPIs, H2RAs are poorly bound to plasma proteins. A small proportion of

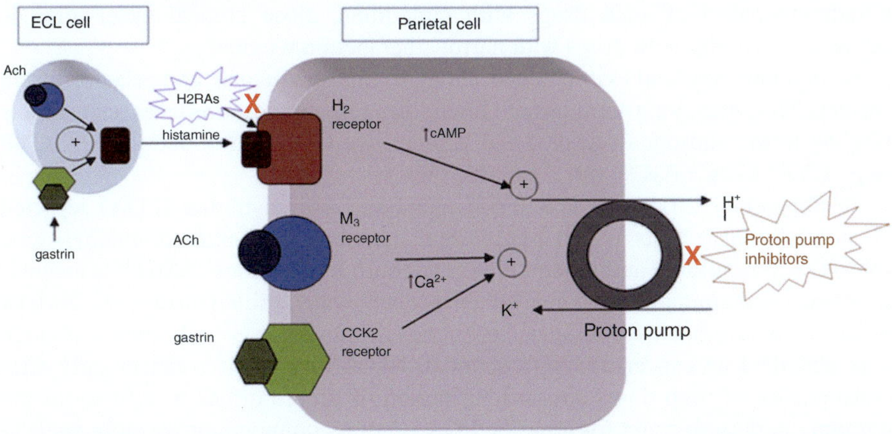

Fig. 5.1 Physiology of gastric acid secretion and H2RA and PPI mechanism of action. There are several stimulants for gastric acid secretion and proton pump, incorporated in apical membrane of a parietal cell, is a final step in those pathways. Acetylcholine, released from vagal nerve during cephalic phase of gastric secretion, leads to Na^+/K^+ ATPase activation via three different pathways. (1) ACh binds to muscarinic M_3 receptor on basolateral membrane of parietal cell which leads to proton pump activation through Ca^{2+} mediated pathway. (2) Muscarinic receptors are also present on ECL cells, which release histamine as a result of muscarinic receptor activation. Histamine thereafter binds to H2 receptors on parietal cell leading to proton pump activation via cAMP mediated pathway. (3) Acetylcholine also stimulates gastrin secretion from G cells in antrum

these drugs is metabolized in liver, only <10% to ~35%. Kidneys excrete both active drugs and their metabolites, therefore dose reduction is necessary in patients with reduced creatinine clearance [1].

Adverse Reactions and Drug Interactions

H2Ras are generally well tolerated, side effects include diarrhea, fatigue, muscular pain, headache, constipation, and drowsiness. Less common side effects include those with strong effect on CNS: slurred speech, headache, confusion, delirium, and hallucinations. Elderly patients are more prone to such adverse events, especially after intravenous administration.

Cimetidine is an exception among H2Ras, it interacts with other medicines due to its high affinity to hepatic oxidase, and it also exerts some serious adverse events. Consequently, its use has decreased significantly [10].

It is well known that cimetidine is a competitive inhibitor of the hepatic oxidase enzymes. This leads to clinically significant interactions with drugs metabolized by the same enzymes. By CYP inhibition cimetidine may cause increased plasma concentration of warfarin, propranolol, β-adrenoceptor blockers, phenobarbital, theophylline, tricyclic antidepressants, various benzodiazepines, estradiol, phenytoin and Ca^{2+} channel blockers and lidocaine. To avoid serious events during co-administration of such drugs with cimetidine, close clinical observation is advised, especially with drugs with narrow therapeutic window.

Cimetidine may lead to impotence and gynecomastia in men, and galactorrhea in women. Moreover, long-term use of cimetidine at higher doses reduces testosterone binding to the androgen receptor and hamper hydroxylation of estradiol by CYP (e.g., CYP1A2, CYP2C9, and CYP2D6) [1].

In September 2019, the U.S. Food and Drug Adminstration (FDA) reported about preliminary tests which found small amounts of *N*-nitrosodimethylamine (NDMA) in ranitidine and several other heartburn medications. NMDA is an environmental contaminant found in vegetables, diary, water, grilled meats [11]. NMDA is classed as a probable carcinogen, but studies in humans are very limited. Although it is classified as cancer-causing chemical, NDMA may cause cancer only after consumption of high doses over a long period of time. Further investigations are currently undergoing and for now, the FDA is not recommending for individuals to stop taking ranitidine, but to consult their doctor should they require prolonged course of acid suppressive therapy [12].

Proton Pump Inhibitors (PPI)

PPIs are among most commonly prescribed medications worldwide. They were long considered to have a very good safety profile. However, in recent years, chronic PPI use has been linked with various concerning side effects, such as increased fracture risk and risk of cardiovascular and cerebrovascular events. It is also known that omeprazole interacts with many clinically important medicines, and clinicians need to be cautious when co-prescribing them. Many of those findings resulted from observational studies, and further investigation is needed to both elucidate mechanisms behind the findings and reveal their clinical relevance.

Indications

PPIs are used to suppress gastric acid secretion in disorders such as:

1. Gastro-oesophageal reflux disease and reflux esophagitis
2. Treatment of peptic ulcer disease, but also ulcer prophylaxis in patients who require long-term NSAID treatment
3. Treatment of non-variceal upper GI bleed (in addition to endoscopic intervention)
4. PPI, in combination with amoxicillin and clarithromycin are standard of care for the eradication of *Helicobacter pylori*
5. PPIs are commonly used to prevent upper GI bleed in susceptible individuals (e.g. elderly persons receiving dual antiplatelet therapy and an anticoagulant or critically ill patients in intensive care units who are known to be susceptible to stress ulcers and upper GI bleed)

Target intraoesophageal pH of above 4 for 16 or more hours/day proved to be sufficient for reflux oesophagitis healing. The target intragastric pH of above 3 for 16 h/day or more needs to be maintained to ensure peptic ulcer healing. All PPIs achieve the aforementioned target pH and are, to date, the best choice therapy in such disorders. However, there is still a small portion of individuals whose symptoms of excess acid secretion return in the number of months after initiating maintenance PPI therapy. This could be due to nocturnal breakthrough acid secretion for which PPIs are ineffective due to their short plasma half life. Tenatoprazole, a drug candidate with sevenfold longer plasma half life, achieves best night time acid suppression, with pH of above 4 for longer period as compared to other PPIs. Though, this property still needs to be investigated for its clinical relevance [13, 14].

Mechanism of Action

PPIs suppress gastric acid production by proton pump inhibition, a common endpoint of different pathways in gastric acid secretion. Figure 5.1 shows the physiology of gastric acid secretion and the mechanism of action of PPIs.

Parietal cell undergoes a transformation from resting to stimulated state after being exposed to ACh, gastrin or histamine. Stimuli lead to additional proton pumps being delivered to apical membrane from cytosol. Proton pump inhibitors are weak bases and prodrugs become activated in acid environment [14]. This characteristic allows them to accumulate in secretory cannaliculus of a parietal cell, as they become trapped in acid environment in ionized state on the luminal side of the parietal cell. Proton pump or Na^+/K^+ ATPase is based on apical membrane of parietal cells. PPIs act by binding covalently to cysteine residue on luminal side of Na^+/K^+ ATPase, which allows them longer duration of action then their relatively short plasma half-life would have. It is an irreversible reaction and the only way to recover from inhibition is de novo Na^+/K^+ ATPase synthesis, which takes up to 36 h [15]. However, not all proton pumps will be active during the 90-min period, which represents PPIs plasma half-life. With once-daily dosing, taken 30–60 min before breakfast, about 70% of pumps are inhibited. Twice daily dosing adds to about 80% pumps being inhibited [14].

Although there are some differences between median pH maintained by a particular PPI, clinically, there is no significant difference in healing of peptic ulcer or reflux oesphagitis, as in, all of them achieve good therapeutic effect [16].

Pharmacokinetics

To preserve PPIs from premature activation in gastric acidic environment and degradation by gastric peptidase there are different delivery formulations available, such as enteric-coated tablets, gelatin capsules, or coated granules supplied as a powder for suspension [17]. PPIs are absorbed in duodenum and their bioavailability varies from 30% to 40% for omeprazole up to 90% for esomeprazole. There are also intravenous formulations of most PPIs available, and they are indicated in non-variceal upper GI bleeds and generally in individuals unable to take oral preparations. In fact, continuous intravenous PPI infusion is the only mode of administration that maintains high pH required for cloth formation in bleeding ulcer [18].

All PPIs are highly bound to plasma proteins, 95–98%. Their plasma half-life is only about 90 min, which represents their disadvantage. First, in order to achieve their maximal effect their administration is meal-dependent—it should be taken 30 min before breakfast. Secondly, not all proton pumps can be inhibited during the 90 min period, as not all of them will be anchored into apical membrane at the time. On addition to that, to achieve their maximal effect, their administration is meal-dependent—PPIs should be taken 30 min before breakfast.

Metabolism All PPIs are to some extent metabolized by CYP2C19 and CYP3A4. Three different phenotypes have been identified: extensive metabolizers (homEM), intermediate (hetEM) and poor metabolizers (PM). Poor metabolizers make up 3% of Caucasians and 15–20% of Asians. Plasma concentration varies significantly among those three phenotypes, for example, the AUC for omeprazole is about 7.5-fold higher in PM than in homEM, about 4.5-fold higher for lansoprazole, and about fourfold higher for rabeprazole [14] Consequently, median intragastric pH varies between different phenotypes, from about 6 in PM to about 3–4 in homEM. As mentioned above, this however does not impact on healing rates of ulcer or oesophagitis between different PPIs [19].

In recent years a significant concern was raised in relation to omeprazole induced CYP2C19 inhibition and consequent interaction with clopidogrel, a widely used antiplatelet that requires activation by the same isoenzime. The effect was noticed in vitro, and although confirmation of its clinical relevance is lacking, it is recommended to use any PPI but omeprazole or esomeprazole in combination with clopidogrel, as they may reduce its effect [17].

Liver Impairment Hepatic impairment leads to an increased plasma concentration and prolonged elimination of PPIs. But esomeprazole proved to be safe in hepatic impairment, unlike other PPIs [20].

Chronic PPI use may lead to bacterial overgrowth in the small intestine due to gastric hypochloremia. A small retrospective observational study published in 2019 found that among patients with liver cirrhosis who were admitted to hospital with hepatic encephalopathy, a higher degree of hepatic encephalopathy affected patients who were taking PPI for at least 30 days prior to hospital admission. Higher ammonia production from bacterial overgrowth may be the reason behind the study findings [21]. However, the study was performed on a small sample, and there were no data about which particular PPI was used or if there was any difference among PPIs used.

Following hepatic metabolism PPIs are excreted via kidneys. There is no need for dose adjustment in patients with renal impairment.

Adverse Drug Reactions

Long-term treatment with PPIs increases risk of iron deficiency anaemia [22]. PPIs lead to hepcidin upregulation and consequent ferroportin inhibition in duodenum, which results in reduced iron absorption [23]. PPIs also may cause gynecomastia [24].

One of the major disadvantages of long-term PPI use is an increased fracture risk. Hip fracture in elderly population is most concerning because it contributes significantly to overall morbidity and mortality worldwide. PPIs decrease bone mineral density by causing hypochlorhydria and consequently reduce Mg^{2+}, Ca^{2+}, and vitamin B12 absorption. On the other hand, PPIs also cause hypergastrinemia, which ultimately leads to hyperparathyroidism and increased osteoclast activity [25]. There are also reports from multiple observational studies about increased risk of cardiovascular and cerebrovascular events in patients with no previous history of MI or CVA, and those events were not related to clopidogrel use. But the causal relationship should be investigated with further studies. It is also worth mentioning that, where possible, PPI cessation needs to be encouraged in patients at risk of *Clostridium difficile* colitis as it is linked with increased risk of the same.

Altogether, PPIs have been considered to have a very good safety profile even in long-term use. However, lately there have been a number of studies linking them to significant adverse events. While further investigation of causal relationship is needed, greater caution should be exercised when prescribing long term PPI therapy and patients should be advised of potential adverse reactions.

Drug–Drug Interactions

By reducing gastric acidity PPIs impair absorption of some medicines. For example, erlotinib, a Tyr-kinase inhibitor, is used in treatment of NSCLC. Studies have proved lower plasma concentrations of erlotinib in concomitant PPI use. However, clinical significance of this interaction is not known. It is advised to avoid this drug combination where risk outweighs the benefit [26]. Bioavailability of ketoconazole and atazanavir is reduced by 50% or more [27].

PPIs decelerate methotrexate clearance after a high-dose methotrexate infusion [28]. Caution should be used whenever PPI is co-prescribed with drug with narrow therapeutic window, e.g., drug monitoring of tacrolimus or phenytoin should be performed if PPI is introduced.

References

1. Hilal-Dandan R, Brunton LL. Drugs affecting gastrointestinal function. In: Goodman and Gilman's manual of pharmacology and therapeutics. McGraw Hill; 2008.

2. Chalasani N, Bonkovsky HL, Fontana R, Lee W, Stolz A, Talwalkar J, et al. Features and outcomes of 899 patients with drug-induced liver injury: the DILIN prospective study. Gastroenterology. 2015;148(7):1340–52.e7.
3. Price AH, Brogden RN. Nizatidine. A preliminary review of its pharmacodynamic and pharmacokinetic properties, and its therapeutic use in peptic ulcer disease. Drugs. 1988;36(5):521–39.
4. Feldman M, Friedman LS, Brandt LJ. Gastrointestinal and liver disease. Pathophysiology/diagnosis/management. 10th ed. Elsevier; 2016.
5. Shamburek RD, Schubert ML. Pharmacology of gastric acid inhibition. Baillieres Clin Gastroenterol. 1993;7(1):23–54.
6. Habibi A, Riley ET. Antihistamines: H1- and H2-Blockers. In: Complications in anesthesia. 2nd ed. Elsevier; 2007. p. 92–93. https://doi.org/10.1016/b978-1-4160-2215-2.50030-2
7. MacFarlane B. Management of gastroesophageal reflux disease in adults: a pharmacist's perspective. Integr Pharm Res Pract. 2018;7:41–52.
8. Lin JH. Pharmacokinetic and pharmacodynamic properties of histamine H2-receptor antagonists. Relationship between intrinsic potency and effective plasma concentrations. Clin Pharmacokinet. 1991;20(3):218–36.
9. Pettit M. Treatment of gastroesophageal reflux disease. Pharm World Sci. 2005;27(6):432–5.
10. Cooke MR, Giovannitti JA. Histamine and histamine antagonists. In: Pharmacology and therapeutics for dentistry. 7th ed. Elsevier; 2017. p. 276–86.
11. Zheng J, Stuff J, Tang H, Hassan MM, Daniel CR, Li D. Dietary N-nitroso compounds and risk of pancreatic cancer: results from a large case-control study. Carcinogenesis. 2019;40(2):254–62.
12. Gagne J. Ranitidine (Zantac) recall expanded, many questions remain (2020). Available at: https://www.health.harvard.edu/blog/ranitidine-zantac-recall-expanded-many-questions-remain-2020040218044. Accessed 18 Dec 2024.
13. Galmiche JP, Bruley Des Varannes S, Ducrotté P, Sacher-Huvelin S, Vavasseur F, Taccoen A, et al. Tenatoprazole, a novel proton pump inhibitor with a prolonged plasma half-life: effects on intragastric pH and comparison with esomeprazole in healthy volunteers. Aliment Pharmacol Ther. 2004;19(6):655–62.
14. Shin JM, Sachs G. Pharmacology of proton pump inhibitors. Curr Gastroenterol Rep. 2008;10(6):528–34.
15. Ban-Hock T, Alderuccio F. Autoantibodies. In: Parietal cell and intrinsic factor autoantibodies. 2nd ed; 2007. p. 8.
16. Lee SY, Shin YW, Hahm KB. Phytoceuticals: mighty but ignored weapons against Helicobacter pylori infection. J Dig Dis. 2008;9(3):129–39.
17. Strand DS, Kim D, Peura DA. 25 Years of proton pump inhibitors: a comprehensive review. Gut Liver. 2017;11(1):27–37.
18. Pang SH, Graham DY. A clinical guide to using intravenous proton-pump inhibitors in reflux and peptic ulcers. Ther Adv Gastroenterol. 2010;3(1):11–22.
19. Klotz U. Clinical impact of CYP2C19 polymorphism on the action of proton pump inhibitors: a review of a special problem. Int J Clin Pharmacol Ther. 2006;44(7):297–302.
20. Sjövall H, Björnsson E, Holmberg J, Hasselgren G, Röhss K, Hassan-Alin M. Pharmacokinetic study of esomeprazole in patients with hepatic impairment. Eur J Gastroenterol Hepatol. 2002;14(5):491–6.
21. Fasullo M, Rau P, Liu DQ, Holzwanger E, Mathew JP, Guilarte-Walker Y, et al. Proton pump inhibitors increase the severity of hepatic encephalopathy in cirrhotic patients. World J Hepatol. 2019;11(6):522–30.
22. Tran-Duy A, Connell NJ, Vanmolkot FH, Souverein PC, de Wit NJ, Stehouwer CDA, et al. Use of proton pump inhibitors and risk of iron deficiency: a population-based case-control study. J Intern Med. 2019;285(2):205–14.
23. Hamano H, Niimura T, Horinouchi Y, Zamami Y, Takechi K, Goda M, et al. Proton pump inhibitors block iron absorption through direct regulation of hepcidin via the aryl hydrocarbon receptor-mediated pathway. Toxicol Lett. 2020;318:86–91.

24. He B, Carleton B, Etminan M. Risk of gynecomastia with users of proton pump inhibitors. Pharmacotherapy. 2019;39(5):614–8.
25. Thong BKS, Ima-Nirwana S, Chin KY. Proton pump inhibitors and fracture risk: a review of current evidence and mechanisms involved. Int J Environ Res Public Health. 2019;16(9):1571.
26. Ohgami M, Kaburagi T, Kurosawa A, Doki K, Shiozawa T, Hizawa N, et al. Effects of proton pump inhibitor coadministration on the plasma concentration of erlotinib in patients with non-small cell lung cancer. Ther Drug Monit. 2018;40(6):699–704.
27. Ogawa R, Echizen H. Drug-drug interaction profiles of proton pump inhibitors. Clin Pharmacokinet. 2010;49(8):509–33.
28. Wang X, Song Y, Wang J, He J, Liu R, Li X, et al. Effect of proton pump inhibitors on high-dose methotrexate elimination: a systematic review and meta-analysis. Int J Clin Pharm. 2020;42:23.

Motility Drugs

6

Rosana Troskot Perić, Nikolina Tolj, Marina Madunić,
and Ana Maria Soldo

Introduction

FGIDs are a large heterogeneous group of digestive disorders characterized by persistent, recurrent symptoms (abdominal pain, defecation disorders, flatulence, etc.) in the absence of clear structural abnormalities (tumors/masses) or biochemical abnormalities [1, 2]. One of the most important functions of the GI system is the movement of food through the GI system. The electrical activity of GI smooth muscle consists of slow waves and spike potentials that represent the true action potential. The gastrointestinal smooth muscle acts as a syncytium, which means that electrical impulses spread along the bundles of the smooth muscle. The following are involved in the regulation of gastrointestinal mobility: the central nervous system (CNS) with parasympathetic and sympathetic innervation, the intestinal nervous system (ENS), various GI reflexes (e.g., within the ENS, reflexes of the gastrocolic, enterogastric or colonoileal type, painful reflexes, defecation reflexes,

R. Troskot Perić (✉)
Department of Gastroenterology and Hepatology, Sveti Duh University Hospital,
Zagreb, Croatia

Faculty of Health Studies, University of Rijeka, Rijeka, Croatia

Zabok General Hospital and the Croatian Veterans Hospital, Zabok, Croatia

N. Tolj
Zabok General Hospital and the Croatian Veterans Hospital, Zabok, Croatia

University of Dubrovnik, Dubrovnik, Croatia

M. Madunić
Zabok General Hospital and the Croatian Veterans Hospital, Zabok, Croatia

A. M. Soldo
Department of Gastroenterology and Hepatology, Sveti Duh University Hospital,
Zagreb, Croatia

M. Banić, D. Erceg (eds.), *Drug Interactions in Gastroenterology*, Clinical
Gastroenterology, https://doi.org/10.1007/978-3-031-69800-2_6

etc.) and various hormones, such as gastrin, cholecystokinin, secretin, motilin, serotonin, etc. [3]. Each part of the GI system (esophagus, stomach, small intestine, colon) has specific motility characteristics, but their common features are contractile activity, tonus, compliance, and transit [4].

Motility drugs (also known as prokinetics) are used in treatment of various gastrointestinal diseases and disorders: gastroesophageal reflux disease (GERD), functional dyspepsia (FD), gastroparesis, bacterial overgrowth syndrome (Small Bowel Bacterial Overgrowth), irritable bowel syndrome (IBS), intestinal pseudo-obstruction, chronic constipation (CC), etc. Most commonly, they are used for the FGIDs, such as the before mentioned FD, IBS, and CC.

FGIDs are thought to be Disorders of Gut-Brain Interaction, where, ENS determines the behavior of the GI musculature, the secretory glands, and the circulatory system of the GI system with specialized cells that act as electrical precursors to smooth muscle cells (Cajal's Interstitial Cells-ICC) [5]. However, in addition to motility disorders, other intertwining factors may be present in the pathogenesis of FGIDs: genetic susceptibility (hereditary predisposition), early environmental exposure, visceral hypersensitivity, mucosal immune barrier disorder, GI microbiome disorder, infections, central dysregulation of pain and motility, and other potential factors [6]. The diagnosis of particular disorders in FGIDs is made based on clinical symptoms that are diverse and often unstable. Therefore, the treatment of these disorders is aimed at relieving the symptoms. For this reason, the prokinetics used are non-selective and come with side effects.

Types of Promotility Drugs

Promotility drugs (also called prokinetics) have proven to be drugs that, in addition to acting on receptors in the GI system, affect other organ systems and cause a number of side effects and possibly, effects opposite to those expected. Promotility drugs can be categorized into several groups, depending on their mechanism of action, and which receptors (or different types of receptors) they act on [7, 8]:

1. Cholinergic Agonists
2. Dopamine Receptor Antagonists
3. Motilin Receptor Agonists
4. Ghrelin Receptor Agonist
5. 5-HT4 Receptor Agonists
6. Other agents

Cholinergic Agonists

Cholinergic agonists act to stimulate M2 muscarinic receptors in GI smooth muscle cells. Cholinesterase inhibitors, such as neostigmine and pyridostigmine, are not used as the treatment of FGIDs and other motility disorders due to their non-selectivity and side effects, which are caused by cholinergic stimulation of muscarinic acetylcholine receptors on smooth muscle and autonomic glands, as well as stimulation of nicotinic acetylcholine receptors on skeletal muscle.

Acotiamide (Z-338)

Acotiamide (Z-338) [7, 9–13] is a novel prokinetic compound which is used for treatment of functional dyspepsia (FD). It is approved in Japan and several other countries but not in the United States. It is a muscarinic (M1 and M2) antagonist and cholinesterase inhibitor. Animal studies have shown that acotinamide improves gastric motility and gastric emptying.

Mechanisms of actions in humans are still needed to clarify whether acotiamide affects GI changes via its effect on gastric emptying alone or in combination with appetite-related hormones such as ghrelin [14]. Clinical trials that have been conducted in Japan, Europe, and the United States showed that acotiamide was efficient in relieving FD symptoms, especially in those patients with postprandial distress syndrome (PDS), subtype of FD; optimal dose is 100 mg t.i.d [11]. Long-term use (continuously during 1 year period) seems to be safe without any (especially cardiovascular) serious side effects, which were confirmed in two open-label trials. It must be noted that the high placebo effect, commonly observed in other trials for FGIDs, is a major limitation for these trials due to open-label study design [15, 16]. Animal studies showed that acotiamide does not have an affinity for dopamine D2 and serotonin 5-HT4 receptors (like other prokinetics such as itopride and mosapride) and, because of that, does not affect QT interval. That means a good cardiovascular safety profile in comparison to other classes of prokinetics [17]. Patients with confirmed GI reflux disease may have concomitant postprandial distress syndrome (PDS) and epigastric pain syndrome (EPS) symptoms where combination therapy like prokinetic plus proton pump inhibitors (PPI) (e.g., acotiamide and rabeprazol) is more effective than rabeprazol monotherapy [12].

Dopamine Receptor Antagonists

Dopamine (D) is a catecholamine neurotransmitter which regulates different functions in the central and peripheral nervous systems [18–20]. The GI tract, spleen, and pancreas produce substantial amounts of dopamine in humans. Five subtypes of dopamine receptors (D1, D2, D3, D4, and D5) are classified in two subfamilies: D1-like subfamily (D1 and D5) and D2-like subfamily (D2, D3, and D4). These two subfamilies differ in structure and action (e.g., stimulation and inhibition of adenylate cyclase, respectively) [19, 20]. Dopamine in GI tract causes inhibition of motility by reducing lower oesophageal sphincter tone, reducing gastric tone and intragastric pressure, and decreasing antroduodenal coordination through the activation of dopamine D2 receptors. This knowledge led to the conclusion that antidopaminergic effects could be a good choice for gastrointestinal prokinetics [20, 21].

Clinical Indications of Antidopaminergic Prokinetics

Two major effects of antidopaminergic prokinetics are anti-dyspeptic and anti-emetic properties. They are used for treatment of upper digestive tract diseases, such as FD, gastroparesis, and prevention of nausea and vomiting (vomiting during pregnancy, cancer chemotherapy vomiting, postoperative vomiting, and vomiting during migraine attack) [20].

Use of antidopaminergic drugs has been reduced after 5-HT3 receptor antagonists introduction (so-called "setrons" such as ondansetron, granisetron, and dolasetron), which were marketed for prevention of chemotherapy-induced nausea and vomiting [22, 23]. However, "setrons" are effective for chemotherapy-induced acute emesis (i.e. emesis occurring within 24–36 h following therapy) but not so effective for delayed emesis (which occur 3–5 days following chemotherapy). In that case, combination therapy with dexamethasone or antidopaminergics is more effective [20, 22, 24].

Extraintestinal Effects of Antidopaminergic Prokinetics

Dopamin-containing neurons are found in central nervous system, minor part in retina and olfactory bulb. Approximately 80% of brain dopaminergic neurons are involved in control of movements and hypothalamic dopaminergic neurons suppress prolactin excretion by activating D2 receptors in pituitary gland. This is why major side effects of antidopaminergic prokinetics include movement disorders and hyperprolactinemia [20, 25]. Extrapyramidal movement disorders include [20, 26]:

1. Akathisia (a feeling of inner restlessness, an urge to move).
2. Drug-induced parkinsonism (muscle rigidity, bradykinesia, and tremor). This side effect is resloved 2–3 months after antidopaminergic drug discontinuation.
3. Dyskinesias or acute dystonic reactions (involuntary muscles contractions resulting in repetitive movements, twisting, and abnormal postures—e.g., facial spasm, torticollis, and trismus). These are the most frequent extrapyramidal side effects for metoclopramide use. Typically occur within 24–48 h of initiating treatment and the incidence rise with higher doses.
4. Tardive dyskinesia (late-onset dyskinesia, occurs after long treatment with antidopaminergic drugs). It is characterized by involuntary movements of the face, tongue, or extremities and occurs for at least 3 months after continuous use of metoclopramide and may not be reversible after discontinuation of metoclopramide.

Several retrospective studies [26–30] showed a significantly increased prevalence and severity of tardive dyskinesia with metoclopramide use and therefore the Food and Drug Administration (FDA) came out with the black-box warning for metoclopramide use in 2009.

The pituitary gland is located outside the blood-brain barrier, and hyperprolactinemia is possible with the use of any antidopaminergic drug, irrespective they affect the central or peripheral D2 receptor. Elevated prolactin (PRL) levels occur within 3 days to 2 weeks after initiation of antidopaminergic prokinetic, but there is still no relationship between antidopaminergic dose and PRL levels and/or symptoms of hyperprolactinemia. However, hyperprolactinemia tends to decrease during chronic use of antidopaminergic drugs, and drug discontinuation usually stops within 1 week [20, 31, 32].

Young women, children, the elderly, diabetics, and patients taking concurrent neuroleptics are at most risk for development of these side effects, especially with higher doses, intravenous application and/or long term use of prokinetics. Genetic factors such as the cytochrome P450 (CYP) enzymes polymorphisms may play a role too [26, 33, 34]. Three most widely used antidopaminergic prokinetics are *metoclopramide*, *domperidone*, and *levosulpiride* [20].

Metoclopramide

Metoclopramide with antydispeptic and antiemetic proportions is used for treatment of gastroesophageal reflux disease and gastroparesis, postoperative or chemotherapy-induced nausea and vomiting. It was first described by Louis Justin-Besaçon and Charles Laville in 1964 and has been available in the USA since 1979 [26]. Metoclopramide is a dopamine D2 (central and peripheral) antagonist with moderate partial 5-hydroxytryptamine-4 (5-HT4) receptor agonist properties and moderate 5-HT3 receptor antagonist properties [20, 26]. It promotes gut motility by increasing lower esophageal sphincter (LES) and gastric tone, increasing intragastric pressure, improving antroduodenal coordination, and accelerating gastric emptying but prokinetic effects are limited to the proximal gut [20, 26, 35]. Initial dose is 5–10 mg orally, 30 min before meals and at bedtime. The dose can be increased up to 20 mg four times daily, which may be limited by its side effects. It is available in a liquid, an orally disintegrating sublingual, intranasal, oral formulation, and injections for subcutaneous and intravenous use [20].

Several randomized clinical trials (RCTs) showed that metoclopramide is effective in short-term therapy up to several weeks, and there is no clinical benefit for chronic use [20, 36]. When the FDA issued a black box warning for tardive dyskinesia with metoclopramide use in 2009, changes in upper FGID treatment were noticed. After the warning, metoclopramide prescription and use decreased with increased rate of adverse event reporting (69.8% of patients received metoclopramide for gastroparesis before warning and only 23.7% after warning), and gastroenterologists prescribed domperidone more often for gastroparesis [37].

Domperidone

Domperidone is a D2 antagonist that acts only on peripheral D2 receptors because it does not cross the blood-brain barrier (unlike metoclopramide), and therefore has fewer CNS side effects. Despite no affect on central D2 receptors it can cause hyperprolactinemia because pituitary gland is outside of blood-brain barrier [8, 20, 31, 32].

Domperidone was directly compared to metoclopramide in a randomized, double-blind multicenter trial. Results showed that they are equally effective in controlling symptoms from diabetic gastroparesis, but CNS side effects were significantly more frequent with the use of metoclopramide [38]. After the FDA black box warning for tardive dyskinesia with metoclopramide use, domperidone appear to be a potential substitute for metoclopramide [39, 40]. Domperidone has been used in more than 20 countries worldwide, but in the United States, it has been approved only on an investigational basis (treatment-refractory gastroparesis) [40].

From a cardiovascular perspective, domperidone has a narrow cardiovascular safety (like cisapride). Domperidone can cause drug-induced long QT syndrome/ torsades de pointes or sudden cardiac death. Etiology of these cardiovascular side effects is multifactorial. Domperidone has affinity for the human ether-a-go-go related gene-hERG/Kv11.1 potassium channels and with other risk factors such as electrolyte disturbances, co-administration of other QT-prolonging medication, drug accumulation due to renal/hepatic impairment or inhibition of cytochrome P450 metabolism, structural heart disease, diabetes, female sex, underlying genetic disposition, older age can cause cardiovascular (CV) side effect. After the previous withdrawal of prokinetic agent cisapride, the USFDA does not have any tolerance to another prokinetic agent with narrow cardiovascular safety [40]. Usual oral dose of domperidone is 10 mg three times a day. The lowest effective dose should be used for the shortest period of time.

Levosulpiride

Levosulpiride is another D2 receptor antagonist with moderate 5HT4 receptor agonist effects in the enteric nervous system. It has been shown to be effective in FD, especially among those with "motility type" dyspepsia because it accelerates gastric emptying. It improves glycemic control over a 6-month period in subjects with diabetic gastroparesis. It has antiemetic effects like metoclopramide or domperidone [41–45]. The enthusiasm for the use of levosulpiride as a prokinetic subsided after the serious cardiovascular and extrapyramidal side effects were reported [46–49].

Itopride

Itopride is a newer D2 receptor antagonist and an acetylcholinesterase inhibitor. It has been investigated in patients with FD, but the results of several studies are conflicting [7, 8, 50, 51, 52]. This was partially due to more liberal inclusion criteria [8, 53]. It is approved for the treatment of FD in Asia and is not available in the United States. The usual oral dose is 50 mg three times a day [7]. A systematic review and meta-analysis that include 29 studies showed that itopride was not superior to domperidone for dyspeptic symptom improvement but the quality of evidence was very low. Itopride is well tolerated, but there is no significant difference in the number of side effects by comparing it with domperidone [54].

Motilin Receptor Agonists

Erythromycin

Erythromycin is a macrolide antibiotic that has motilin-like effects and thus increases gastric emptying by stimulating phase III contractions of the migrating motor complex. In acute gastroparesis, the effect is achieved by short-term intravenous administration of the drug. However, long-term oral administration does not show satisfactory results. An additional limiting factor for the administration of erythromycin and other macrolides is the occurrence of tachyphylaxis [8, 55].

The need for an effective motilin agonist, without the use of antibiotics, led to the development of ***camicinal (GSK962040)*** [56–58]. However, it is important to point out that all of these motilin agonists, which act as prokinetics, have no central anti-emetic effect and are therefore less effective than prokinetics that have central anti-emetic activity [59].

Ghrelin Receptor Agonists

Relamorelin

Relamorelin is a ghrelin receptor agonist that has been studied in patients with diabetic gastroparesis and has shown efficacy in reducing symptoms like nausea, abdominal pain, postprandial fullness, etc. It is administered subcutaneously in different doses (10, 30, or 100 mg 2× daily) [60, 61].

5-HT4 Receptor Agonists

Cisaprid (partial 5-HT4 receptor agonist) and tegaserod (5-HT4/5-HT1 receptor partial agonist and 5-HT2 receptor antagonist), previously used drugs from a group of serotonergic agonists, have been withdrawn because of an increased risk of serious cardiovascular incidents [40, 62].

Prucalopride

In order to avoid significant side effects, more selective 5-HT4 receptor agonists such as prucalopride are introduced. The effects of prucalopride are based on the stimulation of cholinergic activity through the 5-HT4 receptor, the modification of smooth muscle contractility, motor coordination, the acceleration of total intestinal transit, and the stimulation of proximal colon emptying. It is a selective 5-HT4 agonist with very low affinity for other 5-HT receptors or the hERG-K cardiac channels, which makes this drug more potent without cardiotoxic effects. It also has excellent bioavailability with a 24-h half-life [63].

The effect of prucapride on patients with chronic constipation was confirmed in three large, multicenter, randomized, double-blind, placebo-controlled trials of 12 weeks. The results showed significant and consistent improvement of intestinal function over 12 weeks (≥2 spontaneous complete bowel movements-SCBMs), improvement of symptoms, and satisfaction among patients [64–66]. In a study by Cinco et al. [67], women with chronic constipation received 26 g/day of macrogol/polyethylene glycol (PEG) 3350 plus electrolytes or 1–2 mg/day of prucalopride for 4 weeks. In the last week of testing, results showed ≥3 SCBMs weekly were achieved in 67% of PEG 3350 + E subjects and 57% of prucalopride subjects. They have been shown to be equally effective in treating chronic constipation in women who have not responded to treatment with laxatives. PEG 3350 + E is better tolerated than prucalopride, has a wider range of therapeutic indications, and is less expensive. A randomized clinical study was published by Yiannakou et al. [68]. This study included 358 men receiving 1 × 2 mg prucalopride for 12 weeks, and results showed that ≥3 SCBMs/week were achieved in 38% of subjects receiving prucalopride and 18% receiving placebo. Prucalopride was well tolerated and safe.

Prucalopride is approved as a second line of treatment for chronic constipation in men and women, who have previously been unsuccessfully treated with at least two different types of laxatives at the highest recommended doses, for at least 6 months [69]. It is administered orally at a dose of 1–2 mg daily. The drug has also been shown to be safe in people over 65 years of age. The most common side effects of prucalopride are headache, abdominal pain, nausea, and diarrhea. They usually appear at the beginning of treatment and withdraw within a few days [69]. The potential role of prucalopride in other GI motility disorders such as idiopathic gastroparesis is still being investigated [70].

Other selective 5-HT4 agonists, such as ***velusetrag*** and ***naronpride***, are still being tested [8]. The results of the meta-analysis showed that highly selective 5-HT4 agonists (such as prucalopride, velusetrag, or naronapride) have a significant advantage in treatment of chronic constipation over the control group. They are effective in the frequency and consistency of peristalsis, the quality of life associated with constipation, the sum of symptoms, and global assessment. There is no significant difference between efficacy in elderly and younger patients. The most common side effects are headache and diarrhea and they are safe to use [71].

Mosaprid

Mosaprid is a selective 5-HT4 agonist and partial 5-HT3 antagonist used as a prokinetic agent in many Asian countries in the FD therapy. Studies published to date show that mosapride is safe and without cardiotoxicity side effects [8].

Complementary and Alternative Therapies

Management of patients with functional GI disorders with traditional pharmacological therapy sometimes is difficult due to poor efficacy and serious adverse effects of prokinetics (cisapride and tegaserod were withdrawn due to serious side effects). Therefore, herbal medicine may be an attractive alternative because it is based on the perception of its "natural" approach and low risk of side effects [72]. Despite the widespread use of herbal medicine, scientific data indicating clinical efficacy are scarce. Herbal medicine in Japan is very popular and is covered by national health insurance [12].

Rikkunshito

Rikkunshito is a Japanese herbal medicine and it is often prescribed for upper gastrointestinal disorders such as functional dyspepsia (FD), gastroesophageal reflux, and anorexia and is prepared by eight crude drugs: *Atractylodis lanceae rhizoma*, *Ginseng radix*, *Pinellia tuber*, *Hoelen*, *Zizyphi fructus*, *Aurantii nobilis pericarpium*, *Glycyrrhizae radix*, and *Zingiberis rhizome* [73]. In animal models, Rikkunshito is likely mediated via ghrelin levels and through antagonism of 5-HT receptors [74–76]. In treatment-resistant cases, when first-line therapy such as prokinetics, PPIs, and H2 blockers are ineffective patients should be treated with second-line therapies such as antidepressants or a herbal medicine such as Rikkunshito [12].

STW5 (Iberogast®)

STW5 (Iberogast®) is a herbal mixture of nine different herbs, including milk thistle, chamomile, peppermint, and licorice [77]. In healthy volunteers, STW5 stimulates gastric relaxation and antral motility, which may contribute to potential therapeutic effects in FD [78]. Several double-blind multicenter RCTs using STW5 in FD and IBS compared STW5 to placebo and one study compared STW5 to prokinetic cisapride and found statistically significant effects of STW5 on patients' symptoms with a comparable efficacy to a standard prokinetic. Non-interventional and retrospective studies confirmed these effects. Safety studies showed that the incidence of adverse drug reactions was 0.04%. Therefore, SWT5 has a good tolerability which is relevant for long-term treatment [79]. In several countries, STW 5 is approved as the only product both covering functional dyspepsia as well as IBS [79]. Moreover, it is included in the therapy guidelines in Germany for both upper and lower functional gastrointestinal disorders [79, 80]. However, the American College of Gastroenterology and the Canadian Association of Gastroenterology (ACG/CAG) guidelines advise caution due to debatable clinical significance despite statistically significant efficacy [78, 81].

References

1. Drossman DA, Hasler WL. Rome IV—functional GI disorders: disorders of gut-brain interaction. Gastroenterology. 2016;150(6):1257–61. https://doi.org/10.1053/j.gastro.2016.03.035.
2. Drossman DA. Functional gastrointestinal disorders: history, pathophysiology, clinical features and Rome IV. Gastroenterology. 2016;150:1262–79. https://doi.org/10.1053/j.gastro.2016.02.032.
3. Guyton AC, Hall JE, editors. Textbook of medical physiology. 11th ed. Philadelphia: Elsevier Saunders; 2005.
4. Boeckxstaens G, Camilleri M, Sifrim D, Houghton LA, Elsenbruch S, Lindberg G, et al. Fundamentals of neurogastroenterology: physiology/motility—sensation. Gastroenterology. 2016;150:1292–304. https://doi.org/10.1053/j.gastro.2016.02.030.
5. Vanner S, Greenwood-Van Meerveld B, Mawe G, Shea-Donohue T, Verdu EF, Wood J, et al. Fundamentals of neurogastroenterology: basic science. Gastroenterology. 2016;150:1280–91. https://doi.org/10.1053/j.gastro.2016.02.018.
6. Van Oudenhove L, Crowell MD, Drossman DA, Halpert AD, Keefer L, Lackner JM, et al. Biopsychosocial aspects of functional gastrointestinal disorders. Gastroenterology. 2016;150:1355–67. https://doi.org/10.1053/j.gastro.2016.02.027.
7. Camilleri M, Bueno L, Andresen V, De Ponti F, Choi MG, Lembo A. Pharmacological, pharmacokinetic, and pharmacogenomic aspects of functional gastrointestinal disorders. Gastroenterology. 2016;150:1319–31. https://doi.org/10.1053/j.gastro.2016.02.029.
8. Quigley EMM. Prokinetics in the management of functional gastrointestinal disorders. Curr Gastroenterol Rep. 2017;19:53. https://doi.org/10.1007/s11894-017-0593-6.

9. Tack J, Janssen P. Acotiamide (Z-338, YM443), a new drug for the treatment of functional dyspepsia. Expert Opin Investig Drugs. 2011;20(5):701–12. https://doi.org/10.1517/13543784.2011.562890.
10. Kusunoki H, Haruma K, Manabe N, Imamura H, Kamada T, Shiotami A, et al. Therapeutic efficacy of acotiamide in patients with functional dyspepsia based on enhanced postprandial gastric accommodation and emptying: randomized controlled study evaluation by real-time ultrasonography. Neurogastroenterol Motil. 2012;24(6):540–5, e250–1. https://doi.org/10.1111/j.1365-2982.2012.01897.x.
11. Ueda M, Iwasaki E, Suzuki H. Profile of acotiamide in the treatment of functional dyspepsia. Clin Exp Gastroenterol. 2016;9:83–8. https://doi.org/10.2147/CEG.S72172.
12. Yamawaki H, Futagami S, Wakabayashi M, et al. Management of functional dyspepsia: state of the art and emerging therapies. Ther Adv Chronic Dis. 2018;9(1):23–32. https://doi.org/10.1177/2040622317725479.
13. Porika SK, Veligandla KC, Muni SK, Acharya S, Mehta SC, Sharma AD. Real-world, non-interventional, observational study to evaluate effectiveness and tolerability of acotiamide hydrochloride hydrate in treatment of functional dyspepsia. Adv Ther. 2018;35(11):1884–93. https://doi.org/10.1007/s12325-018-0814-x.
14. Yamawaki H, Futagami S, Kawagoe T, Maruki Y, Hashimoto S, Nagoya H, et al. Improvement of meal-related symptoms and epigastric pain in patients with functional dyspepsia treated with acotiamide was associated with acylated ghrelin levels in Japan. Neurogastroenterol Motil. 2016;28(7):1037–47. https://doi.org/10.1111/nmo.12805.
15. Matsueda K, Hongo M, Ushijima S, Akiho H. A long-term study of acotiamide in patients with functional dyspepsia: results from an open-label phase III trial in Japan on efficacy, safety and pattern of administration. Digestion. 2011;84(4):261–8. https://doi.org/10.1159/000332404.
16. Tack J, Pokrotnieks J, Urbonas G, Banciu C, Yakusevich V, Bunganic I, et al. Long-term safety and efficacy of acotiamide in functional dyspepsia (postprandial distress syndrome)—results from the European phase 3 open-label safety trial. Neurogastroenterol Motil. 2018;30(6):e13284. https://doi.org/10.1111/nmo.13284.
17. Matsunaga Y, Tanaka T, Yoshinaga K, Ueki S, Hori Y, Eta R, et al. Acotiamide hydrochloride (Z-338), a new selective acetylcholinesterase inhibitor, enhances gastric motility without prolonging QT interval in dogs: comparison with cisapride, itopride, and mosapride. J Pharmacol Exp Ther. 2011;336(3):791–800. https://doi.org/10.1124/jpet.110.174847.
18. Palermo-Neto J. Dopaminergic systems. Dopamine receptors. Psychiatr Clin North Am. 1997;20(4):705–21. https://doi.org/10.1016/s0193-953x(05)70341-5.
19. Eisenhofer G, Aneman A, Friberg P, Hooper D, Fåndriks L, Lonroth H, et al. Substantial production of dopamine in the human gastrointestinal tract. J Clin Endocrinol Metab. 1997;82(11):3864–71. https://doi.org/10.1210/jcem.82.11.4339.
20. Tonini M, Cipollina L, Poluzzi E, Crema F, Corazza GR, De Ponti F. Review article: Clinical implications of enteric and central D2 receptor blockade by antidopaminergic gastrointestinal prokinetics. Aliment Pharmacol Ther. 2004;19(4):379–90. https://doi.org/10.1111/j.1365-2036.2004.01867.x.
21. Demol P, Ruoff HJ, Weihrauch TR. Rational pharmacotherapy of gastrointestinal motility disorders. Eur J Pediatr. 1989;148(6):489–95. https://doi.org/10.1007/bf00441540.
22. Mitchelson F. Pharmacological agents affecting emesis. A review (Part I). Drugs. 1992;43(3):295–315. https://doi.org/10.2165/00003495-199243030-00002.
23. Walton SM. Advances in use of the 5-HT3 receptor antagonists. Expert Opin Pharmacother. 2000;1(2):207–23. https://doi.org/10.1517/14656566.1.2.207.
24. Roila F, Donati D, Tamberi S, Margutti G. Delayed emesis: incidence, pattern, prognostic factors and optimal treatment. Support Care Cancer. 2002;10(2):88–95. https://doi.org/10.1007/s005200100295.
25. Ben-Jonathan N, Hnasko R. Dopamine as a prolactin (PRL) inhibitor. Endocr Rev. 2001;22(6):724–63. https://doi.org/10.1210/edrv.22.6.0451.
26. Lee A, Kuo B. Metoclopramide in the treatment of diabetic gastroparesis. Expert Rev Endocrinol Metab. 2010;5(5):653–62. https://doi.org/10.1586/eem.10.41.

27. Ganzini L, Casey DE, Hoffman WF, McCall AL. The prevalence of metoclopramide-induced tardive dyskinesia and acute extrapyramidal movement disorders. Arch Intern Med. 1993;153(12):1469–75.
28. Sewell DD, Jeste DV. Metoclopramide-associated tardive dyskinesia. An analysis of 67 cases. Arch Fam Med. 1992;1(2):271–8. https://doi.org/10.1001/archfami.1.2.271.
29. Sewell DD, Kodsi AB, Caligiuri MP, Jeste DV. Metoclopramide and tardive dyskinesia. Biol Psychiatry. 1994;36(9):630–2. https://doi.org/10.1016/0006-3223(94)90077-9.
30. Kenney C, Hunter C, Davidson A, Jankovic J. Metoclopramide, an increasingly recognized cause of tardive dyskinesia. J Clin Pharmacol. 2008;48(3):379–84. https://doi.org/10.1177/0091270007312258.
31. Maddern GJ. Galactorrhoea due to domperidone. Med J Aust. 1983;2(11):539–40. https://doi.org/10.5694/j.1326-5377.1983.tb122658.x.
32. Cho E, Ho S, Gerber P, Davidson AG. Monitoring of serum prolactin in pediatric patients with cystic fibrosis who are receiving domperidone. Can J Hosp Pharm. 2009;62(2):119–26. https://doi.org/10.4212/cjhp.v62i2.440.
33. Miller LG, Jankovic J. Metoclopramide-induced movement disorders. Clinical findings with a review of the literature. Arch Intern Med. 1989;149(11):2486–92. https://doi.org/10.1001/archinte.149.11.2486.
34. Pasricha PJ, Pehlivanov N, Sugumar A, Jankovic J. Drug insight: from disturbed motility to disordered movement—a review of the clinical benefits and medicolegal risks of metoclopramide. Nat Clin Pract Gastroenterol Hepatol. 2006;3(3):138–48. https://doi.org/10.1038/ncpgasthep0442.
35. Albibi R, McCallum RW. Metoclopramide: pharmacology and clinical application. Ann Intern Med. 1983;98(1):86–95. https://doi.org/10.7326/0003-4819-98-1-86.
36. Lata PF, Pigarelli DL. Chronic metoclopramide therapy for diabetic gastroparesis. Ann Pharmacother. 2003;37(1):122–6. https://doi.org/10.1345/aph.1C118.
37. Ehrenpreis ED, Deepak P, Sifuentes H, Devi R, Du H, Leikin JB. The metoclopramide black box warning for tardive dyskinesia: effect on clinical practice, adverse event reporting, and prescription drug lawsuits. Am J Gastroenterol. 2013;108(6):866–72. https://doi.org/10.1038/ajg.2012.300.
38. Patterson D, Abell T, Rothstein R, Koch K, Barnett J. A double-blind multicenter comparison of domperidone and metoclopramide in the treatment of diabetic patients with symptoms of gastroparesis. Am J Gastroenterol. 1999;94(5):1230–4. https://doi.org/10.1111/j.1572-0241.1999.00456.x.
39. Hondeghem LM. Domperidone: limited benefits with significant risk for sudden cardiac death. J Cardiovasc Pharmacol. 2013;61(3):218–25. https://doi.org/10.1097/FJC.0b013e31827afd0d.
40. Giudicessi JR, Ackerman MJ, Camilleri M. Cardiovascular safety of prokinetic agents: a focus on drug-induced arrhythmias. Neurogastroenterol Motil. 2018;30(6):e13302. https://doi.org/10.1111/nmo.13302.
41. Corazza GR, Biagi F, Albano O, Bianchi Porro G, Cheli R, Mazzacca G, et al. Levosulpiride in functional dyspepsia: a multicentric, double-blind, controlled trial. Ital J Gastroenterol. 1996;28(6):317–23.
42. Melga P, Mansi C, Ciuchi E, Giusti R, Sciaba L, Prando R. Chronic administration of levosulpiride and glycemic control in IDDM patients with gastroparesis. Diabetes Care. 1997;20:55–8. https://doi.org/10.2337/diacare.20.1.55.
43. Mansi C, Borro P, Giacomini M, Biagini R, Mele MR, Pandolfo N, et al. Comparative effects of levosulpiride and cisapride on gastric emptying and symptoms in patients with functional dyspepsia and gastroparesis. Aliment Pharmacol Ther. 2000;14(5):561–9. https://doi.org/10.1046/j.1365-2036.2000.00742.x.
44. Mearin F, Rodrigo L, Pérez-Mota A, Balboa A, Jiménez I, Sebastián JJ, et al. Levosulpiride and cisapride in the treatment of dysmotility-like functional dyspepsia: a randomized, double-masked trial. Clin Gastroenterol Hepatol. 2004;2(4):301–8. https://doi.org/10.1016/s1542-3565(04)00059-x.

45. Lozano R, Concha MP, Montealegre A, de Leon L, Ortiz Villalba J, Lee Esteban H, et al. Effectiveness and safety of levosulpiride in the treatment of dysmotility-like functional dyspepsia. Ther Clin Risk Manag. 2007;3(1):149–55. https://doi.org/10.2147/tcrm.2007.3.1.149.
46. Shin HW, Kim MJ, Kim JS, Lee MC, Chung SJ. Levosulpiride-induced movement disorders. Mov Disord. 2009;24(15):2249–53. https://doi.org/10.1002/mds.22805.
47. Kim HJ, Cho JY, Cho YJ, Hong KS. Levosulpiride-induced resting orolingual tremor. Mov Disord. 2009;24(11):1700–1. https://doi.org/10.1002/mds.22578.
48. Agosti S, Casalino L, Bertero G, Burrone A, Brunelli C, Morelloni S. Citalopram and levosulpiride: a dangerous drug combination for QT prolongation. Am J Emerg Med. 2013;31(11):1624.e1–1624.e16242. https://doi.org/10.1016/j.ajem.2013.06.030.
49. Lee HC, Hwang SH, Kang SY. Levosulpiride-associated hemichorea. Yonsei Med J. 2016;57(3):803–5. https://doi.org/10.3349/ymj.2016.57.3.803.
50. Holtmann G, Talley NJ, Liebregts T, Adam B, Parow C. A placebo-controlled trial of itopride in functional dyspepsia [published correction appears in N Engl J Med. 2006 Jul 27;355(4):429]. N Engl J Med. 2006;354(8):832–40. https://doi.org/10.1056/NEJMoa052639.
51. Talley NJ, Tack J, Ptak T, Gupta R, Giguère M. Itopride in functional dyspepsia: results of two phase III multicentre, randomised, double-blind, placebo-controlled trials. Gut. 2008;57(6):740–6. https://doi.org/10.1136/gut.2007.132449.
52. Huang X, Lv B, Zhang S, Fan YH, Meng LN. Itopride therapy for functional dyspepsia: a meta-analysis. World J Gastroenterol. 2012;18(48):7371–7. https://doi.org/10.3748/wjg.v18.i48.7371.
53. Veldhuyzen Van Zanten SJ. Pitfalls in designing trials of functional dyspepsia: the ascent and demise of itopride. Gut. 2008;57(6):723–4. https://doi.org/10.1136/gut.2007.139923.
54. Pittayanon R, Yuan Y, Bollegala NP, Khanna R, Lacy BE, Andrews CN, et al. Prokinetics for functional dyspepsia: a systematic review and meta-analysis of randomized control trials. Am J Gastroenterol. 2019;114(2):233–43. https://doi.org/10.1038/s41395-018-0258-6.
55. Myint AS, Rieders B, Tashkandi M, Borum ML, Koh JM, Stephen S, et al. Current and emerging therapeutic options for gastroparesis. Gastroenterol Hepatol (NY). 2018;14:639–45.
56. Hobson R, Farmer AD, Dewit OE, O'Donnell M, Hacquoil K, Robertson D, et al. The effects of camicinal, a novel motilin agonist, on gastro-esophageal function in healthy humans—a randomized placebo controlled trial. Neurogastroenterol Motil. 2015;27:1629–37. https://doi.org/10.1111/nmo.12663.
57. Chapman MJ, Deane AM, O'Connor SL, Nguyen NQ, Fraser RJ, Richards DB, et al. The effect of camicinal (GSK962040), a motilin agonist, on gastric emptying and glucose absorption in feed-intolerant critically ill patients: a randomized, blinded, placebo-controlled, clinical trial. Crit Care. 2016;20:232. https://doi.org/10.1186/s13054-016-1420-4.
58. Camilleri M. Novel diet, drugs, and gastric interventions for gastroparesis. Clin Gastroenterol Hepatol. 2016;14:1072–80. https://doi.org/10.1016/j.cgh.2015.12.033.
59. Stanghellini V, Chan FK, Hasler WL, Malagelada JR, Suzuki H, Tack J, et al. Gastroduodenal disorders. Gastroenterology. 2016;150:1380–92. https://doi.org/10.1053/j.gastro.2016.02.011.
60. Camilleri M, McCallum RW, Tack J, Spence SC, Gottesdiener K, Fiedorek FT. Efficacy and safety of relamorelin in diabetics with symptoms of gastroparesis: a randomized, placebo-controlled study. Gastroenterology. 2017;153:1240–50.e2. https://doi.org/10.1053/j.gastro.2017.07.035.
61. Tack J, Van den Houte K, Carbone F. Gastroduodenal motility disorders. Curr Opin Gastroenterol. 2018;34:428–35. https://doi.org/10.1097/MOG.0000000000000473.
62. Vijayvargiya P, Camilleri M, Chedid V, Mandawat A, Erwin PJ, Murad MH. Effects of promotility agents on gastric emptying and symptoms: a systematic review and meta-analysis. Gastroenterology. 2019;156:1650–60. https://doi.org/10.1053/j.gastro.2019.01.249.
63. De Maeyer JH, Lefebvre RA, Schuurkes JA. 5-HT4 receptor agonists: similar but not the same. Neurogastroenterol Motil. 2008;20:99–112. https://doi.org/10.1111/j.1365-2982.2007.01059.x.

64. Camilleri M, Kerstens R, Rykx A, Vandeplassche L. A placebo-controlled trial of prucalopride for severe chronic constipation. N Engl J Med. 2008;358:2344–54. https://doi.org/10.1056/NEJMoa0800670.
65. Quigley EM, Vandeplassche L, Kerstens R, Ausma J. Clinical trial: the efficacy, impact on quality of life, and safety and tolerability of prucalopride in severe chronic constipation—a 12-week, randomized, double-blind, placebo-controlled study. Aliment Pharmacol Ther. 2009;29:315–28. https://doi.org/10.1111/j.1365-2036.2008.03884.x.
66. Tack J, van Outryve M, Beyens G, Kerstens R, Vandeplassche L. Prucalopride (Resolor) in the treatment of severe chronic constipation in patients dissatisfied with laxatives. Gut. 2009;58:357–65. https://doi.org/10.1136/gut.2008.162404.
67. Cinca R, Chera D, Gruss HJ, Halphen M. Randomised clinical trial: macrogol/PEG 3350 + electrolytes versus prucalopride in the treatment of chronic constipation—a comparison in a controlled environment. Aliment Pharmacol Ther. 2013;37:876–86. https://doi.org/10.1111/apt.12278.
68. Yiannakou Y, Piessevaux H, Bouchoucha M, Schiefke I, Filip R, Gabalec L, et al. A randomized, double-blind, placebo-controlled, phase 3 trial to evaluate the efficacy, safety, and tolerability of prucalopride in men with chronic constipation. Am J Gastroenterol. 2015;110:741–8. https://doi.org/10.1038/ajg.2015.115.
69. Tack J, Müller-Lissner S, Stanghellini V, Boeckxstaens G, Kamm A, Kamm MA, et al. Diagnosis and treatment of chronic constipation—a European perspective. Neurogastroenterol Motil. 2011;23:697–710. https://doi.org/10.1111/j.1365-2982.2011.01709.x.
70. Carbone F, Van den Houte K, Clevers E, Andrews CN, Papathanasopoulos A, Holvoet L, et al. Prucalopride in gastroparesis: a randomized placebo-controlled crossover study. Am J Gastroenterol. 2019;114:1265–74. https://doi.org/10.14309/ajg.0000000000000304.
71. Shin A, Camilleri M, Kolar G, Erwin P, West CP, Murad MH. Systematic review with meta-analysis: highly selective 5-HT4 agonists (prucalopride, velusetrag or naronapride) in chronic constipation. Aliment Pharmacol Ther. 2014;39:239–53. https://doi.org/10.1111/apt.12571.
72. Suzuki H, Inadomi JM, Hibi T. Japanese herbal medicine in functional gastro-intestinal disorders. Neurogastroenterol Motil. 2009;21(7):688–96. https://doi.org/10.1111/j.1365-2982.2009.01290.
73. Mogami S, Hattori T. Beneficial effects of rikkunshito, a Japanese kampo medicine, on gastrointestinal dysfunction and anorexia in combination with Western drug: a systematic review. Evid Based Complement Alternat Med. 2014;2014:519035. https://doi.org/10.1155/2014/519035.
74. Takeda H, Sadakane C, Hattori T, Katsurada T, Ohkawara T, Nagai K, et al. Rikkunshito, an herbal medicine, suppresses cisplatin-induced anorexia in rats via 5-HT2 receptor antagonism. Gastroenterology. 2008;134(7):2004–13. https://doi.org/10.1053/j.gastro.2008.02.078.
75. Tominaga K, Kido T, Ochi M, Mase A, Okazaki H, Yamagami H, et al. The traditional Japanese medicine rikkunshito promotes gastric emptying via the antagonistic action of the 5-HT(3) receptor pathway in rats. Evid Based Complement Alternat Med. 2011;2011:248481. https://doi.org/10.1093/ecam/nep173.
76. Takeda H, Muto S, Nakagawa K, Ohnishi S, Asaka M. Rikkunshito and ghrelin secretion. Curr Pharm Des. 2012;18(31):4827–38. https://doi.org/10.2174/138161212803216933.
77. Black CJ, Houghton LA, Ford AC. Insights into the evaluation and management of dyspepsia: recent developments and new guidelines. Ther Adv Gastroenterol. 2018;11:1756284818805597. https://doi.org/10.1177/1756284818805597.
78. Pilichiewicz AN, Horowitz M, Russo A, Maddox AF, Jones KL, Schemann M, et al. Effects of Iberogast on proximal gastric volume, antropyloroduodenal motility and gastric emptying in healthy men. Am J Gastroenterol. 2007;102(6):1276–83. https://doi.org/10.1111/j.1572-0241.2007.01142.x.
79. Ottillinger B, Storr M, Malfertheiner P, Allescher HD. STW 5 (Iberogast®)—a safe and effective standard in the treatment of functional gastrointestinal disorders. Wien Med Wochenschr. 2013;163(3–4):65–72. https://doi.org/10.1007/s10354-012-0169-x.
80. Layer P, Andresen V, Pehl C, Allescher H, Bischoff SC, Classen M, et al. S3-Leitlinie Reizdarmsyndrom: Definition, Pathophysiologie, Diagnostik und Therapie. Gemeinsame

Leitlinie der Deutschen Gesellschaft für Verdauungs- und Stoffwechselkrankheiten (DGVS) und der Deutschen Gesellschaft für Neurogastroenterologie und Motilität (DGNM)1 [Irritable bowel syndrome: German consensus guidelines on definition, pathophysiology and management]. Z Gastroenterol. 2011;49(2):237–93. https://doi.org/10.1055/s-0029-1245976.
81. Moayyedi P, Lacy BE, Andrews CN, Enns RA, Howden CW, Vakil N. ACG and CAG clinical guideline: management of dyspepsia [published correction appears in Am J Gastroenterol. 2017 Sep;112(9):1484]. Am J Gastroenterol. 2017;112(7):988–1013. https://doi.org/10.1038/ajg.2017.154.

Mucosal Protective Agents

7

Aleksandar Včev, Tea Omanović Kolarić, and Hrvoje Roguljić

Introduction

Extremely low pH in the gastric lumen requires numerous defense mechanisms to protect the esophagus, stomach and duodenum from harmful effects of this acidic environment. Besides anatomical defense mechanisms, such as lower esophageal sphincter, the diaphragm and angle of HIS, gastric mucosa has also developed several protective mechanisms. All these mechanisms require adequate mucosal blood flow in order to deliver vital nutrients and bicarbonate to gastric superficial cells. The principal defense strategy is the stimulation of mucus and bicarbonate secretion and mucosal blood flow by mucosal prostaglandins PGE_2 and PGI_2. However, some drugs, such as non-steroidal anti-inflammatory drugs (NSAIDs), inhibit the production of prostaglandins and lead to diminished mucosal protection. Various

A. Včev (✉)
Department of Pathophysiology and Physiology with Immunology, Faculty of Dental Medicine and Health, J. J. Strossmayer University of Osijek, Osijek, Croatia

Department of Internal Medicine, University Hospital Center Osijek, Osijek, Croatia
e-mail: aleksandar.vcev@fdmz.hr

T. Omanović Kolarić
Department of Pharmacology and Biochemistry, Faculty of Dental Medicine and Health, J. J. Strossmayer University of Osijek, Osijek, Croatia

Department of Pharmacology, Faculty of Medicine, J. J. Strossmayer University of Osijek, Osijek, Croatia
e-mail: tea.omanovic@mefos.hr

H. Roguljić
Department of Internal Medicine, University Hospital Center Osijek, Osijek, Croatia

Department of Pharmacology, Faculty of Medicine, J. J. Strossmayer University of Osijek, Osijek, Croatia
e-mail: hroguljic@mefos.hr

M. Banić, D. Erceg (eds.), *Drug Interactions in Gastroenterology*, Clinical Gastroenterology, https://doi.org/10.1007/978-3-031-69800-2_7

acid-peptic disorders are also responsible for disturbing mucosal defense strategy and inducing gastric injury. In this chapter, several mucosal protective agents that may diminish mucosal injury caused by gastrointestinal diseases or NSAID administration will be discussed.

Misoprostol

Misoprostol is an orally active semisynthetic methyl prostaglandin E_1 (PGE_1) analog. It has multiple clinical applications. This drug can be used in gastrointestinal conditions (peptic and duodenal ulcer), in clinically justified induction of labor and also as abortifacient in combination with mifepristone. However, numerous side effects and complexity of multiple daily doses limit widespread use of this drug.

Pharmacokinetics

Oral administration of misoprostol is preferred because of rapid absorption and stability of this drug and due to convenience for the patients [1, 2]. Antacids and food can reduce the rate of its absorption, consequently delaying and decreasing peak plasma drug concentrations and therefore diminishing misoprostol effectiveness [3]. After absorption, this drug is de-esterificated to misoprostol-free acid [3]. This acid represents drug's active metabolite. The serum half-life of misoprostol is around 30 min, and the peak of its therapeutic effects occurs within 60–90 min and lasts up to 3 h [3]. Therefore, this drug needs to be administered 3–4 times per day, which in some way limits its clinical use [4]. The active metabolite is excreted mostly in the urine.

Mechanism of Action

Misoprostol exerts several effects on gastric cells. Similar to other local prostaglandins (PGE_2, PGI_2), this synthetic analog of PGE_1 is capable of enhancing mucin and bicarbonate production in gastric superficial epithelial cells and secretion to gastric lumen and also stimulating mucosal blood flow [3, 4] (Fig. 7.1). All these effects are cytoprotective, which means that protective effect of the drug against peptic ulcers occurs at doses that do not reduce acid secretion [5]. Nevertheless, misoprostol also inhibits proton pump by blocking cAMP-dependent pathway, which, in the end, leads to reduction in the concentration of H^+ in gastric lumen, and therefore increase in gastric pH (Fig. 7.1).

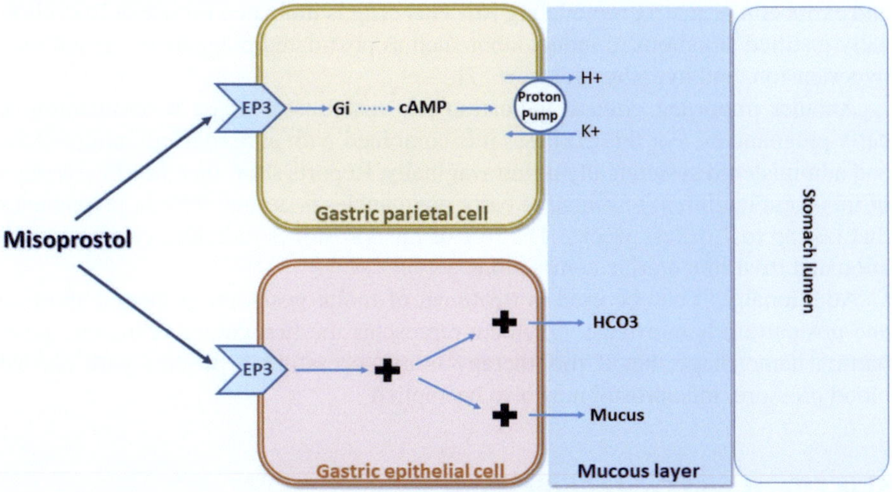

Fig. 7.1 Mechanism of action of misoprostol in gastric parietal and epithelial cell. Misoprostol binds to the EP3 receptor in parietal cell and decreases cAMP production which leads to inhibition of proton pump activity. This drug also binds to EP3 receptor on epithelial cell and enhances the production of bicarbonate and mucus and their secretion to stomach lumen. *EP3* prostaglandin E3 receptor, *Gi* Gi protein, *cAMP* cyclic adenosine monophosphate

Indications and Clinical Uses

Misoprostol, as mentioned earlier has found its role in treating GI peptic diseases. It is often used in order to prevent gastric and duodenal NSAID-induced ulcers. Most important mechanism of action of NSAIDs is inhibition of cyclooxigenase enzymes COX-1 and COX-2. Although this inhibition leads to various therapeutic effects, side effects are also often unavoidable in long-term treatment. COX-1 enzyme is responsible for production of prostanoids involved in gastric epithelial cytoprotection, whereas COX-2 represents the major source of prostanoids in inflammation and cancer [4]. Conclusively, nonselective NSAIDs, that inhibit both COX-1 and COX-2 enzymes diminish the production of gastroprotective prostanoids and finally induce development of gastric and duodenal ulcers. Considering the fact that misoprostol is analog of one specific gastroprotective PGE_1, it is capable of preventing the development of aforementioned NSAID-related side effects. Coadministration of misoprostol (200 mcg four times per day) with non-selective NSAIDs (such as diclofenac) is indicated in patients with a high risk for gastrointestinal bleeding [5]. Effectiveness of misoprostol in this indication was found to be similar to the one of the omeprazole [3]. One large clinical trial demonstrated the evidence that misoprostol diminishes the risk of GI complications in rheumatoid arthritis patients with a high risk of developing gastrointestinal (GI) side effects [5].

Misoprostol may also be used for the induction of labor and ripening of the cervix. It is capable of mimicking the physiological processes that occur in spontaneous labor, which include stimulation of uterine contractions, collagenase activation and extracellular matrix remodeling [6]. This drug is indicated for use only in clinically justified situations to induct labor such as post-dated pregnancies, gestational hypertension, and hypothyroidism [6, 7].

Another important clinical indication for misoprostol usage is termination of early pregnancies. For this purpose, it is combined with antiprogestin mifepristone and administered systemically or intravaginally. Reports show that the effectiveness of this combination in terminating early pregnancies is around 90% in pregnancies that last up to 7 or less weeks. The role of misoprostol is to induce cervical relaxation and rhythmic uterine contractions.

Additionally, it can be used in treatment of molar gestation or missed abortion and postpartum hemorrhage. Oxytocin represents the first choice in treating postpartum hemorrhage, but if this therapy is unsuccessful, in patients with normal blood pressure, misoprostol may also be applied.

Side Effects and Contraindications

Most often side effects due to misoprostol therapy are abdominal pain, cramping pain, diarrhea, nausea, vomiting, flatulence, exacerbations of inflammatory bowel disease, and vaginal bleeding. Diarrhea occurs in up to 30% of patients receiving misoprostol, often in the first 2 weeks of treatment, and if this side effect is affecting the patient's condition severely, drug discontinuation should be considered. Because of the effect of misoprostol on uterus, which includes enhancement of uterus contractility, its administration in pregnant women is contraindicated [3, 5]. Also, it is contraindicated in women with a previous uterine scar due to its linkage to uterine rupture [5]. Before prescribing this drug to women in their childbearing years, proper precautions should be taken: administration of adequate contraceptive measures and a documented negative serum marker of pregnancy within 2 weeks of initiating treatment [5]. When used for the induction of labor severe side effects may occur such as uterine tachysystole, hyperstimulation syndrome, cesarean for nonreassuring fetal heart rate, and meconium staining [6, 8].

Drug–Drug Interactions

Coadministration of misoprostol and other drugs for labor induction, such as oxytocin, should be avoided. Concomitant use of misoprostol and antacids, specifically magnesium-containing ones, may worsen GI toxic effects of misoprostol [9]. Therefore, magnesium-free antacids (aluminum hydroxide, calcium carbonate, and sodium bicarbonate) should be administered in patients requiring this kind of treatment [9].

Sucralfate

Introduction

Sucralfate is FDA-approved mucosal protective agent used mainly in treatment of gastric and duodenal ulcers. This agent represents a complex of sulfated sucrose and sulfated aluminum hydroxide [4, 10].

Pharmacokinetics

Sucralfate is given orally, although its oral absorption is very low, but its main site of action is GI tract, where it resides for a considerable amount of time after ingestion [10]. Because of the fact that main portion of administered sucralfate is unabsorbed it may alter the pharmacokinetics of numerous drugs by reducing their absorption and decreasing the oral bioavailability [10]. Food rich in proteins and phosphate can bind to sucralfate and diminish its therapeutic effect. Therefore, it should be administered on an empty stomach [5]. Sucralfate is excreted by feces.

Mechanism of Action

Several mechanisms of action have been proposed as relevant for sucralfate therapeutic effect, but none of them has been defined as principal. These mechanisms include:

1. Decrease in pepsin concentration
2. Acting as physical barrier between mucosa and luminal contents in form of a polyanion gel
3. Effects on mucus: improvement of mucosal protection from acid by increasing mucous carbohydrate and aluminum content, sulfation, viscosity and hydrophobicity; increase in prostaglandin production which leads to enhancement in mucus production; reduction of ulcerogenesis by preventing the breakdown of mucus by pepsin
4. Increase in bicarbonate production by stomach and duodenum
5. Facilitation of repair by enhancing the binding of growth factors to tissues [11]

Clinical Uses

Sucralfate, an old medication with great affinity for inflamed mucosa can be used for different pathological conditions in GI tract. As a negatively charged molecule, sucralfate has great affinity for positively charged proteins present in mucosal lesions [12]. FDA-approved sucralfate in the treatment of duodenal ulcers. Studies gave advantage to use of sucralfate in prevention of stress ulcers in ventilated patients. Furthermore, sucralfate improves symptoms and heals erosive esophagitis [11]. It is administered four times per day in a dose of 1 g 1 h before meal. Usually, it is used for 6–12 weeks. Topical or rectal usage is also possible like during the treatment of radiation proctitis [13].

Side Effects

As a minimally absorbed drug sucralfate is devoid of systemic adverse effects. Although a special caution is needed in people with renal failure due to possible aluminum accumulation and toxicity. Most common side effect is constipation caused by aluminum salts occurring in up to 2–3%. While less frequent side effects are flatulence, xerostomia, and hypophosphatemia [2, 13].

Bismuth

For centuries, essential or non-essential metal-based drugs were used in medicine. The first known usage of bismuth in the form of a salt was mentioned for skin lesions and syphilis 300 years ago [14]. This non-essential and rare element without any biological role was used for various GI complaints such as stomatitis, gastroenteritis, irritable colon, constipation, diarrhea, flatulence, gastric and duodenal ulcers, and dyspepsia [15]. Nowadays, different forms of bismuth salts, bismuth subcitrate, bismuth subsalicylate, and ranitidine bismuth citrate, are used mainly in the treatment of GI ulcers and *Helicobacter pylori* infection [16].

Pharmacokinetics

Majority of bismuth-containing drugs used in medicine are water-insoluble with low rates of absorption, which is important due to the systemic side effects. Currently, used bismuth salts have absorption rate of around 0.5% while concomitant usage of antacids or thiol-containing drugs decreases bismuth absorption [17]. When absorbed, bismuth binds to plasma proteins and accumulates in the liver. A concentration of bismuth in plasma below 50 ng/L is considered as a safety level while a concentration above 100 ng/L is suggested as a minimal toxicity level. However, bismuth concentration stays under 40 ng/L after single or multiple doses of most often used salt forms [18]. Bismuth is a locally active drug that exerts its effect within the upper GI tract by binding to proteins in the ulcer crater. Unabsorbed bismuth is excreted by stool mostly in the form of the bismuth sulfide, causing the blackening of the stool. Around 90% of absorbed bismuth is excreted by kidneys while biliary secretion is responsible for minority of elimination. Because of the suggested dual elimination pathway, patients with renal impairment or liver disease are in great risk of bismuth accumulation [15].

Mechanism of Action

Exact pharmacodynamic parameters of bismuth are still not fully understood while beneficial effect in the treatment of gastric and duodenal ulcers have been known for a long time. Bismuth salts have gastroprotective effect on the gastric mucosal cells, although bismuth compounds do not have acid neutralizing effect nor inhibit acid secretion. By adherent to ulcerative mucosa, bismuth produces a barrier to aggressive factors within gastric lumen and reduces the accumulation and enzymatic activity of pepsin [19]. Furthermore, bismuth increases production of epidermal growth factor and mucosal prostaglandins which results in increased secretion of alkali compound—bicarbonate [15].

Besides gastroprotective function, a notable antibacterial effect against *H. pylori* makes bismuth one of the treatment options for healing GI ulcers. Bimsuth achieves its antibacterial effect over several different pathways by accumulating on the surface and within *H. pylori*. Forming complexes within bacterial wall and periplasmic space bismuth interferes with adherence of *H. pylori* to gastric mucosa and induces structural degradation of the bacteria. Another important antibacterial mechanism of bismuth is inhibition of several enzymes essential for bacterial colonization and its metabolism. To date, no resistance to bismuth antibacterial effect has been reported [15, 20, 21].

Clinical Uses

Infection with *H. pylori* affects 20–30% of the population in Western world, and it is responsible for the development of peptic ulcer disease. For many years, the strategy to eradicate *H. pylori* has been based on combination of antibiotics and proton pump inhibitors [18]. Due to the increasing resistance of bacteria to antibiotics, first of all, resistance to clarithromycin and metronidazole, new treatment options are introduced such as bismuth-based triple or quadruple therapy. Therefore, current treatment guidelines recommend bismuth-based quadritherapy (a single capsule containing bismuth subnitrate potassium, metronidazole, tetracycline, and omeprazole) as a first-line treatment in regions of high antibiotic resistance (>15%) [16]. Besides *H. pylori*, bismuth exhibits antibacterial effect against other GI pathogens: *E. coli*, *Campylobacter jejuni*, and *Vibrio cholera*; therefore, it is used for different forms of gastroenteritis such as traveler's diarrhea [15].

Side Effects

Bismuth-containing drugs are well-tolerated medications with favorable safety profile in short-term usage. Low uptake of the bismuth by GI tract is one of the main reasons for its low toxicity potential. Most common adverse effect of bismuth usage is blackening of the stool. Furthermore, acute toxicity can be manifested as reversible renal failure [22]. Long-standing use of bismuth salts causes blackening of the tongue and teeth, while the most severe consequence of chronic usage of large quantities of bismuth (>10 g/day) is neurotoxicity. Bismuth encephalopathy is a reversible state characterized by myoclonus, dysarthria, lack of coordination, parkinsonism, seizures, and neuropsychiatric symptoms [18, 23].

References

1. Katzung BG. Basic and clinical pharmacology. 14th ed. McGraw-Hill Education; 2017.
2. Luellmann H, Mohr K, Hein L. Color atlas of pharmacology. 5th ed. Thieme; 2018.
3. Brunton LL, Hilal-Dandan R, Knollmann BC. Goodman and Gillman's the pharmacological basis of therapeutics. McGraw-Hill Education; 2018.
4. Katzun BG, Trevor AJ. Basic and clinical Pharmacology. 13th ed. McGraw-Hill Education; 2015.
5. Dipiro JT, Talbert RL, Yee GC, Matzke GR, Wells BG, Posey ML. Pharmacotherapy: a pathophysiologic approach. 10th ed. McGraw-Hill Education; 2016. p. 2512.
6. Acharya T, Devkota R, Bhattarai B, Acharya R. Outcome of misoprostol and oxytocin in induction of labour. SAGE Open Med. 2017;5:2050312117700809.
7. http://halmed.hr//upl/lijekovi/SPC/Angusta-SPC.pdf.
8. Stephenson ML, Wing DA. Misoprostol for induction of labor. Semin Perinatol. 2015;39(6):459–62.
9. https://www.drugs.com/ppa/misoprostol.html.
10. Sulochana SP, Syed M, Chandrasekar DV, Mullangi R, Srinivas NR. Clinical drug-drug pharmacokinetic interaction potential of sucralfate with other drugs: review and perspectives. Eur J Drug Metab Pharmacokinet. 2016;41(5):469–503.
11. Kudaravalli P, Patel P, John S. Sucralfate. [Updated 2024 Feb 28]. In: StatPearls [Internet]. Treasure Island (FL): StatPearls Publishing; 2024 Jan-. Available from: https://www.ncbi.nlm.nih.gov/books/NBK551527/
12. Savarino E, Zentilin P, Marabotto E, Pellegatta G, Coppo C, Brunacci M, et al. Drugs for improving esophageal mucosa defense: where are we now and where are we going? Ann Gastroenterol. 2017;30(6):585–91.
13. Katzun BG. Basic and clinical pharmacology. 14th ed. McGraw-Hill Education; 2017.
14. Abrams MJ, Murrer BA. Metal compounds in therapy and diagnosis. Science. 1993;261(5122):725–30.
15. Alkim H, Koksal AR, Boga S, Sen I, Alkim C. Role of bismuth in the eradication of Helicobacter pylori. Am J Ther. 2017;24(6):e751–e7.
16. Pellicano R, Zagari RM, Zhang S, Saracco GM, Moss SF. Pharmacological considerations and step-by-step proposal for the treatment of Helicobacter pylori infection in the year 2018. Minerva Gastroenterol Dietol. 2018;64(3):310–21.
17. Koch KM, Kerr BM, Gooding AE, Davis IM. Pharmacokinetics of bismuth and ranitidine following multiple doses of ranitidine bismuth citrate. Br J Clin Pharmacol. 1996;42(2):207–11.
18. Guiard E, Lelievre B, Rouyer M, Zerbib F, Diquet B, Mégraud F, et al. Bismuth concentrations in patients treated in real-life practice with a bismuth subcitrate-metronidazole-tetracycline preparation: the SAPHARY study. Drug Saf. 2019;42(8):993–1003.
19. Beil W, Bierbaum S, Sewing KF. Studies on the mechanism of action of colloidal bismuth subcitrate. II. Interaction with pepsin. Pharmacology. 1993;47(2):141–4.
20. Lambert JR, Midolo P. The actions of bismuth in the treatment of Helicobacter pylori infection. Aliment Pharmacol Ther. 1997;11(Suppl 1):27–33.
21. Ge R, Chen Z, Zhou Q. The actions of bismuth in the treatment of Helicobacter pylori infections: an update. Metallomics. 2012;4(3):239–43.

22. Liu Y, Shen C, Zhang X, Yu H, Wang F, Wang Y, et al. Exposure and nephrotoxicity concern of bismuth with the occurrence of autophagy. Toxicol Ind Health. 2018;34(3):188–99.
23. Ford AC, Malfertheiner P, Giguere M, Santana J, Khan M, Moayyedi P. Adverse events with bismuth salts for Helicobacter pylori eradication: systematic review and meta-analysis. World J Gastroenterol. 2008;14(48):7361–70.

Antimicrobial Drugs

8

Sanja Pleško, Gabrijela Perše, Zrinka Todorić, and Ivana Mareković

Antibacterial Agents

With the introduction of first antibacterial agents in the past century, during World War II began a modern era in medical practice. Nowadays, antibiotics are used almost daily to manage existing infections or as prophylaxis for certain medical conditions and procedures. Antibiotics are generally classified according to their target site and then grouped based on their chemical structure. General mechanism of action is to either inhibit synthesis of bacterial structural components or modify specific metabolic functions that are fundamental for bacterial cell growth and replication [1–3].

Mechanism of Action

Inhibition of Cell Wall Synthesis

The most common mechanism of antibiotic activity is interruption of different stages of bacterial cell wall synthesis. Three major groups of antibiotics that produce this effect are β-lactams, glycopeptides and polypeptides.

Both gram-positive and gram-negative bacteria have cell walls composed primarily of peptidoglycan layer. Peptidoglycan is a polymer composed of disaccharide units consisting of alternating molecules of *N*-acetylglucosamine (NAG) and *N*-acetylmuramic acid (NAM) which are then cross-linked with peptides. This

S. Pleško (✉) · G. Perše · Z. Todorić · I. Mareković
Department for Clinical and Molecular Microbiology, University Clinical Hospital Center Zagreb, Zagreb, Croatia
e-mail: sanja.plesko@kbc-zagreb.hr; gabrijela.perse@kbc-zagreb.hr; zrinka.todoric@kbc-zagreb.hr; ivana.marekovic@kbc-zagreb.hr; imarekov@kbc-zagreb.hr

M. Banić, D. Erceg (eds.), *Drug Interactions in Gastroenterology*, Clinical Gastroenterology, https://doi.org/10.1007/978-3-031-69800-2_8

linkage process is catalyzed by specific enzymes called transpeptidases. These regulatory enzymes are also referred to as penicillin-binding proteins (PBPs), due to their function as receptors for β-lactam antibiotics. When the above mentioned antibiotic binds to specific PBPs in the bacterial cell wall, the assembly of the peptidoglycan layer is disrupted, thus resulting in bacterial cell death by activating a cascade of cell autolysins [2, 4].

Another target for cell wall inhibitors are the termini of the pentapeptide chains. This is the site of action of glycopeptides, highly potent antibiotics which also interfere with peptidoglycan polymerization by binding to 'D-alanine-D-alanine' ending of the peptide sequence [4].

Finally, the remaining mechanism of interference with cell wall synthesis belongs to polypeptides. These antibiotics bind to cytoplasmic membrane and impede its function of active transport and permeability causing cell death [2, 4].

Beta-Lactam Antibiotics

All beta-lactam antibiotics contain beta-lactam ring as a core structure which determines both their activity, but also some types of resistance mechanisms bacteria may develop. They act bactericidal by competitively binding to the PBPs and inhibiting the peptidoglycan assembly in the cell wall of susceptible bacteria.

Different beta-lactams are suitable for intramuscular, intravenous or oral administration. Most of them absorb properly and achieve clinically useful concentrations in serum and most of the tissues such as urine, synovial, pericardial or pleural fluid. Low levels usually achieved in cerebrospinal fluid (CSF) increase in case of meningitis when drug penetration through blood-brain barrier is enhanced due to inflammation process [1, 5].

Beta-lactams are mostly organic acids that are rapidly excreted via tubular secretion by the kidneys. The excretion rate can be decreased by parallel use of probenecid in order to maintain adequate serum and tissue concentrations [1]. Beta-lactams are considered fairly non-toxic agents because peptidoglycan cell wall is a structure unique to bacteria and not found in human cells. The most important adverse effect of these drugs is hypersensitivity reaction, which can range from mild rashes to life-threatening anaphylaxis and angioedema. Blood count abnormalities and neurotoxicity are less common but can occur when inadequately high dosage is applied [1, 3]. Patients allergic to penicillin are usually allergic to cephalosporins as well (especially older-generation compounds), but aztreonam can be safely used in such cases because it shows little to no cross-reactivity [1].

Bacteria employ different resistance mechanism to beta-lactams like efflux of antibiotic out of bacterial cell using active pumps or alteration of PBP receptors, but the major mechanism is production of beta-lactamases, very potent antibiotic-destroying enzymes. The extended spectrum of new beta-lactams has also led to pathogen advancement in terms of resistance, creating extended-spectrum β-lactamases (ESBLs) and carbapenemases active against practically all beta-lactam antibiotics. Currently, there is a whole array of such enzymes (e.g., TEM, SHV, CTX-M, OXA, beta-lactamases, and IMP, VIM, OXA, KPC, CMY and NDM-1 carbapenemases), most of them encoded on bacterial plasmids and easily transferred among different species of bacteria [1].

Penicillins

Penicillins are an extensive group of highly effective beta-lactam antibiotics with acceptable toxicity in humans. These agents are obtained from molds of the genus *Penicillium* (e.g., *Penicillium notatum* and *Penicillium chrysogenum*) [1, 2]. All penicillins share the same basic compound of aminopenicillanic acid with β-lactam ring in its structure. Various biochemical modifications of this precursor result in antibiotics that have improved properties such as increased resistance to gastric acid, enhanced gastrointestinal (GI) tract absorption, resistance to certain penicillinases, or a broader spectrum of activity against bacteria [4].

The clinically important penicillins can be divided into four principal groups:

1. Natural penicillins (penicillin G and penicillin V) have high activity against gram-positive organisms and spirochetes but are susceptible to hydrolysis by β-lactamases.
2. Semisintetic penicillins (e.g., nafcillin, methicillin and oxacillin) possess relative resistance to penicillinase, but lower activity against gram-positive organisms and inactivity against gram-negative organisms.
3. Broad-spectrum penicillins including aminopenicillins, ureidopenicillins and carboxypenicillins have relatively high activity against both gram-positive and gram-negative organisms but are destroyed by β-lactamases.
4. Combinations of β-lactams and β-lactamase inhibitors (e.g., clavulanic acid, tazobactam and sulbactam), which surpass the antibiotic susceptibility to enzymatic decomposition [2, 3].

Cephalosporins

Cephalosporins are another group of mold-derived beta-lactam antimicrobials. They are all derivatives of 7-aminocephalosporanic acid (the β-lactam ring is fused with a dihydrothiazine ring) [4]. Compared to penicillins, cephalosporins have a greater antibacterial spectrum, including gram-negative bacteria, and superior resistance to many β-lactamases. The cephalosporins are divided into four major groups or so-called 'generations' with improved pharmacokinetic features accomplished with each following generation.

First-generation consists of narrow-spectrum antibiotics whose activity is primarily restricted to *Escherichia coli*, *Klebsiella* species, *Proteus mirabilis*, and oxacillin-susceptible gram-positive cocci. Alongside these bacteria, second-generation cephalosporins exert additional activity against *Haemophilus influenzae*, *Enterobacter*, *Citrobacter*, *Serratia* species and some anaerobes, such as *Bacteroides fragilis*. The broad-spectrum, third-generation antibiotics and extended-spectrum, fourth-generation antibiotics are active against most *Enterobacteriaceae* and *Pseudomonas aeruginosa* [4].

Monobactams

Monobactams (e.g., aztreonam) are narrow-spectrum antibiotics that target only aerobic, gram-negative bacteria. The benefit of narrow-spectrum antibiotics is that they can be used to treat susceptible organisms without interfering with patient's physiological, protective microbiota. Despite this advantage, monobactams are not widely prescribed by clinicans [4].

Carbapenems

Carbapenems are another big and important class of β-lactam antibiotics with agents such as imipenem, meropenem and ertapenem. Imipenem was first introduced in clinical practice and has a good coverage of gram-negatives, gram-positives and anaerobes.

However, it is inactivated by renal dehydropeptidase and therefore must be administered together with a peptidase antagonist—cilastatin. The following drug, meropenem, is similar to imipenem in pharmacology and activity but causes less adverse effects since it does not require administration with potentially neurotoxic cilastatin. Ertapenem might be used for some complicated infections, but not those involving *Pseudomonas aeruginosa* and other glucose-nonfermenting gram-negative rods [2, 5].

Because of their broad activity against many groups of bacteria, carbapenems are being favored both as empirical therapy as well as in infections caused by pathogens resistant to other drugs. They owe this preferential status to their great beta-lactamase stability. Unfortunately, due to the emerging population of carbapenemase-producing bacteria, there is an urgent need for new antibiotic development.

Glycopeptides

Glycopeptides, including vancomycin and teicoplanin, also interfere with peptidoglycan polymerization by attaching to pentapeptide side chains. Glycopeptides are poorly absorbed from the gastrointestinal tract so they are most commonly given as parenteral therapy. Their main utility is in treatment of severe systemic infections (sepsis, endocarditis) caused by oxacillin-resistant staphylococci and other gram-positive bacteria resistant to β-lactam antibiotics. Nevertheless, oral form is also available and suitable for treatment of post-antibiotic *Clostridium difficile* colitis. These drugs cannot be used in gram-negative infections because the molecules are too large to penetrate through the outer bacterial membrane pores and reach the peptidoglycan target site. Besides the gram-negatives, some gram-positive bacteria show intrinsic resistance to glycopeptides (e.g., *Erysipelothrix*, *Leuconostoc*, *Lactobacillus* and *Pediococcus*). But what is especially worrisome is an increase in acquired resistance recorded in *Enterococcus faecium* and *Enterococcus faecalis* (vancomycin-resistant enterococci; VRE). There are several genotypes associated with high levels of glycopeptide resistance: vanA, vanB and vanD [1, 4]. Glycopeptides show rather high toxicity, potentially Glycopeptides causing kidney and hearing impairment. Furthermore, vancomycin intravenous infusion must be administered slowly because it might cause histamine rush and series of unpleasant sensations known as 'red man syndrome' [1, 4, 5].

Polypeptides

Polypeptides are considered so toxic that their use is strictly limited to either topical application or systemic treatment of multidrug-resistant (MDR) infections with already limited therapy options. Bacitracin is utilized as local therapy for skin lesions caused by gram-positive bacteria, especially Staphylococcus and group A Streptococcus. On the other hand, polymyxins are selective for gram-negative bacteria where they act by compromising cell permeability and active transport of the phospholipid membrane. Polymyxin E (colistin), available parenterally as colistimethate sodium is the therapy of choice in infections caused by multidrug-resistant *Acinetobacter baumannii*, *Pseudomonas aeruginosa* and carbapenem-resistant Enterobacteriaceae [2, 4, 5].

Inhibition of Protein Synthesis

Apart from cell wall inhibition, antibacterial agents may function as inhibitors of protein synthesis. There are number of antibiotics that use this mechanism; these are aminoglycosides, tetracyclines, glycylcyclines, chloramphenicol, macrolides, lincosamides, streptogramins and oxazolidinones. Every cell depends on continuous protein production for its growth and vitality. Translation of mRNA into the polypeptides that constitute these proteins is a crucial step that occurs at the ribosomes. This large group of antibiotics exerts antimicrobial effects by inhibiting ribosomal action. Once again, the selective toxicity for microbial cells is based on the fact that bacterial ribosomes differ structurally from those of the mammalian. While mammals have an 80S particle, the bacterial ribosome is a 70S particle that consists of two subunits: the 50S (large) and the 30S (small). Although protein synthesis is a complex process involving many enzyme-catalyzed steps, the majority of antibiotics that inhibit bacterial protein synthesis do so by binding to these two subunits. This attachment to the ribosomes has two outcomes: a misreading of the messenger RNA (mRNA), which results in the production of aberrant proteins and interruption of mRNA translation, which prevents polypeptide elongation [3, 4].

Aminoglycosides

Aminoglycosides are a group of bactericidal agents that can easily enter the cytoplasm of vulnerable bacteria and irreversibly bind to 30S ribosomal unit, thus preventing further protein production. The penetration of antibiotics into the bacterial cell is an aerobic, energy-requiring process, meaning aminoglycosides are inactive in anaerobic settings [4].

Aminoglycosides are not resorbed well after oral administration, so they ought to be given by intravenous route. They also hardly cross the blood-brain barrier so when required, intrathecal administration is plausible in treatment of tuberculous meningitis (Streptomycin) or gram-negative neonatal meningitis (Amikacin). They are excreted via the kidneys [1, 5].

The prominent resistance mechanisms are the production of antibiotic-modifying enzymes and alteration of ribosomal target site.

Aminoglycosides exhibit ototoxic, nephrotoxic and even neurotoxic side effects. They should be prescribed cautiously, especially in patients with renal impairment [3, 5].

Tetracyclines

Tetracyclines are antibiotics with potentially the broadest spectrum of activity, but their widespread use has led to resistance expansion, so nowadays they are being used in only few addressed indications. They also act as protein synthesis inhibitors by inhibiting the binding of aminoacyl-tRNA to the 30S ribosomal subunit [2].

Tetracyclines are usually taken orally. They easily penetrate host cells and can inhibit even intracellular bacteria. They are excreted both in stool and urine [1]. Tetracyclines are indicated in treatment of infections caused by *Mycoplasma*, *Chlamydia* and *Rickettsia* species, along with some other gram-positive and gram-negative infections [1, 4].

Resistance in bacteria is common and includes the alteration of ribosomal binding site and active efflux mechanism. Tetracyclines regularly cause adverse effects such as gastrointestinal (GI) tract sensations and much less common hepatotoxicity or photosensitivity. Tetracyclines must be omitted in pregnant women and small children while they interfere with bone development and discolorate the teeth of fetuses and children [1, 3, 5].

Glycylcyclines

Glycylcyclines are synthetic analogs of the tetracyclines and have only one representative in clinical use: tigecycline. It shares the same mechanism of action as tetracyclines but has enhanced affinity for the ribosome and is immune to bacterial efflux or enzymatic alterations [4]. It is available for parenteral use and distributes well in tissues. It is excreted primarily in the bile and also via the kidneys [2]. Tigecycline covers many anaerobic, gram-negative and gram-positive bacteria, including MRSA. It is not active against *Pseudomonas* infections [4, 5].

Chloramphenicol

Chloramphenicol is a very potent antibiotic, but its use is highly restricted due to drugs' severe toxicity. It binds to large 50S ribosomal subunit and disrupts the performance of peptidyl transferase, subsequently preventing peptide elongation [1, 2, 4].

It is generally given orally, but intravenous and even topical preparations are available. Its distribution is extensive in tissues and body fluids, including cerebrospinal fluid (CSF). The drug is inactivated in the liver by conjugation with glucuronic acid and eventually excreted in the urine. Besides bacterial cell metabolism, chloramphenicol affects protein synthesis in human bone marrow cells, thus inducing blood dyscrasias, such as aplastic anemia. The use of chloramphenicol in infants can result in collapse known as 'grey baby syndrome' due to neonatal incomplete liver metabolizing function [1, 2]. Because of these severe adverse effects, it is mainly used in developing countries in treatment of typhoid fever and *H. influenzae* meningitis [5].

Macrolides, Lincosamides and Streptogramins

These three groups of antibacterial agents are chemically distinct, but share many characteristics such as antibacterial spectrum and mechanism as well as cross-resistance. Macrolides bind to the 23S ribosomal RNA (rRNA) in the 50S subunit of the ribosome and hamper the translocation step in protein synthesis [1].

The most prevalent resistance mechanism is a result of the rRNA receptor methylation, and it yields so-called 'MLS (macrolide-lincosamide-streptogramin) resistance'. Other types of resistance mechanisms are unique to macrolides and include active efflux or enzymatic inactivation of antibiotics.

Macrolides are bacteriostatic antibiotics that cover a whole array of microorganisms. Besides their usual utilization in treatment of respiratory infections caused by *H. influenzae*, *M. catarrhalis* and *S. pneumoniae*, they are also active against *M. pneumoniae*, intracellular pathogens such as *Chlamidia*, *Legionella* and *Rickettsia*. Another indication is treatment of *H. pylori* gastritis and boreliosis (*Borrelia burgdorferi*). Because of their great gram-positive coverage, macrolides are being used as an alternative in patients allergic to penicillin.

The side effects of macrolide use are generally mild. The most frequent are gastrointestinal upset (nausea, vomiting and diarrhea) and cholestatic hepatitis caused mainly by erythromycin estolate. More recent agents, clarithromycin and azithromycin, demonstrate much lower incidence of gastrointestinal side effects [5]. Macrolides, taken via oral route or intravenous injection, are well distributed in the body. They are predominantly metabolized in the liver and excreted in the bile. Clindamycin is the most clinically relevant antibiotic which belongs to **lincosamides**. The drug can be given orally or parenterally. Because of its great bone penetration, it is widely used in treatment of osteomyelitis. Excretion is mainly through the liver, bile, and urine. The major therapeutic indication for clindamycin use are anaerobic infections caused by *B. fragilis* and skin or bone infections caused by either susceptible staphylococci or MRSA.

Clindamycin is one of the first and well-known antibiotics that has been associated with *C. difficile* colitis [2].

The only currently available **streptogramin** is quinupristin–dalfopristin, combination of two compounds that act as inhibitors of two consecutive steps in peptide chain extension. This synergistic effect makes these agents bactericidal for many gram-positive cocci, including methicillin-resistant staphylococci and vancomycin-resistant *E. faecium.*

Quinupristin–dalfopristin is administered intravenously and metabolism occurs in the liver [1].

Oxazolidinones

The most clinically relevant drug in this class is linezolid. The drug inhibits initiation of protein synthesis by interfering with translation. Because its activity mechanism is so distinct from any other protein inhibitor, the cross-resistance is not encountered. Linezolid is equally well absorbed and distributed whether taken per os or parenterally. Its use is reserved for cases of pneumonia, sepsis, or skin and soft tissue infections caused by multidrug-resistant isolates: MRSA and VRE [3, 5].

Inhibition of Nucleic Acid Synthesis

Another highly effective mode of action is interruption of nucleic acid synthesis. This antibacterial mechanism is reserved for quinolones, rifamycins, metronidazole, sulfonamides and trimethoprim. Quinolones interfere with the action of DNA gyrase (topoisomerase II), consequently preventing the production and replication of bacterial DNA. Rifamycins are another group of antibiotics that bind to DNA-dependent RNA polymerase and inhibit the synthesis of cell RNA.

Upon entering the bacterial cell, metronidazole is converted to free radical by bacterial nitroreductase, thereby producing cytotoxic product that damages bacterial DNA.

The sulfonamides act as antimetabolic agents that competitively inhibit the production of the folic acid required for nucleotide formation. Since human cells do not synthesize folic acid, sulfonamides only affect microorganisms. They prevent the conversion of *p*-aminobenzoic acid to dihydrofolate. Trimethoprim is another antifolate that inhibits the reduction of dihydrofolate to tetrahydrofolate [3, 4].

Quinolones

Quinolones are large class of comprehensive and widely prescribed antibiotics that act as nucleic acid inhibitors. The first drug of this kind was nalidixic acid which used to serve as a urinary antiseptic, but emerging bacterial resistance placed it out of clinical use. The more recent antibiotics called fluoroquinolones show excellent oral absorption, tissue distribution and activity against both gram-positive and gram-negative bacteria. Because of their extensive excretion into the urine, fluoroquinolones are suitable for treatment of urinary tract infections. Furthermore, they are effective in treatment of lower respiratory tract infections caused by *H. influenzae* and enteritis caused by salmonellae, shigellae, or campylobacters. Some respiratory quinolones such as levofloxacin and moxifloxacin are highly effective against *S. pneumonie* and thus indicated in treatment of community-acquired pneumonia.

The prevalent resistance mechanisms include alteration of the target enzyme and decreased drug intake due to decreased cell wall permeability or active efflux.

The most frequent side effect are GI tract disturbances; neurotoxicity and photosensitivity are observed but less likely to occur. Finally, fluoroquinolones should be avoided in children due to the records of joint damage [3, 5].

Antifungal Agents

Mechanism of Action

Fungi are, like humans, eukaryotes so there are many difficulties in creating a drug that will be successful and with acceptable side effects. The major difficulties in creating a proper antifungal drugs are serious adverse effects because several cellular and molecular processes are similar to human cells, a narrow spectrum, poor penetration, and the selection of resistant strains [6, 7]. With the increasing importance of fungal infections, a number of new antifungal drugs are being developed.

The main groups of antifungal drugs are polyenes, azoles, echinocandins, antimetabolites, allylamines, and grisefulvin, but there are also investigational antifungal agents [4]. Polyenes bind to ergosterol in the cell membrane, so their mode of action is the direct destroy the membrane. This group include amphotericin B as systemic and topical agent, lipid formulations of amphotericin, that are amphotericin B lipid complex or colloidal dispersion and liposomal amphotericin B and nystatin, as topical agent. Azoles are inhibitors of ergosterol synthesis, so they are act on the structure of the cell membrane. Azoles are divided into two subgroups: imidazoles and triazoles [4]. Imidazoles inhibit enzymes necessary for lanosterol metabolism, and the examples are ketokonazole, clotrimazole, econazole, and miconazole as well as others. They can be administered orally and topically. Triazole, such as fluconazole, itraconazole, voriconazole, and posaconazole have the same mechanism of action like imidazoles, but they bind more specific to target enzyme. They can be administered orally or intravenously [4, 6]. Echinocandins inhibit fungal cell wall β-glucan synthesis. The examples are caspofungin, anidulafungin, and micafungin, and they are administered intravenously. Antimetabolite flucytosine is a pyrimidine analog; it inhibits DNA or RNA synthesis, and it is administered orally. Allylamines act on cell membrane. They are inhibitors of ergosterol synthesis, more precisely, they inhibit squalene epoxidase. The examples are naftifine and terbinafine. Naftifine can be administered topically, and terbinafine orally and topically [4, 6]. The site of action for griseofulvin is a nucleus. It interferes with microtubule assembly and inhibits mitosis. Investigational antifungal agents include nikkomycin Z, which is inhibitor of the cell wall synthesis, more precisely, chitin synthesis, sordarin, which inhibits elongation factor 3, and echinocandin aminocandin [4]. Antifungal agents can also be divided, according to application, into systemic and topical agents.

Pharmacokinetics

Polyenes can be administered topically and intravenously [6]. Ampohtericin is used in both ways, and its lipid formulations are used only intravenously. Nystatin is a topical agent and it is used as an oral suspension. It is poorly absorbed via gastrointestinal tract, and it does not absorbed via skin or mucous membrane when applied topically.

Azoles, both imidazoles and triazoles, are used orally or topically, except triazole itraconazole, which can be used only orally [6, 7]. Ketokonazoles is poorly absorbed by the oral route and require an acid gastric pH. It is lipophilic and has a good penetration into fatty tissues and purulent exudates. It is also highly protein bound so its penetration into central nervous system is low [4]. It shows milder adverse effects such as nausea, vomiting, and rash more severe adverse effects like gastric and hepatic toxicity. Fluconazole has excellent oral bioavailability and low toxicity. It is water-soluble, protein binding is low and it is distributed to all organs and tissues, including central nervous system [4]. The side effects are rare, including exfoliative dermatitis or hepatotoxicity. Itraconazole is a lipophilic agent that can be orally administered in capsule or in solution. It requires an acid gastric pH for better absorption and is better on an empty stomach. It is highly protein-bound. Side effects are uncommon, including gastrointestinal intolerance, hypokalemia, edema, rash, and even more rarely hepatotoxicity [4]. Voriconazole has excellent penetration into all tissues and the central nervous system. It is generally well tolerated, but side effect can include transient visual disturbances, hallucinations, confusion, and skin reactions [4, 8]. Posaconazole is available as an immediate-release oral suspension and intravenously. Absorption is enhanced with food intake and is greatest with fatty meals [4]. It is generally well tolerated and the adverse effects include gastrointestinal disturbances, dry mouth, headache, rash, and facial flushing. Hepatotoxicity has also been described [4]. Isavuconazole is water-soluble and can be administered orally or intravenously [4].

Echinocandins are administered intravenously and are highly protein bound. They have well distribution to all organs, although concentrations in cerebrospinal fluid are low. They are well tolerated [4].

Antimetabolite flucytosine is administered orally, it is water-soluble and has excellent bioavailability. It achieves high concentrations in serum, cerebrospinal fluid, and other body fluids [3]. Toxicity occurs in high concentrations and includes bone marrow suppression, hepatotoxicity, and gastrointestinal disturbances [4, 6].

Allylamine terbinafine is administered orally and topically, so it has systemic activity. It is liphophilic, and achieves high concentrations on fatty tissues, skin, hair, and nails. Naftifine is administered topically [4].

Griseofulvin is administered orally. It is well absorbed and concentrated in keratin. It is metabolized in the liver, and metabolites are excreted in the urine. The adverse effects are mild and include nausea, diarrhea, headache, rash, hepatotoxicity, and neurotoxicity [4, 6].

Investigational antifungal agents include nikkomycin Z, and sordarin and azasordarin derivatives are administered orally and possibly be useful in combination with other antifungal agents [4].

Adverse Effects and Toxicity

The toxicity of polyene amphotericin B can be divided into two categories: immediate reactions and delayed side effects. Immediate reactions are related to the infusion of the drug and include flu-like symptoms, fever, chills, vomiting, headache, and muscle spasm. Therefore, premedication with antipyretics or corticosteroids is useful, and slower administration is recommended. Delayed side effects include serious nephrotoxicity, so it is recommended to administer amphotericin B with saline infusions, abnormalities of liver functions, anemia and neurotoxicity. Topically used nystatin rarely causes toxicity, although oral use is often limited by the unpleasant taste [7, 8].

Azoles are generally nontoxic and the most common adverse effects are gastrointestinal disturbances, elevated hepatic enzymes and, rarely, clinical hepatitis. The adverse effects of voriconazole include rash, elevated hepatic enzymes and, transient visual disturbances like blurring and changes in color vision or brightness and photosensitivity dermatitis in chronic oral therapy [7, 8].

Echinocandins are excellent tolerated, but their adverse effects include gastrointestinal disturbances and flushing [8].

The adverse effects of antimetabolite flucytosine include bone marrow toxicity with anemia, leukopenia, and thrombocytopenia. Derangement of liver enzymes and a form of toxic enterocolitis occur rarely [6, 8].

Allylamine terbinafine rarely causes adverse effects. They include headaches and gastrointestinal disturbances [8].

The adverse effects of griseofulvin include an allergic syndrome like serum sickness and hepatitis [8].

Drug Interactions

Azoles have interactions with other drugs because they induce liver cytochrome P450 enzymes. There is a reduced bioavailability of itraconazole when used with rifamycins (rifampin, rifabutin and rifapentine). Fluconazole has the least effect of all the azoles on hepatic microsomal enzymatic system. Voriconazole inhibits CYP3A4, and dose reduction of a number of medications, such as cyclosporine, tacrolimus and HMG-CoA reductase inhibitors, is required with the beginning of voriconazole therapy. Posaconazole increases levels of CYP3A4 substrates, such as tacrolimus and cyclosporine [7, 8].

Echinocandin caspofugin elevates liver enzymes in combination with cyclosporine. Micafungin increases levels of nifedipine, cyclosporine and sirolimus. Anidulafungin does not have significant drug interactions, but histamine release may occur during intravenous administration [6, 8].

Griseofulvin has drug interactions with warfarin and phenobarbital [8].

Systemically Active Antifungal Agents

Polyens

Amhotericin B

Polyens are group of antifungal drugs which basic structure consists of a large lactone ring, a rigid lipophilic chain containing three to seven double bonds, and a flexible hydrophilic portion with several hydroxyl groups. Amphotericin B contains seven conjugated double bonds [4]. Amphotericin B and its lipid formulations are polyene macrolide, a metabolite of *Streptomyces nodosus* [8]. It has at least two different mechanisms of antifungal activity. It forms a complex with ergosterol in cell membrane, and this interaction alters the membrane fluidity and loss of ions and small molecules. It damages the cell, which finally results in leakage of cellular components, and cell death, i.e., amphotericin B is cidal. It has a greater affinity for ergosterol than cholesterol, the predominant sterol in human cell membranes, but it also weakly binds to cholesterol. Because of that, human cells are relatively resistant to complete damage, but thus, they are toxic. The second mechanism of antifungal activity includes membrane damage, which is a result of a cascade of oxidative reactions beginning with amphotericin B itself [4, 7]. It can be administered intravenously as micelles with sodium deoxycholate dissolved in a dextrose solution, but that form has a nephrotoxic side effect, so lipid formulations were developed [4]. They are less toxic and can be used in higher concentrations. It is the most effective drug for life-threatening mycoses. Efficacy depends on the dose and rate of administration, the site of infection, the immune status of the individual, and the susceptibility of the pathogen. Amphotericin B has a broad spectrum and includes most strains of *Candida*, *Cryptococcus neoformans*, *Aspergillus* spp., the Mucormycetes, and the endemic dimorphic pathogens (*Blastomyces dermatitidis*, *Coccidioides immitis*, *Histoplasma capsulatum*, *Paracoccidioides brasiliensis* and *Talaromyces marneffei*). *Aspergillus terreus*, *Fusarium* spp., *Scedosporium* spp., *Lomentospora prolificans*, *Trichosporon* spp. and certain dematiaceous fungi may be resistant. Reduced susceptibility can occur among some strains of *Candida guilliermondi* (further *C.* for *Candida*), *C. glabrata*, *C. krusei*, *C. lusitaniae*, *C. auris* and *C. rugosa* [4]. The primary clinical indications for amphotericin B include invasive candidiasis, cryptococcosis, aspergillosis, mucormycosis, blastomycosis, coccidioidomycosis, histoplasmosis, paracoccidioidomycosis, talaromycosis and sporotrichosis. Amphotericin B is used in combination with flucytosine for treatment of cryptococcosis [4, 7]. It is widely distributed in various tissues and organs. Although penetration of the joints and the cerebrospinal fluid is poor, it is effective in treating infections of the central nervous system. The side effects can be acute or chronic. Acute side effect is manifested by flu-like symptoms. Headaches, nausea, and vomiting are also common. Acute toxicity refers to potential anaphylactic reactions. They can be avoided by prior or simultaneous administration of hydrocortisone or acetaminophen and tolerance occurs during therapy. Chronic side effects are usually nephrotoxicity and related consequences, like azotemia, hypokalemia, and renal tubular acidosis. Headache, nausea, and vomiting are also common. The lipid formulations have reduced toxicity. Drug resistance is rare, but if it occurs, it is a result of alterations in membrane sterols [4, 6, 7].

Nystatin

Nystatin is another polyene, and it is administered topically. It has been developed a lipid formulation for systemic use, but under investigation [4, 6].

Azoles

The group of azoles can be divided into two subgroups, imidazoles and triazoles. Imidazoles have two nitrogens, and triazoles have three nitrogens in the azole ring. Among the imidazoles, only ketoconazole has systemic activity, and the triazoles all have systemic activity. Investigational agents could be divided into the third group, which includes ravuconazole and albaconazole. Their mechanism of action is altering the fungal cell membrane by blocking enzymes included in biosynthesis of ergosterol [4]. In general, they are fungistatic, but depending on the organism and specific azole, they can be fungicidal. They are oral preparations and have a broad spectrum of activity. They are used to treat systemic and localized infections. Imidazoles miconazole and coltrimazole are used topically. Ketoconazole is the most toxic azole. It has a range of side effects and may inhibit the synthesis of testosterone and cortisol, which may result in gynecomastia, decreased libido, impotence, menstrual irregularity, and adrenal insufficiency [7]. It is used for chronic mucocutaneous candidiasis, dermatophytosis, blastomycosis, coccidioidomycosis, paracoccidioidomycosis, and histoplasmosis [7]. Fluconazole has the best penetration of the central nervous system, and it is used for cryptococcal and coccidiodal meningitis. It is also used for treatment of oropharyngeal candidiasis in AIDS patients and candidemia in immunocompetent individuals [6, 7]. Itraconazole is the first choice for histoplasmosis and blastomycosis and for certain cases of coccidioidomycosis, paracoccidioidomycosis, and aspergillosis. It is also used for treatment of chromomycosis and onychomycosis [6, 7]. Voriconazole has a broad spectrum of activity against molds and yeast, for example, *Aspergillus* spp., *Fusarium* spp., and *Scedosporium* spp. [7]. It can cause reversible visual impairment. It can be administered orally and intravenously. Posaconazole has a wide spectrum and has activity against fluconazole-resistant *Candida* spp., aspergillosis, mucormycosis, and other opportunistic invasive molds. The side effects are predominantly result of their ability to inhibit human cytochrome P450 enzymes. Cytochrome P450 enzymes are responsible for drug metabolism, so azoles may have important interactions with other drugs [6, 7]. They can raise serum levels of cyclosporine, phenytoin, oral hypoglycemics, anticoagulants, digoxin and many others [6–8]. Therefore, monitoring of serum levels of both drugs are recommended. All azoles can cause asymptomatic elevations in liver function tests and, rarely, hepatitis.

Ketoconazole

Ketoconazole is imidazole class of antifungal agent, and it is orally or topically administered. Because there are antifungal agents with more potency and less toxicity, it is used as a second line agent for non-life threatening infections [4]. It is effective against endemic dimorphic pathogens, *Candida* spp., *Cryptococcus neoformans*, and *Malassezia* spp., so it is used for nonmeningeal forms of histoplasmosis, blastomycosis, coccidioidomycosis, and paracoccidioidomycosis. It has variable activity against *Pseudallescheria boydii* [4]. If it is used orally, it requires an acid gastric pH. It achieves high concentrations in fatty tissues and purulent exudates due to its lipophilicity. It is highly protein bound (>99%), so it penetrates poorly into central nervous system [4]. The side effects range from nausea, vomiting, and rash to gastric and hepatic toxicity and suppression of endocrine system [4].

Fluconazole

Fluconazole has great oral bioavailability, low toxicity, is easy to apply, and has activity against most yeast-like fungi. It is widely used and is active against *Candida* spp. (*C. krusei* is intrinsically resistant and *C. glabrata* has reduced susceptibility, so it can be treated with higher doses) but only if the patient's hemodynamic stable, *Cryptococcus* spp., *Histoplasma capsulatum*, *Trichosporon* spp., *Coccidioides immitis*, *Paracoccidioides brasiliensis*, and dermatophytes. It has no efficiency against opportunistic molds, including *Aspergillus* spp., *Fusarium* spp., and Mucormycetes [4]. It is used as first-line therapy for candidemia, mucosal candidiasis, and antifungal prophylaxis in immunosuppressed individuals, such as patients with AIDS or transplant recipients, maintenance therapy of cryptococcal meningitis in patients with AIDS, and for the treatment of meningitis caused by *Coccidioides immitis*. It is a second-line agent for treatment of histoplasmosis, blastomycosis, and sporotrichosis [4, 7]. Fluconazole is water-soluble and can be administered orally and intravenously [4, 6]. It has excellent distribution to all organs and tissues, including eyes and central nervous system, because it binds poorly to proteins. It excretes unchanged in urine. Side effects are rare but serious, include exfoliative dermatitis and liver failure [4, 6].

Itraconazole

Itraconazole is a triazole that has a broad spectrum of activity, including against *Candida* spp., *C. neoformans*, *Aspergillus* spp., dermatophytes, dematiaceous molds, *P. boydii*, *Sporothrix schenckii*, and the endemic dimorphic pathogens. It has some activity against some fluconazole-resistant strains of *C. glabrata* and *C. krusei*. The *Mucormycetes*, *Fusarium* spp., and *Lomentospora prolificans* are resistant to itraconazole. It has fungistatic activity against yeast-like fungi and fungicidal activity against *Aspergillus* spp. [4]. Itraconazole can be administered orally in capsule or in solution. Oral absorption requires an acid gastric pH, and is better in fasting state. It is highly protein bound [8]. It is used for treatment of non-life threatening nonmeningeal forms of histoplasmosis, blastomycosis, and paracoccidioidomycosis, maintenance treatment of cryptococcal meningitis, and some forms of phaeohyphomycosis. It is second-line choice for treatment of invasive aspergillosis [4]. The adverse effects are rare and include gastrointestinal disturbances, hypokalemia, edema, rash, and elevated transaminases. Interactions with other agents are common [4].

Voriconazole

Voriconazole is a triazole. It has a broad spectrum activity, including *Candida* spp. (some strains of *C. albicans* and *C. glabrata* have reduced susceptibility). *C. neoformans*, *Trichosporon* spp., *Aspergillus* spp., *Fusarium* spp., dematiaceous fungi, and endemic dimorphic pathogens. It has no activity against the Mucormycetes. It can be administered orally and intravenously [4]. It has excellent penetration into tissues and central nervous system. Voriconazole is a first-line therapy for invasive aspergillosis and has activity against *P. boydii* and *Fusarium* spp. in patient with refractory to other agents or in individuals with brain abscesses caused by *Aspergillus* spp. and *P. boydii* [4]. It is well tolerated but can cause transient visual disturbances, hallucinations or confusion, hepatotoxicity and skin reactions [4, 6, 8]. It may have interactions with other drugs that are metabolized by the hepatic P450 enzymes, such as warfarin and ciclosporins [6, 8].

Posaconazole
Posaconazole is a triazole. It has great efficiency against *Candida* spp., *Cryptococcus* spp., dimorphic fungi and filamentous fungi, including *Aspergillus* spp. and the Mucormycetes [4]. It can be administered orally as an immediate-release suspension and intravenously. Its absorption is enhanced with food intake and is greatest with a concomitant fatty meal [4]. It is used for prophylaxis of invasive fungal infection in individuals with transplants, hematologic malignancies and prolonged neutropenia, oropharyngeal candidiasis, infections refractory to amphotericin B or itraconazole in aspergilossis, fusariosis, chromoblastomycosis, mycetoma and coccidioidomycosis [4, 7, 8]. It is well tolerated, the most common adverse effects include gastrointestinal disturbances, rash, facial flushing, dry mouth and headache [4]. It may be hepatotoxic, and interactions with other drugs that are metabolized by hepatic P450 enzymes, such as tacrolimus or cyclosporine, are common [8].

Isavuconazole
Isavuconazole (Astellas Pharma, Basilea Pharmaceutica) is a triazole. It is water-soluble and can be administered orally or intravenously. It is used for the treatment of candidemia, invasive candidiasis, invasive apsergilossis, and rare mold infections. It has not good activity against *A. niger* and the Mucormycetes [4].

Echinocandins
Echinocandins are novel group of antifungal agents, semisynthetic lipopeptides that inhibit the synthesis of polysaccharide β-glucan, so they inhibit synthesis of the cell wall. They are highly selective because human cells do not contain β-glucan. In fungal cell, β-glucan has a role in maintaining the osmotic integrity of the cell, in cell division, and growth [4]. It has better activity in species in which β-glucan constitute the dominant cell wall glucan component, so it has fungicidal activity against *Candida* spp., excellent activity against fluconazole-resistant strains of *Candida* spp., fungistatic activity against *Aspergillus* spp., and are inactive against *C. neoformans*, *Trichosporon* spp., *Fusarium* spp. and the Mucormycetes [4]. Echinocandins include anidulafungin, caspofungin, and micafungin [8]. They are administered intravenously and are highly (>95%) protein bound. Concentrations in cerebrospinal fluid are low [4]. They are well tolerated and have few drug-to-drug interactions [6].

Caspofungin
Caspofungin is used for treatment of invasive candidiasis, candidemia, invasive aspergillosis refractory to other antifungal agents, and empirical treatment of febrile neutropenia [4, 8]. It is metabolized spontaneously or in liver and may have interactions with cyclosporin and rifampicin. It is well tolerated, the adverse effects are infrequent, and it is administered intravenously [6].

Anidulafungin
Anidulafungin is approved for treatment of esophageal candidiasis and candidemia, and prophylaxis for transplant recipients. It is administered intravenously [4, 6].

Micafungin

Micafungin is used for treatment of esophageal candidiasis and candidemia, prevention of invasive candidiasis, prophylaxis and treatment of neonates, and prophylaxis of transplant recipients. It is metabolized spontaneously or in liver. It may have interactions with cyclosporin and rifampicin. The adverse effects are rare. It is administered intravenously [6, 7].

Aminocandin

Aminocandin inhibit β-glucan synthesis of fungal cell wall, like other ehinocandins. It is an investigational agent [4].

Antimetabolites

Flucytosine (5-fluorocytosine) is a fluorinated derivative of cytosine. It is the only available antimetabolite. Its activity is a result of interference with the synthesis of deoxyribonucleic acid (DNA), ribonucleic acid (RNA), and proteins [4]. Flucytosine enters the fungal cell via cytosine permease and is deaminated to 5-fluorouracil (5-FU) in the cytoplasm. It is converted to 5-fluorouridylic acid, which then competes with uracil in the synthesis of RNA. The result is abnormal protein synthesis and inhibition of DNA synthesis. Human cells lack cytosine permease, so they are protected from toxicity [6, 7]. It is active against *Candida* spp., *C. neoformans*, *Rhodotorula* spp., *Saccharomyces cerevisiae*, and selected dematiaceous molds [4]. Primary resistance is rare, but it can develop during monotherapy among *Candida* spp. (some strains of *C. krusei* and *C. tropicalis* occur innate resistance), and *C. neoformans*. It has no activity against *Aspergillus* spp., Muctomycetes or hyaline molds. It is water soluble, has excellent bioavailability, and is administered orally [4]. It has a good penetration in tissues, cerebrospinal fluid, and serum. It is excreted in the urine [6]. Toxicity is observed in high concentrations and include bone marrow suppression, hepatotoxicity, hair loss, and gastrointestinal disturbances. Monitoring of serum concentrations is preferable [4, 7]. It must be used in combination therapy because resistant strains emerge rapidly, so it is usually used with amphotericin B in the treatment of systemic candidiasis and cryptococcal meningitis [7].

Allylamines

Allylamines are a class of antifungal agents that act on cell wall components, precisely, inhibiting the enzyme squalene epoxidase, which inhibits ergosterol synthesis. Two agents are developed in this group: terbinafine, which has systemic activity, and naftifine, which is a topical agent.

Terbinafine

Terbinafine is an allylamine drug, it blocks ergosterol synthesis by inhibiting squalene epoxidase [7]. It is a lipophilic agent administered orally or topically. It has a broad spectrum of activity, including *Candida* spp., *Malassezia furfur*, *C. neoformans*, *Trichosporon* spp., *Aspergillus* spp., *S. schenckii*, and *T. marneffei*. It achieves high concentrations in fatty tissues, skin, hair, and nails. It can also be used for infections caused by fluconazole-resistant *Candida* spp. in combination with fluconazole. It is given orally to treat dermatophyte infections, including onychomycosis [4, 6]. The adverse effects are rare, including gastrointestinal disturbances, headaches, skin reactions, and loss of sense of taste [7].

Griseofulvin

Griseofulvin inhibit cell growth by disrupting microtubule assembly and inhibit mitosis. It is derived from a species of penicillium [4, 7]. It is well absorbed and concentrates in keratin, in the *stratum corneum*, so it is used as a second-line agent in the treatment of infections caused by dermatophytes [4, 7]. The side effects are mild and include nausea, headache, drowsiness, diarrhea, rash, hepatotoxicity, and neurotoxicity [4]. It is administered orally and requires administration for a long period of time because it is deposited in newly forming skin where it binds to keratin, so allowing the replacement of infected keratin by the new, healthy one, takes a long time [6, 8].

Investigational Antifungal Agents

There are several agents in various stages of clinical evaluation. This group includes a liposomal formulation of nystatin, a novel triazole agent, such as albaconazole and ravuconazole, echinocandin aminocandin, non-echinocandin glucan synthase inhibitor ML-3118, an inhibitor of chitin synthesis nikkomycin Z, that could be used in combination with other inhibitors of cell wall or cell membrane synthesis, and sordarin and azasordarin derivatives, which inhibit elongation factor 3 [4]. The newer agents in each class have a more efficient pharmacokinetic and pharmacodynamic characteristics, decreased toxicity or drug-to-drug interactions, or improved activity against refractory pathogens [4].

Topical Antifungal Agents

A variety of topical antifungal agents are available for the treatment of superficial cutaneous and mucosal fungal infections. Most classes of antifungal agents are available for topical use [4]. For example, in a group of polyenes, topical preparations have amphotericin B, nystatin, and pimaricin, and in a group of allylamines, naftifine and terbinafine. Nystatin is used for the treatment of oral, cutaneous, and mucosal candidiasis and subclinical esophageal candidiasis [4]. Ketoconazole is used primarily as topical therapy for mucocutaneous candidiasis, lymphocutaneous sporotrichosis, and dermatophyte infections. Fluconazole is used for mucocutaneous candidiasis. Itraconazole has activity against mucocutaneous forms of candidiasis. Itraconazole is the treatment of choice for lymphocutaneous sporotrichosis, dermatophytoses, and mucocutaneous candidiasis. It accumulates in keratinized tissue, so it is used for treatment of onychomycosis [4]. Econazole, butoconazole, tioconazole, and terconazole are also available for topical use. Echinocandins micafungin and anidulafungin show activity against mucosal candidiasis in clinical studies. Allylamine naftifine is used as a cream for topical use. Undecylenic acid is available for the treatment of tinea pedis and tinea cruris. Haloprogin and ciclopirox are commonly used in dermatophyte infection [7]. Cutaneous infections and onychomycosis are treated with creams, lotions, ointments, powders, and sprays, and mucosal infections are treated with suspensions, tablets, troches, or suppositories [4]. The choice of topical or systemic therapy depends on the status of the host and the type and extent of infection. For example, most cutaneous dermatophytic infections and oral or vaginal candidiasis will respond to topical therapy, and refractory onychomycoses require systemic therapy.

Combinations of Antifungal Agents

Fungi have become important causes of infections and causes of death. Therefore, the need to discover new drugs and a combination of existing ones reappears. The aim of combination therapy is the treatment of the more difficult-to-treat and refractory mycoses, resulting in a better clinical outcome. The aim of combination therapy is to achieve a more effective synergistic effect and to avoid an antagonistic effect. In antifungal therapy, it is important to consider several mechanisms [4]. Firstly, different stages of the same biochemical pathway can be inhibited. For example, terbinafine and azole both attack the sterol pathway, resulting in inhibition of ergosterol synthesis and disruption of the cell membrane. Secondly, increased penetration of one agent is enabled by another agent. The example is combination of cell membrane disruptor amphotericin B and inhibitor of nucleic acid synthesis flucytosine. Thirdly, inhibition of the transport of one agent out of the cell by another agent. Reserpine inhibits efflux pumps and enhances the activity of the azole. Lastly, simultaneous inhibition of different fungal cell targets can be achieved. An example of this type of combination is inhibition of cell wall synthesis by caspofungin with disruption of cell membrane function by amphotericin B. However, there is always a possibility of antagonism, and it can occur via different mechanisms [4]. The first one is a decrease in the target of one drug due to another. An example is the combination of azole, which depletes the cell membrane of ergosterol, with amphotericin B, whose primary target is ergosterol. The second one refers to the activity of one agent resulting in the modification of the target of another agent. The inhibition of ergosterol synthesis by azole results in accumulation of methylated sterols, to which amphotericin B binds less well. The third mechanism is blocking of the target site of one agent by another. An example is itraconazole, which may be adsorbed to the cell surface and inhibit the binding of amphotericin B to membrane sterols. Despite the above arguments, there are only a few data which has shown the advantages of combination therapy in regard to monotherapy. The strongest data exist for the treatment of cryptococcal meningitis with amphotericin B and flucytosine. Flucytosine with fluconazole or amphotericin B with triazoles is also used for treatment of cryptococcosis. Candidemia is treated with combination of amphotericin B and fluconazole. Refractory oropharyngeal candidiasis may be treated with terbinafine and an azole. Combination therapy for candidiasis is used in meningitis, endocarditis, hepatosplenic infection, and candidiasis recurrent or refractory to monotherapy. Invasive aspergillosis can be treated with combination of voriconazole and anidulafungin. Amphotericin B and rifampin have also been shown to be effective against invasive aspergillosis [4]. However, combination therapy should be used very carefully until more clinical data are available.

Mechanisms of Resistance

Most knowledge about fungal resistance is based on the study of *Candida* spp., which is the most common cause of invasive mycoses. Antifungal resistance genes are not transmissible from cell to cell, like many bacterial resistance genes. The most important mechanism of resistance are multidrug efflux pumps, target alterations, and reduced access to antifungal agents. The resistance usually develops slowly and involves the emergence of intrinsically resistant species or a gradually achieved resistance because of prior exposure [4].

Resistance to polyenes, amphotericin B in particular, is rare. Decreased susceptibility has been reported in *C. lusitaniae*, *C. glabrata*, *C. krusei*, and *C. guilliermondi*. The resistance is usually the result of exposure and primary resistance is less common. The mechanism of resistance is the result of qualitative and quantitative alterations in the fungal cells. Resistant strains have a reduced ergosterol content, and polyene-binding sterols are replaced by less well-binding sterols or masking of ergosterol [4].

Azoles are often used, particularly fluconazole, but resistance appears rarely. *C. krusei* is considered intrisically resistant to fluconazole, and other *Candida* spp. develop resistance very rarely. A cross-reaction resistance between triazoles and fluconazole is also observed. The resistance to fluconazole in isolates of *C. neoformans* is also noted in immunosuppressed patients and individuals with relapsing cryptococcal meningitis. Increased resistance among *Aspergillus* spp. is noticed, maybe as a result of environmental fungicide use. The resistance of azoles in *Candida* spp. can be the result of a modification in the quantity or quality of the target enzymes, reduced access of the drug to the target, and a combination of these mechanisms. The resistance in *A. fumigatus* is a result of both increased drug efflux and alterations in target enzymes. *C. neoformans* develop resistance by efflux pumps and alteration of the target enzyme [4].

Candida spp. rarely shows reduced susceptibility to the echinocandins, but it increases among patients undergoing long-term treatment. The mechanism of resistance is alteration in one enzyme included in glucan synthesis complex that shows a decreased sensitivity to inhibition. The point mutation affects echinocandin susceptibility but retains susceptibility to polyene and azoles [4].

Primary resistance to flucytosine is uncommon. Secondary resistance occurs when it is used as a monotherapy for *Candida* spp. and *C. neoformans* infections. The resistance develops because of decreased uptake of the drug or by loss of enzymatic activity in the pyrimidine pathway [4].

There is a possibility that allylamine terbinafine could be a substrate for efflux pump, but resistance is not shown.

In vitro susceptibility testing is used to determine the activity of antifungal agents. It will provide a reliable estimate of the activity of the antifungal agents, correlate with in vivo activity and predict the outcome, provide a means with which to monitor the development of resistance among a normally susceptible population of organism, and predict the therapeutic potential of novel agents. Although effective agents are used, clinical ineffectiveness may occur. It happens because of complex interaction of the host, drug, and fungal pathogen. The important factors are immune status of the host, site and severity of the infection, presence of a foreign body, such as catheter or vascular graft, activity of the drug, dose and duration, and patient compliance. Also, factors such as age, pre-existing diseases, and socioeconomic status have an impact on the outcome of the treatment [4].

Antiparasitic Agents

Parasites are responsible for a large number of infections in humans. Treatment of these infections is complicated by the fact that parasites are eukaryotic organisms and therefore resemble the human host regarding cell structure and metabolism.

This is the reason why antiparasitic therapy is rather limited, complex and has numerous adverse effects. Furthermore, parasitic diversity, complex life cycles, frequent presence of multiple infections and reinfections all pose a major challenge in management of parasitic infections. Along with antibacterial and antifungal agents, developing safe and efficient antiparasitic drugs must also be based on biochemical differences between the parasite and host to achieve selective toxicity. Although the number of effective antiparasitic agents is rather small, there are some effective antiparasitic agents currently on the market. Generally, they are divided into two large groups: (1) antiprotozoal and (2) antihelminthic agents.

Mechanism of Action

The first large class of drugs are antiprotozoal agents. They are designed to target unicellular organisms which are fast-growing and proliferate rapidly. Most commonly, these agents target nucleic acid synthesis, protein synthesis, or specific metabolic pathways unique to the protozoan parasites. Antihelminthic drugs are targeted at nonproliferating adult organisms with complex life cycles. They have three major target sites: neuromuscular coordination of the parasite within the host, carbohydrate metabolism and microtubular integrity. Most antihelminthic agents act by interfering with one of these biochemical functions of the adult organism [3].

Protozoan infections are especially prevalent in countries of tropical and subtropical areas, where they cause significant morbidity and mortality. Indeed, one of the most common tropical diseases, malaria, is responsible for 350–500 million infections worldwide and approximately one million deaths annually, according to European Centre for Disease Prevention and Control (ECDC) [9]. The disease burden is heaviest in the African region, but the infection can occur worldwide, particularly among travelers. With malaria being a major public health issue affecting millions of people every year, agents used to treat malaria will be discussed in greater detail. In endemic areas such as tropical Africa, the incidence of malaria is higher in children younger than 5 years, due to low acquired immunity.

Antiprotozoal Agents Used to Treat Malaria

There are five medically relevant *Plasmodium* parasites known to cause malaria in humans: *P. vivax*, *P. malariae*, *P. ovale* and *P. knowlesi* account for most cases of uncomplicated disease, while *P. falciparum* is considered the greatest threat because of its high virulence and emerging drug resistance [10, 11].

Medications for malaria prophylaxis and treatment can be divided into several classes: quinoline derivatives, artemisinin derivatives, antifolates and atovaquone-proguanil. The drug of choice to treat malaria is dependent on the *Plasmodium* species, the geographic region of the infecting species, and the severity of the patient's infection.

The most significant quinolone derivatives are chloroquine, quinine, primaquine and mefloquine.

Quinolone Derivatives

The most widely targeted parasitic organelle is food vacuole, the site where host hemoglobin degradation occurs. In the vacuole, parasites convert the host hemoglobin to haem, which is toxic, then polymerize haem into crystalline hemozoin, which is harmless to the parasite. Quinolone derivates act as inhibitors of haem polymerization. This leads to free heme accumulation in erythrocytes, a process that is lethal for parasites [12].

Chloroquine is widely used in treatment of "being" malaria due to susceptible strains of *P. vivax*, *P. ovale* or *P. malariae* and as chemoprophylaxis in areas where *P. falciparum* resistance to chloroquine remains low [5].

Chloroquine can be taken orally or administered parenterally and is usually well tolerated. The drug is rapidly and extensively absorbed from the gastrointestinal tract, then distributed and deposited in the tissues. Chloroquine is 60% bound to nondiffusible plasma constituents and equally metabolized by the kidney and liver [13]. Most common adverse effects are gastrointestinal disorders, visual disturbances and vertigo; even convulsions and transient psychiatric disorders were noted [3].

Drug Interactions Antacids can reduce absorption of chloroquine; an interval of at least 4 h between intake of these agents and chloroquine should be observed. On the other hand, cimetidine can inhibit the metabolism of chloroquine, increasing its plasma level. Concomitant use of cimetidine should therefore be avoided. Chloroquine may enhance the effects of a hypoglycemic treatment, so decrease in doses of insulin or other antidiabetic drugs may be required. Concomitant use of chloroquine with arrhythmogenic drugs and antibacterial moxifloxacin should be avoided because it can increase the risk of ventricular arrhythmias. Another drug to be avoided when used together with chloroquine is mefloquine because of a higher probability of inducing convulsions. Finally, chloroquine increases serum cyclosporine concentration and poses a risk of intoxication [5].

Quinine is another traditional antimalarial agent active against resistant *P. falciparum*. Unfortunately, decrease in the dose responsiveness of *P. falciparum* infections were recorded in regions of Southeast Asia, South America and Africa [14–16].

Furthermore, it has numerous adverse effects such as nausea, vomiting and epigastric distress. Also, quinines should only be administered intravenously when the patient's heart activity is being monitored because of a high risk of cardiac arrhythmias [3].

In other words, whenever it is possible, safer and less toxic agents are prefferred.

Quinine has short mean elimination half-life of 8–12 h. Hepatic biotransformation to hydroxylated metabolites is the primary clearance mechanism for quinine [17].

Drug Interactions Acetazolamide and sodium hydrogen carbonate can increase plasma level of quinine. Concomitant use of quinine with digoxin or mefloquine may increase the risk of cardiotoxicity and should be avoided. On the contrary, quinine decreases anticoagulant activity of heparin so the dose might need to be adjusted [5].

Since its introduction in 1940s, **primaquine** is the only antimalarial drug available to clinicians for the treatment of relapsing forms of malaria. It undergoes unique hepatic biotransformation into toxic oxidative by-products that damage plasmodium mitochondria which leads to parasite death. This specific clearance mechanism makes it suitable for treatment of dormant liver-stage *P. vivax* and *P. ovale* infections, thus preventing recurring parasitaemias. Before starting treatment with primaquine, screening for glucose-6-phosphate dehydrogenase (G6PD)-deficiency must occur because primaquine can cause methemoglobinemia and hemolytic anemia in G6PD-deficient individuals. Primaquine use is also associated with minor gastrointestinal disturbances, such as stomach pain and diarrhea, which are usually dose-dependent and can be minimized when the drug is taken with food. Following gut absorption, primaquine is extensively distributed in tissues without accumulating in erythrocytes. It has a short half-life of approximately 6 h and is quickly metabolized by the liver [3, 5, 12, 18].

Mefloquine is used for treatment and chemoprophylaxis of chloroquine-resistant malaria. Although still effective in most areas, mefloquine-resistant *P. falciparum* strains have appeared in Southeast Asia. Due to possible severe neuropsychiatric adverse events, it is supposed to be used only in cases where there is absence of more appropriate drug. If psychiatric symptoms do occur during treatment, mefloquine therapy should be immediately discontinued. Other side effects include nausea, diarrhea, dizziness, insomnia, and visual and cardiac issues [5].

Mefloquine is available only for oral administration. The absorption is relatively rapid, and apparent volume of distribution is large. The elimination is slow and it takes place in the liver [19].

Drug Interactions Concomitant administration of mefloquine and other related drugs (e.g., quinine, quinidine and chloroquine) may produce electrocardiographic abnormalities and increase the risk of convulsions. If these drugs are to be used in the initial treatment of severe malaria, mefloquine administration should be delayed at least 12 h after the last dose.

In patients taking anticonvulsive therapy, the concomitant use of mefloquine may impair seizure control by lowering the plasma levels of the anticonvulsant. Therefore, these patients should have the blood level of their anti-seizure medication monitored and the dosage adjusted appropriately [5].

Artemisinin Derivatives

Artemisinin is an antimalarial agent naturally produced from Artemisia annua; artesunate and artemether are semisynthetic agents derived from artemisinin. Artemisinin and its derivatives are nowadays the basis of modern malaria therapy worldwide. They are the most potent antimalarials currently available due to various advantages: rapid parasitemia eradication, less toxicity and simple application. They are active against multidrug-resistant falciparum malaria [5].

There are formulations for oral, intravenous, intramuscular and rectal use.

The mechanism of action of these compounds appears to involve the heme-mediated decomposition of the endoperoxide bridge to produce carbon-centered free radicals that damage the parasitic organelles and alkylate parasitic proteins [20].

A major disadvantage of artemisinin-based medications is extremely short half-life of less than 60 min, making them unsuitable for prophylactic or even monotherapeutic use. To overcome this, artemisinins are frequently combined with one of several longer-acting drugs—mefloquine, sulfadoxine/pyrimethamine or lumefantrine—which permit clearance of the residual plasmodium parasites [21]. There are several artemisinin-based combination therapies (ACT) formulations for the treatment of uncomplicated falciparum malaria worldwide [22].

The clinical pharmacology of artemisinin-based combination therapies is highly complex. The short-acting artemisinins and their long-acting counterparts are metabolized and/or inhibit/induce cytochrome P450 enzymes and may thus participate in drug-drug interactions with multiple drugs on the market. Alterations in antimalarial drug plasma concentrations may lead to either suboptimal efficacy or drug toxicity and may compromise treatment [21].

Folic Acid Antagonists

Protozoa are incapable of utilizing exogenous folate and thus are affected by folic acid antagonists the same way as some other microorganisms. The most common antifolate medication used for malaria treatment is the pyrimethamine/sulfadoxin combination. These two compounds act synergistically by inhibiting two consecutive steps in the folic acid pathway. Several serious adverse effects of these drugs are severe allergic reactions, bone marrow suppression, megaloblastic anemia, thrombocytopenia, and many more.

Pyrimethamine and sulfadoxine are considered for treatment and/or prophylaxis only in cases when other antimalarial drugs are unavailable or contraindicated [5].

Atovaquone-proguanil is another fixed combination of synergistic components; atovaquone interferes with cytochrome electron transport system and proguanil inhibits dihydrofolate reductase [10]. It is used for prevention and treatment of uncomplicated cases of resistant falciparum malaria. It is well tolerated and has mild adverse reactions that include rash, nausea and rarely diarrhea [5]. Atovaquone is highly lipophilic and should be taken with fatty food for improved absorption. The primary clearance mechanism occurs in the liver. Proguanil is rapidly and extensively absorbed regardless of food intake. The main route of elimination of proguanil is via renal excretion [23].

Drug Interactions The concomitant use of atovaquone/proguanil with rifamycins or tetracyclin is not recommended because these antibiotics may reduce atovaquone concentration. Proguanil may potentiate the anticoagulant effect of warfarin and other coumarin-based anticoagulants. Before and during proguanil therapy in patients who use these blood thinners, coagulation tests regularly obtained.

Metoclopramide may reduce the bioavailability of atovaquone and it is an option only if other antiemetics are not available.

Other Antiprotozoal Agents

Diloxanide furoate is a luminal amebicidal drug active against cysts of *Entamoeba histolytica* [24]. Mechanism of action is not completely familiar. Diloxanide furoate can be used alone in asyptomatic carriers or in those (patients) who experience non-invasive amoebic colitis. In cases of extraintestinal amebiasis, it should only be used alongside or following exposure to a systemically active agent such as nitroimidazoles (e.g. metronidazole) [24, 25].

It is available for oral administration in tablet form. Its excellent luminal activity arises from its unique metabolism. Diloxanide furoate is a prodrug that is hydrolyzed in the bowel into diloxanide and the ester furoic acid [24]. Parent compound diloxanide is rapidly absorbed and undergoes extensive glucuronidation until it is finally excreted in the urine. Unabsorbed furoic acid obtains high amebicidal intraluminal concentrations for a long period of time before being excreted in the feces [26]. Flatulence is a commonly reported adverse effect, while nausea, vomiting, diarrhea, urticaria and pruritus occur occasionally. There is no record of interactions between diloxanide furoate and either metronidazole or tinidazole [25].

Iodoquinol is another amoebicide that can eradicate cysts and trophozoites of *E. histolytica* in the intestine. Due to its poor gastrointestinal absorption following oral administration, iodoquinol should not be used alone for invasive amebiasis.

Most of the drug is excreted in the feces. It shows activity against *Balantidium coli*, *Dientamoeba fragilis* and *Giardia lamblia* [3].

Iodoquinol is contraindicated in patients with known allergy to either hydroxyquinoline or iodine. Side effects of iodoquinol may include gastrointestinal sensations and, rarely, serious ophthalmological abnormalities including optic atrophy and optic neuritis. Mild to moderate skin reactions may also occur [27]. Clinicians should be aware that this medication may interfere with certain thyroid function tests up to 6 months after discontinuation of therapy [27].

Antimonials. Pentavalent antimonials are antiprotozoal agents that are in use for decades in treatment of leishmaniasis. These agents act by inhibiting enzymes that are essential catalysts in carbohydrate metabolism and consequently block parasitic energy production [3].

There are two important antimonial agents nowadays: meglumine antimoniate and sodium stibogluconate. Their exclusive use is treatment of leishmaniasis, and they successfully treat all forms of disease (cutaneous, mucocutaneous and visceral) [3, 4].

Antimonials are usually administered via intravenous or intramuscular route but can also be administered by intralesional injections to treat localized cutaneous leishmaniasis [28]. Antimonials are extremely toxic to the host, so during therapy, the patient must be closely observed. Toxicity is greatest on cells that are most metabolically active, such as neuronal, renal tubular, intestinal, and bone marrow stem cells. Adverse effects depend on which specific tissue is particularly affected [4]. Pentavalent antimonials are rapidly eliminated via urine.

The antimonials are contraindicated in patients suffering from pneumonia, myocarditis, hepatitis and nephritis as well as in pregnant and breast-feeding women [29]. Concomitant use with drugs which may impair renal function or prolong the QT interval should be carefully evaluated.

Melarsoprol is trivalent arsenical indicated in treatment of late-stage African trypanosomiasis. It is known to disrupt parasitic energy generation by interacting with thiol groups of several crucial enzymes [3]. Although it is effective in all stages of trypanosomiasis, melarsoprol is reserved for cases with central nervous system involvement (stage 2 disease). Occassionally, it can be prescribed for the early or hemolymphatic stage of trypanosomiasis in patients who are refractory to standard therapy with suramin and pentamidine [24, 26].

Melarsoprol is extremely toxic. It has to be given intravenously, and even then, it can cause severe reactions at the injection site such as phlebitis, vein sclerosis, and local necrosis [30]. Nevertheless, the most dangerous complication of melarsoprol therapy is encephalopathic syndrome, which is often times lethal. High-dose systemic corticosteroids and adequate supportive therapy must be initiated if CNS complications are suspected [31].

Melarsoprol is quickly transformed into active metabolites in plasma, having a half-life of under 30 min. The key active metabolite is melarsen oxide, and it is predominantly (80%) excreted through the GI tract. There are no listed interactions of melarsoprol with other drugs [26].

Pentamidine, an aromatic diamidine, demonstrates both antitrypanosomal and antileishmanial activity [32]. It is used in treating the first stage of trypanosomiasis and as a second therapy choice for cutaneous leishmaniasis. Another possible use is treatment or prophylaxis of fungal infection with *Pneumocystis jirovecii* [33]. Pentamidine's mode of action is poorly understood, but it has been proven to interfere with nuclear metabolism producing inhibition of DNA, RNA and protein synthesis, or of topoisomerase activity [34]. Pentamidine metabolism is mainly hepatic, with small amount of drug secreted in the urine slowly for several weeks [34]. It is commercialized as pentamidine isethionate salt and used in form of parenteral therapy or aerosol prophylaxis of *P. jirovecii* infection [33, 34]. Parenteral administration poses a great risk of side effects. These include hypoglycemia, hyperglycemia, pain at the injection site, hypotension, gastrointestinal tract disturbances, reversible nephrotoxicity, elevated serum transaminase levels, electrolyte disturbances, and bone marrow toxicities. Bronchospasm is common when the drug is given by nebulizer. The use of pentamidine with didanosine, foscarnet, erythromycin, or any nephrotoxic drugs should be strictly avoided because potentially *toxic* effects may be *potentiated* [33]. Certain pentamidine prodrugs were synthesised that might have improved oral bioavailability and CNS penetration than pentamidine itself. This could expand clinical use of pentamide, but further research is required [35].

Antiviral Agents

Mechanism of Action

Viruses are obligate intracellular parasites, and because of that, there are few limitations in achieving effective targets. Firstly, antiviral agents must be capable of selectively inhibiting viral functions without damaging the host cell. Secondly, usually, the virus has spread through the body before symptoms occur, resulting in drug ineffectiveness. Thirdly, there are many viruses for which vaccines are not available or not highly effective, and therefore infections cannot be prevented. Lastly, there are increasing numbers of immunosuppressed patients who are at increased risk for infection and virus infection causes significant economic loss because of high morbidity [36]. There are three mechanisms of antiviral agent action: the first one is that they inactivate intact virus, i.e., they are viricidal. This group includes ether, detergents and ultraviolet light, but they are not used for treating patients. In second group, there are antiviral drugs that inhibit viral replication. Steps in viral replication are desired target sites of drug action, such as attachment to host cell receptors, uncoating, genome transcription and replication, maturation, and virion assembly and release, but usually it is difficult to create an agent which will have a virus as a highly specific target and accordingly distinguish viral from host replicative processes. Most of the available drugs were created using these mechanisms. In the third group, there are drugs that do not act directly on the virus but modify host responses, i.e., they enhance host-immune responses and therefore are called immunomodulators [4, 37]. All available antiviral agents are virustatic, so they are active only against replicating viruses. In general, antiviral agents can be divided depending on the site of action in the viral life cycle or the virus against which they are effective. There are six antiviral drugs based on the virus, that is, disease they treat: antiviral drugs for herpesviruses, papillomavirus, influenza viruses, human immunodeficiency virus (HIV), hepatitis B virus (HBV), and hepatitis C virus (HCV) [1]. There are several groups of drugs available to treat herpesvirus infection. In the group of nucleoside analogs, acyclovir, valacyclovir, penciclovir, famciclovir, ganciclovir, and valganciclovir are commonly used. They inhibit nucleic acid replication by inhibiting polymerases essential for nucleic acid replication [36]. Ribavirin and other nucleoside analogs are also used, such as iodoxuridine, trifluorothymidine, and fluorouracil. In the group of nucleotide analogs, cidofovir is used. For papillomaviruses, fluorouracil is used as a topical agent, nucleotide analog cidofovir, and immunomodulators IFN-α and imiquimod. Immunomodulators play an indirect role in preventing infection, acting on the host's immune response. IFN-α stimulates the immune response of the host cell and promotes the resolution of viral infection, and imiquimod stimulates innate responses to attack the virus infection [4]. Influenza A virus can be treated with amantadin, rimantadin, zanamivir, and oseltamivir, and influenza B virus can be treated with zanamivir and oseltamivir. Amantadin and rimantadin participate in conformational change in the hemagglutinin that promotes fusion of the viral envelope with cell membranes [4]. There are several groups of drugs for HIV infections. In the group of nucleoside analogs, azidothymidine is used. Examples of nucleoside reverse transcriptase inhibitors or NRTIs are zidovudine, lamivudine, abacavir, and stavudine. They are competitive inhibitors of HIV-1 reverse transcriptase. They are incorporated into the growing viral DNA chain, which causes premature chain termination due to inhibition of binding with the incoming nucleotide [4]. Nucleotide analog reverse transcriptase inhibitors (NtRTI) include adefovir and tenofovir. The group of nonnucleoside reverse transcriptase inhibitors or nonnucleoside polymerase inhibitors (NNRTIs) are nevirapine, delavirdine, etravirdine, and efavirenz. They bind directly to HIV-1 reverse transcriptase, which results in allosteric inhibition of RNA- and DNA-dependent DNA polymerase activity [4]. Protease inhibitors are the most numerous group and include agents such as fosamprenavir, saquinavir, indinavir, ritonavir, nelfinavir, amprenavir, and darunavir. As the name said, they inhibit HIV protease [4]. There are also a group of entry inhibitors, which include fusion inhibitor enfurvirtide and CCR5 inhibitor maraviroc, and lastly, a group of integrase strand transfer inhibitor, which include integrase inhibitor raltegravir. For the hepatitis B viruses (HBV), NRTIs such as lamivudine are used, but also the agents from the group of NtRTIs, such as adefovir and tenofovir. HBV infections can be treated with guanosine nucleoside analog entecavir or thymidine nucleoside analog telbivudine. For the infections caused by the hepatitis C virus, ribavirin, and pegylated IFN-α may be used (see also Chap. 30). In this chapter, the drugs will be divided based on the mechanism by which they act.

Pharmacokinetics

Antiviral drugs can be administered orally or intravenously; they have different bioavailability and other pharmacokinetics characteristics based on the group of drugs to which they belong. They achieve different levels of concentration in tissue and body fluids. Most of them are metabolized in liver, and excreted in the urine or feces. Nucleoside analog acyclovir has low oral bioavailability (15–20%) and is unaffected by food intake. It can also be administered intravenously. Topical formulations produce high concentrations in herpetic lesions, but systemic concentrations are very low. It is excreted primarily by kidney, by glomerular filtration and tubular secretion. It is administered to all tissues and body fluids. The concentration in cerebrospinal liquid is 20–50% of serum values [4]. Valaciclovir is rapidly converted to acyclovir after oral administration via liver and intestine, which results in three to five times greater serum levels than those achieved with oral acyclovir. Cerebrospinal fluid levels are about 50% of those in serum [38]. Famciclovir is rapidly deacetylated after oral administration and oxidized by first-pass metabolism to penciclovir. The bioavailability of penciclovir from orally administered famciclovir is 70%, and it is excreted primarily in the urine [38]. Ganciclovir may be administered orally, intravenously or via intraocular implant. The bioavailability when administered orally is poor. Cerebrospinal fluid concentrations are approximately 50% of serum concentrations. It is excreted by kidneys and is linearly related to creatinine clearance. Valganciclovir is well absorbed orally and rapidly metabolized in the intestinal wall and liver to ganciclovir. The bioavailability of oral valganciclovir is 60%, and it is recommended that the drug be taken with food. It is excreted by kidneys [38]. Nonnucleoside polymerase inhibitor foscarnet is administered intravenously; it has poor oral bioavailability and is excreted by kidneys. Cerebrospinal fluid concentrations are 43–67% of serum concentrations. The dosage of foscarnet must be titrated according to the calculated creatinine clearance before each infusion [38]. Nucleotide analog cidofovir has poor cerebrospinal fluid penetration and is excreted by kidneys. Intravenously administered cidofovir must be applied with high-dose probenecid, which blocks active tubular secretion and decreases nephrotoxicity [38].

Drug Resistance

The resistance of the drugs developed in a few ways. It is the result of a point mutation within the viral genome [37]. In a group of nucleoside analogs, drug resistance occurs rapidly, therefore, there is a need for combination therapy. It is usually result of a mutation of the polymerase [36]. For example, resistance to acyclovir can be manifested in two ways: by mutation of the thymidine kinase and DNA polymerase [4]. Agents such as foscarnet, cidofovir, and trifluridine do not require activation by viral thymidine kinase and thus have activity against the most acyclovir-resistant strains [38]. On the other side, penciclovir resistance occurred mainly in immunocompromised patients, and a cross-reaction with acyclovir resistance was observed

[37]. In a group of protease inhibitors, drug resistance is a result of mutation of the protease, and it occurs frequently [38]. Anti-influenza drugs, amantadine and rimantadine, develop resistance quickly, and it is the result of an altered hemagglutinin or M2 protein [4]. Mutations in the neuraminidase are a cause of resistance in zanamivir and oseltamivir, but, it is rare [4, 37, 38]. In conclusion, drug resistance in antiviral agents is the result of a change in a protein crucial for drug action.

Adverse Effects and Toxicity

There are several adverse effects and toxicity in the application of antiviral therapy, which range from mild flu-like symptoms to life-threatening conditions. Nevertheless, the benefits of accurate application of antiviral drugs are undeniable. In the group of nucleoside analogs, acyclovir can cause headache, nausea, and diarrhea, and intravenous administration can cause reversible renal toxicity or neurologic disturbances. The adverse effects of valaciclovir are rare and include nausea, vomiting, headache, rash, confusion, hallucinations, and seizures at higher doses. Individuals with AIDS may have gastrointestinal intolerance as well as thrombotic thrombocytopenic purpura and hemolytic-uremic syndrome. High doses in transplant patients may experience confusion and hallucinations [38]. Ganciclovir has mild and severe adverse effects. The mild adverse effects include headache, nausea, diarrhea, fever, rash, insomnia, and peripheral neuropathy. Severe adverse effects include myelosuppression, predominantly neutropenia and thrombocytopenia, and rarely hepatotoxicity. It is mutagenic in mammalian cells [38]. Oral famciclovir is well tolerated and adverse effects include headache, nausea and vomiting. Another nucleoside analog, azydothimidine can cause nausea and myelosupression. Side effects of nucleoside analog reverse transcriptase inhibitors are severe and include lactic acidosis, steatosis, and lipoatrophy [37]. For example, zidovudine can also cause granulocytopenia or anemia, and side effects of stavudine and didanosine include peripheral neuropathy and pancreatitis. Abacavir can cause hypersensitivity in HLA-susceptible individuals. Nucleotide analog reverse transcriptase inhibitors, like tenofovir, can cause renal tubular dysfunction and bone demineralisation [37, 38]. The adverse effects of nonnucleoside polymerase inhibitor, for example, foscarnet, are headache, nausea, vomiting, fatigue, anemia, seizures, and elevation of liver enzymes. The risk of anemia is higher in individuals receiving concurrent zidovudine, and seizures may be increased with concurrent use of imipenem. It has ability to chelate divalent metal ions and they can be incorporated into bone [4, 38]. Because of that, there is a risk of severe hypocalcemia, which is increased with concomitant use of pentamidine. It can also cause nephrotoxicity and electrolyte imbalances. Saline preloading is useful in preventing nephrotoxicity, as does avoidance of concomitant administration of drugs with nephrotoxic potential (e.g., amphotericin B, pentamidine, and aminoglycosides). Other nonnucleoside polymerase inhibitors include nevirapine, delavirdine, etravirine, and efavirenz have serious, potentially life-threatening side effects, including nevirapine rash, hepatitis, and Stevens-Johnson syndrome, for etravirine Stevens-Johnson syndrome, toxic epidermal necrolysis, erythema multiforme, and organ dysfunction, and for efavirenz mood changes, and vivid dreams [37, 38]. Nucleotide inhibitor cidofovir intravenously may be nephrotoxic, which may be reduced with prehydration using normal saline. Other nephrotoxic symptoms include proteinuria, azotemia, metabolic acidosis, and Fanconi's syndrome. It can also cause uveitis, oculary hypotony, and neutropenia [37, 38]. All NRTIs may be associated with mitochondrial toxicity because of inhibition of mitochondrial DNA polymerase gamma. Less frequently, lactic acidosis with hepatic steatosis may occur, which can be fatal. The adverse effects also include rapidly rising aminotransferase levels, hepatomegaly, or metabolic acidodosis. The thymidine analogs zidovudine and stavudine can cause dyslipidemia and insulin resistance. Abacavir or didanosine maybe increase the risk of myocardial infarction [37, 38]. The individuals receiving antiretroviral therapy may have adverse side effects like accumulation of body fat that results in central obesity, dorsocervical fat enlargement (buffalo hump), peripheral and facial wasting, breast enlargement, and a cushingoid appearance, and these effects are associated with the use of protease inhibitors [38]. They have also been associated hyperglycemia and insulin resistance, an increase in triglyceride and low-density lipoprotein levels, an increased risk of intracranial hemorrhage, and with increased spontaneous bleeding in individuals with hemophilia A or B [38]. Saquinavir and ritonavir in combination are associated with QT and PR interval prolongation, so this combination is contraindicated. Atazanavir can cause diarrhea, nausea, vomiting, headache, peripheral neuropathy, nephrolithiasis, prolongation of the PR interval, and rash. In 10% of individuals, indirect hyperbilirubinemia with overt jaundice can occur. Elevation of hepatic enzymes usually occur in individuals with underlying HBV or HCV co-infection. In contrast to the other PIs, atazanavir does not appear to be associated with dyslipidemia, fat redistribution, or the metabolic syndrome [38]. The adverse effects of ritonavir, include headache, nausea, vomiting, diarrhea, altered taste, gastrointestinal disturbances, paresthesias, elevated serum aminotransferase levels, and elevations in serum creatine kinase. Saquinavir can cause gastrointestinal discomfort and rhinitis. When administered in combination with low-dose ritonavir, gastrointestinal toxicity and dyslipidemia are reduced. However, there is an increased risk of QT and PR interval prolongation [38]. Anti-influenza drug oseltamivir can cause nausea, vomiting, and abdominal pain. Headache, fatigue, and diarrhea appear to be more common with prophylactic use. Rash is rare. Zanamivir may cause cough, bronchospasm (occasionally severe), reversible decrease in pulmonary function, and transient nasal and throat discomfort. Therefore, it is not recommended for patients with underlying airway disease [37, 38]. The adverse effects of amantadine and rimantadine can be divided into mild and severe. Mild adverse effects include nausea, anorexia, nervousness, difficulty concentrating, and insomnia [4]. Severe adverse effect may be a result of dopamine neurotransmission like marked behavioral changes, delirium, hallucinations, agitation, and seizures. They may increase with concomitant antihistamines, anticholinergic drugs, hydrochlorothiazide, and trimethoprim-sulfamethoxazole. Anticholinergic activity may be present in acute amantadine overdose [38]. Immunomodulator interferon can cause flu-like symptoms [4].

Drug Interactions

Most antivirial agents have common drug-to-drug interactions and therefore must be applied with caution. Concurrent use of nephrotoxic agents with acyclovir may cause nephrotoxicity. Probenecid and cimetidine decrease acyclovir clearance and increase exposure. Somnolence and lethargy may occur in individuals receiving concomitant zidovudine and acyclovir. Myelosuppression may be additive in patients receiving concurrent zidovudine, azathioprine, or mycophenolate mofetil with ganciclovir. Levels of ganciclovir may increase in individuals concurrently taking probenecid or trimethoprim, and concurrent use of ganciclovir with didanosine may result in increased levels of didanosine [38]. NNRT didanosine absorption interferes with indinavir, delavirdine, atazanavir, dapsone, itraconazole, and fluoroquinolone agents. Therefore, administration should be separated in time. Serum levels of didanosine are increased when co-administered with tenofovir or ganciclovir and are decreased by atazanavir, delavirdine, ritonavir, tipranavir, and methadone [38]. Lamivudine has a greater bioavailability when it is co-administered with trimethoprim-sulfamethoxazole. Lamivudine and zalcitabine may inhibit the intracellular phosphorylation of one another, so their concurrent use should be avoided if possible. Concurrent use of atazanavir, lopinavir, or ritonavir may increase serum levels of tenofovir [38]. Nevirapine is a moderate inducer of CYP3A metabolism, resulting in decreased levels of amprenavir, indinavir, lopinavir, saquinavir, efavirenz, and methadone. Drugs that induce the CYP3A system, such as rifampin, rifabutin, and St. John's wort, can decrease levels of nevirapine, whereas those that inhibit CYP3A activity, such as fluconazole, ketoconazole, and clarithromycin, can increase nevirapine levels [38]. Protease inhibitors are extensively metabolized by CYP3A4. Ritonavir has the most pronounced inhibitory effect, and saquinavir the least. Amprenavir an ritonavir are inducers of specific CYP isoforms. As seen, protease inhibitors have many interactions with other antiretroviral agents and other medications [38]. One interesting fact about ritonavir is that it is a potent CYP3A4 inhibitor, so it is used as a pharmacokinetic enhancer when used in combination with other protease inhibitors. Atazanavir is an inhibitor of CYP3A4 and CYP2C9, so drug-to-drug interactions are frequent. When combined with a proton pump inhibitor, it has a reduced bioavailability, so these combinations are to be avoided. Co-administration with other drugs that inhibit UGT1A1, which is a gene important in the synthesis of enzymes in bilirubin metabolism, such as irinotecan, may increase its levels. Tenofovir and efavirenz should not be co-administered with atazanavir unless ritonavir is added to boost levels. It may cause prolongation of the electrocardiographic PR interval, which is usually inconsequential but may be exacerbated by other causative agents such as calcium channel blockers and may result in AV block QT prolongation [38]. Ritonavir is a potent inhibitor of CYP3A4, resulting in many potential drug interactions with antiretroviral agents. Delavirdine increase its serum level, and tenofovir decreases. Ritonavir increases serum levels of atazanavir, lopanivir, ritonavir, nelfinavir, and saquinavir, and it decreases serum levels of darunavir, delavirdine, didanosine, and etravirine [38]. The concurrent use of saquinavir and ritonavir increase the risk of QT prolongation and PR interval prolongation, so it is contraindicated. When combined with other PI agents, lower doses of ritonavir increase blood levels of latter agents, resulting in lower or less frequent dosing of the other agent. Monitoring of digoxin and theophylline is needed when co-administered with ritonavir [38]. Saquinavir is CYP3A4 inhibitor as well as a substrate. When co-administered with nelfinavir and omeprazole, a decreased dose is required. Liver function tests should be monitored when administered with delavirdine or rifampicin [38].

Groups of Antiviral Agents

Nucleoside Analogs

The majority of available antiviral drugs are in this group of antiviral agents. They inhibit viral polymerases essential for nucleic acid replication or can be incorporated into the nucleic acid and block further synthesis [36]. Nucleoside analogs can block both cellular enzymes and virus-encoded enzymes. Therefore, even the more useful are the latter [36]. Drug resistance can occur rapidly, so the use of combinations of antiviral drugs can delay the emergence of resistant variants. Resistance is usually caused by a mutation of the polymerase. Examples are acyclovir, valacyclovir, penciclovir, famciclovir and ganciclovir [36].

Acyclovir

Acyclovir (ACV or acycloguanosine) has an acyclic side chain instead of sugar and in this way differs from the nucleoside guanosine (hence the name). It has selective action against Herpes simplex virus type 1 and 2 (HSV-2 and HSV-2) and Varicella—zoster virus (VZV), the herpesviruses that encode a thymidine kinase [4]. This enzyme is required to activate the drug by phosphorylation. There is no initial phosphorylation in uninfected cells, so there is no inhibition of cellular DNA synthesis or toxicity [38]. Resistance can occur and can be manifested in two ways, by mutation of either the thymidine kinase, so that activation of ACV cannot occur or by DNA polymerase to prevent ACV binding [4]. It can also be used for the treatment of VZV, but higher doses are required [38]. It is administered orally or by intravenous infusion [37].

Valacyclovir

Valacyclovir is a deoxyguanosine analog. It is the valyl ester derivate of ACV and has better efficiency after oral administration and is rapidly converted into ACV [2]. It is concentrated and persists in the infected cells to a greater extent than ACV. It is used for the treatment of HSV and VZV in higher doses, as well as for Epstein–Barr virus (EBV) and cytomegalovirus (CMV). It is administered orally [4, 37].

Penciclovir

Penciclovir is effective against HSV-1, HSV-2 and VZV and has some activity against EBV and CMV [2]. Resistance occurs mainly in immunocompromised patients, and there is a cross resistance with acyclovir resistance [37].

Famciclovir

Famciclovir is a prodrug derivate of penciclovir, with an increased bioavailability. It is well absorbed orally and is converted to penciclovir in the liver or intestinal lining [4]. It is effective against HSV-1, HSV-2 and VZV [37].

Ganciclovir

Ganciclovir (GCV, dihydroxypropoxymethyl guanine) has a single hydroxymethyl group in the acyclic side chain. Because of that, it has a greater activity against CMV [4]. GCV inhibits all herpesvirus DNA polymerases, which have a greater affinity for the drug than the cellular DNA polymerase [4]. It is active against CMV, Human herpes virus type 6 and 7 (HHV-6 and HHV-7), and HSV-1 and HSV-2. It is used in immunocompromised patients and for the prevention of CMV disease after organ transplantation [37]. It may be administered intraocularly to treat CMV retinitis, either by direct intravitreal injection or by intraocular implant [38]. Toxicity includes myelosuppression, predominantly neutropenia and thrombocytopenia. Ganciclovir is administered intravenously [37].

Valgancyclovir

Valgancyclovir is a valyl ester of GCV. It is a prodrug with a higher tissue concentration. It is administered orally [4]. It is well absorbed and rapidly metabolized in the intestinal wall and liver to ganciclovir. It is recommended to be taken with food. It is eliminated by the kidneys [38].

Ribavirin

Ribavirin is an analog of the nucleoside guanosine. Its base ring is incomplete and open, and it must be phosphorylated intracellularly by host cell enzymes. Ribavirin triphosphate inhibits RNA polymerases, mRNA capping, and other processes important to the replication of many viruses [4]. The oral bioavailability is good, it is recommended to use it with meal with fatty acid, and to avoid co-administration of antacids. The protein binding is very low, and cerebrospinal fluid levels are about 70% those in plasma. It is excreted in the urine. The adverse effects include a dose-dependent hemolytic anemia, fatigue, nausea, pruritus, rash, irritability, insomnia, and depression. Contraindications include anemia, end-stage renal failure, ischemic vascular disease, and pregnancy. It is not recommended to conceive for at least 6 months after therapy [38]. It has activity against a broad range of both DNA and RNA viruses. In children, it can be used to treat respiratory syncytial virus (RSV) infection by administering it in aerosol [4]. In adults, it can be useful against influenza A and B, parainfluenza, paramyxoviruses, HIV-1, and HCV infections. It is administered orally or intravenously. The combined therapy of oral ribavirin and IFN-α and protease inhibitors is more effective than monotherapy with either IFN-α or ribavirin alone in treatment of HCV [38].

Azidothymidine

Azidothymidine (Retrovir®) is a nucleoside analog of thymidine and inhibits the reverse transcriptase of HIV. It is first developed as an anticancer drug. Firstly, it must be phosphorylated by host cell enzymes. It can also be given to pregnant women to prevent transmission to the fetus. Side effects include nausea and myelosuppression. There is extensive development of antiviral drug-resistant strains due to the high error rate of the HIV polymerase. It is administered orally [4].

Idoxuridine, trifluorothymidine, and fluorouracil are analogs of thymidine. They are effective in cells in which extensive DNA replication is taking place, such as in case of HSV infection, and they do not act harmfully in non-growing cells. Fluorouracil is also antineoplastic drug, but it can be used for topical treatment of warts caused by human papillomaviruses. Baloxavir marboxil (BXM, Xofuza®) inhibits the subunit of the influenza polymerase [4].

Nucleoside Reverse Transcriptase Inhibitors (NRTIs)

They are analogs of naturally occurring nucleosides, and they are activated by phosphorylation by cellular enzymes to the triphosphate form. They are used for HIV treatment and post-exposure prophylaxis. This group include zidovudine (AZT), didanosine (ddI), zalcitabine (ddC), stavudine (d4T), lamivudine (3TC), abacavir (ABC), and emtricitabine (FTC). Side effects include lactic acidosis, steatosis, and lipoatrophy. AZT can cause granulocytopenia or anemia, and side effects of d4T and ddI include peripheral neuropathy and pancreatitis. HLA testing is indicated prior to treatment with ABC because of hypersensitivity. These drugs are administered orally [38].

Abacavir

Abacavir (ABC) is a guanosine analog that is well absorbed after oral administration and is unaffected by food. Cerebrospinal fluid levels are approximately one third of those of plasma. Abacavir has a fixed-dose combination with lamivudine and with lamivudine and zidovudine. The adverse effects include headache, fever, nausea, vomiting, fatigue, diarrhea, rash, dyspnea, and rarely pancreatitis. Extra caution is required in individuals with existing cardiac risk factors due to a possible increased risk of myocardial events. Also, abacavir may lower methadone levels [38].

Didanosine

Didanosine (ddI) is a synthetic analog of deoxyadenosine. Oral bioavailability is approximately 40%, and fasting administration is optimal. Cerebrospinal fluid concentrations of the drug are approximately 20% of serum concentrations. The drug is eliminated by both cellular metabolism and renal excretion. The toxicity include dose-dependent pancreatitis, peripheral distal sensory neuropathy, hepatitis, esophageal ulceration, cardiomyopathy, central nervous system toxicity, and hypertriglyceridemia [38].

Lamivudine

Lamivudine (3TC) is a cytosine analog. It has activity against HIV that is synergistic with a variety of antiretroviral nucleoside analogs, including zidovudine and stavudine. It also has activity against HBV. Oral bioavailability is 80% and is not food-dependent. There is a fixed-dose combination of lamivudine with abacavir and zidovudine, either alone or in combination with abacavir. The adverse effects are usually mild and include headache, fatigue, dry mouth, gastrointestinal disturbances, dizziness, and insomnia [38].

Nucleotide Analog Reverse Transcriptase Inhibitor (NtRTI)

Nucleotide analog reverse transcriptase inhibitors (NtRTI) are acyclic phosphonate analogs of adenosine monophosphate, so they contain a phosphate attached to the sugar analog. They are activated by phosphorylation by cellular enzymes to the diphosphate form [37]. They are substrates for DNA polymerases or reverse transcriptase, persist longer in cells and have potency against several types of viruses [4]. Examples are cidofovir, adefovir, adefovir dipivoxil and tenofovir.

Cidofovir

Cidofovir is a cytidine analog. The phosphorylation of cidofovir to the active diphosphate is independent of viral enzymes; thus, activity is maintained against thymidine kinase-deficient or -altered strains of CMV or HSV. Cidofovir-resistant strains tend to be cross-resistant with ganciclovir but retain susceptibility to foscarnet [38]. It is effective against CMV infections in patients with AIDS but also against HPV and polyomaviruses, as well as herpesviruses, adenoviruses, and poxvirus [4].

Adefovir

Adefovir is adenosine analog. It is effective against HBV and HIV. It is administered orally [37].

Adefovir Dipivoxil

Adefovir dipivoxil is a diester prodrug and it is effective against HBV [38].

Tenofovir

Tenofovir competitively inhibits HIV reverse transcriptase and causes chain termination after incorporation into DNA, so it is used for treatment of HIV, and it is also approved for the treatment of patients with HBV infection. Tenofovir disoproxil fumarate is a water-soluble prodrug of active tenofovir. It is administered orally and has a better bioavailability after meal with a fatty acid. It is excreted by kidneys. There is a fixed-dose combination with emtricitabine, either alone or in combination with efavirenz. Emtricitabine and tenofovir are used as preexposure prophylaxis in men who have sex with men for reducing HIV acquisition. The adverse effects include headache, nausea, vomiting, diarrhea, tubular dysfunction, Fanconi's syndrome, and bone demineralization. It may compete with other drugs that are actively secreted by the kidneys, such as cidofovir, acyclovir, and ganciclovir. There is a significant placental passage in humans, so the drug must be administered with caution in pregnant woman [38].

Nonnucleoside Reverse Transcriptase Inhibitors (NNRTIs)

The Nonnucleoside Reverse Transcriptase Inhibitors (NNRTIs) bind directly to HIV-1 reverse transcriptase, resulting in allosteric inhibition of RNA- and DNA-dependent DNA polymerase activity. NNRTIs neither compete with nucleoside triphosphates nor require phosphorylation to be active. The resistance may occur rapidly with monotherapy and can result from a single mutation. There is no cross-resistance between the NNRTIs and the NRTI [38]. Indeed, some nucleoside-resistant viruses display hypersusceptibility to NNRTIs. Resistance appears rapidly if used as monotherapy, but they are useful for the treatment of HIV infection in combination with nucleoside analogs because the mechanism of resistance is different [4, 38]. This group of agents include nevirapine, delavirdine, etravirine, and efavirenz [37, 38].

Nevirapine has excellent oral bioavailability and is not food-dependent. It is highly lipophilic and has 45% levels in cerebrospinal fluid of those in plasma. It does not require phosphorylation for activity and binds directly to reverse transcriptase, so it is a non-competitive inhibitor of reverse transcriptase. It is excreted primarily in urine and metabolized extensively by the CYP3A in the liver. It can be used as a prophylaxis for HIV-positive pregnant women at the onset of labor as a single dose and one more to the neonate within 3 days after delivery [38]. The adverse effects of nevirapine include milder side effects, such as headache, nausea, and usually rash, especially in women, but rash can be accompanied by hepatotoxicity, so liver function tests should be assessed. Life-threatening skin rashes, such as Stevens-Johnson syndrome and toxic epidermal necrolysis, are rare side effects of nevirapine [37, 38].

Nonnucleoside Polymerase Inhibitor

Foscarnet (PFA) is an inorganic pyrophosphate analog [37]. It inhibits viral replication by binding to the DNA polymerase, RNA polymerase, and HIV reverse transcriptase and blocks nucleotide binding [4, 38]. It is used for treatment of CMV retinitis in patients with AIDS, for ganciclovir-resistant CMV, and for aciclovir-resistant HSV and VZV [4, 38]. It has ability to chelate divalent metal ions, and they become incorporated into bone [4]. Its side effects also include nephrotoxicity, resulting in hypercalcemia and hypokalemia. It is administered intravenously [37, 38].

Protease Inhibitors

The HIV protease is responsible for cleaving precursor molecules to produce the final structural proteins of the mature virion core [36]. HIV protease is a good target for antiviral drugs because it is essential in production of a functional virion [4]. As a name says, it works by binding to an active site of the enzyme and inhibiting its action. They prevent the processing of viral proteins into functional conformations, and the result is the production of immature, noninfectious viral particles. Protease inhibitors (PIs) do not need intracellular activation [38]. Drug-resistant strains arise through mutation of the protease [4]. The examples of this group include fosamprenavir, saquinavir, indinavir, ritonavir, nelfinavir, amprenavir, lopinavir, atazanavir, tipranavir, and darunavir [37]. They are active against HIV infection. Side effects include lipodystrophy, hyperlipidemia, and diabetes mellitus [37]. Atazanavir can cause jaundice and elevated total bilirubin. It is administered orally. For the treatment of chronic hepatitis C infection, boceprevir, telaprevir, and simprevir [4].

Atazanavir

Atazanavir is an azapeptide that is administered orally, and it should be taken with a light meal to enhance bioavailability. It requires an acidic medium for absorption, so concurrent proton pump inhibitors are contraindicated. It penetrates well in the cerebrospinal and seminal fluids. It is metabolized by bile [38].

Ritonavir

Ritonavir is administered orally and has a good bioavailability that increases with food. It is metabolized by hepatic enzymes, CYP3A and CYP2D6, and excretes primarily in the feces. It is considered safe during pregnancy [38].

Saquinavire

Saquinavire was originally administered as a hard gel capsule (saquinavir-H®; Invirase®), but oral bioavailability with food was poor. However, reformulation of saquinavir-H in combination with low-dose ritonavir has both improved antiviral efficacy and decreased gastrointestinal adverse effects. Saquinavir should be taken within 2 h after a fatty meal for enhanced absorption. It is highly protein bound, has a large volume distribution, but penetrates poorly into the cerebrospinal fluid. It is excreted in the feces [38].

Anti-influenza Drugs

Anti-influenza drugs include amantadine and rimantadine, which are effective against influenza A virus but not against influenza B virus, and zanamivir and oseltamivir, which are effective against both influenza A and influenza B viruses. There is also an investigational agent, peramivir, for both strains of viruses.

Amantadine and rimantadine are tricyclis amines. They are effective against influenza A, but not influenza B virus [38]. They have effect on endosomal vesicles involved in the uptake of the influenza virus. This effect can inhibit the change in conformation in the hemagglutinin, a surface protein that promotes fusion of the viral envelope with cell membranes. The specificity for influenza A is a result of their ability to bind and block the proton channel formed by the M2 membrane protein of the influenza A virus. It inhibits uncoating of the viral RNA within infected host cells and prevents its replication [4]. They can be used as a prophylactic treatment within 48 h of exposure, and when begun within 1–2 days after the onset of illness, the duration is reduced by 1–2 days. The resistance rapidly occurs, it is a result of single-point mutations. Strains are genetically stable, retain pathogenicity, can be transmitted to close contacts, and may be shed chronically by immunocompromised patients. Cross-resistance does not occur [38].

Amantadine

Amantadine is orally well administered, it is 67% protein bound, an excretes unchanged in the urine. Dose reductions are required in the elderly and in individuals with renal insufficiency [38].

Rimantadine

Rimantadine, an amantadine α-methyl derivative, is administered orally, and it is 40% protein bound, nasal secretion and salivary levels approximate those in the serum, and nasal mucus concentrations are 50% higher than those in plasma. It undergoes extensive metabolism before urinary excretion. Dose reductions are required in the elderly, and in individuals with renal and hepatic insufficiency [38].

Zanamivir (Relenza®) and oseltamivir (Tamiflu®) are sialic acid analogues. They are inhibitors of both influenza A virus and influenza B virus. They act as enzyme inhibitors of the neuraminidase. The neuraminidase inhibitors interfere with the release of progeny virus from infected host cells. The newly released virions clump to each other and to the membrane of the infected cell [4]. They are effective against both influenza A and influenza B viruses [37]. Early administration is very important because replication of the influenza virus peaks at 24–72 h after the onset of illness, so it is recommended to use within 48 h of exposure. It decreases the duration of illness by 1–2 days, the severity is diminished, and the incidence of secondary complications decreases. It can also be used as a prophylaxis, and in this case, it is used once-daily after exposure.

Oseltamivir

Oseltamivir is approved by the FDA for patients 1 year and older, and zanamivir for patients 7 years or older. Oseltamivir is administered orally very well, and it is a prodrug that is activated by hepatic esterases. Plasma protein binding is low, and concentrations in the middle ear and sinus fluids are similar to those in plasma. It is excreted by kidneys in the urine. Probenecid reduces renal clearance of oseltamivir by 50% [38].

Zanamivir

Zanamivir is administered by inhalation or intravenously [37]. Ten to twenty percent of the active compound reaches the lungs, and the remainder is deposited in the oropharynx. Resistance to oseltamivir may be associated with point mutations in the viral hemagglutinin or neuraminidas genes. Rates of resistance to oseltamivir among seasonal H1N1 viruses have risen abruptly and dramatically worldwide, reaching 97.4% in tested strains in the United States from 2008 to 2009. Resistance to oseltamivir in pandemic H1N1 viruses and resistance to zanamivir in seasonal and pandemic H1N1 viruses are rare. All influenza A (H3N2) and influenza B viruses were susceptible to both oseltamivir and zanamivir. Swine-origin influenza A (H1N1) viruses are nearly always susceptible to both oseltamivir and zanamivir [38].

Peramivir

Peramivir is an investigational agent. It is the neuraminidase inhibitor, a cyclopentane analog, and has activity against influenza A and influenza B viruses. The adverse effects include nausea, vomiting, diarrhea, and neutropenia [38]. It is administered intravenously [37].

Immunomodulators

Interferons

Interferons are members of the large cytokine family, and they inhibit viral replication. They bind to cell-surface receptors and initiate a cellular antiviral response and immune response. They are first recognized by their ability to interfere with viral infection in cultured cells (which the name implies). They are produced within hours in response to inducers and are one of the first responders in the defense against viral infection [36]. They are extremely potent. RNA viruses are stronger inducers of IFN than DNA viruses. They major role is in innate immunity, but they also modulate humoral and cellular immunity. They belong into one of three groups: IFN-α, IFN-β and IFN-γ. IFN-α and IFN-β are considered type I or viral IFNs, and they are synthesized by many cell types and bind to specific cell surface receptors on target cells. IFN-γ is type II or immune IFN, and it is produced by lymphocytes, especially T cells and natural killer (NK) cells, and it binds to a different receptor. IFN does not protect the virus-infected cell that produces it. It is not an antiviral agent; it moves to other cells and induces the synthesis of proteins that inhibit viral replication [36]. They are usually host-specific in function but are not specific to a virus. IFN-α is used in treatment of condyloma acuminatum and hepatitis C [2]. Pegylated IFN-α, which is developed by attachment of polyethylene glycol to interferon, has a better efficiency. It is used with ribavirin to treat hepatitis C infection. Side effects include flu-like symptoms [38].

Imiquimod

Imiquimod, a Toll-like receptor ligand, stimulates innate responses to attack the virus infection. It can be used for treatment of papillomaviruses [38].

References

1. Goering RV, Mims CA, Dockrell HM, Zuckerman MA, Chiodini PL. Mims' medical microbiology and immunology. 6th ed. Edinburgh: Elsevier; 2019.
2. Carroll KC, Morse SA, Mietzner TA, Miller S. Jawetz, Melnick & Adelberg's medical microbiology. 27th ed. New York: McGraw-Hill Education; 2016.
3. Kalenić S. Medicinska mikrobiologija. Zagreb: Medicinska Naklada; 2013.
4. Murray PR, Rosenthal KS, Pfaller MA. Medical microbiology. 9th ed. Amsterdam: Elsevier; 2021.
5. Francetić I. Farmakoterapijski priručnik. Zagreb: Medicinska naklada; 2015.
6. Johnson E. Antifungal agents. In: Elliot T, Caesy A, Lambert PA, Sandoe J, editors. Medical microbiology and infection. 5th ed. Hoboken: Wiley-Blackwell; 2011. p. 144–6.

7. Mitchell TG. Medical mycology. In: Brooks GF, Caroll KC, Butel JS, Morse SA, Mietzner TA, editors. Jawetz, Melnick & Adalberg's medical microbiology. 26th ed. New York: McGraw Hill; 2012. p. 704–10.
8. Sheppard D, Lampiris HW. Antifungal agents. In: Katzung BG, Masters SB, Trevor AJ, editors. Basic & clinical pharmacology. 12th ed. New York: McGraw Hill; 2012. p. 849–61.
9. European Centre for Disease Prevention and Control. Fact about malaria [Internet]. https://www.ecdc.europa.eu/en/malaria/facts.
10. Campbell S, Soman-Faulkner K. Antiparasitic drugs. In: StatPearls [Internet]. Treasure Island, FL: StatPearls Publishing; 2020. p. 2021.
11. Gething PW, Elyazar IR, Moyes CL, et al. A long-neglected world malaria map: *Plasmodium vivax* endemicity in 2010. PLoS Negl Trop Dis. 2012;6:e1814.
12. Rathore D, McCutchan TF, Sullivan M, Kumar S. Antimalarial drugs: current status and new developments. Expert Opin Investig Drugs. 2005;14(7):871–83.
13. Ducharme J, Farinotti R. Clinical pharmacokinetics and metabolism of chloroquine. Clin Pharmacokinet. 1996;31:257–74.
14. Pukrittayakamee S, Supanaranond W, Looareesuwan S, Vanijanonta S, White NJ. Quinine in severe falciparum malaria: evidence of declining efficacy in Thailand. Trans R Soc Trop Med Hyg. 1994;88(3):324–7.
15. Jelinek T, Schelbert P, Löscher T, Eichenlaub D. Quinine resistant falciparum malaria acquired in East Africa. Trop Med Parasitol. 1995;46(1):38–40.
16. Segurado AA, di Santi SM, Shiroma M. In vivo and in vitro Plasmodium falciparum resistance to chloroquine, amodiaquine and quinine in the Brazilian Amazon. Rev Inst Med Trop Sao Paulo. 1997;39(2):85–90.
17. Krishna S, White NJ. Pharmacokinetics of quinine, chloroquine and amodiaquine. Clin Pharmacokinet. 1996;30(4):263–99.
18. Hill DR, Baird JK, Parise ME, Lewis LS, Ryan ET, Magill AJ. Primaquine: report from CDC expert meeting on malaria chemoprophylaxis I. Am J Trop Med Hyg. 2006;75(3):402–15.
19. Karbwang J, Na-Bangchang K. Clinical application of mefloquine pharmacokinetics in the treatment of P. falciparum malaria. Fundam Clin Pharmacol. 1994;8(6):491–502.
20. Meshnick SR. Artemisinin: mechanisms of action, resistance and toxicity. Int J Parasitol. 2002;32(13):1655–60.
21. Aweeka FT, German PI. Clinical pharmacology of artemisinin-based combination therapies. Clin Pharmacokinet. 2008;47:91–102.
22. WHO. WHO guidelines for the treatment of malaria. 3rd ed. Geneva: World Health Organization; 2015. http://www.who.int/malaria/publications/atoz/9789241549127/en/. Accessed 14 May 2020.
23. McKeage K, Scott L. Atovaquone/proguanil: a review of its use for the prophylaxis of Plasmodium falciparum malaria. Drugs. 2003;63(6):597–623.
24. Kuhlmann FM, Fleckenstein JM. Antiparasitic agents. In: Infectious diseases. 4th ed. Elsevier; 2017. p. 1345–1372.e2.
25. Diloxanide furoate. In: Meyler's side effects of drugs. 16th ed. Elsevier; 2016. p. 980.
26. McCarthy JS, Wortmann GW, Kirchhoff LV. 41—Drugs for protozoal infections other than malaria. In: Bennett JE, Dolin R, Blaser MJ, editors. Mandell, Douglas, and Bennett's principles and practice of infectious diseases. 8th ed; 2015. p. 510–8.e3.
27. Pediatric Oncall. Child health care. Iodoquinol [Internet]. https://www.pediatriconcall.com/drugs/iodoquinol/674.
28. Benjamin Naman C, Gomes CM, Gupta G. Chapter 9—Phytodrugs and immunomodulators for the therapy of Leishmaniasis. In: Mandal SC, Mandal V, Konishi T, editors. Natural products and drug discovery. Elsevier; 2018. p. 213–75.
29. Sharma S, Anand N. Chapter 15—Organometallics. In: Sharma S, Anand N, editors. Pharmacochemistry library, vol. 25. Elsevier; 1997. p. 384–92.
30. Lejon V, Bentivoglio M, Franco JR. Chapter 11—Human African trypanosomiasis. In: Garcia HH, Tanowitz HB, Del Brutto OH, editors. Handbook of clinical neurology, vol. 114. Elsevier; 2013. p. 169–81.

31. Bouteille B, Dumas M. Human African trypanosomiasis. In: Aminoff MJ, Daroff RB, editors. . Encyclopedia of the neurological sciences: Academic; 2003. p. 587–94.
32. Werbovetz K. Diamidines as antitrypanosomal, antileishmanial and antimalarial agents. Curr Opin Investig Drugs. 2006;7(2):147–57.
33. Ryan ET. 296—Antiparasitic agents. In: Long SS, Prober CG, Fischer M, editors. Principles and practice of pediatric infectious diseases. 5th ed. Elsevier; 2018. p. 1567–87.e2.
34. Rex JH, Stevens DA. 39—Drugs active against fungi, pneumocystis, and microsporidia. In: Bennett JE, Dolin R, Blaser MJ, editors. Mandell, Douglas, and Bennett's principles and practice of infectious diseases. 8th ed; 2015. p. 479–94.e4.
35. Kotthaus J, Kotthaus J, Schade D, et al. New prodrugs of the antiprotozoal drug pentamidine. ChemMedChem. 2011;6(12):2233–42.
36. Butel J. Pathogenesis and control of viral diseases. In: Brooks GF, Caroll KC, Butel JS, Morse SA, Mietzner TA, editors. Jawetz, Melnick & Adalberg's medical microbiology. 26th ed. New York: McGraw Hill; 2012. p. 441–9.
37. Nastouli E. Antiviral agents. In: Elliot T, Caesy A, Lambert PA, Sandoe J, editors. Medical microbiology and infection. 5th ed. Hoboken: Wiley-Blackwell; 2011. p. 147–53.
38. Safrin S. Antiviral agents. In: Katzung BG, Masters SB, Trevor AJ, editors. Basic & clinical pharmacology. 12th ed. New York: McGraw Hill; 2012. p. 861–91.

Anti-inflammatory Drugs and the Gastrointestinal Tract

9

Mladen Merćep

Abbreviations

5-ASA	5-aminosalicylic acid
6-TGNs	6-Thioguanine nucleotides
AZA	Azathioprine
BDP	Beclomethasone dipropionate
CD	Crohn's disease
COX-2	Cyclooxygenase 2
DMARDs	Disease-modifying anti-rheumatic drug
GI	Gastrointestinal tract
HGPRT	Hypoxanthine-guanine phosphoribosyltransferase
IBD	Inflammatory bowel disease
JAK	Janus tyrosine kinase
LPAM	Lymphocyte Peyer patch adhesion molecule
LTB4	Leukotriene B4
MadCAM-1	Mucosal addressing cell adhesion molecule-1
MTX	Methotrexate
NF-κB	Nuclear factor κB
NSAIDs	Nonsteroidal anti-inflammatory drugs
PAF	Platelet-activation factor
PML	Progressive multifocal leukoencephalopathy
PPAR-γ	Peroxisome proliferator-activated receptor gamma
PPI	Proton pump inhibitors

M. Merćep (✉)
Department of Translational Research, Mediterranean Institute of Life Sciences-MedILS, Split, Croatia

Department of Biotechnology, University of Rijeka, Rijeka, Croatia
e-mail: mladen.mercep@medils.hr; mladen.mercep@uniri.hr

M. Banić, D. Erceg (eds.), *Drug Interactions in Gastroenterology*, Clinical Gastroenterology, https://doi.org/10.1007/978-3-031-69800-2_9

Th1	T helper cells 1
Th17	T helper cells 17
TYK2	Tyrosine kinase 2
UC	Ulcerative colitis
VCAM-1	Vascular cellular adhesion molecule 1
VLA-4	Very late antigen-4

Inflammation can affect any part of the gastrointestinal (GI) tract. The largest number of anti-inflammatory drugs are used to treat inflammatory bowel disease (IBD). Therefore, medications used for the treatment of IBD, including aminosalicylates (5-ASA), corticosteroids (CS), immunomodulating drugs, Janus kinase inhibitors, and biologic agents such as TNF-α (Tumor Necrosis Factor-Alpha), integrin, and interleukin blockers together with the nonsteroidal anti-inflammatory drugs (NSAIDs) will be briefly reviewed here. Medications used to treat other inflammatory conditions of the GI tract will be presented within the specific drug class.

IBD is a term that covers two chronic and relapsing inflammatory conditions of the gastrointestinal tract—Crohn's disease (CD) and ulcerative colitis (UC). The symptoms of IBD are linked to the signs of the underlying gut inflammation and disturbance of small and large bowel physiological functions leading to the appearance of pain, cramps, diarrhea, rectal bleeding, fever, weight loss, and fatigue. CD and UC have similar clinical manifestations, and it is not always easy to distinguish one from the other. However, they differ by the affected area of the GI tract, pathohistological findings, the extent of the gut wall involvement, and the extraintestinal manifestations [1]. Factors that enable CD and UC differentiation are shown in Table 9.1.

Differentiation between the two conditions is crucial since it has significant bearing on the appropriate treatment and the disease prognosis since the main drivers differ in various patients.

CD in itself is a clinically heterogeneous disease with variable presentation and progression. It is possible to distinguish five types of CD, i.e., gastroduodenal CD, jejunoileitis, ileitis, ileocolitis, and granulomatous Crohn's colitis when analyzing the affected area of the GI tract. Furthermore, by analyzing the histological appearance of the Paneth cells' secretory granule morphology, two subtypes of CD with distinct pathognomonic and clinical features could be distinguished. This stratification makes sense since Paneth cells are important mediators of innate immune system response by producing antimicrobial peptides such as a-defensins and lysozymes and their effects on the intestinal microbiome. Subtype 1 is characterized by the abnormal histological appearance of Paneth cells associated with genetic defects, such as *NOD2 R702W*, *NOD2 L1007fsXinsC*, and *ATG15L1 T300A* changes, altered and specific immune cell activation that reflects itself in the perturbed Paneth cell morphology, reduced epithelioid granuloma incidence, and shorter post-resection time to the disease recurrence. Subtype 2 is characterized by normal Paneth cells appearance. However, the number of epithelioid granulomas is significantly

Table 9.1 Differentiation of Crohn's disease and ulcerative colitis

	Crohn's disease	Ulcerative colitis
Affected area	Any part of the GI tract from the mouth to the anus	Limited to the colon
Disease spread	Discontinuous with the uninvolved tissue interspersed with the inflamed areas	Continuous from the rectum up
	Rectum rarely involved	Rectum almost always involved
	When the colon is affected, it is usually right sided	Usually left sided
Gross rectal bleeding	Rare except when the colon is affected	Always present
Fistulas	Common	Absent
Abscess formation	Common	Uncommon
Gut wall involvement	Transmural—can affect all layers of the bowel walls	Mucosa only
Epithelioid granulomas in the gut wall or lymph nodes	Present in 25–50% of cases	Absent
X-ray findings	Serosal surface irregular	Serosal surface smooth
Surgical removal	Does not cure	Cures
Extraintestinal manifestations such as sclerosing cholangitis and autoimmune hepatitis	Weak association	Strong association
Risk of colon cancer	Slightly increased	Significantly increased
Response to antibiotics	Yes	No

increased, there are no signs of immune system activation, and the post-resection time to recurrence is prolonged [2].

Better clinical and molecular understanding of CD and UC is necessary to achieve an untenable jet goal of disease prevention or cure through therapy personalization. A good example is anti-TNF-α monoclonal antibodies' effects on induction and maintenance of remission in CD. Remission is achieved in about 70% of the patients with CD, but 23–46% of patients lose the therapeutic response and experience disease flare 12 months from the remission [3, 4]. The fact that 30% of the patients do not experience it and more than 50% are not controlled 1 year later indicates the need to gain additional insights into disease pathophysiology and develop novel drugs targeting other disease-driving pathways.

The etiology of IBD is not known. However, it is considered to result from gut homeostasis perturbance, leading to an abnormal immune response toward environmental factors that may include host microbiota in the susceptible hosts [5].

5-Aminosalicylic Acid (5-ASA) Drugs

The four prominent representatives of the 5-ASA drugs are sulfasalazine, mesalazine, olsalazine, and balsalazide (see also Chap. 28). 5-ASA drugs are the mainstay of the first-line therapy for induction and maintenance of remission in patients with mild-to-moderate UC [6–8].

The remarkable story of the 5-ASA drugs discovery goes back to the discovery of sulfasalazine which was approved for medical use in the USA in 1950 and is on the World Health Organization's List of Essential Medicines. It is a disease-modifying anti-rheumatic drug (DMARDs). It is used to treat other types of inflammatory arthritis, such as psoriatic arthritis and reactive arthritis as well [9]. The work on its discovery was started by Nanna Svartz at the Karolinska Hospital in the late 1930s. It was assumed at that time that bacteria were the root cause of rheumatoid arthritis and UC. To improve rheumatoid arthritis treatment, she worked on combining the sulfonamide antibacterial drugs—sulfanilamide or sulfapyridine with various salicyl preparations that have anti-inflammatory activity. It was found that a conjugate prodrug compound, named sulfasalazine, in which sulfapyridine was linked to the 5-ASA (also known as mesalazine or mesalamine) by an azo group (Fig. 9.1), was effective in treating rheumatoid arthritis and UC. Colonic bacterial azoreductases break down sulfasalazine into sulfapyridine and mesalazine [10]. The discovery of sulfasalazine significantly changed UC patients' fate by offering them a real therapeutic option for the first time [9]. The significance of sulfasalazine discovery in the treatment of UC became evident when it was found that sulfasalazine was effective in the induction of the disease remission and prevention of UC relapses [11]. In contrast, corticosteroids are useful in the induction of remission but are entirely ineffective in preventing UC relapses [12, 13].

A major step forward in understanding the mode of sulfasalazine action was made in 1977 when Khan and colleagues treated UC patients by applying retention enemas of sulfasalazine and its two building blocks—sulfapyridine and mesalazine. Significant and equipotent histological improvements were observed with the sulfasalazine and mesalazine, but not with sulphapyridine. The results showed that mesalazine is the active therapeutic moiety of sulfasalazine [14]. Additional improvements and developments came from a better understanding of efficacy, drug safety profiling, and pharmacokinetic behavior.

Although sulfasalazine has excellent anti-inflammatory activity, its clinical usefulness is reduced by dose-dependent frequency and potentially serious adverse effects. At the recommended dose of 500 mg tablets 4–6 times daily, the most common adverse reactions that occur in about one-third of the patients are headache, nausea, vomiting, gastric distress, anorexia, and oligospermia with sperm motility impairment that usually reverses within 2–3 months from the drug discontinuation [15]. Less frequent adverse reactions that appear with a frequency of one in every 30 patients or less are hypersensitivity reactions (skin rash, pruritus, and urticaria), fever, Heinz body anemia, hemolytic anemia, and cyanosis due to the amino-sulfapyridine binding to hemoglobin. Rare but severe side effects include aplastic anemia, agranulocytosis, and erythema multiforme (Stevens-Johnson syndrome).

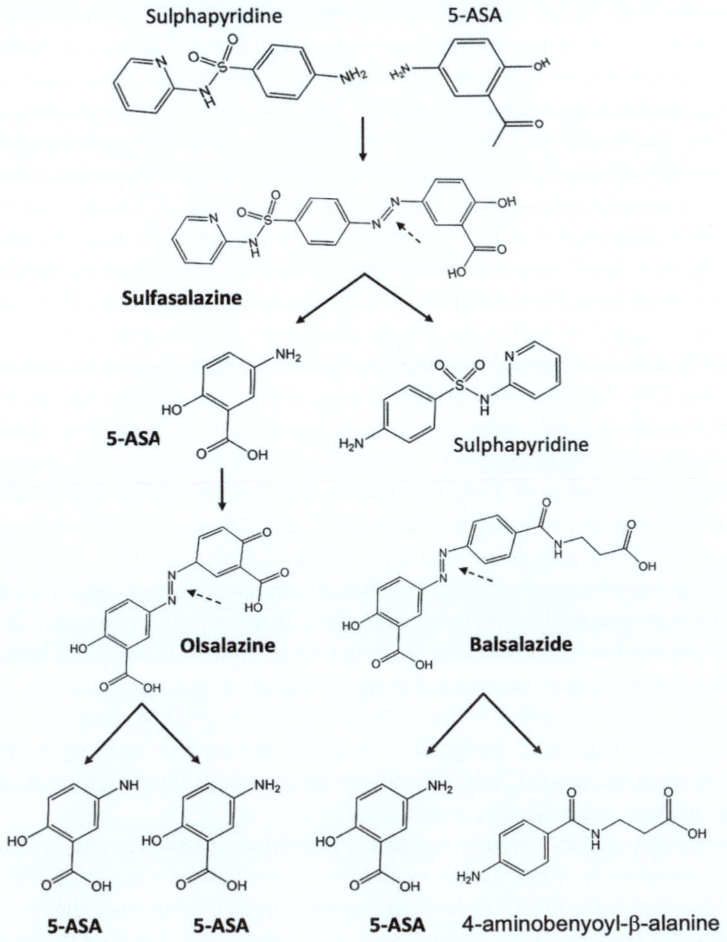

Fig. 9.1 Development of 5-ASA drugs. Historical development of 5-ASA drugs is shown. Azoreductases from the gut bacteria cleave 5-ASA prodrugs at the sites indicated with a dashed arrow and release active 5-ASA

Patients should initially be monitored for nephrotoxicity 2–3 months from the initiation of therapy and then annually after that. They should also be instructed to take adequate fluid intake since sulfasalazine can cause crystalluria, crystal formation, and kidney stone formation. Furthermore, sulfasalazine can cause yellow-orange discoloration of urine and other body fluids [16, 17]. Sulfasalazines' side effects are primarily due to the high plasma sulfapyridine concentrations that are present in patients taking higher doses of sulfasalazine or in genetically predisposed individuals (slow acetylators) [18, 19]. As described in the following paragraph, mesalazine is poorly absorbed from the colon and cannot therefore have the side effects associated with sulfapyridine.

Following oral intake, sulfasalazine is poorly absorbed in the jejunum, and the majority applied dose passes into the colon. Even the fraction of sulfasalazine absorbed in the small intestine ultimately ends up in the large intestine since absorbed sulfasalazine is mainly excreted into bile, and only a fraction is excreted in the urine. Sulfasalazine in the colon is reduced by bacterial azoreductases to sulfapyridine and mesalazine. Sulfapyridine is rapidly absorbed from the colon, inactivated to *N*-acetyl-sulfapyridine via *N*-acetyltransferase 2 (NAT2) in the liver, subsequently hydroxylated and conjugated with glucuronide, and excreted in the urine with only small amounts remaining in the stool. In contrast, mesalazine is poorly absorbed from the colon and is largely excreted in the stool. However, when mesalazine is applied orally by simple tablets or capsules, most of the drug is absorbed in the small bowel and the therapeutic concentrations cannot reach the distal colon [20]. Systemically absorbed and colonic mesalazine are inactivated to *N*-acetyl-5-aminosalicylic acid via *N*-acetyltransferase 1 (NAT1) in the live and colonic mucosa, respectively [21].

As shown by Khan et al. [14], mesalazine is active following its topical application by enema and is primarily responsible for the efficacy of sulfasalazine. It does not have the side effects associated with sulfapyridine [22]. Oral drug delivery is preferred for the treatment of IBD, and clinical efficacy could be improved by maintaining the high mucosal 5-ASA concentrations in all colonic segments [23]. Due to the rapid absorption of mesalazine from the small intestine, simple tablets or capsule formulations cannot deliver a therapeutic dose of mesalazine to the colon. To solve this problem, a number of formulations and new prodrugs, such as olsalazine and balsalazide (Fig. 9.1), designed to increase mesalazine delivery to the distal colon have been developed [24]. The newly developed products have a much better safety profile and are generally well tolerated.

Mesalazine must be coated or contained in unique capsules to ensure drug delivery to the intestine or colon. These mesalazine formulations were designed to maximize the fraction of the orally applied drug in the colon and minimize the systemically absorbed drug fraction. This requirement stems from the fact that the mesalazine efficacy in UC and CD requires the presence of relatively high free drug concentrations at the site of inflammation [25, 26] and CD [27, 28]. New formulations with targeted delivery, mostly in the terminal ileum and colon, were enabled by developing polymers that dissolve above a specific trigger pH. By selecting particular polymers that dissolve at different pH levels and by varying their ratios in the coating compositions, one can get delayed-release drug forms that release the active drug starting from mid-jejunum (Claversal®) or terminal ileum onwards (Asacol®, Asacol HD®, Claversal®, and Delzicol®) (Table 9.2). By combining the pH-dependent approach through the appropriate coating with the use of different core matrices such as pH-independent polymer Eudragit NE (Salofalk/Apriso) or hydrophilic/lipophilic matrix core known as Multiple matrix (MMX®) (Merzavant XL/Lialda), drugs with delayed- and sustained-release of active compound are obtained. A somewhat different mechanism of drug delivery was used to create the controlled-release formulation used in Pentasa®. The tablets do not have any coating, and they disintegrate in the stomach, releasing many ethylcellulose-coated micro granules.

Table 9.2 Commercial products of orally acting mesalazines

Trade name	Formulation	Mesalazine availability
Delayed-release formulations		
Asacol	Eudragit S coating	Terminal ileum, colon
Asacol HD	Eudragit S and L for the outer coat and Eudragit S for the inner coating	Terminal ileum, colon
Claversal	Eudragit L100 coating	Mid-jejunum, ileum
Delzicol	Eudragit S coating	Terminal ileum, colon
Controlled-release formulations		
Pentasa	Ethylcellulose-coated micro granules compressed into tablets	Stomach, duodenum, jejunum, ileum, colon
Delayed- and sustained-release formulations		
Salofalk/Apriso	Eudragit NE and L	Terminal ileum, colon
Mezavant XL/ Lialda	Eudragit S and L	Terminal ileum, colon

Mesalazine is slowly released by diffusion through the insoluble polymer coat that provides the drug in all parts of the gut, both in the small and the large bowel. The advantage of the before-mentioned formulation is the possibility of treating CD of the small bowel and UC in the colon [29].

The drug formulations described here release mesalazine in the indicated parts of the GI tract based on the pH-dependent dissolution and release of the active drug at the desired site of the GI tract. Their characteristics are briefly illustrated and described. **Asacol**, delayed-release tablets. Its coating dissolves at pH $\geq$ 7.0 and is indicated for mild-to-moderate active UC and remission maintenance [30]; **Asacol HD**, delayed-release tablets with two layers of coating. The outer coating comprises two polymers, Eudragit L, which dissolves at pH $\geq$ 6, and Eudragit S which dissolves at pH $\geq$ 7. Their ratio is not disclosed. Therefore, it is reasonable to infer that it starts to break at pH > 6. Once the external coating is dissolved, the dissolution of the internal layer starts at pH $\geq$ 7. It is indicated for the treatment of moderately active UC in adults [31]; **Claversal**, film-coated tablets. Its protective coating starts to dissolve at pH > 6. It is indicated for the treatment of acute disease and remission maintenance in UC and the treatment of active CD [32]; **Delzicol**, delayed-release capsules that begin to dissolve at pH $\geq$ 7.0. It is indicated both for the treatment of active disease and maintenance of UC remission [33]; **Pentasa**, slow-release tablets without gastro-resistant coating. It is indicated for the treatment of mild-to-moderate exacerbations and the maintenance of remission of UC [34]; **Apriso** (in the USA) or **Salofalk** (rest of the world), delayed and extended-release capsules for once-daily dosing. Gastric resistance is achieved by coating with Eudragit L and sustained release from a matrix core with the pH-independent polymer, Eudragit NE. It is indicated for treating acute, mild-to-moderate UC and maintaining UC remission [35, 36]; **Merzavant XL** (Europe)/**Lialda** (USA), gastro-resistant, sustained-release tablets coated with a polymer film consisting of Eudragit L and S with an undisclosed ratio that breaks down at pH > 6. The inner core is a hydrophilic/lipophilic matrix core that forms a viscous gel with the intestinal fluid that slows the mesalazine release. This delivery system is known as MultiMatrix technology (MMX®, a registered trademark of Cosmo Technologies Ltd., and MMX Multi Matrix System, a registered trademark of Cosmo S.p.A.). It is used for the targeted delivery of other drugs as well [37]. Merzavant XL/Lialda is intended for once-daily dosing for the treatment of acute mild-to-moderate UC and maintenance of remission [38–40].

The second approach in ensuring the delivery of sufficient quantities of mesalazine to the colon was the continuation of the original mesalazine conjugate prodrugs used in creating sulfasalazine. The binding of mesalazine to sulfapyridine through the azo group in sulfasalazine creates a compound that is poorly absorbed in the small intestine and from which active compound is released by bacteria in the colon. Two such compounds were created—olsalazine and balsalazide (Fig. 9.1). They are generally well tolerated with few side effects.

Olsalazine consists of two mesalazine molecules bound together by an azo bond between their amino groups. The complex is poorly absorbed but two mesalazine molecules are released when bacterial azoreductases in the distal small bowel and colon split the azo bond. Olsalazine was approved by the Food and Drug Administration (FDA) in 1990 [24]. Olsalazine almost doubled the colonic concentrations of mesalazine compared with equimolar doses of either Pentasa or Salofalk. Since mesalazine is released mainly in the colon from which systemic absorption in low, olsalazine treatment is at the same time associated with lower serum concentrations and urinary excretions than the other two drug mesalazine preparations. The low systemic load of 5-ASA provided by olsalazine reduces the potential risk of nephrotoxicity during long-term treatment [41].

Balsalazide was first synthesized in 1983, and the FDA approved it in 2000. It consists of mesalazine bound to an inactive carrier moiety, 4-aminobenzoyl-beta-alanine, and has low systemic bioavailability. When it arrives in the colon, it is cleaved by bacterial azoreductases to the active 5-ASA and an inactive carrier moiety [24, 42]. The tolerability of balsalazide is similar to that of mesalazine but better than that of sulfasalazine at therapeutically relevant dosages [43].

Although the 5-ASA drugs have been in clinical use for about 80 years, their mode of anti-inflammatory action is not known. Mesalazine inhibits the production of several proinflammatory mediators (prostaglandins, leukotrienes, thromboxanes, nitric oxide, and platelet-activation factor (PAF)) and function of mucosal lymphocytes, macrophages, neutrophils, natural killer (NK) cells, and mast cells. It also acts as a scavenger of reactive oxygen species, inhibitor of nuclear factor kB (NF-kB) activation [44], and agonist of peroxisome proliferator-activated receptor gamma (PPAR-γ) nuclear receptor [45]. Through inhibition of NF-kB and PPAR-γ stimulation, 5-ASA drugs inhibit the production of proinflammatory cytokines and adhesion molecules involved in migration of the inflammatory cells [43].

Corticosteroids Used in the Treatment of IBD

Glucocorticoids are one of the most active anti-inflammatory compounds. It is not entirely understood how they exert anti-inflammatory activity, but it is known. Glucocorticoids bind to the cytoplasmic glucocorticoid receptors and inhibit many inflammatory processes, including inflammatory cell activation, cytokine production, and expression of adhesion molecules on endothelial and epithelial cells. They are used for the short-term treatment of practically all skin, eye, airways, and gastrointestinal tract inflammatory conditions. Inhalation corticosteroids, in particular, play a crucial role in the treatment of allergic rhinitis and asthma. Glucocorticoids are further used in the treatment of inflammatory conditions of the gastrointestinal tract with dedicated formulations developed to treat eosinophilic esophagitis and IBD [46].

Numerous side effects accompany the excellent anti-inflammatory activity of glucocorticoids in various diseases. At least one adverse event may appear in up to 90% of the patients taking glucocorticoids for more than 60 days, especially in patients taking high doses [47]. Glucocorticoids affect almost all major organ systems, including the immune system (thymus involution and susceptibility to infections), skin (acne, skin thinning and bruising, delayed wound healing, hirsutism, and hair loss), eyes (glaucoma and cataract formation), brain (mood changes, depression, concentration, and memory impairment), gastrointestinal, cardiovascular (hypertension, coronary heart disease, ischemic heart disease, and heart failure), endocrine (glucocorticoid-induced hyperglycemia, dyslipidemia, weight gain, cushingoid features, adrenal suppression, and growth suppression), and musculoskeletal (osteoporosis and osteonecrosis, muscle weakness and atrophy) system [48]. Careful dosing and limiting the treatment duration could reduce the risk of these side effects. Furthermore, several dedicated formulations aimed at minimizing systemic glucocorticoid exposure while locally maintaining sufficient therapeutic concentrations were developed and will be briefly reviewed here.

The glucocorticoids used in the treatment of the gastrointestinal tract are represented by the first-generation glucocorticoids such as prednisone, methylprednisolone, and hydrocortisone that have pronounced systemic side effects, and by the second-generation glucocorticoids such as prednisolone that are designed to have reduced adverse activity with similar or better efficacy driven by a higher affinity for the glucocorticoid receptors (see also Chap. 28). The most relevant second-generation glucocorticoids used in treating inflammation in the gastrointestinal tract are budesonide and beclomethasone dipropionate (BDP). Their usefulness is further increased by developing several drug delivery systems designed to allow targeted delivery of active substances. When applied topically or as a novel oral form, their efficacy is similar to standard glucocorticoids but is associated with less adrenal suppression [22].

Oral Preparations of Budesonide

Budesonide is a second-generation glucocorticoid with an affinity for glucocorticoid receptors that is about 200-fold higher than that of cortisol and 15-fold that of prednisolone. The topical potency of budesonide is approximately fivefold better than that of prednisone. Budesonide in the systemic circulation is subject to high first-pass metabolism (80–90%) and high plasma clearance. The plasma elimination half-life is between 2.0 and 3.6 h. The high potency and low systemic bioavailability represent glucocorticoids with better safety profile [49].

The oral formulations for targeted delivery of budesonide to various parts of the gastrointestinal tract are Jorveza®, Budenofalk®, Entocort EC®, and Budesonide MMX®.

Jorveza® —mouth dissolving tablet for the treatment of eosinophilic esophagitis, a rare and chronic debilitating condition characterized by eosinophilic esophagitis that initially leads to dysphagia and later leads to the esophagus narrowing as a consequence of chronic inflammation and scarring. The tablet is dissolved when placed on the tongue and pressed against the mouth's roof. The dissolved budesonide effectively treats acute exacerbations caused by the ingestion of intolerant substance(s). It is also used for remission maintenance. Relatively frequent side effects are fungal infections of the mouth, pharynx, and esophagus [50].

Budenofalk® gastro-resistant granules are indicated for the once-daily treatment of mild-to-moderate CD of ileum and ascending colon and the maintenance of remission for up to 3 months of treatment. Budesonide-containing granules are coated with acid-resistant polymers that dissolve at pH $\geq$ 6.4 with active substance release starting in the ileum and continuing parts of the colon [51].

Entocort EC® capsules have a protective coating designed to dissolve when they reach the duodenum. The pill contains granules in which budesonide is enclosed by ethylcellulose. Budesonide is slowly diffusing from the insoluble ethylcellulose matrix in the ileum and ascending colon. It is indicated for the treatment of active mild-to-moderate CD involving the ileum and ascending colon. Therapeutic effects similar to oral prednisolone are better than the mesalazine slow-release formulation. Only about 10% of the applied dose is systemically available but due to the high first-pass metabolism effect and short plasma elimination half-life. Glucocorticoid-related adverse effects are significantly less frequent during short-term therapy with budesonide than with prednisolone [52].

Budesonide MMX® (Cortiment MMX® (Europe)/Uceris® (USA)) uses the same technology used for the extended delivery of mesalazine in Merzavant XL/Lialda preparations. The tablet is enteric coated to protect dissolution until exposure to a pH $\geq$ 7 in the small intestine. The coating encloses a matrix that, in contact with the gut juices, forms a gel-like substance. When the coating layer disintegrates, budesonide is slowly released from the core matrix throughout the ascending, transverse, and descending colon. It is indicated for remission induction in patients with active mild-to-moderate UC, especially in patients in which mesalazine therapy is not sufficient. It has a very good tolerability profile similar to that of a placebo [53].

Oral Preparations of Beclomethasone Dipropionate

The gastrointestinal-specific formulation of second-generation corticosteroid beclomethasone dipropionate is Clipper®. The tablets have a gastro-resistant coating that dissolves above pH 6.0 and releases the BDP in the ileum and proximal colon. The released BDP is hydrolyzed by esterases in tissue and intestinal juices to the active metabolite, beclometasone-17-monopropionate (B-17-MP) with 30 times higher affinity for the glucocorticoid receptors than BDP. Absorbed BDP has high plasma clearance with the terminal elimination of half-lives of 0.5 h for BDP and 2.7 h for the B-17-MP [54]. It is approved for the treatment of patients with mild-to-moderate UC who do not respond to mesalazine [54–56] with therapeutic effectiveness in two-third of active UC patients [57]. Clipper® is as effective as oral prednisone in the treatment of patients with mild-to-moderate UC but with a safety profile that is similar to mesalamine adverse events [56].

In the treatment of IBD, topically acting glucocorticoids are indicated for the treatment of mild-to-moderate UC and remission induction in the mild CD of the terminal ileum and ascending colon. Their efficacy in these conditions is similar to the activities of topical mesalazine preparations. However, they are not recommended as a maintenance therapy since they do not reduce the risk of disease relapse [13]. Systemic glucocorticoids (e.g., methylprednisolone at 60 mg/day or hydrocortisone at 100 mg q6h) are recommended treatments for acute severe UC. These glucocorticoids or topically acting oral glucocorticoids could be used for remission induction in mild-to-moderate UC unresponsive to combined oral and topical mesalazine [6–8, 58].

Small Molecular Weight Inhibitors

Immunomodulating Drugs

Thiopurine class of drugs are analogues of the naturally occurring purine bases, hypoxanthine and guanine (see also Chap. 28). They compose several agents of which azathioprine (Imuran® and Azasan®), 6-mercaptopurine (6-MP) (Purinethol® and Purixan®), and 6-thioguanine (6-TG) (Tabloid®) are used in clinical practice.

Thiopurines are prodrugs that must undergo extensive metabolic transformations to generate pharmaceutically active compounds. The first step is converting azathioprine (AZA) after oral administration and absorption by sulfhydryl-containing compounds such as glutathione and cysteine to 6-mercaptopurine (6-MP). Alternatively, 6-TG could be administered orally and used immediately for the conversion to the active compounds. The full description of the metabolic transformations of 6-MP and 6-TG required for the generation of active compounds is beyond this chapter's scope. Therefore, only the essential enzymes and end products will be described. Key active end products are 6-thioguanine nucleotides (6-TGNs), methylated metabolites, 8-aza guanine, and 6-thio-guanosine-5′-triphosphate (6-thio-GTP). Two enzymes, hypoxanthine-guanine phosphoribosyltransferase (HGPRT) and thiopurine *S*-methyltransferase (TPMT), play a crucial role. While 6-MP conversion by HGPRT to 6-thioinosine 5′-monophosphate (6-TIMP) requires two additional enzymatic modifications for its transformation to the 6-thioguanosine-5′-monophosphate (6-TGMP), 6-TGMP could be produced from 6-TG in a one-step reaction. Several kinases and reductases further metabolize the 6-TGMP to produce deoxy-6-thioguanosine-5′-triphosphate (dGs). Incorporation of the aberrant purine deoxyguanosine triphosphate, dGs, in DNA activates the mismatch repair system and induces S phase cell-cycle arrest and apoptosis through the unsuccessful cycles of DNA repair synthesis. An additional cytotoxic effect is related to incorporating 8-aza guanine into RNA and interference with protein synthesis. Metabolic conversion by TPMT is responsible for the generation of methylated products, especially 6-methyl-mercaptopurine (6-MeMP) which are potent inhibitors of de novo purine synthesis and inhibition of cell proliferation. The additional active compound generated by metabolizing the thiopurines is 6-thio-guanosine triphosphate (6-T-GTP). 6-T-GTP acts as a competitive antagonist of guanosine GTP that plays essential roles in many signaling pathways mediated by G-protein coupled receptors or small GTPases. It was shown that 6-T-GTP binds to and inhibits Rac1 GTPase, a member of the Rho family of small GTP-biding proteins that plays a vital role in MEK/NF-kB activation in CD28 co-stimulation of T cells. Inhibition of Rac1 downregulates expression of B-cell lymphoma extra-large (Bcl-xL) protein belonging to the Bcl-2 family. Bcl-xL is a transmembrane mitochondrial protein that inhibits apoptosis by binding and sequestering the proapoptotic proteins BAX and BAK, thereby maintaining the mitochondrial membrane permeability and preventing the release of cytochrome c. Its downregulation liberates proapoptotic proteins, BAX and BAK that enable the change of mitochondrial membrane potential, cytochrome *c* release, subsequent activation of the caspase cascade, and execution of the intrinsic apoptotic cell-death pathway. Immunosuppressive effects of thiopurines result from the incorporation of 6-TGNs in cellular DNA, inhibition de novo purine synthesis, and induction of activated CD4+ lymphocytes apoptosis ending in inhibition of immune cell proliferation and apoptotic cell death of activated T cells [59–61].

Clinical use of thiopurines is linked with several side effects such as nausea and vomiting, diarrhea, loss of appetite, rash, fever, tiredness, muscle aches, dizziness, and low blood pressure. Treatment with thiopurines could be terminated in about one-third of patients due to side effects such as the appearance of leucopenia, hepatotoxicity, pancreatitis, and gastric intolerance [62]. Due to their genotoxic effects, thiopurines are associated with the induction of cancers such as lymphoma, leukemia, hepatosplenic T-cell lymphoma (HSTCL), and skin cancer in long-term survivors. Thiopurines are classified as human carcinogens, and AZA has a black box warning for cancer development. Additional serious side effects associated with the long-term use include myelosuppression, severe pancytopenia, life-threatening macrophage activation syndrome (MAS), and even death, especially in the genetically predisposed individuals lacking TPMT or nucleotide diphosphatase nudix hydrolase 15 (NUDT15) [61, 63].

To mitigate the potential for the development of side effects and ensure therapeutic, it is desirable to personalize the AZA therapy by performing the TPMT/NUDT15 testing prior to the start of therapy and monitoring 6-TGNs and 6-MeTIMP levels in red blood cells while on treatment. The importance of 6-TGNs and 6-MeMP monitoring is best demonstrated by the improvement of therapeutic outcomes in 90% of patients where the dosing was directed by the monitoring results compared with the 33% improvement in those not guided [64]. It is advisable to monitor their levels 4–6 weeks after the start of thiopurine therapy and 4–6 weeks after any dose adjustment. In approximately 15–20% of the patients, thiopurine hypermethylation occurs. In these patients, the ratio of 6-MeMP to 6-TGNs is greater than 11. A good therapeutic range of TGNs is 235–450 pmol/8 × 10^8 red blood cells (RBCs). Patients with thiopurine hypermethylation are at an increased risk of therapeutic failure due to the subtherapeutic concentrations of TGNs, and a higher risk of hepatotoxicity due to the 6-MeMP >5700 pmol/8 × 10^8 RBCs. Hypermethylation could be corrected by the coadministration of xanthine oxidase inhibitor allopurinol and the administration of 25–50% AZA or MP standard monotherapy doses [62].

Thiopurines are a mainstay of treatment for inflammatory diseases, with AZA being the class' preferred member. Thiopurines are one of the pillars of therapy for CD and moderate-to-severe UC but are also used to treat autoimmune disorders, leukemia, solid tumors, and organ transplantations [63]. Thiopurines have a slow onset of action. It takes 12–16 weeks to manifest their therapeutic effects. Therefore, they are not used as a monotherapy to induce remission in patients with active moderate-to-severe CD or UC. However, they are recommended for the treatment of patients with steroid-dependent CD and UC with the hope of withdrawing steroids and maintaining remission. It is also recommended to continue treating CD patients in long-term remission on thiopurine maintenance therapy since the risk of relapse is higher when the treatment is discontinued [7, 8]. If the patient is in clinical remission, discontinuation of the treatment should be considered after 4 years of therapy due to the increased risk of skin cancer and lymphoma appearance, particularly in patients above 50 years of age [65]. When the maintenance therapy with thiopurines is discontinued, the 1-year clinical relapse rates are 23% in CD and 12% in UC [66].

Methotrexate (MTX) is a competitive inhibitor of dihydrofolate reductase that inhibits purine nucleotides and thymidylate production and interferes with DNA synthesis, repair, and cellular replication (see also Chap. 28). It is believed that this is the mechanism responsible for its antineoplastic activities. MTX is used at much lower doses in the treatment of psoriasis and rheumatoid arthritis. Weekly application of low-dose MTX is the cornerstone of rheumatoid arthritis and severe psoriasis treatment if first-line therapy has failed or patients do not tolerate those treatments. The mechanism of its anti-inflammatory activity is not known [67]. However, the anti-inflammatory mechanism is probably quite different from the mechanism in malignant diseases. The concomitant use of folic or folinic acid has no or mild-to-moderate effect on the MTX anti-inflammatory activity [68]. Several MTX biological effects may contribute to its anti-inflammatory activity, such as increased adenosine release at the inflamed sites and reduction of leukocyte accumulation [69], immune suppression through the action of regulatory T cells (Treg) [70], inhibition of TNF-α [71], IL-1β and adhesion molecules E-selectin and VCAM-1 expression [72], rheumatoid factor production suppression [73], and inhibition of leukotriene B4 (LTB4) synthesis. LTB4 is a potent chemoattractant of neutrophils and macrophages that activate leukocytes and prolong their survival [74].

The use of MTX is associated with potentially severe side effects, including hepatotoxicity, bone marrow suppression, and lung and kidney toxicities. Especially worrisome is the fact that liver fibrosis and cirrhosis may not be preceded by symptoms or abnormal liver function tests in the psoriasis population. Therefore, it is advisable to conduct periodic liver biopsies in psoriatic patients with long-term MTX treatment. It is essential to carefully monitor patients for signs of liver, kidney, bone marrow, and lung toxicity by performing regular biochemical tests of their function and looking for symptoms of dry, nonproductive cough. Severe, occasionally fatal, and acute skin reactions were observed following single or multiple doses of methotrexate that may reverse with discontinuation of therapy. Potentially fatal opportunistic infections, especially *Pneumocystis carinii* pneumonia, can occur during treatment with MTX. A further severe complication of MTX treatment is the appearance of malignant lymphomas that may regress following the discontinuation of MTX treatment or require appropriate lymphoma treatment. Since MTX can cause fetal death and/or congenital anomalies, women of childbearing age must have a pregnancy test before starting MTX. Those women should take one of the most reliable contraceptive methods such as an oral contraceptive pill, intrauterine device, or contraceptive injection. Pregnancy should be avoided for a minimum of 3 months after therapy for male patients and at least one ovulatory cycle after treatment for female patients [67].

There is no agreement on the use of MTX for the induction of remission in CD patients. However, MTX can be considered in a moderate-to-severe steroid-dependent CD when alternative options cannot be used. MTX is recommended for remission maintenance in patients with steroid-dependent CD with weekly intramuscular administration of 15 mg MTX [7]. Methotrexate monotherapy should not be used for induction or maintenance of remission in UC. Its concomitant use with biological drugs to maintain remission in UC is not recommended either [8].

Cyclosporine and **tacrolimus** are potent immunosuppressive drugs that block the activation of T cells (see also Chap. 28). Cyclosporine and tacrolimus inhibit calcineurin phosphates by binding to cyclophilin or the 12-kDaFK506 binding protein (FKBP-12). The complexes inhibit calcineurin phosphate-mediated dephosphorylation and subsequent translocation of the nuclear factor of activated T cells (NF-AT). NF-AT inhibition lowers the production of IL-2 and expression of IL-2 receptor transcription and prevents activation of T lymphocytes [75].

The cyclosporine and tacrolimus treatments are associated with numerous side effects such as neurotoxicity, nephrotoxicity, hypertension, hyperglycemia, gastrointestinal disturbances, increased susceptibility to infections, and development of lymphoma and other malignancies [76, 77].

They are cornerstones of immunosuppressive therapy to prevent solid organ transplant rejection and the treatment of allograft rejection. Cyclosporine and tacrolimus could be used in severe UC unresponsive to corticosteroids and biologic agents [8].

Janus Kinase Inhibitors

Janus kinase inhibitors are the latest addition to the list of drugs approved for the treatment of IBD (see also Chap. 29). The importance of developing drugs targeting additional inflammatory mechanisms is best illustrated by the fact that 25–40% of UC patients fail primary or secondary therapy, and up to 10% eventually undergo a colectomy [78].

Janus kinase inhibitors are orally acting anti-inflammatory drugs that inhibit one or more of the Janus tyrosine kinase (JAK) family members. There are four JAK kinases—JAK1, JAK2, JAK3, and tyrosine kinase 2 (TYK2). One of the JAK kinases is associated with particular cytokine receptors. Ligand binding induces dimerization of a given receptor and activation of associated JAK kinase through auto- and trans-phosphorylation, creating docking sites for receptor-specific signal transducer activator of transcription (STAT) factor. JAK kinase phosphorylates the docked STAT factor, which then forms homo- or heterodimers. The dimer translocates to the nucleus where they regulate gene expression of the respective cytokine target genes. Due to the complexity of the JAK-STAT pathways, and the fact that a particular JAK kinase associates with multiple cytokine receptors, inhibition of the JAK kinases simultaneously affects the signaling of multiple cytokines. This is advantageous in the treatment of IBD since multiple cytokine pathways involved in colitis could be simultaneously targeted [79].

The four approved JAK inhibitors are tofacitinib, upadacitinib, baricitinib, and filgotinib. As powerful immunomodulators, all of them carry a risk of lymphoma and other malignancies, development of serious infection tuberculosis (TB) and bacterial, invasive fungal, viral, and other opportunistic infections leading to hospitalization or death. Patients should be screened for latent tuberculosis and treated if positive prior to the initiation of the JAK kinase inhibitors treatment. Active tuberculosis monitoring should be continued during treatment even if the initial latent tuberculosis test is negative, and the treatment must be interrupted if a serious infection develops. An additional serious adverse event associated with the JAK kinase inhibitors is the development of thrombosis, especially lung embolism [80].

Tofacitinib was initially approved in 2012. It is an orally active pan-JAK inhibitor with a higher affinity for JAK1 and JAK3 than JAK2 or TYK2. It blocks the downstream effects of cytokines, such as IL-6, IL-2, IL-4, IL-7–IL-9, IL-12, IL-15, IL-21, IL-23, IL-27, IL-35, interferons, proliferation, differentiation, and function of multiple cell types implicated in the UC pathophysiology [81].

The most frequent adverse events reported in more than 5% of the treated UC patients include upper respiratory tract infection, headache, rash, diarrhea, herpes zoster, elevated cholesterol, and creatine phosphokinase levels.

Tofacitinib is approved for treating adult patients with moderately to severely active rheumatoid arthritis and psoriatic arthritis who had an inadequate response or intolerance to MTX. It was the first JAK inhibitor approved for treating adult patients with moderately to severely active UC [80]. Tofacitinib offers an additional therapeutic option for UC patients that cannot be controlled with aminosalicylates, corticosteroids, immunosuppressants, or biologics [78]. It is currently recommended for the UC remission maintenance and treatment of patients who did not respond to the infliximab treatment [8]. Due to the convenient oral route of application, rapid onset of action even in severe UC, acceptable safety profile, and lack of immunogenicity, it could change the current UC treatment paradigms [81].

Baricitinib and **upadacitinib** are JAK inhibitors approved in 2018 [82] and 2019 [83], respectively, to treat rheumatoid arthritis who had an inadequate response to one or more TNF-α antagonists or other DMARDs. The clinical trials of their use in the treatment of other inflammatory diseases, including IBD, are ongoing.

Filgotinib is an orally active, selective inhibitor of the JAK1 tyrosine kinase approved for the treatment of adults with moderate-to-severe rheumatoid arthritis in patients in the EU and Japan. It could be used alone or in combination with MTX in patients in which one or more DMARDs failed or were not tolerated enough. It is under review by the European Medicines Agency for the treatment of adults with moderately to severely active UC who did not respond, lost the response to, or were intolerant to conventional therapy or biologic. The most common side effects are nausea, dizziness, upper respiratory, and urinary tract infections. There are also concerns that it could reduce fertility in men [84].

Biologics in the Treatment of IBD

Three types of biologics are used in the treatment of IBD (see also Chaps. 13 and 29):

1. TNF-α inhibitors
2. Integrin blockers
3. Interleukin blockers

TNF-Alpha Inhibitors

Both CD and UC are associated with the increased production of TNF-α in the inflamed gut tissue which plays an important role in their pathogenesis [85]. It was only natural to explore their effectiveness in treating these conditions once the first inhibitors of TNF-α were produced. They revolutionized the treatment not only of Crohn's disease and UC but also other chronic inflammatory diseases. The FDA-approved inhibitors of TNF-α are etanercept, infliximab, adalimumab, certolizumab pegol, and golimumab. They are recombinant proteins belonging to the biological class of medicines.

Infliximab (Remicade®) was the first TNF-α inhibitor approved for use in clinical practice. On August 24, 1998, it received FDA marketing authorization for the treatment of CD [86]. It narrowly beat the etanercept that was approved on November 2, 1998 for the treatment of rheumatoid arthritis [87]. Infliximab is a chimeric murine-human monoclonal antibody (mAb) consisting of TNF-α specific light and heavy chain variable region (V) genes from murine hybridoma joined with the human kappa light chain constant region and human IgG1 heavy chain constant region genes, respectively [88]. Replacement of the murine sequences with their human counterparts reduces the immunogenicity of the infliximab and increases its therapeutic usefulness. Infliximab binds specifically both soluble and cell-surface bound forms of TNF-α and blocks its interaction with the TNF-α receptors. Infliximab was initially developed for the treatment of sepsis syndrome but was found to have a remarkable anti-inflammatory effect in a child with severe Crohn's colitis [89]. Infliximab is currently approved for use in the treatment of adult and pediatric CD, adult and pediatric UC, and rheumatoid arthritis in combination with methotrexate, ankylosing spondylitis, plaque psoriasis, and psoriatic arthritis [90].

Etanercept (Enbrel®) is quite different from the other TNF-α inhibitors. It is a fusion protein between the two extracellular, TNF-α binding parts of the receptor p75 receptor (TNFR2) and the Fc portion of human IgG1 [91]. Soluble truncated TNFR2 is present in body fluids, and it is thought to be involved in the negative regulation of TNF-α in various conditions. It binds circulating TNF-α and prevents interactions with its cell surface receptors. It is on the World Health Organization Model List of Essential Medicines [92]. It is approved to treat rheumatoid arthritis, juvenile rheumatoid arthritis, ankylosing spondylitis, psoriasis, and psoriatic arthritis [93]. When tested in CD, surprisingly, it was not effective in treating moderate-to-severe CD [94] providing the first indication that the mechanisms of TNF-α inhibition in rheumatoid arthritis and CD by etanercept and other TNF-α inhibitors are different. An additional surprise came when patients with rheumatoid arthritis, psoriasis, psoriatic arthritis, ankylosing spondylitis, pemphigus, alopecia areata, and vitiligo-treated with TNF-α inhibitors for 15 years were compared with the patients that did not receive TNF-α inhibitors. It was found that patients treated with etanercept had an increased risk of de novo diagnosis of IBD, primarily CD. There was no such risk for a new CD with golimumab or certolizumab pegol and only a slight increase with infliximab and adalimumab [95].

Adalimumab (Humira®), as for "human monoclonal antibody in rheumatoid arthritis") was the first fully human monoclonal antibody approved, as well as the first phage display-derived antibody that gained FDA approval in 2002. It was developed from a high-affinity mouse monoclonal antibody using guided selection and stepwise mutagenesis of the complementarity-determining regions (CDR). In this process, immunoglobulin heavy and light chains from the starting hybridoma were paired with human light and heavy chains, respectively, into a single-chain variable fragments (scFv) phage display library. The best binding scFv were selected, and their human heavy and light chains were recombined with human light and heavy chains into a second library that was rescreened for the best biding of TNF-α. The best binding scFv were combined with V_L kappa and V_H IgG1 immunoglobulin chains in a third library for yet another selection process. The best-binding antibodies were subjected to stepwise CDR mutagenesis to obtain high-affinity human antibodies [96]. Adalimumab binds on the same epitope on TNF-α that mediates its binding to the TNF-α receptors and subsequently inhibits binding of TNF-α to its receptors [97, 98]. Adalimumab is approved for the treatment of rheumatoid arthritis, juvenile idiopathic arthritis, ankylosing spondylitis, psoriasis, psoriatic arthritis, CD, UC, hidradenitis suppurativa, and noninfectious uveitis [99].

Certolizumab pegol (Cimzia®) is a humanized antigen-binding fragment (Fab′) of a monoclonal antibody. The starting point for its production was a high-affinity anti-TNF-α-specific hybridoma from which both variable light (VL) and variable heavy (VH) chains were cloned and inserted into the human framework sequences of the constant's parts of the kappa light and CH1 domain of the heavy chain so that only remaining parts of the original murine antibody and the CDRs. After successive rounds of selection and CDR mutagenesis, a high-affinity humanized Fab′ was selected. Since the Fab′ fragments have a short half-life in circulation, certolizumab was pegylated by the attachment of two cross-linked PEG chains to its hinge region to improve its pharmacokinetic properties [100]. Unlike other biological TNF-α inhibitors that are produced in eucaryotic expression systems, certolizumab Fab′ is manufactured in *Escherichia coli*. It binds to and neutralizes both soluble and membrane-associated human TNF-α [101]. Certolizumab is approved for the treatment of adult patients with moderately to severely active CD who have had an inadequate response to conventional therapy and for the remission maintenance, moderately to severely active rheumatoid arthritis, psoriatic arthritis, moderate-to-severe plaque psoriasis, ankylosing spondylitis, and active nonradiographic axial spondyloarthritis with objective signs of inflammation. It is still not approved for the treatment of UC [102].

Golimumab (Simponi®) is a fully human anti-TNF-α IgG1κ monoclonal antibody obtained from the humanized transgenic mice. It was selected as a high-affinity hybridoma made by immunization of HuMab transgenic mice with the human TNF-α. These mice produce fully human mAbs due to murine IgM and κ-light chains' deletions and the transgenic introduction of human heavy chain minilocus containing human IgM and IgG heavy chains locus together with the variable kappa chains [103]. Golimumab is approved for treating moderately to severe rheumatoid arthritis combined with methotrexate, psoriatic arthritis, and ankylosing spondylitis in adults to treat moderate-to-severe CD and the maintenance of remission. It is also indicated for treating patients with moderately to severe corticosteroid-dependent UC or patients with insufficient therapeutic response or intolerance to oral aminosalicylates, oral corticosteroids, AZA, or 6-mercaptopurine and for remission maintenance [104]. It is administered by subcutaneous (SC) injection and was the first patient-administered anti-TNF-α drug [105].

The safety profiles of the approved anti-TNF-α drugs are similar. Their use is associated with the reactivation of tuberculosis (TB) and hepatitis B (HBV). The screening for latent TB and HBV infection should be done before the therapy initiation. They could also lead to severe and potentially deadly conditions such as bacterial sepsis, invasive fungal infections such as histoplasmosis, opportunistic infections, lymphoma, and other malignancies such as hepatosplenic T-cell lymphoma, and hepatotoxicity. Heart failures, cytopenias, lupus-like syndrome, exacerbations, and new onset of demyelinating disease could also occur. Patients should be carefully monitored for the signs and symptoms of these diseases. Their use is contraindicated in patients with moderate-to-severe heart failure or severe hypersensitivity reaction to the drug. Furthermore, these patients should not be vaccinated with a live vaccine; and in pediatric patients, all vaccinations should be completed before the therapy initiation [90, 102, 106].

TNF-α inhibitors are recommended for remission induction in patients with moderate-to-severe active CD who have not responded to conventional therapy and for remission maintenance in patients who achieved remission with anti-TNF-α agents. While it is recommended to combine infliximab with a thiopurine for remission induction, TNF-α monotherapy is recommended for remission maintenance. Infliximab is also recommended for the induction and maintenance of remission in CD perianal fistulae [7]. In mild-to-moderate ulcerative colitis, adalimumab self-administration could be considered. In contrast, in the treatment of moderately to severely active ulceratives, TNF-α could be used as a monotherapy or in combination with thiopurines or methotrexate both for remission induction and maintenance. Furthermore, in hospitalized patients with acute severe UC who do not respond to intravenous corticosteroids, the use of infliximab or cyclosporine is advised [8].

It is expected that about one-third of patients with CD will fail the initial anti-TNF-α therapy [101], and an additional 10–20% of patients lose the response each year requiring either a dose increase or a switch of therapy [107].

Integrin Blockers

When integrin blockers were introduced in the clinical practice for the treatment of IBD, integrin blockers were a new therapeutic option for treating patients who failed classical therapy with corticosteroids and immunomodulators TNF-α-biological blockers. They were developed based on the concept that integrin blocking will prevent the migration of the activated T cells into the diseased tissues and will reduce the ensuing immunopathology. Since monoclonal antibodies have high specificity, they offer a remarkable opportunity to target T cells' tissue-specific recruitment at the site of inflammation [108]. Two integrin blockers—natalizumab and vedolizumab—are approved for clinical use.

Natalizumab was initially approved to treat multiple sclerosis and CD in 2004 [109]. It is an IgG4 humanized monoclonal antibody that binds the α4 subunit of α4β1 (very late antigen-4 (VLA-4)) and α4β7 (lymphocyte Peyer patch adhesion molecule (LPAM)) integrins. VLA-4 is expressed on T and B lymphocytes, natural killer cells, monocytes, basophils, and eosinophils. VLA-4 mediates these cells' interaction with the vascular cellular adhesion molecule 1 (VCAM-1) expressed on endothelium at sites of inflammation [108]. α4β7 is expressed on lymphocytes and binds specifically to the mucosal addressing cell adhesion molecule-1 (MadCAM-1) expressed on high endothelial venules of mucosal lymphoid organs. It is responsible for T cell homing into gut-associated lymphoid tissues. T cells' intestinal specificity is established in the mesenteric lymph node by the upregulation of α4β7 when the T cell cognate antigen is presented on retinoic acid-producing CD103 dendritic cells [110].

Unfortunately, natalizumab was associated with the appearance of progressive multifocal leukoencephalopathy (PML). PML is a rare, often fatal demyelinating disorder caused by the reactivation of the John Cunningham (JC) polyomavirus. It is most often observed in people infected with the human immunodeficiency virus (HIV) but was also observed in people on long-term immunosuppressive treatment with methotrexate, cyclophosphamide, azathioprine, anti-CD11a mAb efalizumab (withdrawn from the market since), and the anti-CD20 mAb rituximab [111, 112]. The presence of anti-JC virus antibodies significantly increases PML development risk. While the risk of PML development in anti-JC virus antibody-positive patients is estimated to be 3.87 per 1000 treated patients, the estimated incidence in JC-antibody-negative patients was 0 cases per 1000 treated patients [113]. Due to the adverse benefit-to-risk ratio, natalizumab is no longer available for IBD treatment. Natalizumab is one of the most potent drugs for treating multiple sclerosis. It is currently available only through the TOUCH® prescribing program as a monotherapy treatment for a relapsing form of multiple sclerosis [114].

Vedolizumab is a humanized anti-α4β7 integrin IgG1 monoclonal antibody that blocks its interaction with MAdCAM-1. It is thought that the α4β7 interaction with MAdCAM-1 is an important factor in underlying inflammatory response in CD and ulcerative colitis. While MAdCAM-1 is expressed mainly on the gut endothelial cells, α4β7 integrin is expressed on the surface of gut homing memory T and B cells. It is not expressed on neutrophils, eosinophils, monocytes, or platelets. Vedolizumab inhibits the migration of T lymphocytes into the inflamed gut tissue. It does not activate or induce cytokine production from T lymphocytes, has no effect on the function of regulatory T cells, or does it induce antibody-dependent cytotoxicity [115].

Vedolizumab has quite a good safety profile. The most common adverse reactions are upper respiratory tract infection, nasopharyngitis, headache, arthralgia, nausea, pyrexia, fatigue, cough, bronchitis, influenza, back pain, rash, pruritus, sinusitis, oropharyngeal pain, and pain in extremities [116]. Vedolizumab has no inhibitory effect on the adaptive or innate immune responses systemically. Therefore, no systemic opportunistic infections are observed [117]. Furthermore, vedolizumab does not affect the interaction of α4β1 and VCAM-1 and does not increase the risk of developing PML [116].

Vedolizumab is recommended for induction of response and remission in adult patients with moderately to severely active CD or UC with an inadequate response, intolerance, or failed conventional therapy and/or anti-TNF-α therapy, or have corticosteroid dependent CD. Vedolizumab is also recommended for maintaining clinical remission in CD patients who achieved remission with vedolizumab but not for perianal fistula healing [7, 8, 116].

Interleukin Inhibitors

Interleukin inhibitors are the third class of biologics used to treat IBD. At the moment, ustekinumab is the only drug in this class that has been FDA-approved for IBD treatment [118].

Ustekinumab is a human IgG1 kappa monoclonal antibody specific for the p40 protein subunit shared by the IL-12 and IL-23 (IL-12/23) cytokines [118]. They are members of the IL-12 family of cytokines consisting of four members, IL-12, IL-23, IL-27, and IL-35. IL-12/23 are produced by antigen-presenting cells such as macrophages and dendritic cells. While the most critical function attributed to IL-12 is the regulation of the Th1 effector differentiation, IL-23 is a crucial driver for the development and differentiation of Th17 cells. Both Th1 and Th17 cells have direct pro-inflammatory activities by producing cytokines such as IFN-g and TNF-α or IL-17 and IL-22, respectively. Furthermore, they also amplify the inflammatory responses by inducing the production of other inflammatory mediators such as IL-1β, IL-6, and TNF-α from DCs and macrophages [119].

IL-12/23 are heterodimeric cytokines consisting of the p40 subunit combined with the p35 subunit in IL-12 and the p19 subunit in IL-23. The posttranslational association of their subunits forms the active cytokines. IL-12 and IL-23 exert their biological effects by specific binding to their respective receptors. While the IL-12 receptor is composed of IL-12Rβ1 and IL-12Rβ2 [120], IL-23 interacts with a receptor consisting of the IL-12Rβ1 subunit and the IL-23-specific subunit IL-23R [121]. The binding of ustekinumab to the p40 subunits of the IL-12/23 cytokines prevents their interaction with the shared cell-surface receptor chain IL-12Rβ1 subunit and disrupts IL-12/23 signaling and cytokine cascades. IL-12/23 plays an essential role in the inflammatory response seen in CD. Furthermore, p40 gene deletion or treatment with the blocking antibodies was protective in the murine models of colitis [118]. Therefore, it was natural to test the therapeutic effects of IL-12/23 blockade with ustekinumab in CD. Ustekinumab had a significant impact on disease activity in CD patients with moderately to severely active disease and in the maintenance of remission in patients with positive therapeutic responses [122]. Ustekinumab is also undergoing clinical trials to treat UC [123].

Ustekinumab is approved for the treatment of moderate-to-severe plaque psoriasis and psoriatic arthritis. It is also approved for induction of remission in moderately to severely active CD with inadequate response to conventional therapy with corticosteroids and immunomodulators or in patients with an insufficient response to anti-TNF-α therapy. Ustekinumab is recommended to maintain clinical remission in CD patients who achieved remission with ustekinumab. However, it is not recommended for CD patients with a complex perianal fistula or in CD patients who have failed anti-TNF-α therapy [7, 118].

As with other immunomodulators described earlier, the use of ustekinumab is also associated with the risk of developing serious infections, tuberculosis, malignancy, or hypersensitivity reactions. The most common side effect affecting more than 3% of the treated patients during the induction of the remission phase is vomiting. The most common adverse events during remission maintenance are upper respiratory tract infections, infections of the genitourinary tract, injection site erythema, and pruritus [118].

NSAID and Gastrointestinal System

Nonsteroidal anti-inflammatory drugs (NSAIDs) are among the most prescribed medications in the world due to their analgesic, antipyretic, and anti-inflammatory effects. They are used for the short-term treatment of headaches, gout, acute musculoskeletal pain due to injuries, dental and postoperative pain, and fever control. They are also used long-term to treat conditions such as rheumatoid arthritis, osteoarthritis, other forms of arthritis, thrombosis, prevention of cardiovascular events, and colon cancer. Extended use of NSAIDs is linked with adverse gastrointestinal events, kidney damage, and cardiovascular events [124].

NSAID-related gastrointestinal adverse events could affect any part of the gastrointestinal tract and can be divided into several categories:

1. Nuisance symptoms such as regurgitation, heartburn, belching, epigastric discomfort, bloating, nausea, dyspepsia, and abdominal pain. Nuisance symptoms affect approximately 10–20% of patients taking NSAIDs.
2. Superficial mucosal lesions such as punctate subepithelial hemorrhages, erosions, and ulcerations. These could be acutely detected endoscopically in as many as 80% of the patients taking NSAIDs.
3. Gastroduodenal ulceration and its serious GI complications such as bleeding, perforation, and death. These complications occur in 1–2% of individuals taking NSAIDs regularly. Other less commonly recognized serious complications of NSAID use include pill esophagitis, small-bowel ulceration, small-bowel strictures, colonic strictures, diverticular disease, and exacerbations of inflammatory bowel disease [125, 126].
4. NSAID-related enteropathy is common and most frequently presents as anemia. Pump inhibitors (PPI) exacerbate NSAID-related enteropathy by causing small intestine gram-negative dysbiosis, increased ulcerations, and occult blood bleeding. As many as 70% of long-term users of NSAIDs have small intestinal inflammation, and 30% have erosions or ulcers [127].

Serious gastrointestinal complications could appear without warning signs, and it is crucial to analyze the risks of their appearance and plan the mitigating actions prior to initiation of the NSAID treatment. The definite risk factors for the development of NSAIDs ulcer complications are age over 65 years, history of prior ulcer disease, previous gastrointestinal bleeding, high-dose or the concurrent use of multiple NSAIDs, concomitant anticoagulation, corticosteroid, selective serotonin reuptake inhibitors, or oral bisphosphonates use, and duration of therapy longer than 3 months. Possible risk factors include conditions such as rheumatoid arthritis requiring NSAID treatment, female sex, smoking, alcohol, and *Helicobacter pylori* infections [125, 127].

Several actions could limit NSAID-related gastrointestinal adverse events. The most obvious ones are NSAID selection, dose adjustment, and shortening the treatment duration. If therapeutically appropriate, the use of paracetamol [128] or COX-2 selective drugs such as celecoxib should be considered. They have a lower risk of developing gastric ulcers. However, COX-2 selective inhibitors increase the risk of myocardial infarction and stroke. The risk of NSAID-related gastrointestinal adverse events could also be reduced by the PPI, synthetic prostaglandin analog misoprostol, or stimulant of the intracellular prostaglandin production rebamipide. In contrast, antibiotics such as metronidazole or rifaximin or probiotics such as *Lactobacillus casei* and *Lactobacillus gasseri* could reduce NSAID-enteropathy [127].

References

1. Ghosh S, Shand A, Ferguson A. Ulcerative colitis. BMJ. 2000;320:1119–23.
2. VanDussen KL, Liu TC, Li D, et al. Genetic variants synthesize to produce paneth cell phenotypes that define subtypes of Crohn's disease. Gastroenterology. 2014;146:200–9.
3. Molnár T, Farkas K, Nyári T, Szepes Z, Nagy F, Wittmann T. Frequency and predictors of loss of response to infliximab or adalimumab in Crohn's disease after one-year treatment period—a single center experience. J Gastrointestin Liver Dis. 2012;21:265–9.
4. Ben-Horin S, Chowers Y. Review article: Loss of response to anti-TNF treatments in Crohn's disease. Aliment Pharmacol Ther. 2011;33:987–95.
5. Jairath V, Feagan BG. Global burden of inflammatory bowel disease. Lancet Gastroenterol Hepatol. 2020;5:2–3.
6. Lamb CA, Kennedy NA, Raine T, et al. British Society of Gastroenterology consensus guidelines on the management of inflammatory bowel disease in adults. Gut. 2019;68:s1–s106.
7. Torres J, Bonovas S, Doherty G, et al. ECCO guidelines on therapeutics in Crohn's disease: medical treatment. J Crohns Colitis. 2020;14:4–22.
8. Feuerstein JD, Isaacs KL, Schneider Y, et al. AGA clinical practice guidelines on the management of moderate to severe ulcerative colitis. Gastroenterology. 2020;158:1450–61.
9. Plosker GL, Croom KF. Sulfasalazine: a review of its use in the management of rheumatoid arthritis. Drugs. 2005;65:1825–49.
10. Svartz N. Salazopyrin, a new sulfanilamide preparation. A. Therapeutic results in rheumatic polyarthritis. B. Therapeutic results in ulcerative colitis. C. Toxic manifestations in treatment with sulfanilamide preparations. Acta Med Scand. 2009;110:577–98.
11. Dissanayake AS, Truelove SC. A controlled therapeutic trial of long-term maintenance treatment of ulcerative colitis with sulphasalazine (Salazopyrin). Gut. 1973;14:923–6.
12. Truelove SC, Witts LJ. Cortisone and corticotrophin in ulcerative colitis. Br Med J. 1959;1:387–94.
13. Lennard-Jones JE, Misiewicz JJ, Connell AM, Baron JH, Jones FA. Prednisone as maintenance treatment for ulcerative colitis in remission. Lancet. 1965;1:188–9.
14. Azad Khan AK, Piris J, Truelove SC. An experiment to determine the active therapeutic moiety of sulphasalazine. Lancet. 1977;2:892–5.
15. O'Moráin C, Smethurst P, Doré CJ, Levi AJ. Reversible male infertility due to sulphasalazine: studies in man and rat. Gut. 1984;25:1078–84.
16. Azulfidine (sulfasalazine tablets) [package insert]. Pfizer. U.S. Food and Drug Administration. LAB-0241-3.0. Revised 2009. https://www.accessdata.fda.gov/drugsatfda_docs/label/2009/007073s124lbl.pdf. Accessed 20 May 2019.
17. Durando M, Tiu H, Kim JS. Sulfasalazine-induced crystalluria causing severe acute kidney injury. Am J Kidney Dis. 2017;70:869–73.

18. Lennard-Jones JE, Powell-Tuck J. Drug treatment of inflammatory bowel disease. Clin Gastroenterol. 1979;8:187–217.
19. D'Incà R. 5-ASA colonic mucosal concentrations resulting from different pharmaceutical formulations in ulcerative colitis. World J Gastroenterol. 2013;19:5665.
20. Myers B, Evans DN, Rhodes J, et al. Metabolism and urinary excretion of 5-amino salicylic acid in healthy volunteers when given intravenously or released for absorption at different sites in the gastrointestinal tract. Gut. 1987;28:196–200.
21. Vree TB, Dammers E, Exler PS, Sörgel F, Bondesen S, Maes RA. Liver and gut mucosa acetylation of mesalazine in healthy volunteers. Int J Clin Pharmacol Ther. 2000;38:514–22.
22. Linn FV, Peppercorn MA. Drug therapy for inflammatory bowel disease: Part I. Am J Surg. 1992;164:85–9.
23. Frieri G, Giacomelli R, Pimpo M, et al. Mucosal 5-aminosalicylic acid concentration inversely correlates with severity of colonic inflammation in patients with ulcerative colitis. Gut. 2000;47:410–4.
24. Desreumaux P, Ghosh S. Review article: Mode of action and delivery of 5-aminosalicylic acid—new evidence. Aliment Pharmacol Ther. 2006;24:2–9.
25. Schroeder KW, Tremaine WJ, Ilstrup DM. Coated oral 5-aminosalicylic acid therapy for mildly to moderately active ulcerative colitis. N Engl J Med. 1987;317:1625–9.
26. Hanauer S, Schwartz J, Robinson M, et al. Mesalamine capsules for treatment of active ulcerative colitis: results of a controlled trial. Pentasa Study Group. Am J Gastroenterol. 1993;88:1188–97.
27. Gendre JP, Mary JY, Florent C, et al. Oral mesalamine (Pentasa) as maintenance treatment in Crohn's disease: a multicenter placebo-controlled study. The Groupe d'Etudes Thérapeutiques des Affections Inflammatoires Digestives (GETAID). Gastroenterology. 1993;104:435–9.
28. Singleton JW, Hanauer SB, Gitnick GL, et al. Mesalamine capsules for the treatment of active Crohn's disease: results of a 16-week trial. Pentasa Crohn's Disease Study Group. Gastroenterology. 1993;104:1293–301.
29. Rasmussen SN, Bondesen S, Hvidberg EF, et al. 5-Aminosalicylic acid in a slow-release preparation: bioavailability, plasma level, and excretion in humans. Gastroenterology. 1982;83:1062–70.
30. Asacol [package insert]. Mason, OH: Warner Chilcott (under licence from Medeva Pharma Suisse AG); 2010.
31. ASACOL HD [package insert]. Madison, NJ: Allergan USA, Inc. (under licence from Medeva Pharma Suisse AG); 2020.
32. Claversal [package insert in German: Gebrauchsinformation]. Wayne, PA: Shire US (Pentasa is a registered trademark of Ferring B.V.); 2013.
33. Delzicol [package insert]. Madison, NJ: Allergan USA; 2020.
34. Pentasa [package insert]. Wien, Austria: Merck GmbH; 2019.
35. Salofalk tablets [package insert]. Freiburg, Germany: Dr. Falk Pharma; 2012.
36. Apriso [package insert]. Morrisville, NC: Salix Pharmaceuticals; 2008.
37. Nardelli S, Pisani LF, Tontini GE, Vecchi M, Pastorelli L. MMX® technology and its applications in gastrointestinal diseases. Ther Adv Gastroenterol. 2017;10:545–52.
38. Merzavant XL [package insert]. London, England: Shire Pharmaceutials Ltd.; 2020.
39. Lialda [package insert]. Wayne, PA: Shire US (under licence from Giuliani S.p.A., Milan, Italy); 2010.
40. Hinojosa J, Navas V, Saro C. Pharmacokinetics: efficacy and safety of MMX mesalamine formulation for treating ulcerative colitis. Rev Colomb Gastroenterol. 2014;29:46–54.
41. Staerk Laursen L, Stokholm M, Bukhave K, Rask-Madsen J, Lauritsen K. Disposition of 5-aminosalicylic acid by olsalazine and three mesalazine preparations in patients with ulcerative colitis: comparison of intraluminal colonic concentrations, serum values, and urinary excretion. Gut. 1990;31:1271–6.
42. Perrotta C, Pellegrino P, Moroni E, et al. Five-aminosalicylic acid: an update for the reappraisal of an old drug. Gastroenterol Res Pract. 2015;2015:1–9.

43. Muijsers RBR, Goa KL. Balsalazide: a review of its therapeutic use in mild-to-moderate ulcerative colitis. Drugs. 2002;62:1689–705.
44. Bantel H, Berg C, Vieth M, Stolte M, Kruis W, Schulze-Osthoff K. Mesalazine inhibits activation of transcription factor NF-kappaB in inflamed mucosa of patients with ulcerative colitis. Am J Gastroenterol. 2000;95:3452–7.
45. Rousseaux C, Lefebvre B, Dubuquoy L, et al. Intestinal antiinflammatory effect of 5-aminosalicylic acid is dependent on peroxisome proliferator-activated receptor-gamma. J Exp Med. 2005;201:1205–15.
46. Dubois-Camacho K, Ottum PA, Franco-Muñoz D, et al. Glucocorticosteroid therapy in inflammatory bowel diseases: from clinical practice to molecular biology. World J Gastroenterol. 2017;23:6628–38.
47. Curtis JR, Westfall AO, Allison J, et al. Population-based assessment of adverse events associated with long-term glucocorticoid use. Arthritis Rheum. 2006;55:420–6.
48. Oray M, Abu Samra K, Ebrahimiadib N, Meese H, Foster CS. Long-term side effects of glucocorticoids. Expert Opin Drug Saf. 2016;15:457–65.
49. Abdalla MI, Herfarth H. Budesonide for the treatment of ulcerative colitis. Expert Opin Pharmacother. 2016;17:1549–59.
50. Jorveza [summary of product characteristics]. Freiburg, Germany: Dr. Falk Pharma GmbH; 2020.
51. Budenofalk [summary of product characteristics]. Freiburg, Germany: Dr. Falk Pharma GmbH; 2019.
52. McKeage K, Goa KL. Budesonide (Entocort EC Capsules): a review of its therapeutic use in the management of active Crohn's disease in adults. Drugs. 2002;62:2263–82.
53. Hoy SM. Budesonide MMX(®): a review of its use in patients with mild to moderate ulcerative colitis. Drugs. 2015;75:879–86.
54. Clipper [package insert]. Manchester, UK: Chiesi Limited; 2019.
55. Zhao X, Li N, Ren Y, et al. Efficacy and safety of beclomethasone dipropionate versus 5-aminosalicylic acid in the treatment of ulcerative colitis: a systematic review and meta-analysis. PLoS One. 2016;11:e0160500.
56. Rizzello F, Mazza M, Salice M, et al. The safety of beclomethasone dipropionate in the treatment of ulcerative colitis. Expert Opin Drug Saf. 2018;17:963–9.
57. Nunes T, Barreiro-de Acosta M, Nos P, et al. Usefulness of oral beclometasone dipropionate in the treatment of active ulcerative colitis in clinical practice: the RECLICU Study. J Crohns Colitis. 2010;4:629–36.
58. Salice M, Rizzello F, Calabrese C, Calandrini L, Gionchetti P. A current overview of corticosteroid use in active ulcerative colitis. Expert Rev Gastroenterol Hepatol. 2019;13:557–61.
59. Nelson JA, Carpenter JW, Rose LM, Adamson DJ. Mechanisms of action of 6-thioguanine, 6-mercaptopurine, and 8-azaguanine. Cancer Res. 1975;35:2872–8.
60. Tiede I, Fritz G, Strand S, et al. CD28-dependent Rac1 activation is the molecular target of azathioprine in primary human CD4+ T lymphocytes. J Clin Invest. 2003;111:1133–45.
61. Cara CJ, Pena AS, Sans M, et al. Reviewing the mechanism of action of thiopurine drugs: towards a new paradigm in clinical practice. Med Sci Monit. 2004;10:RA247–54.
62. Warner B, Johnston E, Arenas-Hernandez M, Marinaki A, Irving P, Sanderson J. A practical guide to thiopurine prescribing and monitoring in IBD. Frontline Gastroenterol. 2018;9:10–5.
63. Imuran (azathioprine) [product information]. Roswell, GA: Sebela Pharmaceuticals; 2018. https://www.accessdata.fda.gov/drugsatfda_docs/label/2018/016324s039lbl.pdf.
64. Smith M, Blaker P, Patel C, et al. The impact of introducing thioguanine nucleotide monitoring into an inflammatory bowel disease clinic. Int J Clin Pract. 2013;67:161–9.
65. Beigel F, Steinborn A, Schnitzler F, et al. Risk of malignancies in patients with inflammatory bowel disease treated with thiopurines or anti-TNF alpha antibodies. Pharmacoepidemiol Drug Saf. 2014;23:735–44.
66. Kennedy NA, Kalla R, Warner B, et al. Thiopurine withdrawal during sustained clinical remission in inflammatory bowel disease: relapse and recapture rates, with predictive factors in 237 patients. Aliment Pharmacol Ther. 2014;40:1313–23.

67. Methotrexate Tablets [product information]. Huntsville, AL: Dava Pharmaceuticals; 2016. https://www.accessdata.fda.gov/drugsatfda_docs/label/2016/008085s066lbl.pdf.
68. Chan ES, Cronstein BN. Methotrexate—how does it really work. Nat Rev Rheumatol. 2010;6:175–8.
69. Cronstein BN, Naime D, Ostad E. The antiinflammatory mechanism of methotrexate. Increased adenosine release at inflamed sites diminishes leukocyte accumulation in an in vivo model of inflammation. J Clin Invest. 1993;92:2675–82.
70. Deaglio S, Dwyer KM, Gao W, et al. Adenosine generation catalyzed by CD39 and CD73 expressed on regulatory T cells mediates immune suppression. J Exp Med. 2007;204:1257–65.
71. Neurath MF, Hildner K, Becker C, et al. Methotrexate specifically modulates cytokine production by T cells and macrophages in murine collagen-induced arthritis (CIA): a mechanism for methotrexate-mediated immunosuppression. Clin Exp Immunol. 1999;115:42–55.
72. Dolhain RJ, Tak PP, Dijkmans BA, De Kuiper P, Breedveld FC, Miltenburg AM. Methotrexate reduces inflammatory cell numbers, expression of monokines and of adhesion molecules in synovial tissue of patients with rheumatoid arthritis. Br J Rheumatol. 1998;37:502–8.
73. Alarcón GS, Schrohenloher RE, Bartolucci AA, Ward JR, Williams HJ, Koopman WJ. Suppression of rheumatoid factor production by methotrexate in patients with rheumatoid arthritis. Evidence for differential influences of therapy and clinical status on IgM and IgA rheumatoid factor expression. Arthritis Rheum. 1990;33:1156–61.
74. Sperling RI, Coblyn JS, Larkin JK, Benincaso AI, Austen KF, Weinblatt ME. Inhibition of leukotriene B4 synthesis in neutrophils from patients with rheumatoid arthritis by a single oral dose of methotrexate. Arthritis Rheum. 1990;33:1149–55.
75. Barbarino JM, Staatz CE, Venkataramanan R, Klein TE, Altman RB. PharmGKB summary: cyclosporine and tacrolimus pathways. Pharmacogenet Genomics. 2013;23:563–85.
76. Neoral Soft Gelatin Capsules (cyclosporine capsules) [package insert]. East Hanover, NJ; Novartis; 2009. https://www.accessdata.fda.gov/drugsatfda_docs/label/2009/050715s027,050716s028lbl.pdf.
77. Prograf (tacrolimus) [package insert]. Deerfield, IL: Astellas Pharma. 2012. https://www.accessdata.fda.gov/drugsatfda_docs/label/2012/050709s031lbl.pdf.
78. Magro F, Estevinho MM. Is tofacitinib a game-changing drug for ulcerative colitis. United European Gastroenterol J. 2020;8:755–63.
79. Soendergaard C, Bergenheim FH, Bjerrum JT, Nielsen OH. Targeting JAK-STAT signal transduction in IBD. Pharmacol Ther. 2018;192:100–11.
80. Xeljanz (tofacitinib) [package insert]. North Chicago, IL: Pfizer; 2018. https://www.accessdata.fda.gov/drugsatfda_docs/label/2018/203214s018lbl.pdf.
81. Fernández-Clotet A, Castro-Poceiro J, Panés J. Tofacitinib for the treatment of ulcerative colitis. Expert Rev Clin Immunol. 2018;14:881–92.
82. Olumiant (baricitinib) [package insert]. Indianapolis, IN: Eli Lilly; 2018. https://www.accessdata.fda.gov/drugsatfda_docs/label/2018/207924s000lbl.pdf.
83. Rinvoq (upadacitinib) [package insert]. North Chicago, IL: Abvie. 2019. https://www.accessdata.fda.gov/drugsatfda_docs/label/2019/211675s000lbl.pdf.
84. Filgotinib (Jyseleca) [EPAR—Medicine overview]. Corrintohill, Ireland: Gilead Sciences Ireland; 2020. https://www.ema.europa.eu/en/medicines/human/EPAR/jyseleca.
85. Fuss IJ. Is the Th1/Th2 paradigm of immune regulation applicable to IBD. Inflamm Bowel Dis. 2008;14(Suppl 2):S110–2.
86. Melsheimer R, Geldhof A, Apaolaza I, Schaible T. Remicade® (infliximab): 20 years of contributions to science and medicine. Biologics. 2019;13:139–78.
87. Etanercep [product approval information]. Seattle, WA: Immunex Corporation; 1998. https://www.accessdata.fda.gov/drugsatfda_docs/appletter/1998/etanimm110298L.htm.
88. Knight DM, Trinh H, Le J, et al. Construction and initial characterization of a mouse-human chimeric anti-TNF antibody. Mol Immunol. 1993;30:1443–53.
89. Derkx B, Taminiau J, Radema S, et al. Tumour-necrosis-factor antibody treatment in Crohn's disease. Lancet. 1993;342:173–4.

90. Infliximab [package insert]. Horsham, PA: Janssen Biotech; 2013. https://www.accessdata.fda.gov/drugsatfda_docs/label/2013/103772s5359lbl.pdf.
91. Enbrel [product approval]. Seattle, WA: Immunex Corporation; 1998. https://www.accessdata.fda.gov/drugsatfda_docs/label/1998/etanimm110298lb.pdf.
92. World Health Organization Model List of Essential Medicines—21st list. 2019. https://www.who.int/publications/i/item/WHOMVPEMPIAU2019.06.
93. Enbrel [package insert]. Thousand Oaks, CA: Amgen Inc.; 2020. https://www.accessdata.fda.gov/drugsatfda_docs/label/2020/103795s5574s5577lbl.pdf.
94. Sandborn WJ, Hanauer SB, Katz S, et al. Etanercept for active Crohn's disease: a randomized, double-blind, placebo-controlled trial. Gastroenterology. 2001;121:1088–94.
95. Korzenik J, Larsen MD, Nielsen J, Kjeldsen J, Nørgård BM. Increased risk of developing Crohn's disease or ulcerative colitis in 17 018 patients while under treatment with anti-TNFα agents, particularly etanercept, for autoimmune diseases other than inflammatory bowel disease. Aliment Pharmacol Ther. 2019;50:289–94.
96. Osbourn J, Groves M, Vaughan T. From rodent reagents to human therapeutics using antibody guided selection. Methods. 2005;36:61–8.
97. Frenzel A, Schirrmann T, Hust M. Phage display-derived human antibodies in clinical development and therapy. MAbs. 2016;8:1177–94.
98. Hu S, Liang S, Guo H, et al. Comparison of the inhibition mechanisms of adalimumab and infliximab in treating tumor necrosis factor α-associated diseases from a molecular view. J Biol Chem. 2013;288:27059–67.
99. Humira FDA approval history. https://www.drugs.com/history/humira.html.
100. Fleischmann R, Shealy D. Developing a new generation of TNFalpha antagonists for the treatment of rheumatoid arthritis. Mol Interv. 2003;3:310–8.
101. Melmed GY, Targan SR, Yasothan U, Hanicq D, Kirkpatrick P. Certolizumab pegol. Nat Rev Drug Discov. 2008;7:641–2.
102. Cimzia (certolizumab pegol) [prescribing infomration]. Smyrna, GA: UCB; 2019. https://www.cimzia.com/themes/custom/cimzia/docs/CIMZIA_full_prescribing_information.pdf.
103. Weiner LM. Fully human therapeutic monoclonal antibodies. J Immunother. 2006;29:1–9.
104. Simponi (golimumab) [media-center]. Horsham, PA: Johsnon-Johnson; 2013. https://www.jnj.com/media-center/press-releases/simponi-golimumab-receives-fda-approval-for-ulcerative-colitis.
105. Mazumdar S, Greenwald D. Golimumab. MAbs. 2009;1:422–31.
106. Humira (adalimumab) [package insert]. North Chicago, IL: AbbVie; 2020. https://www.accessdata.fda.gov/drugsatfda_docs/label/2020/125057s415lbl.pdf.
107. Allez M, Vermeire S, Mozziconacci N, et al. The efficacy and safety of a third anti-TNF monoclonal antibody in Crohn's disease after failure of two other anti-TNF antibodies. Aliment Pharmacol Ther. 2010;31:92–101.
108. Stefanelli T, Malesci A, De La Rue SA, Danese S. Anti-adhesion molecule therapies in inflammatory bowel disease: touch and go. Autoimmun Rev. 2008;7:364–9.
109. TYSABRI (natalizumab) [approval letter]. Cambridge, MA: Biogen; 2004. https://www.accessdata.fda.gov/drugsatfda_docs/appletter/2004/125104_0000_ltr.pdf.
110. Kempster SL, Kaser A. α4β7 integrin: beyond T cell trafficking. Gut. 2014;63:1377–9.
111. Langer-Gould A, Atlas SW, Green AJ, Bollen AW, Pelletier D. Progressive multifocal leukoencephalopathy in a patient treated with natalizumab. N Engl J Med. 2005;353:375–81.
112. Tan CS, Koralnik IJ. Progressive multifocal leukoencephalopathy and other disorders caused by JC virus: clinical features and pathogenesis. Lancet Neurol. 2010;9:425–37.
113. Bloomgren G, Richman S, Hotermans C, et al. Risk of natalizumab-associated progressive multifocal leukoencephalopathy. N Engl J Med. 2012;366:1870–80.
114. TYSABRI (natalizumab) [package insert]. Cambridge, MA: Biogen; 2020. https://www.tysabri.com/content/dam/commercial/tysabri/pat/en_us/pdf/tysabri_prescribing_information.pdf.
115. Wyant T, Yang L, Fedyk E. In vitro assessment of the effects of vedolizumab binding on peripheral blood lymphocytes. MAbs. 2013;5:842–50.

116. ENTYVIO (vedolizumab) [package insert]. Deefield, IL: Takeda Pharmaceuticals; 2014. https://www.accessdata.fda.gov/drugsatfda_docs/label/2014/125476s000lbl.pdf.
117. Fedyk ER, Wyant T, Yang LL, et al. Exclusive antagonism of the α4 β7 integrin by vedolizumab confirms the gut-selectivity of this pathway in primates. Inflamm Bowel Dis. 2012;18:2107–19.
118. STELARA (ustekinumab) [package insert]. Horsham, PA: Janssen Biotech; 2016. https://www.accessdata.fda.gov/drugsatfda_docs/label/2016/761044lbl.pdf.
119. Interleukin 12/interleukin 23 pathway: biological basis and therapeutic effect in patients with Crohn's disease. World J Gastroenterol. 2018;24(36):4093.
120. Presky DH, Yang H, Minetti LJ, et al. A functional interleukin 12 receptor complex is composed of two beta-type cytokine receptor subunits. Proc Natl Acad Sci USA. 1996;93:14002–7.
121. Parham C, Chirica M, Timans J, et al. A receptor for the heterodimeric cytokine IL-23 is composed of IL-12Rbeta1 and a novel cytokine receptor subunit, IL-23R. J Immunol. 2002;168:5699–708.
122. Feagan BG, Sandborn WJ, Gasink C, et al. Ustekinumab as induction and maintenance therapy for Crohn's disease. N Engl J Med. 2016;375:1946–60.
123. Hanžel J, D'Haens GR. Anti-interleukin-23 agents for the treatment of ulcerative colitis. Expert Opin Biol Ther. 2020;20:399–406.
124. Scheiman JM. NSAID-induced gastrointestinal injury: a focused update for clinicians. J Clin Gastroenterol. 2016;50:5–10.
125. Lichtenstein DR, Syngal S, Wolfe MM. Nonsteroidal antiinflammatory drugs and the gastrointestinal tract. The double-edged sword. Arthritis Rheum. 1995;38:5–18.
126. Wolfe MM, Lichtenstein DR, Singh G. Gastrointestinal toxicity of nonsteroidal antiinflammatory drugs. N Engl J Med. 1999;340:1888–99.
127. Tai FWD, McAlindon ME. NSAIDs and the small bowel. Curr Opin Gastroenterol. 2018;34:175–82.
128. Gastrointestinal safety of paracetamol: is there any cause for concern. Expert Opin Drug Saf. 2004;3(4):269.

Part III

Basics of Drug Interactions

Adverse Drug Reactions and Drug Interactions

10

Damir Erceg, Nikola Raguž-Lučić, and Sabina Steiner Srdarević

Introduction

The brief information regarding pharmacogenomics in BMJ, mistakenly substituted adverse drug reactions (ADRs) with drug interactions, while writing about cause for two million patients hospitalized in USA annually [1]. In the response of above-mentioned article, Khan explained that drug interactions are subset of ADRs, but the reverse is not possible [2, 3]. There are many terms embraced as drug interactions including drug-drug interaction, our topic in this chapter. Interactions with food and herbal products are the topics in the other chapters.

ADRs were defined in that time as "a response to drug which is harm and unwanted and which is related at usual dose range" [4]. Some of very important events as drug abuse, treatment failures, medication errors (MEs), noncompliance

D. Erceg (✉)
Srebrnjak, Children's Hospital, Zagreb, Croatia

School of Medicine, Catholic University of Croatia, Zagreb, Croatia

Department of Pharmacology and Biochemistry, Faculty of Dental Medicine and Health Osijek, J. J. Strossmayer University of Osijek, Osijek, Croatia

Department of Pharmacology, Faculty of Medicine, J. J. Strossmayer University of Osijek, Osijek, Croatia
e-mail: derceg@bolnica-srebrnjak.hr

N. Raguž-Lučić
Department of Pharmacology, Faculty of Medicine, J. J. Strossmayer University of Osijek, Osijek, Croatia

Department of Pharmacology and Biochemistry, Faculty of Dental Medicine and Health Osijek, J. J. Strossmayer University of Osijek, Osijek, Croatia

S. Steiner Srdarević
Department of Pharmacology and Biochemistry, Faculty of Dental Medicine and Health Osijek, J. J. Strossmayer University of Osijek, Osijek, Croatia

M. Banić, D. Erceg (eds.), *Drug Interactions in Gastroenterology*, Clinical Gastroenterology, https://doi.org/10.1007/978-3-031-69800-2_10

were not included at that time in definition of ADRs [5–7]. Due to nonstandardized using of safety terms, it was a difficult to compare different studies and calculate incidence rates. This story represent a short introductory statement and was a starting point of a terms and standardization in pharmacovigilance (PV).

Terms in PV

Adverse Events

Adverse events (AE) is an untoward medical occurrences after exposure to a medicine, which is not necessarily caused by that medicine. Also, it could be each unfavorable and unintended sign symptom, temporally associated with medication regardless the relationship of the event [5–7]. AEs and adverse drug events (ADEs) are synonyms.

AEs can be classified related to seriousness (serious and nonserious), causality assessment (certainly, definitely, probably, likely, or not related) and expectedness (expected and unexpected) (Fig. 10.1). According to severity, we can divide AEs into three categories: mild, moderate, and severe.

The event can be categorized as serious adverse events (SAEs) in following situations:

- If requires hospitalization, or prolonged existing hospitalization
- Is life threatening
- Results in death
- Causes congenital malformation/birth defect
- Result in significant or persistent incapacity/disability, or
- Is judged as medically important

All clinical trials have the potential to produce AEs. AEs occurring in clinical studies, have to be reported to the sponsor of pharmaceutical product. The sponsor also notifies all participating sites of the AEs, as well as both the investigators' and the sponsors' judgment of the seriousness of the AEs. All investigators and sponsor

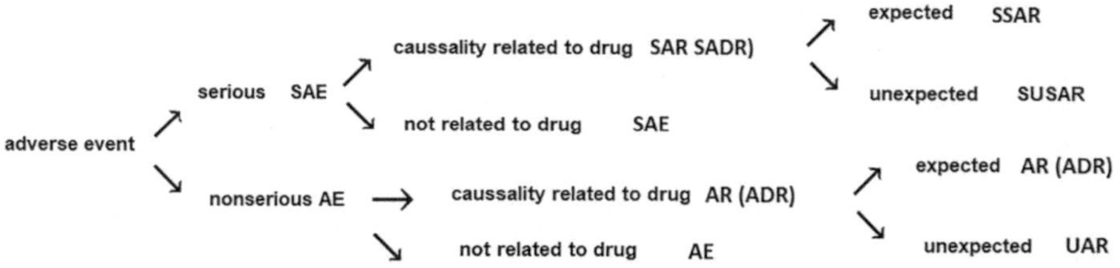

Fig. 10.1 Classification of AE regarding seriousness, causality assessment, and expectedness. *AE* adverse event, *AR* adverse reactions, *ADR* adverse drug reactions, *SAE* serious adverse event, *SAR* serious adverse reactions, *SADR* serious adverse drug reactions, *UAR* unexpected adverse reactions, *SSAR* suspected serious adverse reactions, *SUSAR* suspected unexpected serious adverse reactions

have access to study data that might suggest potential problems with the study treatment. All AEs that are serious and unexpected (SUSAR) should be a subject of expediated reporting to regulatory authority. The life threatening or fatal SAE should be reported immediately to sponsor (entire 24 h). The regulatory authorities should be informed by the sponsor within 7 days after the first alert. The sponsor has to submit a final a report in eight additional calendar days. All other serious and unexpected reports that are not life threatening or fatal have to be submitted in 15 calendar days. Besides expedited reporting, periodic or aggregate reports have to be submitted by sponsor to relevant regulatory authority, reviews the cumulative safety data from different sources.

Adverse Drug Reactions

Adverse reaction (ARs) and adverse drug reaction (ADRs) are synonyms. There are many various definitions of ADRs. Ferner et al. suggested following definition: "Medicines have unintended side effects, and if any of these is harmful, the patient has an adverse drug reaction" [8]. ADRs can be AE with causal link to a drug. Rawlins and Thompson suggested basic classifications of ADRs, divided into two groups: type A as a predictable and dose dependent and type B with opposite characteristics [9]. Same authors later invented mnemonic names: type A—"Augmented" and type B— "Bizarre." Other authors added new categories with mnemonic names: as "type C (continuous) and type E (end of use, i.e., withdraw), type F as failure, and type G for genetic/genomic" [9].

Vervloet et al. suggested that risk factors for ADRs could appear in general population (overdose, ADR, DDI), or in a specific susceptible population (intolerance, idiosyncrasy, drug allergy, pseudoallergic reactions) [10]. Also, the other classification divide ADRs in the following types: expected and unexpected reactions (Fig. 10.1). The expected reaction are usually extensions of treatment effects and the result of interactions with known drugs. The unexpected reaction is related to anaphylaxis, allergic reactions, prescription errors, idiosyncratic reactions as, DDI with unknown drug combination and critical care environment.

Aronson and Ferner were introduced new classifications of ADRs DoTS according to dose, time, and susceptibility which they occur. The many factors can alter susceptibility of patients giving mnemonic I GASPED (**I**mmunological, **G**enetic, **A**ge, **S**ex, **P**hysiology, **E**xogenous influences, and **D**iseases). Influence of these factors are depended on the dose and explain difference between patients affected and nonaffected by ADRs [11].

Drug-Drug Interactions

Drug-drug interactions (DDIs) are a measurable modification in magnitude or duration of the pharmacological response of one drug, due to the presence of another drug that is pre- or coadministered [12]. The drug interactions usually mean drug-drug interactions, but patient's response to a drug can be modified by food, drink, herbal, environmental factors, and so on (see also Chaps. 14, 15, and 16) [13]. Drugs may also interact with diseases, potentially worsening their symptoms (see also Chap. 17). Also, DDIs are responsible for 10% cases in emergency department as well as 3–5% of MEs [14]. DDIs occur when the effect of one drug is altered in the presence of another drug. DDIs account 6–30% of all ADRs, according to one source [13]. DDIs account for more than 20% of ADRs in general population, about 10% of the cases in emergency department and contribute 3–5% of the ME in-patients according to other sources [14, 15]. The variations in drug pharmacokinetic parameters, altered by enzymes- and transporters-mediated DDIs, can significantly change the drug efficacy or toxicity. The most prominent cause of DDIs is based on drug metabolism due to inhibition and induction of metabolic enzymes and transporters (CYP 3A4 and UGT) [16]. Potential DDIs can be predicted from the known pharmacological effects of the drug. The list of potential DDIs includes at least 2500 drug pairs, but according to other source is more than double [17, 18]. The drugs with wide therapeutic windows are usually not involved in clinically significant DDIs. Some patients' groups (extensive or poor metabolizers of a CYP isoenzyme) can be involved in clinically significant DDIs. There are scarce data regarding the actual contribution DDIs to ADRs. The most studies are focused on hospital population. The protective data from large hospital populations estimated between 16.6% and 59.1% of ADRs needing hospital care are related to DDIs [16, 19]. Also, other authors reported that 5–15% of elderly patients suffer clinically significant ADRs due to DDIs, while the number of elderly patients exposed to a potential DDI is estimated to be between 35% and 60% [20, 21]. DDIs are important in clinical practice, because they considered as preventable drug-related problems (DRPs). Sometimes DDIs can be beneficial and have therapeutic advantage in many conditions like cancer, HIV, epilepsy, or heart disease. In many cases, DDI involve an effect of one drug on the action of another (victim or perpetrator) without reciprocal effects. They can be commonly divided in three main categories as pharmaceutical, pharmacokinetic, or pharmacodynamic [21] (Fig. 10.2).

Pharmaceutical interactions are also called direct interaction, and they occur before administration to patients (e.g., precipitation as a consequence of mixing

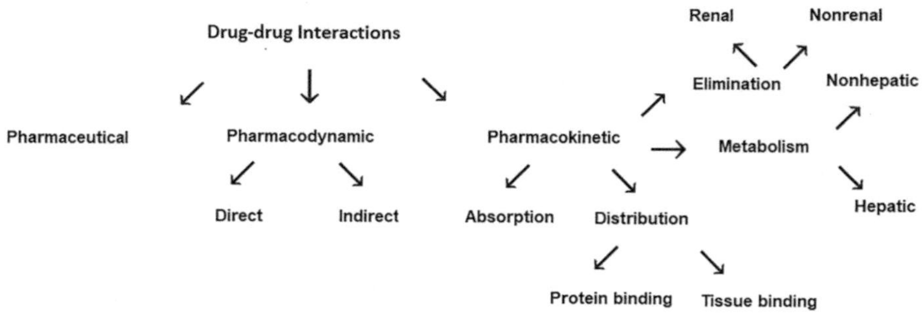

Fig. 10.2 Classification of DDIs

different drug in syringe). Pharmacokinetic interactions interfere with pharmacokinetic processes. Pharmacokinetic interactions are results of changes in ADME (absorption, distribution, metabolism, or elimination) of another drug. They are expressed as a change in kinetic parameters such as peak serum concentration, AUC (area under curve), or $t_{1/2}$. The most common type of pharmacokinetic interactions are metabolic interactions with cytochrome P450 isoenzymes (CYPs) in a main role.

The altered effects of one drug by the presence of another, without pharmacokinetic changes are pharmacodynamic interactions. Pharmacodynamic interactions are those where the effects of one drug change by the presence of another, without alterations in drug kinetics. The competition at the level of drug receptors can, in some cases, be responsible for pharmacodynamic DDIs. In the other cases, reasons are interference with physiology and other indirect mechanisms Additive or synergistic interactions can cause an increase in pharmacological effects, but antagonistic interactions that cause a decrease. DDI can be associated with length and cost of hospitalization [22]. Prescribing of more drugs is often necessary practice, usually in older people. It was shown that the incidence of potential DDIs rapidly increase with higher number of drug taken by [23]. Harmful DDI occur in following conditions [24]:

- High first-pass metabolism (extensive metabolism in GI tract and sensitive to metabolic induction or inhibition).
- Steep dose-response curve (a significant increase in plasma concentrations as a result a small increase of the dose).
- One route of elimination (e.g., renal or hepatic metabolism) (drug can cause a significant increase in plasma concentration).
- Narrow therapeutic window (toxic effect can be caused by small changes in plasma concentration as well as treatment failure).

Medication Errors (MEs)

MEs can be defined as "a failures in the treatment process that leads to, or has the potential to lead to, harm to the patient" [25]. A systematic literature review found 26 different terminologies employed for a medication error [26]. There are different classifications and according to that prevention's measures. MEs can be classified according to stages during medication process The classification and prevention at any stage during the medication process (choosing, prescribing, manufacturing, dispensing, administering, or monitoring) is broad definition suggested by National Coordinating Council for Medication Error Reporting and Prevention (NCC MERP) [27]. MEs can be classified according to numerous approaches [25, 28]. One of them consider the types of errors occurring during the process [28, 29]:

- Errors based on knowledge—for example, administration of penicillin, without checking of patient history due to allergy. Prevention methods be informed about the prescription medicine and patient using computerized prescribing systems, and cross-checking.

- Errors based on rule—for example, injecting analgetic drug ketoprofen into the lateral thigh instead of the buttock. Prevention methods: education help and propter rule.
- Errors based on action (slips)—for example, picking up a bottle containing chlorpropamide instead chlorpromazine. Prevention methods: computerized reminders, the use of checklists, and bar code system.
- Errors based on memory (lapses) —for example, giving some drug, knowing the patient is allergic, but forgetting. Prevention methods: computerized prescribing systems, cross-checking.

Pharmacovigilance (PV)

Pharmacovigilance (PV) or drug safety has a very important role in healthcare system regarding monitoring, collecting, detecting, assessing as well as preventing ADRs of pharmaceutical products. PV takes care about detection of statistical signal from different sources of data. All pharma companies routinely search their safety databases for occurrences of ADRs. Also, a few main regulatory databases allow analysis of adverse events. AEs, MEs, and product complaints resulting in AE submitted to the FDA becomes a part of safety database called FAERS (FDA Adverse Event Reporting System). This database support postmarketing surveillance program for biologic products and drugs covering about third all pharmaceutical products in the world. In Europe, the suspected ADRs are submitted electronically to EudraVigilance Data Analysis System (EVDAS) by pharmaceutical companies that are marketing authorization holders (MAHs) and national drug regulatory authorities. This database is maintained by European Medicines Agency (EMA) maintained this database and performs risk-benefit evaluation of medicine during development and after authorization in EU. In Japan, the Pharmaceutical and Medical Devices Agency (PMDA), collects ADR reports in Japanese Adverse Drug Event Report Database (JADER).

Finally, VigiBase is the World Health Organization's (WHO's) global database with individual safety reports (ICSR) submitted since 1968. This largest database in the world, with more 20 million reports of suspected ADRs, is maintained by Uppsala Monitoring Centre (UMC), Sweden. UMC has collaboration with other safety databases and exchange the safety data as a part of WHO's program for International Drug Monitoring. These databases have different operational characteristics for frequency of updates (quarterly in FAERS, daily in EVDAS), mode of access and available information. There is possibility to monitor more safety databases for signal of disproportionate reporting (SDRs) compared with internal database. In one of comparative disproportionality analysis across different safety databases, very similar low SDRs was noticed [30–32].

Discussion

There is so much confusion about terminology used in medication safety despite growing interest in few last decades [33, 34]. According to Nebeker et al. potential terminology problems in part comes from the regulatory and clinical context that are much narrower than patient safety and improvement of quality. The use of these terms in the new and broader context revealed inconsistent safety terminology [35]. Yu et al. confirmed those claims [36]. They made electronical search of 160 web sites related to medication safety [36]. There are 25 different safety terms including 119 definitions across 33 web sites. Burkle et al. performed a search of literature for relevant safety terms and found results in line with previous authors. They found out at least 12 distinct definitions for ADRs, 9 definitions for AEs, and 5 definitions for MEs [37]. There are many more terms used in literature (i.e., AE, side effects, error, adverse event, near miss, potential ADEs, ADRs, drug medication events, medication incident, or sentinel event). Many definitions were refined after that [5, 6]. Also, many diagrams trying to explain associations between AEs, ADRs, and MEs have been published [33, 38, 39]. The interpretation of relationship between different terms like MEs, ADRs, AEs, and DDIs are in Fig. 10.3.

Terms such as AE and ADR that initially come from safety, and PV can help physicians relate to medications and some conditions. The International Conference on Harmonizations (ICH) is responsible for harmonization of technical requirements and bringing together regulatory authorities such as US FDA, EMA, PMDA, and the WHO. They define AEs as "any untoward medical occurrence that may present during treatment with a pharmaceutical product but which does not necessarily have a causal relationship with this treatment" [40]. This definition provides context for the ADRs. The principal difference between AE and ADR is shown in Fig. 10.3. The causal relationship is suspected for the ADRs but is not required for AEs [41]. ADRs are a subset of AEs reports. A side effect usually describes secondary effect of a medication that is not related to desirable therapeutic effect. This term should generally be avoided in favor of ADR according to recommendations. ADRs may results from MEs but most do not. Most MEs do not harm patients. According to Bates, less than 1% of MEs result in harm [38]. About 25% of AEs are due to

Fig. 10.3 AEs, ADRs, MEs, and DDIs

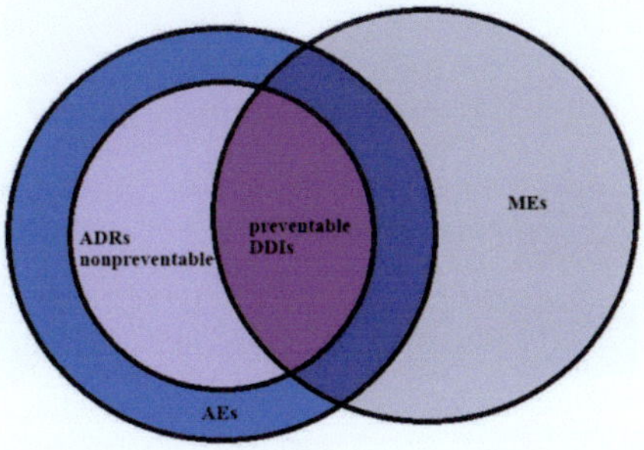

MEs [35]. In some cases, errors like a missed dose of drug carry on minimal potential for harm. There are many types of error with significant risk to patients but are escaped before reaching the patient, like potential ADEs, near misses, and so on [42]. Terms ADE and AE are synonyms without causal relationship between drug and event according to FDA [43]. Their use is consistent in PV and patient safety communities.

A causality assessment made by Naranjo was designed to evaluate AEs. This assessment is not appropriate to assess DDIs due to the use of some questions. Horn et al. developed the Drug Interaction Probability Scale (DIPS) with the aim to assess DDIs [44]. The knowledge of pharmacologic characteristics of both drug is necessary in proper assessment of DDI. This questionnaire assists physicians in suitable assessment of DDIs as well as good guide in preparing or evaluation DDIs case reports.

The incidence of potential DDIs is invariably higher in comparison with actual DDIs. The clinically recognizable or actual DDIs are the visible part of an iceberg (between a third or fifth of its total volume), while potential DDIs are "submerged" (rest of it) [45]. Actual DDIs are responsible for emergency room visits, admissions to hospital, and rehospitalizations. The published studies reported variable incidence regarding the type of patients included in the studies. More than 20% of the reported ADRs are related to DDIs. Many of these cases were serious, and some of them were fatal. The risk factors for DDIs are summarized in Fig. 10.4. Among them, polypharmacy is certainly one of the most important risk factor for ADRs [46,

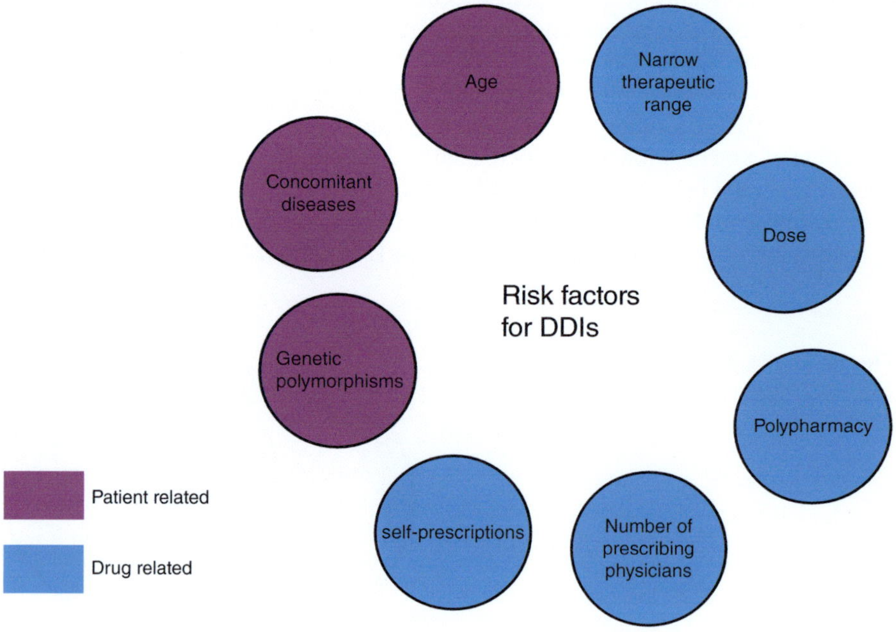

Fig. 10.4 Risk factors for DDIs

47], as well as DDIs [48, 49]. The number of medication concomitantly used increase a risk for DDIs, according to Goldberg. The incidence of DDIs is 13% (if patients use two drugs), in comparison with 38% when patients taking four drugs. Further increase of incidence to 82% appear when patient is coadministered with seven or more drugs [50]. Bjerrum et al. analyzed prescription data retrieved from prescription database covering prescriptions to all inhabitants in one region in Denmark [51]. During the observation period of 1 year, there are three almost equal groups: population with two or more medications (polypharmacy), population with monotherapy as well population did not take any drug. Combinations of drugs with potential interactions were designated based on documentation quality and severity of interactions in three categories: major, moderate, or minor. In population with polypharmacy average number of medications were 3.4 with range between 2 and 23.

Twenty-nine percent of patients exposed to more drugs simultaneously were not treated with medications with potential DDIs. Only 6% of individuals received potentially interacting drugs. The high age, a followed by numbers of prescribing physicians, numbers of simultaneously used medications, and small female share are patients factors connected with growing of interaction risk. This is one example, where prescription data can be helpful in identifying risk patients for drug interactions. Mainly, drugs with a narrow therapeutic window are the most involved in DDIs. Most of interactions are serious with many fatal cases. Also, reduced efficacy or therapeutic failure are often underestimated as an important part of DDIs. The several sources of available safety information for health professionals intended to prevent DDIs: Stockley's Drug Interactions, Micromedex Healthcare Series, SFINX-system, Lexi-Interact, Physicians' Desk Reference, Drug Interactions Checker, Drug Interaction Facts, and so on. Some sources are available online, on paper, or both. The Summary Product Characteristics (SPC) of the drugs and available data in national formularies (e.g., VIDAL, BNF) are other source of safety information [46]. Computerized systems are effective in the reduction of potential DDIs as well as the use of DDI alert systems. The prescribing physician in addition to that must be aware of proper risk-benefit evaluation.

Conclusion

Drugs are associated with significant safety risks including MEs, AEs, ADRs, DDIs, and other repercussions of medications use. It was hard to compare numerous studies and calculate incidence rates due to nonstandard usage different safety terms before standardization of terminology. The risk factors for DDIs are polypharmacy, high age of patients, narrow therapeutic index, as well as genetics. DDIs account for more than 20% of ADRs in general population, ADRs can be result of DDIs, but reverse is not possible. Furthermore, consequences of DDIs can be treatment failure or higher toxicity, increased hospitalization, morbidity, even death. DDIs are responsible for a significant amount of the healthcare cost regarding to DRPs. The estimated mean of health care cost due to nonoptimized medication used was 528.4 billion USD in 2016 [52].

References

1. Tanne JH. The new word in designer drugs. BMJ. 1998;316:1930.
2. Khan SA. Descriptions of adverse drug events should be standardised. BMJ. 1999;318:7176.
3. Lazarou J, Pomeranz BH, Corey PN. Incidence of adverse drug reactions in hospitalized patients: a metaanalysis of prospective studies. JAMA. 1998;279:1200–5.
4. Vervloet D, Durham S. ABC of allergies: adverse reactions to drugs. BMJ. 1998;316:1511–4.
5. Pharmacovigilanvce glossary. https://www.emwa.org/media/2640/pv-sig-glossary-august-2017.pdf. Accessed 31 Jan 2021.
6. E6 (R2) Step 2b Addendum—Good clinical practice (europa.eu). 2015. https://www.ema.europa.eu/en/documents/scientific-guideline/guideline-good-clinical-practice-e6r2-4-step-2b_en.pdf. Accessed 31 Jan 2021.
7. Glossary of pharmacovigilance terms. https://www.who-umc.org/global-pharmacovigilance/publications/glossary. Accessed 21 Jan 2021.
8. Ferner RE, McGettigan P. Adverse drug reactions. BMJ. 2018;363:k4051. https://doi.org/10.1136/bmj.k4051.
9. Aronson JK, Ferner RE. Clarification of terminology in drug safety. Drug Saf. 2005;28(10):851–70. https://doi.org/10.2165/00002018-200528100-00003.
10. Vervloet D, Durham S. Adverse reactions to drugs. BMJ. 1998;316(7143):1511–4. https://doi.org/10.1136/bmj.316.7143.1511.
11. Ferner R, Aronson J. Susceptibility to adverse drug reactions. Br J Clin Pharmacol. 2019;85(10):2205–12. https://doi.org/10.1111/bcp.14015.
12. Neis AS. Practical principles. In: Hardman JG, Limbird LE, Gilman GA, editors. Goodman & Gilman's the pharmacological basis of therapeutics. 10th ed. New York: McGraw-Hill (Medical Publishing Division); 2001. p. 45–66.
13. Drug interactions and adverse reactions. In: Ionescu C, Caira MR, editors. Drug metabolism. Dordrecht: Springer; 2005. https://doi.org/10.1007/1-4020-4142-X_8. Accessed 31 Jan 2021.
14. Leape LL, Bates DW, Cullen DJ, Cooper J, Demonaco HJ, Gallivan T, et al. Systems analysis of adverse drug events. ADE Prevention Study Group. JAMA. 1995;274(1):35–43.
15. Roscetti R, Morgutti M, Menniti-Ippolito F, et al. Suspected adverse drug events requiring emergency department visits or hospital admissions. Eur J Clin Pharmacol. 1999;54(12):959–63.
16. Pirmohamed M, James S, Meakin S, Green C, Scott AK, Walley TJ, et al. Adverse drug reaction as cause of admission to hospital: prospective analysis of 18 820 patients. BMJ. 2004;329:15–9.
17. Baxter K. Stockley's drug interactions. London: Pharmaceutical Press; 2008.
18. Magro L, Moretti U, Leone R. Epidemiology and characteristics of adverse drug reactions caused by drug-drug interactions. Expert Opin Drug Saf. 2012;11(1):83–94. https://doi.org/10.1517/14740338.2012.631910.
19. Leone R, Magro L, Moretti U, Cutroneo P, Moschini M, Motola D, Tuccori M, Conforti A. Identifying adverse drug reactions associated with drug-drug interactions: data mining of a spontaneous reporting database in Italy. Drug Saf. 2010;33(8):667–75. https://doi.org/10.2165/11534400-000000000-00000.
20. Davies EC, Green CF, Taylor S, et al. Adverse drug reactions in hospital in-patients: a prospective analysis of 3695 patient episodes. PLoS One. 2009;4(2):E4439.
21. Doucet J, Chassagne P, Trivalle C, et al. Drug-drug interactions related to hospital admissions in older adults: a prospective study of 1000 patients. J Am Geriatr Soc. 1996;44:944–8.
22. Lindley CM, Tully MP, Paramsothy V, Tallis RC. Inappropriate medication is a major cause of adverse drug reactions in elderly patients. Age Ageing. 1992;21:294–300.

23. Grattagliano I, Portincasa P, D'Ambrosio G, Palmieri VO, Palasciano G. Avoiding drug interactions: here's help. J Fam Pract. 2010;59:322–9.
24. IUPHAR. Pharmacology Education Project. Drug interactions. https://www.pharmacologyeducation.org/clinical-pharmacology/drug-interactions. Accessed 31 Jan 2021.
25. Aronson JK. Medication errors: what they are, how they happen, and how to avoid them. QJM. 2009;102(8):513–21. https://doi.org/10.1093/qjmed/hcp052.
26. Lisby M, Nielsen LP, Brock B, Mainz J. How are medication errors defined? A systematic literature review of definitions and characteristics. Int J Qual Health Care. 2010;22:507–18.
27. National Coordinating Council for Medication Error Reporting and Prevention. What is a medication error? New York, NY: National Coordinating Council for Medication Error Reporting and Prevention; 2015. http://www.nccmerp.org/about-medication-errors. Accessed 31 Jan 2021.
28. Ferner RE, Aronson JK. Clarification of terminology in medication errors: definitions and classification. Drug Saf. 2006;29:1011.
29. Aronson JK. Medication errors. Focus Farmacovigilanza. 2008;53(9):1.
30. Vogel U, van Stekelenborg J, Dreyfus B, Garg A, Habib M, Hosain R, Wisniewski A. Investigating overlap in signals from EVDAS, FAERS, and VigiBase®. Drug Saf. 2020;43:351. https://doi.org/10.1007/s40264-019-00899-y.
31. Candore G, Juhlin K, Manlik K, Thakrar B, Quarcoo N, Seabroke S, et al. Comparison of statistical signal detection methods within and across spontaneous reporting databases. Drug Saf. 2015;38(6):577–87.
32. EFPIA. Report to the EMA: joint industry position paper on current challenges and experiences with signal detection in EudraVigilance with proposal for the future. Brussels: EFPIA Pharmacovigilance Expert Group; 2019.
33. Ackroyd-Stolarz S, Hartnell N, Mackinnon NJ. Demystifying medication safety: making sense of the terminology. Res Social Adm Pharm. 2006;2(2):280–9. https://doi.org/10.1016/j.sapharm.2006.01.001.
34. Otero MJ, Schmitt E. Clarifying terminology for adverse drug events. Ann Intern Med. 2005;142:77.
35. Nebeker JR, Barach P, Samore MH. Clarifying adverse drug events: a clinician's guide to terminology, documentation and reporting. Ann Intern Med. 2004;140:795–801.
36. Yu KH, Nation RL, Dooley MJ. Multiplicity of medication safety terms, definitions and functional meanings: when is enough? Qual Saf Health Care. 2005;14:358–63.
37. Bürkle T, Müller F, Patapovas A, et al. A new approach to identify, classify and count drug-related events. Br J Clin Pharmacol. 2013;76(Suppl 1):56–68. https://doi.org/10.1111/bcp.12189.
38. Bates DW, Leape LL, Petrycki S. Incidence and preventability of adverse drug events in hospitalized adults. J Gen Intern Med. 1993;8:289–94.
39. Aronson JK, Ferner RE. Clarification of terminology in drug safety. Drug Saf. 2005;28:851–70.
40. Clinical safety data management: definitions and standards for expedited reporting. London: European Agency for the Evaluation of Medicinal Products, Human Medicines Evaluation Unit; 1995. www.emea.eu.int/pdfs/human/ich/037795en.pdf. Accessed 31 Jan 2021.
41. Dal Pan DJ, Lindquist M, Gelperin K. Postmarketing spontaneous pharmacovigilance reporting system. In: Storm BL, Kimmel SE, Hennessy S, editors. Pharmacoepidemiology, vol. 6. Wiley; 2020. p. 169–203.
42. Schaaf T, Van der Lucas DA, Hale AR, editors. Near miss reporting as a safety tool. Oxford: Butterworth-Heinemann; 1991.
43. US FDA. Guideline for postmarketing reporting of adverse drug experiences. Rockville, MD; 1992. https://www.fda.gov/media/83280/download. Accessed 31 Jan 2021.
44. Horn JR, Hansten PD, Chan LN. Proposal for a new tool to evaluate drug interaction cases. Ann Pharmacother. 2007;41(4):674–80. https://doi.org/10.1345/aph.1H423.
45. Turabian JL. Approach to the epidemiology of drug interactions in primary health care. Epidemol Int J. 2019;3(2):000126.

46. Nguyen JK, Fouts MM, Kotabe SE, Lo E. Polypharmacy as a risk factor for adverse drug reactions in geriatric nursing home residents. Am J Geriatr Pharmacother. 2006;4:36–41.
47. Leendertse AJ, Egberts AC, Stoker LJ, van den Bemt PM. Frequency of and risk factors for preventable medication-related hospital admissions in The Netherlands. Arch Intern Med. 2008;168:1890–6.
48. Viktil KK, Blix HS, Moger TA, Reikvam A. Polypharmacy as commonly defined is an indicator of limited value in the assessment of drug-related problems. Br J Clin Pharmacol. 2007;63:187–95.
49. May FE, Stewart RB, Cluff LE. Drug interactions and multiple drug administration. Clin Pharmacol Ther. 1977;22:322–8.
50. Goldberg RM, Mabee J, Chan L, Wong S. Drug-drug and drug-disease interactions in the ED: analysis of a high-risk population. Am J Emerg Med. 1996;14:447–50.
51. Bjerrum L, Lopez-Valcarcel BG, Petersen G. Risk factors for potential drug interactions in general practice. Eur J Gen Pract. 2008;14(1):23–9. https://doi.org/10.1080/13814780701815116.
52. Watanabe JH, McInnis T, Hirsch JD. Cost of prescription drug-related morbidity and mortality. Ann Pharmacother. 2018;52(9):829–37. https://doi.org/10.1177/1060028018765159.

11 Types of Drug Interactions

Martina Smolić, Kristina Bojanić, Kristina Duspara, and Sonja Vukadin

Due to easy access to numerous medicines and widely prevalent polypharmacy, the harm caused by drug-drug interactions and unsafe healthcare systems has grown to be a significant global health issue [1]. Although there is no consensus definition for polypharmacy, it can be defined as concurrent use of multiple medications, often routine use of five or more medications. This includes over-the-counter, prescription and/or traditional and complementary medicines [2].

M. Smolić (✉) · S. Vukadin
Department of Pharmacology, Faculty of Medicine, J. J. Strossmayer University of Osijek, Osijek, Croatia

Department of Pharmacology and Biochemistry, Faculty of Dental Medicine and Health Osijek, J. J. Strossmayer University of Osijek, Osijek, Croatia
e-mail: martina.smolic@mefos.hr; martina.smolic@fdmz.hr; sonja.sarcevic@mefos.hr; sonja.vukadin@fdmz.hr

K. Bojanić
Department of Biophysics and Radiology, Faculty of Dental Medicine and Health Osijek, J. J. Strossmayer University of Osijek, Osijek, Croatia

Department of Biophysics and Radiology, Faculty of Medicine Osijek, J. J. Strossmayer University of Osijek, Osijek, Croatia

Department of Radiology, University Hospital Center Osijek, Osijek, Croatia
e-mail: kristina.bojanic@fdmz.hr; kristina.bojanic@mefos.hr; kristina.bojanic@dzo.hr

K. Duspara
Department of Pharmacology, Faculty of Medicine, J. J. Strossmayer University of Osijek, Osijek, Croatia

Department of Pharmacology and Biochemistry, Faculty of Dental Medicine and Health Osijek, J. J. Strossmayer University of Osijek, Osijek, Croatia

Public Health Institution, Tuzla, Bosnia and Herzegovina
e-mail: kristina.duspara@fdmz.hr; kristina.duspara@mefos.hr

M. Banić, D. Erceg (eds.), *Drug Interactions in Gastroenterology*, Clinical Gastroenterology, https://doi.org/10.1007/978-3-031-69800-2_11

It is important to empasize the difference between adequate and inadequate polypharmacy [3]. If patients benefit from multiple medications prescribed based on the best available evidence (e.g., secondary prevention of myocardial infarction with beta-blockers in combination with statins, an antiplatelet agent or/and ACE inhibitor), this can be defined as adequate polypharmacy. In contrast, inadequate polypharmacy can be defined as the unreasonable prescribing of numerous medicines exposing patients to a high risk of adverse events [1, 3].

Polypharmacy, which is common in elderly patients, increases the risk of drug-drug interactions substantially [4]. *Drug-drug interaction* is a change in the effect of one drug (enhancing or decreasing the effect) with simultaneous or earlier administration of another drug [5]. Drug-drug interactions are oftentimes intentionally provoked in the treatment of certain conditions, such as tuberculosis and other complex infections, hypertension or bronchial asthma in order to achieve a cumulative effect, but drug interactions can also cause adverse events or reduce the therapeutic effect itself. Such modification of drug activity may be a result of pharmacokinetic changes, pharmacodynamical changes or a combination of both [6]. Pharmacokinetic interaction, in general, can be described as a change in the metabolic process of a drug at the level of absorption, distribution, metabolism or excretion (*ADME*) [5]. Pharmacodynamic interactions are defined as additive, synergistic or antagonistic [5].

In a long list of drug interactions, clinically significant are mostly those of the drugs with the following characteristics:

1. Narrow therapeutic window (a small reduction in plasma concentration leads to the loss of therapeutic effect, while its increase leads to toxic effect).
2. Exponential concentration-response curve (a small change in drug concentration leads to an exponential change in its effect).
3. Significant first-pass metabolism. Induction or inhibition of enzymes involved in first-pass metabolism can significantly alter the drug's plasma concentration and clinical effect.
4. Simple eliminatory mechanism through cytochrome metabolism or renal clearance which can be affected by another drug and lead to an increase of drug concentration in plasma [7].

Pharmacokinetic Interactions

Pharmacokinetic drug interactions are the results of modification in the absorption, distribution, metabolism or elimination of a drug.

Drug-Drug Interactions Due to Changes in Absorption

Agents that can affect gastrointestinal absorption of another drug are drugs that are absorbed from a large surface, agents with the tendency to bind or to produce chelated compounds (e.g., resins, antacids and calcium-containing food), agents altering gastric pH (Proton Pump Inhibitors-PPIs) and gastrointestinal motility (e.g., metoclopramide or antimuscarinics) or agents affecting transport proteins such as P-glycoprotein and organic anion transporters in the intestine.

In order to understand the process of absorption better, it is necessary to distinguish between the velocity of absorption and the degree of absorption. A decrease in the velocity of absorption usually does not lead to a clinically significant decrease in drug bioavailability, unlike a reduction in the degree of absorption which can result in subtherapeutic drug plasma concentration. Similarly, an increase in the extent of absorption can lead to drug toxicity. By increasing gastric pH, antacids decrease the gastrointestinal absorption of digoxin, ketoconazole, quinolone antibiotics and tetracyclines.

Clinicians need to advise their patients not to take calcium-containing food or beverages (e.g., milk or mineral water) with tetracyclines, quinolones, levothyroxine, or bisphosphonates due to formation of complexes. Ca^{2+} can slow down and inhibit their absorption [4].

P-glycoprotein (P-gp, ABCB1) is a multidrug resistance transporter expressed in tissue barriers of many organs, such as the placenta, liver, kidney, intestine, blood-brain barrier, testis, lymphocytes and tumor cells, where it influences net absorption of drugs [4]. Certain drugs act as P-gp inducers, e.g., St. John's wort extract (hyperforin), antiretroviral drug (efavirenz) or anticonvulsants (phenobarbital, phenytoin, carbamazepine and primidone), whereas other drugs are its inhibitors, e.g., antimycotics (itraconazole and ketoconazole), macrolide antibiotics (erythromycin and claritromycin) and antiarrhythmic drugs (amiodarone, propafenone and quinidine). Their concomitant use may result in absorption changes of a particular drug [4].

Reduced subcutaneous drug-drug interactions due to changes in absorption can be induced by simultaneous application of vasoconstrictor. This principle is used in local anesthetic applications by adding adrenaline in order to restrict lidocaine absorption and in that way prolonging its effect on a tissue. A similar effect can be provoked by the addition of a cardiac depressant with a consequent decrease in tissue perfusion (e.g., β blockers) [6].

Drug Interactions Due to Changes in Drug Distribution and Binding

A change in drug-drug interactions due to changes in absorption distribution can be a result of competition for binding sites on plasma proteins, drug displacement from tissue binding sites or changes in tissue barriers such as inhibition of P-glycoprotein in the blood-brain barrier.

Good examples of drug-drug interactions based on plasma protein binding site competition are methotrexate, warfarin, phenytoin and sulfonylureas which all can be displaced by sulfonamides from their binding sites on albumin. Salicylates and other nonsteroidal anti-inflammatory drugs (NSAIDs) can displace oral anticoagulants and oral antidiabetics.

Drug distribution changes occur when one medicine modulates the compartment in which another medicine is distributed. An example of this kind of interaction is the administration of a diuretic which by reducing intravascular volume increases lithium and aminoglycoside concentration in plasma and can lead to their toxic effects [6].

Drug-Drug Interactions Due to Changes in Metabolic Clearance

Drug-drug interactions due to changes in metabolic clearance are the result of concurrent administration of a drug inductor or inhibitor of metabolizing enzymes in the liver, predominantly cytochrome P450 isoenzymes (CYP450) with another drug. This kind of drug-drug interaction is well-documented and has a significant clinical impact. Examples of agents that act as CYP450 *inducers* are barbiturates, carbamazepine, phenytoin, rifampicin, rifabutin, polycyclic hydrocarbons in cigarette smoke and troglitazone. By inducing CYP450, these drugs accelerate the metabolism of other drug substrates of the same CYP450 isoenzime when used simultaneously. On the other hand, examples of CYP450 *inhibitors* are allopurinol, androgens, amiodarone, ciprofloxacin, enoxacin, erythromycin, cimetidine, omeprazole, diltiazem, disulfiram, fluconazole, itraconazole, quinaconazole, miconazole, fluvoxamine, fluoxetine, paroxetine, furanocoumarins in grapefruit juice, isoniazid, metronidazole, mexiletine, ritonavir, verapamil, sulfonamides, zafirlukast zileuton, all of which can cause a significant increase in plasma concentration of drugs metabolized by the same isoenzyme. Higher sensitivity to inhibitory effects is characteristic of CYP3A4, a dominant isoenzyme of CYP450 [6, 8, 9].

Reduced blood flow (e.g., with propranolol use) through the liver can cause a reduction in the clearance of other drugs which are metabolized in the liver, especially drugs with flow-dependent hepatic clearance, such as morphine and verapamil [6].

A modified form of drug-drug interaction based on metabolic clearance is when a certain drug is responsible for impeding the metabolism of an endogenous substance resulting in increased stores of endogenous substances. Administration of another drug can cause extensive endogenous substance release and may have an unexpected action as a result. Sensitization of patients taking monoamine oxidase (MAO) inhibitors to sympathomimetics (e.g., amphetamine and phenylpropanolamine) is a good example of this kind of interaction. Severe hypertensive reaction to regular doses of cold remedies, decongestants and appetite suppressants can lead to severe hypertensive reactions in these patients [6].

Drug-Drug Interactions Due to Changes in Renal Excretion

The excretion of weak acids or weak bases by kidneys can be changed by other drugs that alter urinary pH. Urine acidification increases weak base excretion and decreases weak acid excretion, while urine alkalinisation does the opposite [7]. Administration of acetazolamide can cause neurotoxicity by pursuing weak acid drugs to concentrate in the CNS. In this instance, plasma pH should be increased (e.g., with sodium bicarbonate) to avoid such adverse events [7].

Active secretion into the renal tubules is an important elimination pathway and inhibition of transporters involved in this process can lead to increased serum drug concentrations. Examples of drugs partially eliminated by P-glycoprotein in tubules are digoxin, cyclosporin, dabigatran, colchicine, daunorubicin and tacrolimus. Inhibitors of P-glycoprotein are amiodarone, clarithromycin, erythromicin, ketoconazole, ritonavir and quinidine, and they can increase the plasma concentration of the aforementioned drugs. Another example of such interaction is a reduction of the uricosuric effect of probenecidcaused by salicylates (interaction is likely with more than 1.5 g of salicylate per day) [9]. But also, probenecid can interfere with renal excretion of other weak acids (e.g., penicillin, which in this case, is intentionally used in clinical practice to prolong penicillin plasma half-life) and, in general, with drugs that undergo active tubular secretion [9].

Pharmacodynamic Interactions

Drug interaction in which one drug influences another drug's effects directly [4] and without influencing its pharmacokinetics is called pharmacodynamic drug interaction. Human genome sequencing proved to be very useful in predicting drug effects. A diversity in enzyme system, G proteins and membrane receptors are the cause of individual reactions to drugs [7] and as such can play a role in predisposition to drug interactions too. Pharmacodynamic drug interactions are difficult to investigate because the drug mechanism of action needs to be well-known in order to clarify which drug can reduce or potentiate the effect of another one [4].

Pharmacodynamic drug interactions occur at three different levels: the receptor, signaling pathway or effector level and can result in three different outcomes: additive effect, synergism or antagonism. The additive effect is predictable by simply adding up the effects of the two drugs. An example of this kind of interaction is the simultaneous use of paracetamol and ibuprofen—when taken together, each of them achieves its full effect. On the other hand, an undesirable additive effect is respiratory and CNS depression with concurrent use of opioids and benzodiazepines [10].

When two combined drugs have different mechanisms of action, their simultaneous administration results in either synergism or antagonism [11]. Examples of synergistic drug interaction are combinations of chemotherapeutic agents in the treatment of a complex infection (e.g., infective endocarditis) or malignancy (many treatment protocols include several drugs). In clinical practice, synergistic drug interactions are oftentimes desirable. When two drugs achieve synergistic pharmacological effects, a lower dose of each of them can be used in a particular clinical setting, thereby reducing the side effects [10]. Antagonism is achieved when one drug impedes the pharmacological effect of another one. An example of this is the concurrent use of ibuprofen and acetylsalicylic acid (ASA). The mechanism behind this antagonism is a reversible binding of ibuprofen to COX-1, which prevents ASA from acetylating COX-1. Consequently, inhibition of COX-1-mediated thromboxane A2 synthesis by ASA is prevented, leading to an increased cardiac risk in patients with known cardiovascular disease [4].

Many of the commonly used medications interact with a wide range of other medications, and this needs to be kept in mind when adding a new medicine to a patient's existing therapeutic regimen (Table 11.1).

Table 11.1 Some clinically relevant interactions [5, 6, 9]

Drug	Clinically documented interactions
Antacids	Atazanavir: ↓ gastrointestinal absorption
	Indinavir: ↓ gastrointestinal absorption
	Digoksin: ↓ gastrointestinal absorption
	Iron: gastrointestinal absorption with calcium-containing antacids
	Itraconazole: ↓ gastrointestinal absorption
	Ketoconazole: ↓ gastrointestinal absorption
	Quinolones: ↓ gastrointestinal absorption
	Salicylates: only at high doses of salicylate, the renal clearance of salicylate could be reduced as a result of increased urine pH
	Tetracyclines: ↓ gastrointestinal absorption
	Thyroxine: gastrointestinal absorption
	General instruction: to be used 2 h apart from other drugs
Anticoagulants oral	Acetaminophen: ↑ effect of anticoagulants
	Acetylsalicylic acid: bleeding (from the stomach) [6]
	Aminogluthimide: ↑ anticoagulant metabolism
	Amiodarone: ↓ elimination of anticoagulants
	Antibiotics: ↑ warfarin levels [6]
	Antifungals (azole): e.g., ketoconazole, itraconazole, voriconazole or posaconazole are ↓ apixaban, dabigatran, edoxaban, rivaroxaban and potential elimination of warfarin
	Barbiturates: ↑ anticoagulant metabolism
	Carbamazepine: ↑ anticoagulant elimination
	Cimetidine: ↓ warfarin levels
	Clopidogrel: ↓ warfarin levels
	Disulfiram: ↓ warfarin levels
	Efavirenz: ↓ warfarin levels
	Fluconazole: ↓ warfarin levels
	Fluoxetine: ↓ warfarin levels
	Gemfibrozil: not specified
	Lovastatin: ↓ warfarin levels
	Macrolides: ↓ caused by clarithromycin and erythromycin
	Metronidazole: ↓ warfarin levels
	Miconazole: ↓ warfarin levels
	NSAIDs: ↓ platelet function and gastrointestinal erosions
	Propafenone: ↓ elimination of anticoagulants
	Quinidine: ↓ apixaban, dabigatran, edoxaban and rivaroxaban system of elimination
	Ritonavir:: ↓ apixaban, dabigatran, edoxaban and rivaroxaban system of elimination
	Salicylates: ↓ platelet only with acetylsalicylic acid
	Simvastatin: ↓ warfarin metabolism
	Sulfonamides: ↓ inhibition of warfarin
	Trimethoprim-sulfamethoxazole: ↓ warfarin metabolism
	Verapamil: ↓ apixaban, dabigatran, edoxaban and rivaroxaban
	Phenytoin: ↑ anticoagulant metabolism
	Primidone: ↑ anticoagulant metabolism
	Rifabutin: ↑ elimination of oral anticoagulants
	Rifampin: ↑ elimination of oral anticoagulants
	Steroids (anabolic): ↑ effect of anticoagulants
	St. John's wort: ↑ elimination of oral anticoagulants

(continued)

Table 11.1 (continued)

Drug	Clinically documented interactions
Azole antifungals	*Drugs that may have effect on azole antifungals*:
	Barbiturates: ↑ metabolism of itraconazole and ketoconazole
	H2-receptor antagonists: ↓ metabolism of itraconazole and ketoconazole
	Proton pump inhibitors: ↓ absorption of itraconazole and ketoconazole
	Rifampin: ↑ metabolism of itraconazole, ketoconazole and voriconazole
	Effect of azole antifungals on other drugs:
	Carbamazepine: ↓ metabolism of carbamazepine
	Cisapride: ↓ metabolism of cisapride, possible occurrence of ventricular arrhythmias
	Cyclosporine: ↓ metabolism of cyclosporine
	HMG-CoA reductase inhibitors: ↓ metabolism of statins
	Opioid analgesics: ↓ elimination of alfentanil, fentanyl, methadone, oxycodone and sufentanil
	Phenytoin: ↓ metabolism of phenytoin using fluconazole, probably the same effect as voriconazole
	Pimozide: ↓ metabolism of pimozide
Bile acid-binding resins	Acetaminophen: ↓ gastrointestinal absorption
	Digitalis glycosides: ↓ gastrointestinal absorption (possibly also digoxin)
	Furosemide: ↓ gastrointestinal absorption
	Methotrexate: ↓ gastrointestinal absorption
	Mycophenolate: ↓ gastrointestinal absorption
	Thiazide diuretics: ↓ gastrointestinal absorption
	Thyroid hormones: ↓ thyroid absorption
Barbiturates	Antivirals: ↑ metabolism of antivirals amprenavir, atazanavir, boceprevir, darunavir, delavirdine, fosamprenavir, indinavir, nelfinavir, ritonavir, saquinavir, simeprevir and telaprevir with barbiturates
	β-Blockers: ↑ metabolism of β-blockers
	Calcium channel blockers: ↑ metabolism calcium channel blockers
	CNS depressants: additive depression effect on central nervous system
	Corticosteroids: ↑ metabolism of corticosteroids
	Doxycycline: ↑ doxycycline metabolism
	Estrogens: ↑ estrogen metabolism
	Kinase inhibitors: ↑ metabolism of kinase inhibitors
	Opioid analgesics: ↑ elimination of alfentanil, fentanyl, methadone, oxycodone and sufentanil
	Phenobarbital: ↓ phenobarbital's effect (e.g., propranolol, quinidine and cyclosporine) [9]
	Phenothiazine: ↑ phenothiazine metabolism
	Phenytoin: ↑ phenytoin metabolism
	Quinidine: ↑ quinidine metabolism
	Valproic acid: ↓ phenobarbital metabolism

(continued)

Table 11.1 (continued)

Drug	Clinically documented interactions
β-Blockers	*Drugs with possible ↑ β-blocker effect*:
	Amiodarone: ↓ β-blockers metabolism via CYP2D6 (*)
	Cimetidine: ↓ β-blockers metabolism primarily cleared via the liver (propranolol). There is lesser effect or no effect on those β-blockers cleared via kidneys
	Diphenhydramine: ↓ β-blockers metabolism via CYP2D6 (*)
	Haloperidol: ↓ metabolism of β-blockers metabolized by CYP2D6 (*)
	Quinidine: ↓ metabolism of β-blockers metabolized by CYP2D6 (*)
	Selective serotonin reuptake inhibitors (SSRIs): some SSRIs (fluoxetine and paroxetine) inhibit CYP2D6 and result in ↑ concentrations of some β-blockers (*)
	Terbinafine: ↓ metabolism of β-blockers metabolized by CYP2D6 (*)
	*Carvedilol, metoprolol, nebivolol, propranolol and timolol
	Drugs that may ↓ β-blocker effect:
	Nonsteroidal anti-inflammatory drugs (NSAIDs): indomethacin and other prostaglandin inhibitors ↓ antihypertensive effects
	Enzyme inducers: phenytoin, barbiturates and rifampicin ↑ metabolism of β-blockers
Calcium channel blockers	*Drugs with possible effects on calcium channel blockers*:
	Cimetidine: ↓ calcium channel blockers metabolism
	Carbamazepine: ↑ calcium channel blockers metabolism, also ↓ metabolism of carbamazepine using diltiazem and verapamil
	Kinase inhibitors: ↓ calcium channel blockers metabolism with ceritinib, dasatinib, imatinib, idelalisib and lapatinib. Also ↓ metabolism of kinase inhibitors by diltiazem, nicardipine and verapamil
	Macrolide antibiotics: ↓ metabolism of calcium channel blockers with macrolide antibiotics
	Phenytoin: ↑ metabolism of calcium channel blockers
	Rifampin: ↑ metabolism of calcium channel blockers
	Effects of calcium channel blockers (diltiazem, nicardipine and verapamil) on other drugs:
	Cyclosporine: ↓ elimination of cyclosporine
	Sirolimus: ↓ elimination of sirolimus
	Statins: ↓ elimination of statins
	Tacrolimus: ↓ tacrolimus elimination
	Theophylline: ↓ theophylline metabolism

(continued)

Table 11.1 (continued)

Drug	Clinically documented interactions
Carbamazepine	*Possible effects of carbamazepine on other drugs*:
	Corticosteroids: ↑ corticosteroid metabolism
	Estrogens: ↑ metabolism of estrogens
	Haloperidol: ↑ metabolism of haloperidol
	Sirolimus: ↑ metabolism of sirolimus
	Tacrolimus: ↑ metabolism of tacrolimus
	Theophylline: ↑ metabolism of theophylline
	Possible effects of other drugs on carbamazepine:
	Amiodarone and dronedarone: ↑ metabolism of amiodarone and dronedarone, also ↓ metabolism of carbamazepine
	Antivirals: amprenavir, atazanavir, boceprevir, darunavir, delavirdine, fosamprenavir, indinavir, nelfinavir, ritonavir, saquinavir, simeprevir and telaprevir ↓ metabolism of carbamazepine. Also ↑ metabolism of antivirals by carbamazepine
	Cimetidine: ↓ metabolism of carbamazepine
	Cyclosporine: possible ↓ metabolism of carbamazepine. Also ↑ cyclosporine metabolism
	Danazol: ↓ metabolism of carbamazepine
	Fluvoxamine: ↓ metabolism of carbamazepine
	Isoniazid: ↓ carbamazepine metabolism
	Macrolide antibiotics: ↓ carbamazepine metabolism
	Nefazodone: ↓ carbamazepine metabolism
	Rifampin: ↑ carbamazepine metabolism
	Selective serotonin reuptake inhibitors (SSRIs): fluoxetine and fluvoxamine ↓ carbamazepine metabolism
	St. John's wort: ↑ metabolism of carbamazepine
Cimetidine	Benzodiazepines: ↓ metabolism of some benzodiazepines, excluded: lorazepam, oxazepam and temazepam
	Carmustine: ↑ suppression of bone marrow
	Lidocaine: ↓ metabolism of lidocaine
	Phenytoin: ↓ phenytoin metabolism
	Procainamide: ↓ renal excretion of procainamide
	Quinidine: ↓ metabolism of quinidine
	Theophylline: ↓ theophylline metabolism
Cisapride	Macrolide antibiotics: clarithromycin and erythromycin ↓ cisapride metabolism, possible ventricular arrhythmias
	Amiodarone and dronedaron: ↓ cisapride metabolism
	Antiviral: ritonavir ↓ cisapride metabolism
	Cobicistat: ↓ metabolism of cisapride
	Conivaptan: ↓ metabolism of cisapride
	Cyclosporine: ↓ metabolism of cisapride

(continued)

Table 11.1 (continued)

Drug	Clinically documented interactions
Cyclosporine	Aminoglycosides: probability of nephrotoxicity
	Amphotericin B: probability of nephrotoxicity
	Cidofovir: possible additive nephrotoxicity
	Statins: ↓ metabolism of statins. Myopathy and rhabdomyolysis were noted in patients taking statins and cyclosporine
	Drugs that may increase the cyclosporine effect:
	Amiodarone and dronedarone: ↓ cyclosporine elimination
	Androgens: ↑ serum cyclosporine concentration
	Antiviral ritonavir: ↓ metabolism of cyclosporine
	Kinase inhibitors: ↓ metabolism of cyclosporine with ceritinib, dasatinib, imatinib, idelalisib and lapatinib. Cyclosporine ↓ metabolism of kinase inhibitors
	Macrolide antibiotics: clarithromycin and erythromycin ↓ metabolism of cyclosporine
	Nefazodone: ↓ cyclosporine metabolism
	Drugs that may decrease the cyclosporine effect:
	Bosentan: ↑ cyclosporine elimination
	Dexamethasone: ↑ cyclosporine metabolism
	Efavirenz: ↑ cyclosporine metabolism
	Etravirine: ↑ cyclosporine metabolism
	Nevirapine: ↑ cyclosporine metabolism
	Phenytoin: ↑ cyclosporine metabolism
	Rifampin: ↑ cyclosporine elimination
	Kinase inhibitors: ↓ metabolism of cisapride with ceritinib, dasatinib, imatinib, idelalisib and lapatinib
	Selective serotonin reuptake inhibitors (SSRIs): fluvoxamine ↓ cisapride metabolism
	St. John's wort: ↑ cyclosporine elimination
Estrogens	Ampicillin: impaired enterohepatic estrogen circulation, possible ↓ in efficacy as an oral contraceptive. Similar effect to some other oral antibiotics
	Corticosteroids: ↓ corticosteroid metabolism (increased corticosteroid effect). Dexamethasone may ↑ estrogen metabolism
	Griseofulvin: possible ↓ in efficacy as an oral contraceptive by an unknown mechanism
	Phenytoin: ↑ metabolism of estrogen, possible ↓ in efficacy as an oral contraceptive
	Primidone: ↑ metabolism of estrogen, possible ↓ in efficacy as an oral contraceptive
	Rifabutin: ↑ metabolism of estrogen, possible ↓ in efficacy as an oral contraceptive
	Rifampin: ↑ metabolism of estrogen, possible ↓ in efficacy as an oral contraceptive
	St. John's wort: ↑ metabolism of estrogen, ↓ in efficacy as an oral contraceptive

(continued)

Table 11.1 (continued)

Drug	Clinically documented interactions
HMG-CoA reductase inhibitors (statins)	Amiodarone and dronedarone: ↓ statins metabolism
	Antivirals (ritonavir) ↓ statins metabolism
	Bosentan: ↑ statin metabolism
	Carbamazepine: ↑ statins metabolism
	Clofibrate: ↑ risk of myopathy
	Cobicistat: ↓ statins metabolism
	Conivaptan: ↓ statins metabolism
	Cyclosporine: ↓ statins metabolism, ↑ risk of myopathy
	Kinase inhibitors: ↓ statins metabolism by ceritinib, dasatinib, imatinib, idelalisib and lapatinib
	Macrolide antibiotics: ↓ statins elimination and metabolism
	Nefazodone: ↓ statin metabolism
	Phenytoin: ↑ statin metabolism
	Rifampin: ↑ statin metabolism
	St. John's wort: ↑ statin metabolism
Iron	Methyldopa: ↓ methyldopa absorption
	Mycophenolate: ↓ mycophenolate absorption
	Quinolones: ↓ absorption of ciprofloxacin and other quinolones
	Tetracyclines: ↓ absorption of tetracyclines, decreased efficacy of iron
	Thyroid hormones: ↓ thyroxine absorption
MAOIs (monoamine oxidase inhibitors)	Anorexiants: ↓ hypotensive effect (e.g., combining with benzphetamine, diethylpropion, mazindol, phendimetrazine or phentermine)
	Antidiabetics: ↓ hypoglycemic, but additive effect
	Dextromethorphan: lethal effects (hyperpyrexia, coma)
	Mirtazepin: avoid use
	Nefazodone: avoid use
	Opioid analgesics: ↑ hypertension, excitation or rigidity
	Phenylephrine: ↓ hypotensive effect
	SSRIs: avoid use
	Sibutramine: avoid use
	Sympathomimetics: ↑ hypertensive effect
	Tramadol: avoid use
	Venlafaxine: avoid use
Nonsteroidal anti-inflammatory drugs (NSAIDs)	ACE inhibitors (ACEIs): ↓ antihypertensive response
	Acetylsalicylic acid: avoid concurrent use with ibuprofen due to ↓ ASA effect
	Angiotensin II receptor blockers (ARBs): ↓ antihypertensive effect
	Antidepressants (e.g., citalopram): bleeding in the gastrointestinal tract [10]
	Antihypertensives: ↑ blood pressure [6]
	Furosemide: ↓ diuretic, antihypertensive and natriuretic effect of furosemide
	Hydralazine: ↓ antihypertensive effect of hydralazine
	Methotrexate: possibly ↑ toxicity of methotrexate (primarily at anticancer doses of methotrexate)
	Selective serotonin reuptake inhibitors (SSRIs): ↑ risk of bleeding due to platelet inhibition
	Triamterene: concomitant use of triamterene and indomethacin could ↓ renal function not only in patients but also in healthy subjects

(continued)

Table 11.1 (continued)

Drug	Clinically documented interactions
Paracetamol (acetaminophen)	Phenytoin: ↓ the effectiveness of paracetamol. ↑ risk of hepatotoxicity
	Isoniazid: ↑ risk of hepatotoxicity
	Carbamazepine: ↑ risk of hepatotoxicity
	Warfarin: increasing the risk of bleeding at a dose >2 g/day
	Zidovudine: possible onset of neutropenia, hepatotoxicity
Probenecid	Clofibrate: ↓ glucuronide conjugation of clofibric acid
	Methotrexate: ↓ renal methotrexate excretion, possible methotrexate toxicity
	Pralatrexate: ↓ renal pralatrexate excretion, possible pralatrexate toxicity
	Penicillin: ↓ renal penicillin excretion
	Salicylates: ↓ uricosuric effect of probenecid (probability of interaction with more than 1.5 g of salicylate daily)
Salicylates	Carbonic anhydrase inhibitors: ↑ acetazolamide serum concentrations; ↑ salicylate toxicity due to decreased blood pH
	Corticosteroids: ↑ salicylate elimination, possible additive toxic effect on gastric mucosa
	Heparin: concomitant use of aspirin ↑ bleeding tendency, other salicylates are excluded
	Methotrexate: ↓ renal methotrexate clearance, increases methotrexate toxicity (particularly using anticancer doses)
	Selective serotonin reuptake inhibitors (SSRIs): ↑ risk of bleeding due to platelet inhibition
Theophylline	Beta-blockers: ↓ theophylline bronchodilation effect, especially with noncardioselective β-blockers
	Macrolide antibiotics: clarithromycin and erythromycin ↓ theophylline metabolism
	Smoking: ↑ metabolism of theophylline
	Tacrine: ↓ metabolism of theophylline
	Ticlopidine: ↓ metabolism of theophylline
	Zileuton: ↓ metabolism of theophylline

Combined Interactions

Drug interaction at any level must be taken seriously. Creating a list of pharmacodynamic and pharmacokinetic drug interactions and involving those results in electronic prescribing systems is one way to prevent such adverse clinical outcomes [4]. Taking two or more drugs with toxic effects on the same organ, e.g., nephrotoxic drugs, results in an additive effect and can cause severe side effects even when subdosing drugs [5]. In practice, combined drug interactions are rare (3–5% clinically significant), but this percentage can become higher in polypharmacy [5].

Interactions of Herbal Medication with Other Drugs

Herbal products can lead to clinically important interactions (Table 11.2). See more in Chap. 14, "Interactions of Drugs and Herbs in Gastroenterology".

Ginkgo biloba can cause bleeding, especially with the concurrent use of acetylsalicylic acid and oral anticoagulants [5, 12].

Table 11.2 Serious clinical interactions of herbal products containing St. John's wort and certain drugs [5, 6, 9]

Drug	Clinically documented interactions
Anticonvulsants (e.g., carbamazepine, phenobarbiton and fenitoin)	↓ Serum levels of anticonvulsants
Anticoagulants—oral (e.g., warfarin)	↓ Serum levels of oral anticoagulants
Cyclosporine	↓ Serum levels cyclosporine, higher risk of an implant rejection
Digoxin	↓ Serum levels of digoxin
HIV-protease inhibitors (e.g., indinavir, ritonavir, saquinavir and nelfinavir)	↓ Serum levels of HIV-protease inhibitors, possible ↓ effect in HIV-suppression
Nonnucleoside reverse transcriptase inhibitors (e.g., delavirdine, efavirenz and nevirapine)	↓ Serum levels nonnucleoside reverse transcriptase inhibitors, possible ↓ effect of HIV-suppression
Oral contraceptives	↓ Serum levels of oral contraceptives, possible ↓ contraceptive effect
Serotonin reuptake inhibitors (SSRIs) (e.g., citalopram, fluoxetine, fluvoxamine, paroxetine, sertraline and nefazodone)	Possible ↑ serum levels of SSRIs, ↑ serotonergic effect
Tacrolimus	↓ Serum levels of tacrolimus, higher risk of implant rejection
Triptans (sumatriptan, naratriptan, rizatriptan and zolmitriptan)	Possible ↑ serum levels of triptans, ↑ serotoninergic effect

The active components of *grapefruit juice* (furanocoumarins that inhibit CYP 3A4 and some other unknown substances that inhibit p-glycoprotein) cause an increase in the plasma concentration of macrolide antibiotics, terfenadine, midazolam, triazolam, felodipine, nifedipine, nimodipine, ethinylestradiol, cyclosporine and statins [5, 13].

St. John's wort (*Hypericum perforatum*) leads to clinically important interactions with a number of drugs. A marker of standardization for currently marketed products of St. John's wort was thought to be hypericin. Recent studies suggest that hyperforin is the major ingredient responsible for CYP and P-gp-inducing activity of St. John's wort. The interactions may be pharmacokinetic, accelerating metabolism (inducing cytochrome P-450 isoenzymes in the liver, especially CYP 3A4, but also 1A2 and 2C9 as well as P-gp) and pharmacodynamic (serotonin reuptake inhibitors and migraine treatment drugs) [13, 14]. Case reports involving the use of St. John's wort have shown that herbal medication containing St. John's wort could have serious clinical interactions with several groups of traditional drugs such as anticonvulsants, oral anticoagulants, immunosuppressants, oral contraceptives, anticancer and cardiovascular drugs [16]. Studies suggest that concurrent use of the herb resulted in subtherapeutic levels of digoxin, oral contraceptives, cyclosporine, HIV protease and nonnucleoside reverse transcriptase inhibitors, warfarin, irinotecan, theophylline and anticonvulsants, which in several cases resulted in life-threatening events [15].

References

1. WHO. Medication safety in polypharmacy. WHO; 2019.
2. Masnoon N, et al. What is polypharmacy? A systematic review of definitions. BMC Geriatr. 2017;17(1):230.
3. Scottish Government Model of Care Polypharmacy Working Group. Polypharmacy guidance. 2nd ed. Edinburgh: Scottish Government; 2015.
4. Cascorbi I. Drug interactions—principles, examples and clinical consequences. Dtsch Arztebl Int. 2012;109(33–34):546–55; quiz 556.
5. Francetic I, Vitezić D. Clinical pharmacology. 2nd ed. Zagreb: Medicinska Naklada; 2014.
6. Katzung BG, Kruidering-Hall M, Trevor AJ. Katzung & Trevor's pharmacology: examination & board review. 12th ed. Adobe Garamond Pro by Cenveo® Publisher Services.
7. James R, et al. Rang & Dale's pharmacology. 9th ed. Elsevier; 2019.
8. Tannenbaum C, Sheehan NL. Understanding and preventing drug-drug and drug-gene interactions. Expert Rev Clin Pharmacol. 2014;7(4):533–44.
9. Katzung BG. Basic & clinical pharmacology. 14th ed. McGraw-Hill Education; 2017.
10. Cokol M, et al. Systematic exploration of synergistic drug pairs. Mol Syst Biol. 2011;7:544.
11. van den Berg JP, et al. Pharmacokinetic and pharmacodynamic interactions in anaesthesia. A review of current knowledge and how it can be used to optimize anaesthetic drug administration. Br J Anaesth. 2017;118(1):44–57.
12. Hoban CL, Byard RW, Musgrave IF. Analysis of spontaneous adverse drug reactions to echinacea, valerian, black cohosh and ginkgo in Australia from 2000 to 2015. J Integr Med. 2019;17(5):338–43.
13. Fasinu PS, Rapp GK. Herbal interaction with chemotherapeutic drugs—a focus on clinically significant findings. Front Oncol. 2019;9:1356.
14. Asher GN, Corbett AH, Hawke RL. Common herbal dietary supplement-drug interactions. Am Fam Physician. 2017;96(2):101–7.
15. Nicolussi S, et al. Clinical relevance of St. John's wort drug interactions revisited. Br J Pharmacol. 2020;177(6):1212–26.
16. Mannel, M. Drug interactions with St John's wort. Drug Safety. 2004;27:773–97. https://doi.org/10.2165/00002018-200427110-00003

Enzymes and Transporters Involved in Drug Interactions

12

Ines Bilić Ćurčić, Vjera Ninčević, Tomislav Kizivat, and Nikola Raguž-Lučić

Drug Interactions in Drug Metabolism

Introduction

Cytochrome P450 (CYP450) superfamily enzymes involved in drug metabolism are classified as phase I metabolism enzymes and are available in above 50 forms: 57 functional genes and 58 pseudogenes, responsible for the metabolism of the

I. Bilić Ćurčić (✉)
Department of Pharmacology, Faculty of Medicine, J. J. Strossmayer University of Osijek, Osijek, Croatia

Department of Endocrinology, University Hospital Center Osijek, Osijek, Croatia
e-mail: ibcurcic@mefos.hr

V. Ninčević
Department of Pharmacology, Faculty of Medicine, J. J. Strossmayer University of Osijek, Osijek, Croatia

Department of Pharmacology and Biochemistry, Faculty of Dental Medicine and Health, J. J. Strossmayer University of Osijek, Osijek, Croatia
e-mail: vnincevic@mefos.hr; vnincevic@fdmz.hr

T. Kizivat
Clinical Institute of Nuclear Medicine and Radiation Protection, University Hospital Center Osijek, Osijek, Croatia

Department for Nuclear Medicine and Oncology, Faculty of Medicine, Josip Juraj Strossmayer University of Osijek, Osijek, Croatia
e-mail: tkizivat@mefos.hr

N. Raguž-Lučić
Department of Pharmacology, Faculty of Medicine, J. J. Strossmayer University of Osijek, Osijek, Croatia

Department of Pharmacology and Biochemistry, Faculty of Dental Medicine and Health Osijek, J. J. Strossmayer University of Osijek, Osijek, Croatia

M. Banić, D. Erceg (eds.), *Drug Interactions in Gastroenterology*, Clinical Gastroenterology, https://doi.org/10.1007/978-3-031-69800-2_12

majority of therapeutic drugs (see also Chap. 4). CYP family polymorphisms are the key players in the fate of drugs (see also Chap. 13).

CYP Enzymes

The usual classification of the drug metabolism is presented in phase I reactions (oxidation, reduction and hydrolysis) and phase II conjugation reactions with glutathione, acetylation, glucuronidation, methylation or sulfoconjugation and N-acylation. CYPs predominantly catalyze phase I reactions usually converting the original drug into a more polar metabolite through the introduction or detection of a functional group (-OH, -NH2- and -SH). Since phase I enzymes are involved in the biotransformation of more than 75% of the prescribed drugs, their polymorphisms can significantly affect plasma concentrations and consequently alter drug effects [1–3]. CYPs can be found in the membrane of the endoplasmic reticulum in the liver, as well as in the lung, brain, lymphocytes, kidney, intestine and placenta. The majority of CYP enzymes are primarily located in the centrilobular area of the liver [4], endoplasmic reticulum and mitochondria. The mitochondria enzymes are usually involved in the synthesis of steroids and fatty acids, while enzymes in the endoplasmic reticulum generally metabolize exogenous compounds, primarily drugs and chemicals [2]. Besides drug catabolism, CYPs are also accountable for activation of prodrugs such as cancer therapeutics and antipsychotics The evaluation of the metabolic pathways of a large number of different drugs revealed that about 50% are metabolized by CYP3A4, 20% by CYP2D6, 15% by CYP2C9 and CYP2C19 and the remaining by CYP2E1, CYP2A6 and CYP1A2 [1]. These enzymes are mainly responsible for the deactivation of exogenous chemicals by enhancing the polarity of lipid-soluble substances to become more water-soluble, thus facilitating the excretion of drugs. Many phase I products are not excreted rapidly and therefore undergo phase II metabolism conjugation reactions with glucuronic acid, sulfuric acid or glutathione-binding endogenous substrates such as glucuronic acid, sulfuric acid or amino acids to newly incorporated functional groups forming more water-soluble conjugates than the original metabolite. Enzymes of both metabolism phases exhibit genetic variability contributing to the variable pharmacokinetics, and overall bioavailability of the active substance, affecting drug effectiveness and toxicity. The most important enzymes involved in drug metabolism are CYP2C9, CYP2C19, CYP2D6 and CYP3A4. It should be noted that CYP3A4 alone is responsible for the metabolism of more than 50% of all drugs that are metabolized in the liver, while CYP1A2 and CYP2C9 are included in the metabolism of the most clinically important drugs.

Polymorphisms in cytochrome P450 genes can affect the function of the enzymes altering capacity and velocity of drug metabolism. Depending on a genotype and phenotype, we can differentiate:

- poor metabolizer (PM),
- intermediate metabolizer (IM),

- extensive metabolizer (EM),
- ultrarapid metabolizer (UM).

Phenotyping implicates the administration of a test drug whose metabolism depends only on the enzyme involved, tracked by the evaluation of the metabolic ratio (MR), defined as the ratio of the unaltered medicine to its metabolite measured in urine or serum [2, 3].

Around 59% of drugs investigated in adverse drug reaction (ADR) studies are metabolized by polymorphic phase I enzymes and 86% of them belonging to CYPs, while only 20% of drugs are non-polymorphic enzyme substrates [5].

Genetic polymorphisms can have a major influence on clinical practice and should be considered especially in case of unexpected adverse events. Intermediate and poor metabolizers could be more susceptible to serious side effects due to drug accumulation; however, if a parent drug is in question, efficacy could be lower due to slow metabolism. With the possibility of genotyping for relevant polymorphisms in major drug-metabolizing enzymes, we could predict patients' responses, avoid adverse drug reactions and improve treatment with the ultimate goal of achieving personalized treatment [2].

The CYP2C19 is mainly involved in the metabolism of acidic drugs including clopidogrel, propranolol, omeprazole, diazepam, antidepressants and antiepileptics. The four clinical phenotypes associated with CYP2C19 activity (PM, IM, NM and UM) are closely related to genetic markers that may help to implement individualized therapeutic approaches in determining drug dosage. The specific polymorphisms of the gene encoding CYP2C19-allele *2 and *3 lead to the PM. Previously identified genetic polymorphisms CYP2C19 are mainly the consequences of the single-point mutation. The combined frequency of the *2 and *3 alleles is approximately 95% in Caucasians. Furthermore, CYP2C19 *17 polymorphic allele responsible for enhanced enzyme activity phenotypically may be associated with EM. Genetic variability has an important influence on the activation of clopidogrel prodrugs and the pharmacokinetics of voriconazole with clinically relevant consequences. There are more and more indicators of greater risk of bleeding with clopidogrel in UM due to accelerated drug activation; thus, it is important to perform the testing for the CYP2C19 *17 allele, since its effectiveness may be increased, thereby increasing the risk of bleeding. The study on the metabolism of the proton pump inhibitor (PPI) through the system cytochrome P-450 in the liver has gained importance in recent years. The patients can be classified as poor metabolizers and heterozygous and homozygous extensive metabolizers based on key enzymes involved in the metabolism of these drugs, CYP2C19 and CYP3A4. In gastroenterology, in the treatment of inflammatory bowel disease, one should be particularly aware of possible interactions with methotrexate since PPI can inhibit the secretion and lead to toxicity of said immunosuppressant, which is generally actively secreted in the distal tubules of the kidneys. Therefore, it would be better to replace the IPP with the H2 blocker in those cases. In addition, in homozygous CYP2C19 extensive metabolizers, it is not possible to achieve adequate suppression of gastric acid with the administration of a standard dose of omeprazole and lansoprazole (IPP) [1, 3].

Omeprazole in PMs has a significantly prolonged half-life. In patients, heterozygous for an abnormal *CYP2C19* allele treatment rate for *Helicobacter pylori* infections was significantly improved with concomitant treatment with omeprazole and amoxicillin [6].

The CYP2C9 enzyme is included in the oxidative metabolism of numerous drugs: anticonvulsants, antidiabetics, anticoagulants, antiepileptics, nonsteroidal antirheumatics, antimicrobials and angiotensin II receptor blockers, including tolbutamide, phenytoin, losartan, S-warfarin and nonsteroidal *anti*-inflammatory drugs. Individuals with slow or discontinued CYP2C9 activity may experience toxic side effects (diclofenac and phenytoin) or life-threatening bleeding (warfarin). More than 50 different alleles of the CYP2C9 enzyme are known, and the most important are the alleles *2 and *3 due to their association with reduced drug-substrate metabolism [1, 3].

The enzyme CYP2D6 participates in the hepatic metabolism of around 25% of all drugs used in clinical practice, mainly including basic treatment options such as antidepressants, antipsychotics, beta-blockers and opioid analgesics. The CYP2D6 genetic polymorphism is associated with four types of phenotypes which mutually differ according to the capacity to metabolize the drug, i.e., AM, IM, EM and UM. The gene encoding CYP2D6 is highly polymorphic and more than 95% of the phenotype can be predicted with only nine alleles: the alleles of CYP2D6 *3, *4, *5 and *6 that are nonfunctional alleles; alleles *10, *17 and *41 that have a reduced function and alleles *1 and *2 that are fully functional. Among the most common PM phenotypes, allele *4 is the most frequent one (70%), then allele *5 (26%) and the third one is allele *3 (3%). The alleles *17 and *41 are usually associated with the IM phenotype. It is important to choose adequate alleles to be tested. The recommendation is to pharmacogenetically determine the phenotype of postmenopausal patients treated with tamoxifen. In comparison with NMs CYP2D6, PMs and IMs have reduced endoxifen concentrations leading to an increased risk of breast cancer recurrence and poor survival. In PMs, the current recommendation is to use other hormonal therapies such as aromatase inhibitors [7, 8]. This particular enzyme is also responsible for the O-demethylation conversion of codeine to morphine. NM patients convert enough codeine to morphine in order to achieve the desired analgesic effect. In PM and IM phenotypes, insufficient pain relief is likely to occur, while the patients with UM phenotype are at increased risk of side effects such as drowsiness and respiratory depression due to higher systemic concentrations of morphine. One of the extreme examples of the potential danger of genetic variances was seen in several deaths of infants due to respiratory depression in breastfeeding mothers who were taking codeine, and phenotypically were UM [3].

The enzyme family CYP3A, CYP3A4 and CYP3A5 are involved in the oxidative metabolism of many drugs such as analgesics, antiarrhythmics, anticonvulsants, antihistamines, lipid-lowering drugs, anticancer and antimicrobial drugs, lidocaine, paracetamol, etc. The CYP3A4 predominantly can be found in the enterocytes (82%), followed by CYP2C9 (14%) and other CYPs [9, 10]. The highest expression of CYP3A enzymes is in the duodenum [11]. In some clinical trials, it was shown that inhibition of CYP3A4 by itraconazole and its metabolites enlarged the oral bioavailability of the sedative midazolam in the gut [12]. Inhibition of CYP3A4 by macrolide antibiotic (troleandomycin) increases gut oral bioavailability and area under the curve (AUC) of the opioid drug alfentanil [13]. The CYP3A4 is strongly influenced by environmental factors such as food or smoking and by various medicines taken at the same time, such as azole compounds, antibiotics, antiepileptics and cyclosporine. For example, citruses such as grapefruit already have inhibitory effects on the intestinal level of CYP3A4, but also on the transmitter of the drug, P-glycoprotein. CYP3A5 is active in 3–15% of the white population, while its frequency in Asia is 30% and 65–85% in the African population. The activity of CYP3A5 can overcome drug interactions at the level of CYP3A4 [3].

The variability of CYP gene polymorphisms varies interindividually and depends greatly on ethnicity. Genotyping as part of pharmacogenetics has great potential to optimize treatment efficacy and minimize adverse events of future and current therapeutical modalities.

Drug Interactions in Drug Transporters

Introduction

In order to achieve the therapeutic effect of a drug, several conditions need to be fulfilled. After application and possible metabolic activation, the drug molecules should reach the target site of action, bind to the target molecule and cause a specific action. During this process, a drug passes through the cell membrane governed by the transporters, binds to the receptors, couples with the ending receptors and only then shows pharmacological activity. In the drug delivery process, two major superfamilies of membrane transporters are known as key players: ATP binding cassette (ABC) and solute carrier (SLC) (see also Chap. 4).

Effects on Drug Absorption

Depending on the direction of transfer through the cell membrane, the transporters are divided into transporters that influx or export efflux substrates from cells. Most of the membrane proteins ABC are primary active transporters, utilizing the energy of *adenosine triphosphate* (ATP) binding and hydrolysis enabling the transport of substrates across membranes, either for uptake or export, often against the diffusion gradient. The best-known membrane transmitter in the superfamily ABC is P-glycoprotein (P-gp, ABCB1 gene encoded). The function of transporters, besides the genetic variability, also depends on the concomitant use of other drug-substrates that can inhibit, but also induce their activity, which is crucial in order to predict the potential interaction of concomitant drugs [3]. Drug transporters can be found on the apical and basal membrane surface of the enterocytes. On the apical side of the enterocytes, Pgp and the breast cancer resistance protein (BCRP) are expressed as well as organic anionic transporter polypeptide 1A2 (OATP1A2) [14, 15]. The role of Pgp and BCRP is to mediate the efflux of drugs from the cytosol to the intestinal lumen, while in contrast, 1A2 functions as a drug influx transporter [16–19]. Drug-drug interactions (DDIs) have a great influence on the inhibition and induction of enterocyte transporters, consequently affecting drug absorption. For example, erythromycin inhibition of Pgp decreased the secretion of talinolol (beta receptor antagonist investigated for gastrointestinal motility disorders) in the intestinal lumen and enlarged its oral bioavailability [20]. On the other hand, induction of Pgp by rifampicin leads to reduced oral bioavailability of talinolol [21]. When inhibiting BCRP, also an efflux transporter, the oral bioavailability of drugs could be increased. For example, inhibition of the BCRP by fostamatinib enhanced the oral bioavailability of rosuvastatin [22]. In contrast, influx transporter OATP1A2 shifts drugs from the intestinal lumen to the cytosol and its inhibition by naringin from grapefruit juice leads to a reduction in the oral bioavailability of the fexofenadine [23].

Effects on Drug Distribution

Introduction

Three barriers, blood-brain barrier, placenta, and cancer cell membrane, are different from "normal" tissues in the human body, in part by the expression of specific transporter proteins. This specificity is responsible for the different distribution of drugs across these barriers compared to the distribution in other body tissues and niches. Therefore, site-specific transporter-mediated drug-drug interactions are likely to occur.

Blood-Brain Barrier

The blood-brain barrier is constructed of a lipophilic environment and is highly controlled by tight junctions between endothelial cells which protect CNS from drugs, and other molecules, by preventing paracellular diffusion [24]. To enter, the CNS drugs must be transported by passive diffusion, by active or facilitated transport [25]. Small lipophilic molecules are most likely transported through blood-brain barrier by passive diffusion, while other drugs that do not have those properties must be actively transported by transporter proteins [26]. The blood-cerebrospinal fluid barrier also contains transporter proteins that control the permeability of the choroid plexus membrane to drugs.

Two main superfamilies of transporter proteins ATP-binding cassette (ABC) and solute carrier (SLC) are found on the blood-brain barrier and could have a significant role in altering the pharmacodynamics of drugs to CNS [24]. ABC superfamily consists of predominantly efflux transporters that push molecules out of cells (i.e., P-gp, BCRP and MRP1-MRP6), while the SLC superfamily consists of mostly influx transporters involved in the uptake of molecules to the cell (i.e., OAT, OCT,

OCTN and ENT). The solute carrier superfamily (SLCO) family includes organic anion-transporting polypeptides (i.e., OTP1A2, OATPB1, OATP3A1 and OATP4A1) and L-type amino acid transporter (LAT1) [24].

At the moment, there is limited information on the localization and expression of transport proteins on the blood-brain barrier considering their effect on the pharmacokinetics of CNS active drugs. Modulation of P-gp expressed on the blood-brain barrier can alter distribution characteristics of medications causing either enhancement or reduction of CNS uptake and causing clinically significant drug-drug interaction. Moreover, certain CNS illnesses such as epilepsy or genetic polymorphisms in genes can alter the expression of P-gp on blood-brain barrier. The induction of transporter proteins that mediate the efflux of CNS drugs can result in a considerable reduction of drug concentrations. A similar effect can be caused by inhibition of uptake transporters, i.e., OATP. On the other side, induction of CNS uptake transporters such as OATP or inhibition of efflux proteins such as P-gp can result in higher CNS exposure to drugs causing accumulation and increased adverse effects and potential toxicity [24]. Among the most extensively studied drug-drug interactions on P-gp proteins is the Non-steroidal anti-inflammatory drugs (NSAID) and opioid drugs interaction, both drugs that are often administered together for pain relief. NSAID increases the expression of P-gp on blood-brain barrier, thus increasing efflux and limiting the effect of opioids on CNS [27].

Specificities of blood-brain barrier are very important to consider in the light of recent expansion of herbal medicines usage over-the-counter drugs. These drugs usually are not taken into consideration even though some have proven effects on blood-brain barrier and blood-cerebrospinal fluid transporters. Some of these drugs include Kava kava, St. John Wort, Echinacea, *Gingko biloba*, ginseng, ginger, green tea and garlic.

Placenta

For decades, it was assumed that the human placenta acted like a barrier, keeping the fetus away from xenobiotics circulating in mothers' blood. The thalidomide incident changed that concept. With time, it had become clear that the placenta allows most xenobiotics to pass, but it also has a significant metabolizing capacity itself [28].

From the beginning of development, the placenta has two main parts. First is the fetal part developing from the chorion and second the maternal part from the uterine epithelium and stroma that form decidua, each of these two parts having its separate circulation. Transfer of nutrients, oxygen and other molecules from the mother to the child is carried through the placental barrier which is composed of the trophoblastic cells, sub-trophoblastic tissue and fetal capillary walls. Conditions and composition of the placental barrier change from fertilization toward birth, thus affecting and changing the transfer of drugs and other molecules [28]. There are two main ways for the molecules to pass through the placental barrier: firstly, through free diffusion for the small lipophilic, uncharged molecules and secondly, through a network of transporters [29]. Drugs that can change any of these conditions may affect the transfer of other drugs, but it is also important to consider the metabolic function of the placenta and the possible effects of drugs on cytochrome P450 and UGTs expressed in the placenta [30].

ABC superfamily of transporters is mostly expressed on the maternal side of the placenta and plays a major role in the efflux of xenobiotics from the fetus. Members of this family expressed are P-gp, breast cancer resistance protein (BCRP) and in lesser measure multidrug resistance protein (MRP) 1–3 and 5. P-gp can be inhibited by therapeutic compounds cyclosporin A and verapamil, thus decreasing its function and increasing concentrations of HIV-protease inhibitors, immunosuppressive drugs and antibiotics in the fetus, as its function is to remove them from the placenta to the mother's blood. Substrates of BCRP include nitrofurantoin and glyburide, and its inhibitors are ritonavir, saquinavir, cyclosporine A and omeprazole [30].

SLC superfamily transporters expressed in the placenta involved in drug transfer include organic anion transporting polypeptides, organic cation transporters (OCT), organic anion transporters, monoamine transporters (MT) and equilibrate nucleoside transporters. Potential drug-drug interference is possible with OCT and MT. OCT substrates include verapamil, quinidine and possibly metformin, which can be inhibited by cimetidine. MT substrates are amphetamines, and inhibitors of MT are a variety of antidepressants [30].

Cancer Cells

Multidrug resistance is a serious pharmacotherapeutic problem that hinders the success of anticancer drugs. A common mechanism for this is overexpression of ABC efflux transporters such as P-gp, MRP and BCRP in cancer cells. These proteins mostly act as efflux transporters keeping cancer cells free or lowering concentrations of some anticancer drugs [31].

As a high-capacity transport protein, P-gp is involved in the transport of a wide range of pharmacologically and structurally diverse drugs including chemotherapeutics, antiretroviral drugs, cardioactive drugs, immunosuppressants and others. Some other drugs inhibit the activity of P-gp, such as verapamil, cyclosporin, ketoconazole, quinidine [32] and, in some cases, thyronine kinase inhibitors [33], thus possibly increasing the activity of anticancer drugs in cancer cells, but because of wide expression of P-gp in other tissues also causing adverse effects. It is important to note that herbal drugs including silymarin, ginseng, piperin, capsaicin and others have been reported to inhibit the activity of P-gp, while some others such as St. John's wort are typical inducers of P-gp [32].

Effects on Drug Excretion

Introduction

There are two major pathways of drug elimination from the body. First is through renal clearance into the urine and the second one is clearance through the liver into bile and feces. Part of this clearance happens through passive diffusion, but the majority occurs through active transport governed by membrane transporters. Activation or inactivation of these transporters can be a potential medium for drug-drug interactions.

Effects on Renal Excretion

Excretion of drugs through renal clearance is an important path of drug elimination. Of the top 200 drugs prescribed in the US, around 32% are eliminated through renal clearance with more than 25% of the absorbed dose excreted unchanged [34]. Renal excretion is a result of three processes occurring concurrently in the nephron, glomerular filtration which is a passive process, tubular secretion and tubular reabsorption involving a variety of transporters located on basolateral and luminal membranes. These transporters are located on the proximal tubule and work together to eliminate drugs from the bloodstream [35].

Major transporters participating in tubular secretion of cationic drugs include organic cation transporter (OCT2) on the basolateral membrane and the apical membrane multidrug and toxin extrusion proteins 1 and 2-K (MATE1 and MATE2-K). Also, expressed on the apical membrane is P-gp in charge of the excretion of larger and more hydrophobic cations. MRP2 and MRP4 are expressed on the apical membrane, and organic cation transporters 1 and 3 (OAT1 and OAT 3) are expressed on the basolateral membrane, which are engaged in the secretion of anion drugs [35].

Transporter-mediated drug-drug interactions are becoming more recognized as an important modifier of the pharmacodynamics and pharmacokinetics of drugs. Moreover, inhibition of renal drug transporters can cause significant changes in pharmacodynamics, resulting in clinically important drug-drug interaction, but also it can cause abnormal drug accumulation in renal tubular cells, thus causing drug-induced nephrotoxicity [35].

Interactions involved with OCT2 and MATE1/2-K transporters involve lowering of metformin clearance caused by cimetidine, pyrimethamine and dolutegravir [36]. Cisplatin nephrotoxicity is also an important side effect connected to OCT and MATE transporters in the kidney, and some studies have shown that administering OCT2 selective inhibitors such as cimetidine can lead to partial protection from cisplatin nephrotoxicity [37].

Probenecid is a prototype inhibitor drug for the OAT transporters. Its inhibition of renal anion secretion has been used clinically to enhance the activity of antibiotics and reduce renal accumulation and nephrotoxicity of some antiviral drugs. It has also been shown that probenecid decreases renal clearance of furosemide, fexofenadine and cidofovir [35].

Efflux pump transporter P-gp has been involved in many reports of transporter-mediated drug-drug interactions. Best-studied interactions involve digoxin, whose excretion is inhibited by quinidine.

Biliary Drug Excretion

Numerous metabolites, xenobiotics and drugs are transported from the bloodstream through the sinusoidal membrane of hepatocytes to intracellular space with transporter-mediated processes.

Organic cation transporters, OTAP-C and OTAP8, are exclusively expressed in the basolateral membrane of hepatocytes, while other members of OTAP family transporters that are found in hepatocytes (OTAP-A, OTAP-B, OTAP-D and OTAP-E) can be found in other tissues. These transporters play a central role in organic anion drug clearance from the liver [38]. Substrates for OTAP are bile salts, organic anions and statins, while inhibitors of these transporters are itraconazole, nefazodone, nifedipine, diazepam and sulfasalazine [39].

Organic anion transporter in the liver, mainly, OCT1 is expressed at the basolateral membrane of hepatocytes, but also in the small intestine and proximal tubules of the kidney. This transporter plays a role in the uptake of small organic cations such as tetraethylammonium, nicotinamide and dopamine in the liver and subsequent excretion to bile [38].

The basolateral membrane of hepatocytes contains several members of MRP transporters (MRP1/3/5 and 6). Proteins from this superfamily (ABC) are also expressed in the canalicular transport system and represent a majority of transport proteins in this localization. Most important transporters expressed in the canalicular transport system are MDR1/p-gp, MDR3, MRP2/CMOAT, BSEP/SPGP and BCRP [38]. Some substrates for these transporters are sulfated drugs, anticancer drugs and rosuvastatin, and inhibitors of these transporters are cyclosporine, propranolol, furosemide, ketoconazole, NSAID, verapamil and others [39].

References

1. Elizabeta T, Dragan P, Stipan J, Mario Š. In: Mbilmuk P, editor. Medicinska biokemija i laboratorijska medicina u kliničkoj praksi. 2nd ed. Zagreb: Medicinska Naklada; 2018. p. 827.
2. Bozina N, Bradamante V, Lovrić M. Genetic polymorphism of metabolic enzymes P450 (CYP) as a susceptibility factor for drug response, toxicity, and cancer risk. Arh Hig Rada Toksikol. 2009;60(2):217–42.
3. Nada B. Farmakogenomika u personaliziranoj medicini. 1st ed. Zagrebu MfSu, Zagreb Kbc, editors. Zagreb: Medicinska naklada; 2019. p. 280.
4. Zhou M, Maitra SR, Wang P. The potential role of transcription factor aryl hydrocarbon receptor in downregulation of hepatic cytochrome P-450 during sepsis. Int J Mol Med. 2008;21(4):423–8.

5. Phillips KA, Veenstra DL, Oren E, Lee JK, Sadee W. Potential role of pharmacogenomics in reducing adverse drug reactions: a systematic review. JAMA. 2001;286(18):2270–9.
6. Klotz U, Schwab M, Treiber G. CYP2C19 polymorphism and proton pump inhibitors. Basic Clin Pharmacol Toxicol. 2004;95(1):2–8.
7. (EBCTCG) EBCTCG. Aromatase inhibitors versus tamoxifen in early breast cancer: patient-level meta-analysis of the randomised trials. Lancet. 2015;386(10001):1341–52.
8. Pagani O, Regan MM, Walley BA, Fleming GF, Colleoni M, Láng I, et al. Adjuvant exemestane with ovarian suppression in premenopausal breast cancer. N Engl J Med. 2014;371(2):107–18.
9. Galetin A, Gertz M, Houston JB. Contribution of intestinal cytochrome p450-mediated metabolism to drug-drug inhibition and induction interactions. Drug Metab Pharmacokinet. 2010;25(1):28–47.
10. Paine MF, Hart HL, Ludington SS, Haining RL, Rettie AE, Zeldin DC. The human intestinal cytochrome P450 "pie". Drug Metab Dispos. 2006;34(5):880–6.
11. Shen DD, Kunze KL, Thummel KE. Enzyme-catalyzed processes of first-pass hepatic and intestinal drug extraction. Adv Drug Deliv Rev. 1997;27(2–3):99–127.
12. Templeton I, Peng CC, Thummel KE, Davis C, Kunze KL, Isoherranen N. Accurate prediction of dose-dependent CYP3A4 inhibition by itraconazole and its metabolites from in vitro inhibition data. Clin Pharmacol Ther. 2010;88(4):499–505.
13. Kharasch ED, Walker A, Hoffer C, Sheffels P. Intravenous and oral alfentanil as in vivo probes for hepatic and first-pass cytochrome P450 3A activity: noninvasive assessment by use of pupillary miosis. Clin Pharmacol Ther. 2004;76(5):452–66.
14. Vaessen SF, van Lipzig MM, Pieters RH, Krul CA, Wortelboer HM, van de Steeg E. Regional expression levels of drug transporters and metabolizing enzymes along the pig and human intestinal tract and comparison with Caco-2 cells. Drug Metab Dispos. 2017;45(4):353–60.
15. Kalliokoski A, Niemi M. Impact of OATP transporters on pharmacokinetics. Br J Pharmacol. 2009;158(3):693–705.
16. Wilkens S. Structure and mechanism of ABC transporters. F1000Prime Rep. 2015;7:14.
17. Ni Z, Bikadi Z, Rosenberg MF, Mao Q. Structure and function of the human breast cancer resistance protein (BCRP/ABCG2). Curr Drug Metab. 2010;11(7):603–17.
18. Obaidat A, Roth M, Hagenbuch B. The expression and function of organic anion transporting polypeptides in normal tissues and in cancer. Annu Rev Pharmacol Toxicol. 2012;52:135–51.
19. Roth M, Obaidat A, Hagenbuch B. OATPs, OATs and OCTs: the organic anion and cation transporters of the SLCO and SLC22A gene superfamilies. Br J Pharmacol. 2012;165(5):1260–87.
20. Schwarz UI, Gramatté T, Krappweis J, Oertel R, Kirch W. P-glycoprotein inhibitor erythromycin increases oral bioavailability of talinolol in humans. Int J Clin Pharmacol Ther. 2000;38(4):161–7.
21. Westphal K, Weinbrenner A, Zschiesche M, Franke G, Knoke M, Oertel R, et al. Induction of P-glycoprotein by rifampin increases intestinal secretion of talinolol in human beings: a new type of drug/drug interaction. Clin Pharmacol Ther. 2000;68(4):345–55.
22. Elsby R, Martin P, Surry D, Sharma P, Fenner K. Solitary inhibition of the breast cancer resistance protein efflux Transporter results in a clinically significant drug-drug interaction with Rosuvastatin by causing up to a 2-fold increase in statin exposure. Drug Metab Dispos. 2016;44(3):398–408.
23. Bailey DG, Dresser GK, Leake BF, Kim RB. Naringin is a major and selective clinical inhibitor of organic anion-transporting polypeptide 1A2 (OATP1A2) in grapefruit juice. Clin Pharmacol Ther. 2007;81(4):495–502.
24. Kibathi LW, Bae S, Penzak SR, Kumar P. Potential Influence of Centrally Acting Herbal Drugs on Transporters at the Blood–Cerebrospinal Fluid Barrier and Blood–Brain Barrier. Eur J Drug Metab Pharmacokinet. 2018;43(6):619–35.
25. Chaves C, Shawahna R, Jacob A, Scherrmann JM, Declèves X. Human ABC transporters at blood-CNS interfaces as determinants of CNS drug penetration. Curr Pharm Des. 2014;20(10):1450–62.
26. Zhao Z, Nelson AR, Betsholtz C, Zlokovic BV. Establishment and dysfunction of the blood-brain barrier. Cell. 2015;163(5):1064–78.

27. Sanchez-Covarrubias L, Slosky LM, Thompson BJ, Zhang Y, Laracuente ML, DeMarco KM, et al. P-glycoprotein modulates morphine uptake into the CNS: a role for the non-steroidal anti-inflammatory drug diclofenac. PLoS One. 2014;9(2):e88516.
28. Koren G, Ornoy A. The role of the placenta in drug transport and fetal drug exposure. Expert Rev Clin Pharmacol. 2018;11(4):373–85.
29. Young AM, Allen CE, Audus KL. Efflux transporters of the human placenta. Adv Drug Deliv Rev. 2003;55(1):125–32.
30. Rubinchik-Stern M, Eyal S. Drug Interactions at the human placenta: what is the evidence? Front Pharmacol. 2012;3:126.
31. Choi YH, Yu AM. ABC transporters in multidrug resistance and pharmacokinetics, and strategies for drug development. Curr Pharm Des. 2014;20(5):793–807.
32. Fasinu PS, Rapp GK. Herbal interaction with chemotherapeutic drugs-a focus on clinically significant findings. Front Oncol. 2019;9:1356.
33. Wu S, Fu L. Tyrosine kinase inhibitors enhanced the efficacy of conventional chemotherapeutic agent in multidrug resistant cancer cells. Mol Cancer. 2018;17(1):25.
34. Morrissey KM, Stocker SL, Wittwer MB, Xu L, Giacomini KM. Renal transporters in drug development. Annu Rev Pharmacol Toxicol. 2013;53:503–29.
35. Yin J, Wang J. Renal drug transporters and their significance in drug-drug interactions. Acta Pharm Sin B. 2016;6(5):363–73.
36. Yin W, Xu S, Wang Z, Liu H, Peng L, Fang Q, et al. Recombinant human GLP-1(rhGLP-1) alleviating renal tubulointestitial injury in diabetic STZ-induced rats. Biochem Biophys Res Commun. 2018;495(1):793–800.
37. Sleijfer DT, Offerman JJ, Mulder NH, Verweij M, van der Hem GK, Schraffordt Koops HS, et al. The protective potential of the combination of verapamil and cimetidine on cisplatin-induced nephrotoxicity in man. Cancer. 1987;60(11):2823–8.
38. Tsuji A. Transporter-mediated drug interactions. Drug Metab Pharmacokinet. 2002;17(4):253–74.
39. Kolarić TO, Ninčević V, Smolić R, Smolić M, Wu GY. Mechanisms of hepatic cholestatic drug injury. J Clin Transl Hepatol. 2019;7(1):86–92.

Pharmacogenomics of Drugs Used in Gastroenterology

13

Lidija Bach-Rojecky and Dragan Primorac

Introduction

Drugs used in gastroenterology include several classes of drugs with the application either in the prevention or treatment of disorders of the gastrointestinal tract. Functional gastrointestinal disorders represent the most common diagnoses in gastroenterology and are characterized by motility disturbances and visceral hypersensitivity. Among those, functional dyspepsia and irritable bowel syndrome are the most widely present and affect up to 20% of the general population around the world [1]. The most difficult to treat because of the complex immuno-pathophysiology are inflammatory bowel diseases such as ulcerative colitis and Crohn's disease. Because of the immunological background, the current treatment strategies are mostly oriented to modulation of the excessive intestinal immune response and reduction of mucosal inflammation.

L. Bach-Rojecky
Faculty of Pharmacy and Biochemistry, University of Zagreb, Zagreb, Croatia
e-mail: lbach@pharma.hr

D. Primorac (✉)
St. Catherine Specialty Hospital, Zagreb, Croatia

School of Medicine, University of Split, Split, Croatia

Eberly College of Science, State College, Penn State University, University Park, PA, USA

The Henry C. Lee College of Criminal Justice and Forensic Sciences, University of New Haven, West Haven, CT, USA

Faculty of Medicine, J.J. Strossmayer University of Osijek, Osijek, Croatia

School of Medicine, University of Rijeka, Rijeka, Croatia

Faculty of Dental Medicine and Health, J.J. Strossmayer University of Osijek, Osijek, Croatia

Medical School REGIOMED, Coburg, Germany

M. Banić, D. Erceg (eds.), *Drug Interactions in Gastroenterology*, Clinical Gastroenterology, https://doi.org/10.1007/978-3-031-69800-2_13

Some of the medicines, such as antacids, blockers of histamine H2 receptors, some proton pump inhibitors, and laxatives, are available without a prescription. Others, such as immunomodulators and biologicals, carry significant risks, and patients should be monitored to prevent or treat adverse effects and toxicities. Efficacy and safety for some of the drugs could be predicted based on certain patient- and/or drug-related risk factors. The influence of genetic variations as inherent risk factors for drug efficacy and safety is intensively investigated. For some drugs used to treat certain nonmalignant disorders of the gastrointestinal tract, such as proton pump inhibitors, 5-HT3 antagonists and thiopurines, the international expert consortium (The Clinical Pharmacogenetics Implementation Consortium) has published evidence-based guidelines and recommended optimization of the pharmacotherapy according to patient genotype (Table 13.1).

While we are waiting for more proof of genetic polymorphisms and their influence on the efficacy and safety of a broader range of drugs, pharmacogenomics has yet to enter the clinical practice and become a cornerstone for personalized therapy [5].

Table 13.1 Drugs with clinical guidelines linking the results of pharmacogenetic tests to specific therapeutic recommendations (according to CPIC)

Drug class/drugs of interest	Gene/ polymorphism	Phenotype	Clinical significance	Ref.
Proton pump inhibitors: Omeprazole Esomeprazole Lansoprazole Pantoprazole	*CYP2C19* *1*/17** *CYP2C19* *17*/17**	Rapid metabolizers Ultrarapid metabolizers	Increased metabolism to inactive compounds - possible therapeutic failure CPIC recommends increase in starting dose by 100% (ultrarapid metabolizers), increase in dose by 50%-100% for the *Helicobacter pylori* eradication (rapid and normal metabolizers)	Lima et al. [2]
Antiemetics 5-HT3 antagonists: Ondansetron, tropisetron	*CYP2D6* **1/*1xN* **1/*2xN* **2/*2xNc*	Ultrarapid metabolizers	Increased metabolism to less active compounds when compared to normal metabolizers is associated with decreased response to ondansetron and tropisetron *CPIC recommends an alternative drug (granisetron)*	Bell et al. [3]

(continued)

Table 13.1 (continued)

Drug class/drugs of interest	Gene/ polymorphism	Phenotype	Clinical significance	Ref.
Thiopurines: Azathioprine Mercaptopurine Thioguanine	*TPMT* **1/*2, *1/*3A, *1/*3B, *1/*3C, *1/*4, *2/*8, *3A/*7 *3A/*3A, *2/*3A, *3A/*3C, *3C/*4, *2/*3C, *3A/*4*	Intermediate metabolizers Poor metabolizers	Increased risk of thiopurine-induced hematotoxicity. *CPIC recommends starting with reduced starting doses* (30–80% of normal dose) Greatly increased risk of thiopurine-related myelosuppression. *CPIC recommends alternative nonthiopurine immunosuppressant therapy*	Relling et al. [4]
	NUDT15 **1/*2, *1/*3 *2/*5, *3/*6 *2/*2, *2/*3, *3/*3*	Intermediate metabolizers Poor metabolizers	Increased risk of thiopurine-related myelosuppression *CPIC recommends starting with reduced starting doses* (30–80% of a normal dose) Greatly increased risk of thiopurine-related myelosuppression. *CPIC recommends alternative nonthiopurine immunosuppressant therapy*	Relling et al. [4]

CPIC Clinical Pharmacogenetics Implementation Consortium

Proton Pump Inhibitors

Proton pump inhibitors (PPIs) are the most effective class of gastric acid-suppressing drugs, diminishing the basal and stimulated production of acid by around 90% and are among the highest-selling drugs in the world. They are used in the therapy of gastroesophageal reflux disease, gastric and peptic ulcers, and Zollinger-Ellison syndrome, as well as for treatment and prevention of gastrotoxic effects associated with chronic use of nonsteroidal anti-inflammatory drugs. Furthermore, they are an obligatory part of eradication therapy for *Helicobacter pylori* infection because they increase the pH, thus providing optimal conditions for the antibiotic drugs' actions. PPIs are well-tolerated drugs; however, prolonged use has been linked to less common adverse events including infections, hypomagnesemia, kidney disease, osteoporosis, bone fractures, and dementia [6].

Six PPIs are available: omeprazole and esomeprazole, lansoprazole and dexlansoprazole, pantoprazole, and rabeprazole. They share a common mechanism of action on H^+/K^+-ATPase but differ in pharmacokinetic properties which finally can impact their efficacy and safety. PPIs are rapidly absorbed from the small intestine and metabolized by hepatic CYP2C19 and to a lesser extent by CYP3A4. The exception is rabeprazole which mostly undergoes a nonenzymatic reduction in the liver, with only 10% of the parent compound being metabolized by CYP enzymes. Different factors may affect the response to PPI, such as the patient's age, and other medications, as well as variations in the *CYP2C19* gene, which is highly polymorphic [7]. The most common polymorphism, with allele frequencies of ~15% in Caucasians and Africans and 29–35% in Asians, is *CYP2C19*2* (c.681G > A, rs4244285), which generates a nonfunctional protein. Poor (PM) and intermediate metabolizers (IM), which carry two copies or one copy of a nonfunctional allele, respectively, share an impaired possibility to metabolize PPIs and, therefore, have increased PPIs' plasma concentrations compared to normal metabolizers. On the other hand, the *CYP2C19*17* allele (c.-806C>T, rs12248560) results in increased activity, with allele frequencies of ~3–21% in different ethnic groups. Individuals with one or two increased function alleles (*1/*17, *17/*17) are categorized as rapid (RM) and ultrarapid metabolizers (UM) and are at increased risk of therapy failure due to increased PPIs clearance [8]. This is especially important when the strongest PPI antisecretory activity is needed, like in the eradication of *Helicobacter pylori* infection. Currently, Royal Dutch Pharmacogenetics Working Group provides dose recommendations for four PPIs: omeprazole, esomeprazole, pantoprazole, and lansoprazole. They recommend a dose increase of 400%, 200%, 100–200%, and 50–100% for pantoprazole, lansoprazole, omeprazole, and esomeprazole, respectively, in the case of UM/RM phenotypes in *Helicobacter pylori* eradication therapy [6]. Recommendations for a dose decrease in IM/PM phenotypes for any of the PPIs are not provided. Additionally, CPIC published clinical guidelines for the same PPIs and recommended dose adjustments for UM/RM, but also for IM and PM (suggesting reduction in daily dose by 50% for those on chronic therapy and *CYP2C*2/*2*, **3/*3*, **2/*3*,**2/*9*, **3/*9*, **1/*2*, **1/*3*, **2/*17*, **3/*17* carriers (2).

Antiemetic Drugs

Serotonin (5-HT3) receptors antagonists are the cornerstone of prophylactic therapy for chemotherapy-induced, radiation-induced, as well as postoperative nausea and vomiting. They can be divided into two generations—the first is represented by dolasetron, granisetron, ondansetron, tropisetron, azasetron, and ramosetron (the last two being licensed in Southeast Asia only), while palonosetron represents the second generation. In comparison to the first-generation, 5-HT3 receptor antagonists, palonosetron has a higher potency, a significantly longer half-life, and a different molecular interaction with 5-HT3 receptors. All drugs are well-tolerated, with a headache, occasional diarrhea, and constipation being the most reported [9]. Intravenous ondansetron administration has been connected with a dose-dependent risk for QT interval prolongation.

5-HT3 receptor antagonists have different pharmacological characteristics, including differences in receptor binding affinity, biotransformation pathways, plasma half-lives, and duration of effect. 5-HT3 antagonists are metabolized via CYP 3A4, CYP1A2, and CYP2D6 to inactive metabolites. Ondansetron is mostly metabolized via CYP3A4, while CYP2D6 mediates approximately 30% of total ondansetron metabolism. On the contrary, around 91% of tropisetron metabolism is carried out by CYP2D6 with a minor contribution from CYP3A4 [10]. *CYP2D6* is highly polymorphic with over 100 known allelic variants and subvariants identified. *CYP2D6* allele frequencies have been shown to vary substantially among world populations, with some allelic variants being detected only in a certain ethnic group [11].

Variation in CYP2D6 activity can impact the pharmacokinetics of ondansetron and tropisetron, ultimately affecting their efficacy. Individuals carrying duplications of functional alleles (*1/*1xN, *1/*2xN, and *2/*2xN; N—the number of *CYP2D6* gene copies) have the phenotype of ultrarapid metabolizers (UMs). Those patients have decreased exposure and a reduced response to ondansetron and tropisetron, as measured by an increased number of vomiting episodes compared to CYP2D6 normal metabolizers (NMs). For those patients, granisetron is a drug of choice, since it is metabolized via CYP3A4 and CYP1A2 [3].

For individuals with intermediate or poor CYP2D6 phenotype, potentially elevated blood levels of ondansetron might suggest a greater risk for torsades de pointes; however, there are no clinical data to support this. The synonymous variant rs1045642 in the *ABCB1* gene (encoding ATP-dependent drug efflux pump for xenobiotic compound) may affect ondansetron efficacy, where the G allele is associated with a reduced response to ondansetron, with more vomiting episodes following acute drug application [12]. Other genetic polymorphisms with potential impact on 5-HT3 receptor antagonists are still a matter of investigation.

Drugs Used for Inflammatory Bowel Diseases

Ulcerative colitis and Crohn's disease represent two subtypes of inflammatory bowel disease (IBD)—a chronic inflammatory intestinal condition with increasing prevalence around the world. It is estimated that over one million residents in the USA and 2.5 million in Europe suffer from IBD [13]. The pathogenesis of both conditions involves intestinal epithelial barrier defects, dysregulated immune responses, with strong influence of genetic predisposition. The goals of pharmacological therapy for IBD are focused on the reduction of inflammation, on controlling acute exacerbations, maintaining remission, treating specific complications, and reducing the risk of colorectal cancer. Treatments depending on the disease type and severity and therapy goals may include 5-aminosalicylic acid drugs (5-ASA), corticosteroids, immunosuppressants (such as thiopurines and methotrexate), and biological drugs—monoclonal antibodies (anti-TNF—infliximab, adalimumab, anti-adhesion molecule—vedolizumab, and ustekinumab) [14, 15].

5-Aminosalicylic Acid Drugs

First-line therapy for mild-to-moderate ulcerative colitis usually involves mesalazine, sulfasalazine, and balsalazide. They reduce inflammation of colonic mucosa through a variety of anti-inflammatory mechanisms, such as the activation of peroxisome proliferator-activated receptors-γ (PPAR-γ), inhibition of cyclooxygenase and lypoxygenase enzymes and eicosanoid synthesis, reduction of NF-κB activation, etc. [16]

Sulfasalazine is a combination of 5-aminosalicylic acid and sulfapyridine linked together by an azo bond which is reduced by gut bacteria in the colon, thus releasing active 5-ASA and sulfapyridine. While 5-ASA is responsible for the efficacy of sulfasalazine, sulfapyridine is the main cause of side effects. Sulfapyridine undergoes fast absorption from the colon and biotransformation to N-acetyl-sulfapyridine by N-acetyltransferase 2 (NAT2) [17]. This process is significantly reduced in slow acetylators (carriers of two variant alleles *NAT2*5B*, **6A*, **7B* or **5*, **6*, and **7*) compared to both normal and rapid acetylators (*NAT2*4/*4*), thus possibly increasing the risk of dose-related sulfapyridine-induced side effects, such as headache, nausea, fatigue, and allergic reactions [18]. However, the clinical significance of the slow acetylator phenotype for the safety of sulfasalazine is not confirmed. Furthermore, one study suggested that in the Chinese Han population, *HLA-B*13:01* might be associated with a sulfasalazine-induced rash with eosinophilia and systemic symptoms, thus predicting the risk of those potentially serious adverse effects. More information is needed for other patient populations and related risks [19]. Additionally, drug monographs include warnings regarding sulfasalazine use in patients with glucose-6-phosphate dehydrogenase deficiency, but the evidence indicates that there is no hemolytic effect at therapeutic dosages [20].

Glucocorticoids

Because of their anti-inflammatory action and impact on the immune system, glucocorticoids (GCs), such as budesonide, prednisolone, and beclomethasone dipropionate, are often used for the induction of remission in patients with moderate or severe disease activity. About 28% of patients become steroid-dependent, and budesonide and prednisolone are not effective in maintaining remission. However, GCs are not equally effective in all patients, and some of them do not respond to treatment because of GC resistance.

The mechanisms of GC resistance in IBDs may be associated with single nucleotide polymorphisms (SNPs) in the *NR3C1* gene (rs6189, rs6190, rs6195, and rs41423247) resulting with changed receptor structure and transduction. Although a meta-analysis that included the mostly Caucasian population found no association, the analysis of the presence of the combination of more than one SNP could show risk associations of these variants with GC resistance [21]. Other genes possibly associated with GC resistance are those encoding for enzymes involved in the proteasomal degradation of the GC receptors, such as steroid sulfatase and MDM2 oncogene E3 ubiquitin-protein ligase, but more studies are needed to further investigate possible connections [22].

Thiopurines

Immunosuppressant drugs azathioprine (AZA) and its active metabolite mercaptopurine (6-MP) are used as monotherapy in the maintenance, but not in the induction of remission in Crohn's disease. In 20–30% of patients thiopurine treatment causes various side effects, such as nausea, vomiting, anorexia, weight loss, headache, fatigue, stomatitis, alopecia, arthralgia, muscular weakness, rash, or pancreatitis. More serious adverse effects are dose-dependent, and include hepatotoxicity, myelosuppression, and the risk of opportunistic infections [23]. In order to predict the risk for toxicities, the concentration of 6-thioguanine nucleotides (TGN) can be measured in the erythrocytes and dosage adjusted accordingly. Furthermore, a change in the activity of thiopurine-s-methyltransferase (TPMT) contributes significantly to the risks for myelotoxicity. TPMT catalyzes the conversion of 6-MP to an inactive methyl-mercaptopurine base and is also involved in the generation of immunosuppressive and potentially hepatotoxic methylmercaptopurine nucleotides from the thioinosine monophosphate. Another important enzyme in thiopurine metabolism is a nucleoside diphosphatase, nudix hydrolase 15 (NUDT15), which catalyzes the conversion of cytotoxic metabolites thioguanine triphosphates (TGTP) to the less toxic thioguanine monophosphates. Activities of both TPMT and NUDT15 seem to be an important factor in the prediction of the risk of thioguanine-induced myelosuppression (TIM). While TPMT deficiency due to genetic polymorphisms is the main cause of thiopurine intolerance in Europeans and Africans, *NUDT15* gene polymorphisms can explain the risks for TIM in Asians and Hispanics [4].

Individuals with two loss-of-function *TPMT* alleles (**3A/*3A*, **2/*3A*, **3A/*3C*, **3C/*4*, **2/*3C*, and **3A/*4* dyplotypes) have very high concentrations of TGN metabolites due to slow 6-MG metabolism (phenotype of slow metabolizers). In those individuals, thiopurines should be avoided because of the increased risk of myelosupression[4]. Additionally, carriers of *TPMT *1/*2*, **1/*3A*, **1/*3B*, **1/*3C*, and **1/*4* dyplotypes (intermediate metabolizers), have one normal function allele and one no function allele and are at increased risk of TIM. Reduced starting dose (30–80% of the normal dose) and regular hematological monitoring of patients are suggested by the guidelines[4]. Pretreatment testing of TPMT is recommended by the US Food and Drug Administration to identify patients at risk of TIM. However, *TPMT* variants are only found in 25% of patients of European ancestry affected by TIM, suggesting the contribution of other genetic and environmental factors.

Two loss-of-function *NUDT15* alleles (**2/*2*, **2/*3*, and **3/*3* dyplotypes) correlate to poor metabolizer phenotype, and are also associated to an increased risk of thiopurine-related leukopenia, neutropenia, and myelosuppression and should avoid the use of thiopurines, while NUDT15 intermediate metabolizers (**1/*2*, **1/*3*) should start the therapy with 30–80% lower than normal dose. In contrast to *TPMT* genotype-guided dose adjustment, the clinical implementation of *NUDT15* variants in thiopurine dosing is relatively recent and its exact contribution in predicting the risk of TIM is less clear [4, 24].

Thiopurine-induced pancreatitis (TIP) is an idiosyncratic drug reaction with unknown pathophysiology which often causes drug withdrawal. Recent studies showed a higher prevalence of TIP in individuals with the *HLA-DQA1*02:01-HLA-DRB1*07:01* haplotypes. Patients heterozygous at rs2647087 have a 9% risk of developing pancreatitis, whereas homozygotes have a 17% risk. However, due to a benign course and reversibility of the occurring symptoms, routine screening is not considered cost-effective at present [25].

Methotrexate

Methotrexate (MTX) in a single weekly low dose is an effective immunosuppressive treatment for the induction and maintenance of remission of Crohn's disease if thiopurines are contraindicated. Its use in higher doses is limited by unpredictable efficacy and toxicity (bone marrow suppression, pulmonary fibrosis, hepatotoxicity, nausea, vomiting, etc.). Most pharmacogenetic studies are performed on a high dose of MTX, used either on oncologic or rheumatological patients. MTX cellular pathways are complex and involve a number of enzymes. Therefore, it could be expected that functional genetic variation in genes encoding these proteins has an impact on MTX efficacy and safety [26]. In contrast to a number of studies on patients with oncological indications as well as rheumatoid arthritis, only sparse studies are available that examine the association between specific polymorphisms and the clinical efficacy of MTX in patients with Chron's disease, but with inconclusive results [27].

Biologicals

Biological therapy targets specific inflammatory pathways after binding to receptors or soluble molecules (see also Chap. 9). Biologicals significantly improved the treatment outcomes of IBD, because of a better quality of patients' life, reduced number of hospitalizations, improved mucosal healing, and reduced risks of drugs' side effects. The anti-TNF agents (like, infliximab and adalimumab) serve as a mainstay biological therapy, which inhibit the pro-inflammatory activity of the cytokine TNFα thus controlling exaggerated immune respone. Vedolizumab exerts gut-selective anti-inflammatory activity because it prevents the migration of T-cells to inflamed gastrointestinal tissue. Ustekinumab targets cytokines IL-12 and IL-23 involved in inflammatory and immune responses [28].

Anti-TNF: Monoclonal antibodies to TNF-α are used to treat moderate-to-severe IBD. Since around 30% of patients do not respond to the treatment, the ability to predict anti-TNF nonresponders by evaluating potential genetic markers, could improve therapeutic outcomes.

One study suggested that variants in toll-like receptor 4 (*TLR*, rs55030728), FC fragment of IgG receptor IIIa (*FCGR3A*, rs396991), TNF receptor superfamily 1A (*TNFRS1A*, rs4149570), interferon-gamma (*IFNγ*, rs2439561), interleukin-6 (*IL-6*, rs10499563), and interleukin-1B (*IL-1B*, rs4848306) could be associated to better treatment response to anti-TNF, in contrast to *TLR2* rs3804099 and *TLR9* rs352139 SNPs that might be associated with a weaker response [29].

The *TNF-α* gene contains several SNPs, wuth potential relevance for the response of anti-TNF treatment. One meta-analysis showed that certain *TNF-α* gene polymorphisms could predict therapeutic response because, because in individuals with the −308 G/G genotype and −857 C/C genotype, better anti-TNF response was observed [30].

However, the level of clinical evidence is not high enough to recommend testing of specific genetic markers to predict therapeutic outcome to anti-TNF drugs, at least not before testing in larger cohorts over longer time periods [28].

Vedolizumab is a humanized monoclonal antibody that specifically binds to α4β7 integrin, blocking its interaction with MAdCAM-1 on the intestinal endothelial cell. It is licensed for the treatment of moderate-to-severe ulcerative colitis as well as Crohn's disease in case of a failure of TNF-antagonists. Although one study found higher α4β7 expression on CD4+ T cells and natural killer cells in responders to vedolizumab, the study sample was small, and this observation needs further validation as a potential predictor for vedolizumab clinical response [31].

Ustekinumab is a monoclonal antibody which binds with high affinity to the p40 subunit of human interleukin 12 and 23 (IL12 and IL23) and is indicated for the treatment of adult patients with plaque psoriasis and psoriatic arthritis, but also for Crohn's disease and more recently for active moderate-to-severe ulcerative colitis. It is licensed for the induction and maintenance of remission in moderate-to-severe Chron's disease in patients who are resistant to TNF antagonists [32]. Although some genetic studies demonstrated possible associations of particular SNPs with the efficacy of ustekinumab in psoriatic patients [33], such studies are lacking in patients with IBD.

References

1. Oshima T, Miwa H. Epidemiology of functional gastrointestinal disorders in Japan and in the world. J Neurogastroenterol Motil. 2015;21(3):320–9. https://doi.org/10.5056/jnm14165.
2. Lima JJ, Thomas CD, Barbarino J, et al. Clinical Pharmacogenetics Implementation Consortium (CPIC) Guideline for CYP2C19 and Proton Pump Inhibitor Dosing. *Clin Pharmacol Ther*. 2021;109(6):1417–1423. https://doi.org/10.1002/cpt.2015.
3. Bell GC, Caudle KE, Whirl-Carrillo M, et al. Clinical pharmacogenetics implementation consortium (CPIC) guideline for CYP2D6 genotype and use of ondansetron and tropisetron. Clin Pharmacol Ther. 2017;102(2):213–8. https://doi.org/10.1002/cpt.598.
4. Relling MV, Schwab M, Whirl-Carrillo M, et al. Clinical pharmacogenetics implementation consortium guideline for thiopurine dosing based on TPMT and NUDT15 genotypes: 2018 update. Clin Pharmacol Ther. 2019;105(5):1095–105. https://doi.org/10.1002/cpt.1304.
5. Primorac D, Bach-Rojecky L, Vađunec D, et al. Pharmacogenomics at the center of precision medicine: challenges and perspective in an era of big data. Pharmacogenomics. 2020;21(2):141–56. https://doi.org/10.2217/pgs-2019-0134.
6. El Rouby N, Lima JJ, Johnson JA. Proton pump inhibitors: from CYP2C19 pharmacogenetics to precision medicine. Expert Opin Drug Metab Toxicol. 2018;14(4):447–60. https://doi.org/10.1080/17425255.2018.1461835.

7. Hagymási K, Müllner K, Herszényi L, Tulassay Z. Update on the pharmacogenomics of proton pump inhibitors. Pharmacogenomics. 2011;12:873–88. https://doi.org/10.2217/pgs.11.4.
8. Scott SA, Sangkuhl K, Shuldiner AR, et al. PharmGKB summary: very important pharmacogene information for cytochrome P450, family 2, subfamily C, polypeptide 19. Pharmacogenet Genomics. 2012;22(2):159–65. https://doi.org/10.1097/FPC.0b013e32834d4962.
9. Navari RM. 5-HT3 receptors as important mediators of nausea and vomiting due to chemotherapy. Biochim Biophys Acta. 2015;1848:2738–46. https://doi.org/10.1016/j.bbamem.2015.03.020.
10. Huddart R, Altman RB, Klein TE. PharmGKB summary: ondansetron and tropisetron pathways, pharmacokinetics and pharmacodynamics. Pharmacogenet Genomics. 2019;29(4):91–7. https://doi.org/10.1097/FPC.0000000000000369.
11. Gaedigk A, Sangkuhl K, Whirl-Carrillo M. Prediction of CYP2D6 phenotype from genotype across world populations. Genet Med. 2017;19(1):69–76. https://doi.org/10.1038/gim.2016.80.
12. He H, Yin JY, Xu YJ, et al. Association of ABCB1 polymorphisms with the efficacy of ondansetron in chemotherapy-induced nausea and vomiting. Clin Ther. 2014;36(8):1242–1252.e2. https://doi.org/10.1016/j.clinthera.2014.06.016.
13. Kaplan GG. The global burden of IBD: from 2015 to 2025. Nat Rev Gastroenterol Hepatol. 2015;12(12):720–7. https://doi.org/10.1038/nrgastro.2015.150.
14. Torres J, Mehandru S, Colombel JF, Peyrin-Biroulet L. Crohn's disease. Lancet. 2017;389(10080):1741–55. https://doi.org/10.1016/S0140-6736(16)31711-1.
15. Ungaro R, Mehandru S, Allen PB, et al. Ulcerative colitis. Lancet. 2017;389(10080):1756–70. https://doi.org/10.1016/S0140-6736(16)32126-2.
16. Perrotta C, Pellegrino P, Moroni E, De Palma C, Cervia D, Danelli P, Clementi E. Five-aminosalicylic acid: an update for the reappraisal of an old drug. Gastroentl Res Practice. 2015;2015:456895. https://doi.org/10.1155/2015/456895.
17. Kuhn UD, Anschütz M, Schmücker K, et al. Phenotyping with sulfasalazine—time dependence and relation to NAT2 pharmacogenetics. Int J Clin Pharmacol Ther. 2010;48(1):1–10. https://doi.org/10.5414/cpp48001.
18. McDonagh EM, Boukouvala S, Aklillu E. PharmGKB summary: very important pharmacogene information for N-acetyltransferase 2. Pharmacogenet Genomics. 2014;24(8):409–25. https://doi.org/10.1097/FPC.0000000000000062.
19. Yang F, Gu B, Zhang L, Xuan J, et al. HLA-B*13:01 is associated with salazosulfapyridine-induced drug rash with eosinophilia and systemic symptoms in Chinese Han population. Pharmacogenomics. 2014;15(11):1461–9. https://doi.org/10.2217/pgs.14.69.
20. Youngster I, Arcavi L, Schechmaster R, et al. Medications and glucose-6-phosphate dehydrogenase deficiency: an evidence-based review. Drug Saf. 2010;33(9):713–26. https://doi.org/10.2165/11536520-000000000-00000.
21. Chen HL, Li LR. Glucocorticoid receptor gene polymorphisms and glucocorticoid resistance in inflammatory bowel disease: a meta-analysis. Dig Dis Sci. 2012;57(12):3065–75. https://doi.org/10.1007/s10620-012-2293-2.
22. Montero-Meléndez T, Llor X, García-Planella E, et al. Identification of novel predictor classifiers for inflammatory bowel disease by gene expression profiling. PLoS One. 2013;8(10):e76235. https://doi.org/10.1371/journal.pone.0076235.
23. Frei P, Biedermann L, Nielsen OH, Rogler G. Use of thiopurines in inflammatory bowel disease. World J Gastroenterol. 2013;19(7):1040–8. https://doi.org/10.3748/wjg.v19.i7.1040.
24. Luber RP, Honap S, Cunningham G, Irving PM. Can we predict the toxicity and response to Thiopurines in inflammatory bowel diseases? Front Med (Lausanne). 2019;6:279. eCollection 2019. https://doi.org/10.3389/fmed.2019.00279.
25. Heap GA, Weedon MN, Bewshea CM, et al. HLA-DQA1-HLA-DRB1 variants confer susceptibility to pancreatitis induced by thiopurine immunosuppressants. Nat Genet. 2014;46(10):1131–4. https://doi.org/10.1038/ng.3093.
26. Lamb CA, Kennedy NA, Raine T, et al. British Society of Gastroenterology consensus guidelines on the management of inflammatory bowel disease in adults. Gut. 2019;68(Suppl 3):s1–s106. https://doi.org/10.1136/gutjnl-2019-318484.

27. Herrlinger KR, Cummings JR, Barnardo MC, et al. The pharmacogenetics of methotrexate in inflammatory bowel disease. Pharmacogenet Genomics. 2005;15(10):705–11. https://doi.org/10.1097/01.fpc.0000172242.19675.33.
28. Wang C, Baer HM, Gaya DR, et al. Can molecular stratification improve the treatment of inflammatory bowel disease? Pharmacol Res. 2019;148:104442. https://doi.org/10.1016/j.phrs.2019.104442.
29. Bek S, Nielsen JV, Bojesen AB. Systematic review: genetic biomarkers associated with anti-TNF treatment response in inflammatory bowel diseases. Aliment Pharmacol Ther. 2016;44(6):554–67. https://doi.org/10.1111/apt.13736.
30. Tong Q, Zhao L, Qian X-D. Association of TNF-α polymorphism with the prediction of response to TNF blockers in spondyloarthritis and inflammatory bowel disease: a meta-analysis. Pharmacogenomics. 2013;14(14):1691–700. https://doi.org/10.2217/pgs.13.146.
31. Boden EK, Shows DM, Chiorean MV, Lord JD. Identification of candidate biomarkers associated with response to vedolizumab in inflammatory bowel disease. Dig Dis Sci. 2018;63(9):2419–29. https://doi.org/10.1007/s10620-018-4924-8.
32. Kotze PG, Ma C, Almutairdi A, Panaccione R. Clinical utility of ustekinumab in Crohn's disease. J Inflamm Res. 2018;11:35–47. https://doi.org/10.2147/JIR.S157358.
33. Prieto-Pérez R, Llamas-Velasco M, Cabaleiro T, et al. Pharmacogenetics of ustekinumab in patients with moderate-to-severe plaque psoriasis. Pharmacogenomics. 2017;18(2):157–64. https://doi.org/10.2217/pgs-2016-0122.

14 Interactions of Drugs and Herbs in Gastroenterology

Agostino Di Ciaula, David Q.-H. Wang, and Piero Portincasa

Introduction

Herbal therapy is one of the most common alternative and complementary treatments for human disease. It is now used widely in Western Countries, and scientists are becoming more interested in the therapeutic effects of herbs on various human diseases. Herbal medicine is often used with prescribed and nonprescribed drugs [1]. In the field of gastroenterology, herbs are mainly used for treating inflammatory bowel disease (IBD) [2–5], nonalcoholic fatty liver disease (NAFLD) [6–9], and dysfunctional digestive disorders such as dyspepsia, irritable bowel syndrome (IBS) [10, 11], and gastro-esophageal reflux [12].

The number of users of herbal medicines or dietary supplements ranges from 5.9 to 48.3% in European Countries [13]. In the USA, a National survey in the year 2012 showed that 42% of adults with gastrointestinal disorders used complementary and alternative medicine [14].

A recent prospective, cross-sectional study, conducted in an EU Country (Serbia), revealed that 10.4% of patients used herbs for various gastrointestinal disorders,

A. Di Ciaula
Clinica Medica "A. Murri", AOUC Policlinico, Bari, Italy

D. Q.-H. Wang
Department of Medicine and Genetics, Division of Gastroenterology and Liver Diseases, Marion Bessin Liver Research Center, Einstein-Mount Sinai Diabetes Research Center, Albert Einstein College of Medicine, Bronx, NY, USA
e-mail: david.wang@einsteinmed.org

P. Portincasa (✉)
Clinical Medica "A. Murri", Department of Precision and Regenerative Medicine and Ionian Area (DiMePre-J), University of Bari Medical School, Bari, Italy
e-mail: piero.portincasa@uniba.it

M. Banić, D. Erceg (eds.), *Drug Interactions in Gastroenterology*, Clinical Gastroenterology, https://doi.org/10.1007/978-3-031-69800-2_14

mainly for constipation (44% of cases) and dyspepsia (23%). This study also shows that in the majority of cases, patients used herbal medicine following the recommendation of pharmacists or as self-prescription, and rarely after a medical prescription [15].

An increasing use of herbal medicine has also been noticed in children and adolescents, due to the high prevalence of dysfunctional gastrointestinal disorders such as IBS, constipation, and infantile colic [16]. These users usually believe that herbal medicine is "natural and safe" [17], are dissatisfied with traditional therapies, or fear the side effects of drugs [18]. In the case of IBD [19] or IBS [10], combination therapy of drugs with herbs might show better outcomes than single therapy. In fact, herbal medicine contains a mixture of biologically active plant constituents, since their synergistic effects may be greater than the sum of the effects of a single component.

Although one drug usually contains a single active compound, herbal medicine is often composed of numerous pharmacologically active ingredients. This difference is important when the increased risk of herb-drug interactions is identified. Several interactions between herbs and drugs exist, but the risk for their side effects is largely unknown. In particular, interaction may develop with warfarin, antidepressants, digoxin, antidiabetics, corticosteroids, theophylline, cyclosporin, and/or phenytoin. Such interactions may lead to either potentiated or decreased therapeutic effects of drugs, and in turn, altered effectiveness and safety of these drugs, in particular during long-term medications [20, 21]. Ordinary people believe that medical treatments with herbs are intrinsically safe because they are "natural." However, this concept is not supported by the literature. There is evidence showing herb-drug interaction-induced side effects and toxicity in the liver, kidneys, and/or heart during short-term or long-term treatment, particularly in patients with polytherapy.

Combined treatments of herbs with drugs, on the other hand, might ameliorate therapeutic outcomes in specific clinical conditions. This effect is due to positive synergies of actions potentiating the pharmacokinetic and pharmacodynamic effects of drugs.

The increasing use of herbs in the management of common gastrointestinal diseases requires physicians and the public to pay special attention to possible herb-drug interaction-induced toxicity. This could greatly minimize unnecessary harmful side effects, and therefore would further protect patients against these toxicity and side effects.

This chapter will provide an adequate understanding of mechanisms responsible for herbs and drug interaction in order to minimize risks and to ameliorate the therapeutic efficacy of both principles, in particular during polytherapy and in subjects with chronic gastrointestinal diseases.

Main Mechanisms of Herb-Drug Interaction

Several aspects might render the ultimate interpretation of herb-drug interaction rather complex. The therapeutic effect of drugs can be magnified or decreased, leading to potential undesired outcomes.

Medicinal herbs may comprise mixtures of biologically active compounds as well as variable amounts of ingredients. Similar herbal extracts, furthermore, can imply different preparation methods or can originate from different parts of plants. These aspects make a comprehensive evaluation of interactions rather difficult.

In clinical trials, for example, this variability can explain poorly comparable results. Systematic reviews and meta-analyses can better address the clinical outcome of herbal medications in specific diseases, although true herb-drug interactions are usually poorly explored.

Most of the evidence about herb-drug interactions derives from case reports and from in vitro or animal models. In some cases, sound evidences are available [22, 23]. However, case reports lack pharmacokinetic trials, have poor translational value, and clinical relevance of interactions. In addition, the effects of herb-drug interaction might differ in ethnic groups, due to gene polymorphisms of metabolic enzymes influencing complex pathways [24].

Concomitant administration of herbs may affect drug transport, metabolism, or excretion, due to altered pharmacokinetic/pharmacodynamic pathways [25–27].

Pharmacokinetic interactions may alter the absorption, distribution, metabolism, and excretion of drugs due to changes in Cmax, Tmax, and/or area-under-curve (AUC). Interactions mainly involve the interplays between cytochrome P450, UDP-glucuronyltransferases (UGTs), and drug transporter proteins. These mechanisms are more often reported but are more difficult to characterize [24].

Pharmacodynamic interactions imply the effects of one drug changed by the presence of another substance at its action site. Notably, the pharmacokinetic interactions between herbs and drugs will also influence the pharmacodynamic interactions, which include competitive or noncompetitive antagonism and synergism or additive effects. Changes can affect drug efficacy or toxicity. Beneficial effects due to the interactions between herbs and drugs are also possible [28]. Pathways include improved drug bioavailability, prolonged therapeutic effects, and additive or synergistic effects [27].

As foods, ingested herbal pharmaceuticals may produce systemic effects through gastrointestinal absorption, and portal tract delivery to the liver. In the liver, herbal components undergo metabolization and are eventually transferred to the systemic circulation.

During this process, herbs may influence (enhance or reduce) the absorption of drugs in the gastrointestinal tract, can modulate carrier proteins (by inhibiting efflux transporters and/or stimulating uptake transporters), and affect (decrease or induction) intracellular metabolic enzymes, mainly CYP450 enzymes.

Herb-drug interactions can also occur at the level of the kidney and/or other target organs.

In vivo and in vitro studies describe several interplays between herbs and intestinal and/or hepatocellular transporters [24, 29].

Some herbs can increase the intestinal absorption of drugs by opening the tight junctions between the gut epithelial cells [27, 30–32]. The monocellular layer of enterocytes is one component of the gut barrier [33], together with Goblet cells (which produce mucus), Tufts cells (with chemosensory function) [34], and Paneth cells (which produce antimicrobial peptides) [35]. This cellular barrier has physical, electrical, and chemical properties. The layer is impermeable to most solutes, and solutes need a specific transporter to cross the barrier and a mechanism involving transcellular pathways.

P-glycoprotein (P-gp) regulates drug permeation through the intestinal barrier and, therefore, the amount of drug reaching the liver [36]. P-gp is a protein located in many tissues such as the intestine, liver, kidney, and brain. In the gastrointestinal tract, P-gp is found in the apical domain of human ileum and colon cells, and its expression progressively decreases in the jejunum, duodenum, and stomach [24]. In addition, liver and kidney P-gp regulate the excretion of drugs from the hepatocytes and renal tubules, respectively. Notably, medicinal herbs modulate [37] (mainly inhibit [38, 39]) P-gp activity [24].

In the liver, herb-drug interactions depend strongly on the presence of cytochrome P450 enzymes (CYPs), which play a critical role in the biotransformation, inactivation, and clearance of a number of both drugs [40] and herbs [41]. CYPs promote biotransformation reactions through oxidation, reduction, hydrolysis, and hydration. Phase I biotransformation reactions include the introduction of a hydrophilic functional group into molecules or the introduction of new functional groups of molecules. Phase II biotransformation reactions include sulfation, methylation, acetylation, glutathione conjugation, fatty acid conjugation, and glucuronidation [24]. Herbs, besides enzyme induction, can inhibit CYP450 enzymes through competitive/noncompetitive inhibition or inductive effects, which are mediated through the nuclear receptor pregnane X receptor (PXR). PXR is a metabolic "sensor" that regulates a number of processes by modulation of gene expression of specific transporter proteins and cytochrome P450 (CYP) family members. In particular, PXR can play a key role in both CYP and P-gp induction. In this respect, herbs can act as an endogenous activating ligand for PXR.

Thus, herbs able to activate PXR (Table 14.1) can strongly influence drug metabolism and biotransformation processes during combination therapies [24, 43, 54–56].

Finally, herbs can markedly affect the therapeutic outcomes of orally ingested drugs by changes in gastrointestinal motility. For example, *Ginkgo biloba* leaf extract, ginger, *Piper methysticum*, *Echinacea purpurea*, *Hypericum perforatum*, and *Cassia angustifolia* accelerate gastrointestinal transit and reduce the contact time between the drug and gut epithelium, affecting drug absorption [24].

Table 14.1 Most commonly employed herbs able to activate the nuclear receptor PXR

• *Andrographis paniculata* [42]
• *Argemone mexicana* [38]
• *Astragalus membranaceus* [43]
• *Coleus forskohlii* [44]
• *Crataegus monogyna* (hawthorn) [45]
• Culinary herbs and spices [46]
• Curcumin [47]
• *Eschscholzia californica* (California Poppy) [48]
• *Fritillariae cirrhosae* [43]
• Gancao (Glycyrrhizae Radix) [49, 50]
• Gan Cao [44]
• Ging hao [44]
• Glycyrrhizin [51]
• Gugu lipids [44]
• Hypoxis [44]
• *Momordica charantia* [38]
• Kava [44]
• *Phellodendron amurense* [43]
• *Phyllanthus amarus* [38]
• Quiercitin [44]
• *Sarothamnus scoparius* [43]
• *Schisandra sphenanthera* [50]
• *Sophorae flavescentis* [43]
• *Silybum marianum* [52]
• St. John's Wort [53]
• Sutherlandia [44]
• *Tithonia diversifolia* [38]

Herb-Drug Interactions Relevant in Gastroenterology

Clinicians frequently face questions regarding the efficacy and safety of herbal medicines. This problem is mainly due to the unsatisfactory efficacy of traditional drugs (in particular, in functional gastrointestinal disorders and metabolic diseases), auto-medications, and the need for combined treatments in the management of disorders of multifactorial origin (i.e., functional disorders, dyspepsia, and nonalcoholic fatty liver disease (NAFLD)). Several medicinal plants are therefore traditionally used for the treatment of chronic gastrointestinal disorders.

In addition, comorbidities often require polytherapy, and this is true, especially in the elderly and patients with chronic diseases. Under this scenario, the likelihood of pharmacologic interactions increases in patients taking both drugs and herbs. An additional factor is that patients may forget to report herbal medicine use, which is considered "natural" and therefore "non-pharmacological" therapies.

It is important to spread adequate knowledge about potential herb-drug interactions, especially for main herbs employed in highly prevalent gastrointestinal disorders. A discussion about the main conditions relevant in this context appears in the following paragraphs.

Constipation

Patients with constipation frequently use herbs. In a recent real-life survey in Serbia, 44% of consumers of herbal products for gastrointestinal disorders had constipation and mainly used Buckthorn (*Rhamnus frangula*, Rhamnaceae), Senna (Cassia sp., Fabaceae), or dietary fibers [15].

Laxative or bulk-forming herbs (Table 14.2) usually accelerate intestinal transit, and changes can potentially interfere with drug absorption in the intestine [24].

Rhubarb (*Rheum rhabarbarum*) is a plant of the genus *Rheum* in the family *Polygonaceae*. It is a herbaceous perennial growing from short, thick rhizome roots, and stems contain anthraquinones such as emodin, rheican, and resveratrol. Rhubarb can be toxic if leaves are eaten, due to its high content of calcium oxalate in the form of intracellular sharp projections called raphides. If the plant is chewed, the raphides are injected into the gastrointestinal mucosa along with proteolytic enzymes, which can cause localized irritation and swelling. Rhubarb induces CYP3A and CYP2D6 enzymes, a step potentially affecting the intracellular concentration of drugs metabolized by these enzymes [57, 58]. In the study from Gao et al. [58], wine-processed rhubarb induced CYP1A2 activity, and both the processed rhubarbs inhibited the CYP2C6 activity and induced CYP2E1. Cooked rhubarb induced CYP3A1 activity. Both the processed rhubarbs reduced the absorbance and bioavailability but increased the clearance of saxagliptin, a dipeptidyl peptidase 4 (DPP-4) inhibitor (used as initial pharmacologic therapy for the treatment of type 2 diabetes or as a second agent in those who do not respond to a single agent such as a sulfonylurea). In the animal models, Rhubarb decreased the bioavailability of cyclosporine [59] and increased the exposure to methotrexate [60]. The clinical relevance of these interactions, however, is still undetermined.

Inflammatory Bowel Disease (IBD)

IBD patients may decide to use complementary and alternative medicines because of unsatisfactory responses to drugs or fears about side effects in these chronic relapsing disorders [3]. However, a recent survey in Hungary found that IBD patients use herbs less frequently, compared with patients with other

Table 14.2 Most popular herbs used for constipation

– Anthranoid-containing senna (*Cassia senna* and *C. angustifolia*)
– Anthranoid-containing cascara sagrada (*Rhamnus purshiana*)
– Dried exudate from the aloe vera (*Aloe barbadensis*) leaf
– Anthranoid-containing plants: frangula (*Rhamnus frangula*), yellow dock (*Rumex crispus*), and Chinese rhubarb (*Rheum officinale*)

gastrointestinal diseases and controls. In the majority of cases, medicinal plants are taken together with conventional standard-dose medications [61]. Although real-life evidence is limited, positive outcomes exist following treatments of IBD with the most commonly used herbs (Table 14.3). Best evidence exists for *Aloe vera* [61],

Table 14.3 Most popular herbs used in patients with inflammatory bowel diseases and reported herb-drug interactions

Herb	Possible drug-herb interaction (s)
Aloe vera	Altered drug concentration due to inhibition of CYP3A4 and CYP2D6 [62]. P-gp activation [36]. Improved bioavailability of vitamins C and E [63]. Possible increased effect of glibenclamide
Andrographis paniculata	Altered drug concentration due to inhibition of CYP1A2, CYP2C9, CYP3A4 [64, 65], and UGT2B7 [66]. CYP1A1 induction [67]. Interference with aminophylline [68], azathioprine, 6-MP, prednisone [21], platelet aggregation [69, 70], and hypotensive drugs [71, 72]. Interaction with naproxen (synergistic anti-arthritic activity) [73] and nabumetone (decreases anti-arthritic activity) [74]
Artemisia absinthium (wormwood)	CYP2B6 and CYP3A4 induction [75]. Drugs to prevent seizures [76]. Possible interference with warfarin (increased risk of bleeding) [77]
Barley foodstuff	None reported
Bilberry	None reported
Boswellia serrata	Altered activity of the organic anion transporter OATP1B3 and the multidrug-resistant protein MRP2 [78]. Inhibition of P-gp. Possible interaction with azathioprine, 6-mercaptopurine, corticosteroids, and platelet aggregation [21]
Chamomile	Cyclosporin [79]
Curcumin (turmeric)	Inhibition of CYP3A4 [80], CYP1A2 [81], and CYP2D6 [82]. Induction of CYP2A6 [81]. Modulation of P-gp [24]. Interactions with camptothecin [83], mechlorethamine [83], paclitaxel [84], doxorubicin [83], cyclophosphamide [83], cyclosporin A 157–160), sulfasalazine [85], methotrexate [86–89], norfloxacin [90], amphotericin B [91], celiprolol and midazolam [92], verapamil [93], tacrolimus [94], acetaminophen [95], ibuprofen [95], and aspirin [95]
Oenotherabiennis (evening primrose oil)	Increased levels of antiretrovirals [96]. Possible interaction with warfarin, aspirin, and nonsteroidal anti-inflammatory drugs [97]. Sodium valproate (decrease of seizure threshold and decreased therapeutic effectiveness) [98]
Ginger	Cyclosporin [21], dabigatran [99], paracetamol [100], and warfarin [101]
Harpagophytum procumbens (devil's claw)	Cyclosporin [21]. Morphin (synergistic antinociceptive effect) [102]
Plantago ovata (blond psyllium)	Reduced bioavailability of several drugs (i.e., lithium, digoxin, and levothyroxine) following a combined administration [103]. Possible beneficial effects on levodopa pharmacodynamics [28]
Tripterygium wilfordii (thunder god vine)	Inhibition of CYP3A4, CYP2C19, CYP2D6, CYP1A2, and CYP2E1 [104]. Azathioprine, 6-MP, and prednisone [105]
Ulmus rubra (slippery elm bark)	Interference with drug absorption due to the mucilage layer in the gut [21]

Plantago ovata [3, 106], and curcumin [107–109] (Fig. 14.1) in the maintenance therapy in patients with ulcerative colitis [5]. *Andrographis paniculata* (Indian Echinacea), *Boswellia serrata*, and topical Xilei-San are beneficial in active ulcerative colitis [110], while wheatgrass juice is effective in proctitis [5]. Wormwood [111] and *Tripterygium wilfordii* [112–114] play a role in Chron's disease [3, 5, 110,

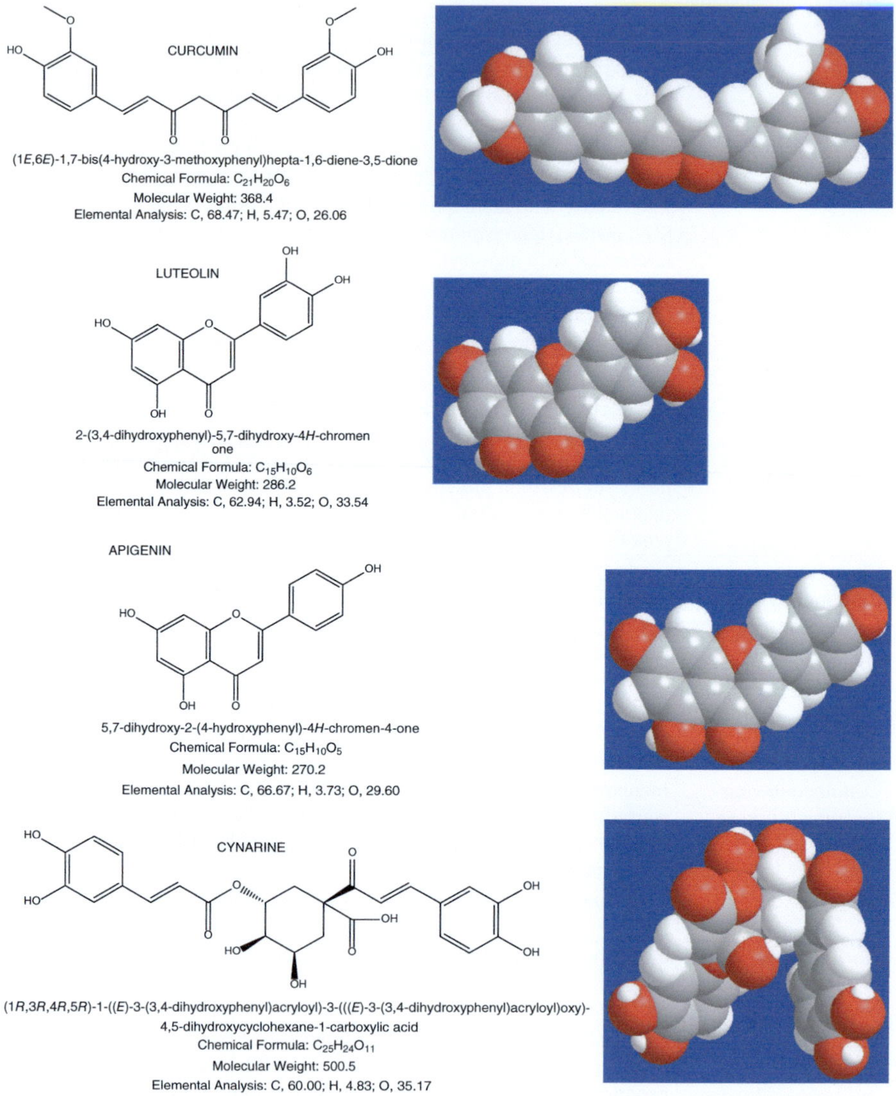

Fig. 14.1 Chemical structure, name, formula, molecular weight, elemental analysis, and 3D structure of specific molecules: curcumin, luteolin, apigenin, cynarine, silybin, and omeprazole. In the 3D structure, elements are indicated in grey (carbon, C), white (hydrogen, H), red (oxygen, O), blue (nitrogen, N), and yellow (sulphur, S)

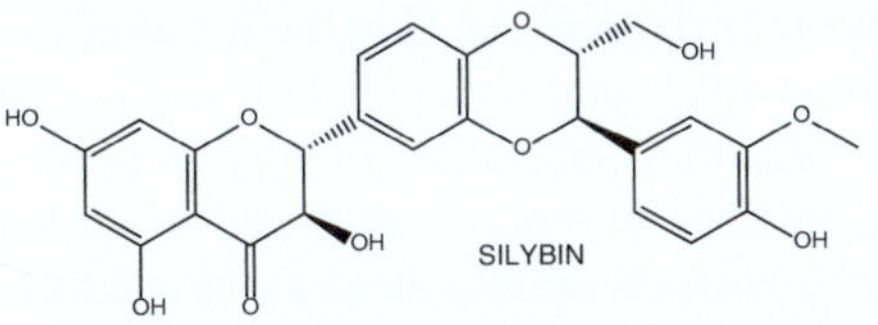

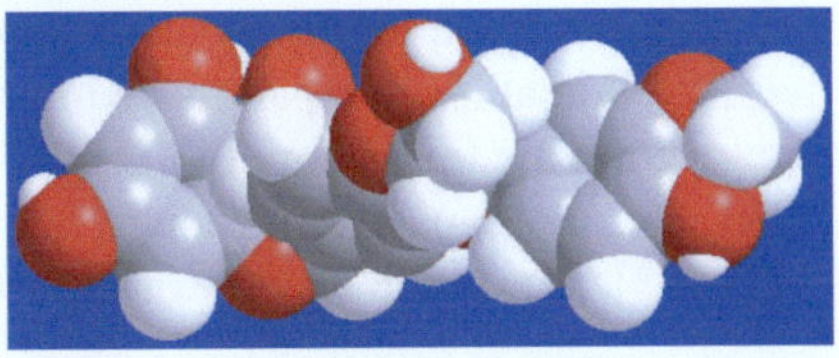

(2*R*,3*R*)-3,5,7-trihydroxy-2-((2*R*,3*R*)-3-(4-hydroxy-3-methoxyphenyl)-2-(hydroxymethyl)-2,3-dihydrobenzo[*b*][1,4]dioxin-6-yl)chroman-4-one
Chemical Formula: $C_{25}H_{22}O_{10}$
Molecula Weight: 482.4r
Elemental Analysis: C, 62.24; H, 4.60; O, 33.16

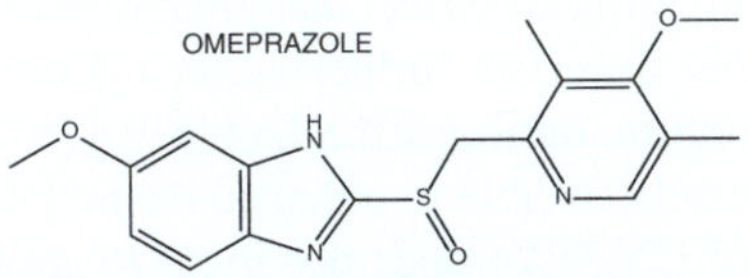

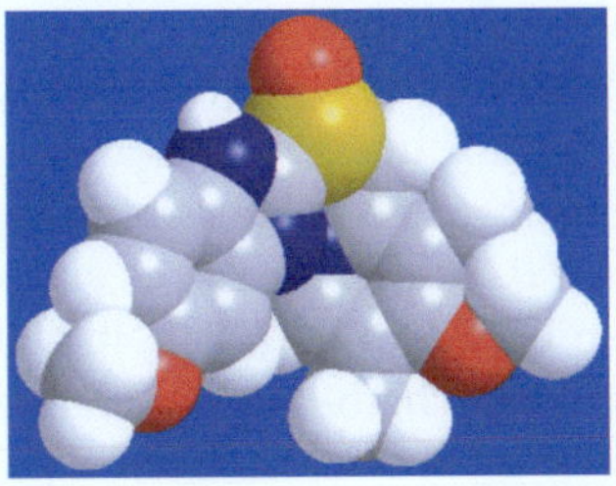

6-methoxy-2-(((4-methoxy-3,5-dimethylpyridin-2-yl)methyl)sulfinyl)-1*H*-benzo[*d*]imidazole
Chemical Formula: $C_{17}H_{19}N_3O_3S$
Molecular Weight: 345.4
Elemental Analysis: C, 59.11; H, 5.54; N, 12.17; O, 13.90; S, 9.28

Fig. 14.1 (continued)

113, 114]. The biologically active herbs act mainly through antibacterial, antioxidant, anti-cytokine, antispasmodic, and neuro-modulatory effects.

Herb-drug interactions imply different mechanisms (Table 14.3). Among the most popular herbs for IBD, aloe juice inhibits CYP3A4 and CYP2D6 in vitro. This effect can alter the intracellular concentration of metabolized drugs [62]. In addition, aloe can activate P-gp and, therefore, plays a critical role in the intestinal transport of drugs [36]. Furthermore, the *Aloe vera* leaf can enhance drug permeation across the intestinal barrier (i.e., increase drug absorption), due to the opening of tight junctions between the epithelial cells [30]. *Aloe vera* also improved the bioavailability of vitamins A and E [63].

Plantago ovata is a common source of psyllium, a dietary indigestible fiber that may be fermented into butyrate (a short-chain fatty acid) by butyrate-producing bacteria. The seed and husks of *Plantago ovata* (blond psyllium), mixed with water to form a gel, increase the viscosity of stools acting as a laxative. The use of *Plantago ovata* in IBD (mainly ulcerative colitis [106]) depends on the production of the short-chain fatty acid butyrate (a cytokine inhibitor with anti-inflammatory effects) during fermentation in the gut [106]. Evidence concerning interactions between *Plantago ovata* and drugs is scarce. Results are variable and mainly document a reduced bioavailability of several drugs (i.e., lithium, digoxin, and levothyroxine) following a combined administration [103]. In an animal model, the oral administration of *Plantago ovata* husk modified the pharmacodynamics of levodopa, with potential beneficial effects in patients with Parkinson's disease (improvement of levodopa kinetic profile with higher final concentrations, longer plasma half-life, and lower Cmax) [28].

Curcumin is one of the main elements of the herb turmeric. Curcumin was effective at a clinical level in patients with irritable bowel syndrome [11, 115] and is also employed in the treatment of IBD [107–109] due to its anti-inflammatory properties [116], and the capacity to reduce mucosal injuries in the animal model of colitis [117–123]. Curcumin might exert its beneficial effects mainly through the modulation of I-kappa B kinase activity, driven by the inhibition of nuclear factor-κB (NF-kB) and pro-inflammatory cytokines (tumor necrosis factor-alpha and interleukin 1β and 6) [124–127].

A number of animals and *in vitro* studies reported interactions of curcumin with several drugs (Table 14.3). However, in the majority of cases, the clinical relevance of this herb-drug interaction is unknown and deserves further studies. However, herb-drug interactions are possible, since curcumin inhibits CYP3A4 [80], CYP1A2 [81], and CYP2D6 [82] enzymes and, conversely, is able to enhance the activity of the enzyme CYP2A6 [81]. The inhibition of CYP3A4 does not seem to result in clinically relevant herb-drugs interactions in healthy volunteers [128], and the clinical relevance of the interactions with CYP1A2, CYP2D6, and CYP2A6 is still uncertain and needs to be further explored by appropriate therapeutic trials.

Of note, curcumin can increase serum levels of sulfasalazine up to 3.2 times the therapeutic doses, due to an inhibitory effect on a protein involved in the uptake modulation of this drug [85]. In vitro, *Andrographis paniculata* (Indian Echinacea) inhibits CYP1A2, 2C9, 3A4 [64, 65], and UDP-glucuronosyltransferase (UGT) 2B7 [66] and induces CYP1A1 [67]. The documented interactions between these enzymes and Indian Echinacea might potentially affect the intracellular concentrations of metabolized drugs.

In rats, in particular, the labdane diterpenoid andrographolide affects the metabolism of aminophylline, increasing the risk of side effects from this drug [68]. Experimental observations also indicate that Andrographis extracts could inhibit platelet aggregation [69, 70] and may have hypotensive effects [71, 72] which will increase the effect of blood pressure-lowering drugs. In animals, *Andrographis paniculata* is able to interact with Naproxen, leading to a synergistic anti-arthritic activity [73], and with nabumetone, with a significant decrease in the anti-arthritic activity of this drug [74]. In the majority of cases, however, the ultimate clinical relevance of such effects is not properly known.

Boswellia serrata (containing constituents such as β-boswellic acid, acetyl-β-boswellic acid, 11-keto-β-boswellic acid, and acetyl-11-keto-β-boswellic acid) is used in IBD patients (mainly with ulcerative colitis [129, 130]). *Boswellia serrata* acts as a noncompetitive inhibitor of 5-lipoxygenase and, in turn, inhibits the production of inflammatory leukotrienes [131, 132].

The major component of *Boswellia serrata*, i.e., boswellic acid, is a 5-lipoxygenase inhibitor with anti-inflammatory [133] and antimicrobial activities [134].

Due to its immune-stimulating capacity [135, 136], Boswellia might decrease the therapeutic efficacy of other drugs employed in the treatment of IBD such as azathioprine, 6-mercaptopurine, and corticosteroids. This theoretical hypothesis, however, needs to be adequately tested.

It has been reported in vitro that 11-keto-beta-boswellic acid (KBA) and 3-acetyl-11-keto-beta-boswellic acid (AKBA) can modulate the activity of the organic anion transporter OATP1B3 and the multidrug-resistant protein MRP2 [78], with uncertain clinical relevance. Furthermore, Boswellia extracts and keto-boswellic acids inhibit the activity of P-gp, thus affecting drug transport through the intestinal wall [137]. Finally, Boswellia extracts exert an inhibitory effect on platelet aggregation [138], potentially increasing the risk of bleeding when used with anti-coagulants or antiplatelet drugs.

Wormwood (*Artemisia absinthium*) mainly contains absinthin, absinthic acid, absinthol, dihydroartemisinin, and thujone [139–141], and its use has been purposed in patients with Chron's disease due to anti-inflammatory properties [111]. In the human liver microsome, wormwood can induce CYP2B6 and CYP3A4 [75], affecting serum concentrations of drugs metabolized by these enzymes. Wormwood may also decrease the effects of medications used to prevent seizures [76].

Tripterygium wilfordii (thunder god vine) has shown anti-inflammatory and immunosuppressive properties through a decreased expression of cytokines including COX-1, COX-2, PGE2, IL-1, Il-2, IL-17, IFN-gamma, 5-lipoxygenase, TNF-alpha, NF-kappa B, and iNOS [142–144]. This herb has been used to prolong remission in Chron's disease [3, 5, 110, 112–114], and at high doses may have an immunosuppressive effect when used with azathioprine, 6-MP, and corticosteroids [105].

Liver Diseases

Herbal medicines can be used in various liver diseases, including hepatitis and liver cancer [145, 146]. Products are especially prescribed for the treatment of liver diseases of metabolic origin, and, in particular, in patients with NAFLD (Table 14.4) [6–8, 208, 209].

Artichoke (*Cynara cardunculus* var. Scolymus) is a variety of a species of thistle cultivated as a food. Bioactive agents contained in artichoke are apigenin and luteolin (Fig. 14.1) and the potent antioxidant cynarine (Fig. 14.1). The active compounds contained in artichoke exhibit hypoglycemic, cholesterol-lowering, choleretic, anti-cholestatic, and hepatoprotective effects [210–212]. Other hepatoprotective effects may include anti-obesity and antioxidant ability following a high-fat diet [211]. Patients with NAFLD often use artichoke leaf extract [209]. No significant herb-drug interaction has been reported following the administration of artichoke extracts which, conversely, seem to be beneficial, particularly in the presence of specific gene polymorphisms, in reducing insulin resistance and ameliorating glucose and lipid metabolism [213, 214].

Silymarin is the extract of *Silybum marianum* (milk thistle). Silybin is the principal active compound of silymarin and has been used in several chronic liver diseases (including liver cancer) due to its antioxidant, immune-modulating, anti-inflammatory, antifibrotic, and liver regenerating properties [145, 146], as well as antisteatogenic effect [215–217]. Although this herbal medicine seems to have

Table 14.4 Most popular herbs used in patients with liver diseases and reported herb-drug interactions

Herb	Possible drug-herb interaction (s)
Artichoke (*Cynara scolymus*, Asteraceae)	None reported
Bayberry (Myrica)	CYP2C9 and CYP3A4 enzyme inhibition [147]. Doxorubicin (synergistic effect) [148]
Berberine	Competitive binding on CYP3A and CYP2D [149]. Sulfonylureas [149], metformin [150], statins (cardiotoxicity) [151], losartan [152], macrolides (cardiotoxicity) [153], ketoconazole [154], and cyclosporin [155]
Cinnamon	Inhibition of CYP450 2C9, 3A4, 2A6, and 2D [156, 157]. Statins (drug-induced hepatitis) [158]. Pioglitazone [159]. Dabigatran [99]
Crataegus monogyna (hawthorn)	CYP3A4 induction by activating PXR [45]. Antiplatelets, anticoagulants (inhibition of thromboxane A2 biosynthesis) [160]. Digoxin [161]
Curcumin (turmeric)	Inhibition of CYP3A4 [80], CYP1A2 [81], and CYP2D6 [82]. Induction of CYP2A6 [81]. Modulation of P-gp [24]. Interactions with camptothecin [83], mechlorethamine [83], paclitaxel [84], doxorubicin [83], cyclophosphamide [83], cyclosporin A [162–165], sulfasalazine [85], methotrexate [86–89], norfloxacin [90], amphotericin B [91], celiprolol and midazolam [92], verapamil [93], tacrolimus [94], acetaminophen [95], ibuprofen [95], and aspirin [95]
Danning Pian	None reported
Flaxseed	None reported
Garlic	Inhibition of CYP 2C9 and 2C19 enzymes [166, 167]. Possible effects on CYP 3A4 (contrasting evidences) [166, 167]. P-gp induction [168]. Possible interference with warfarin/platelet aggregation due to increased fibrinolytic activity and diminished human platelet aggregation [169, 170]. Protease inhibitors (darunavir and saquinavir [171, 172])
Green tea	Inhibition of CYP 3A4 enzyme [173, 174]. Modulation of UGT enzymes [175] Atorvastatin [176], amoxicillin [177], bortezomib [178], tamoxifen [179], verapamil [180], irinotecan [181], acetaminophen (increased liver toxicity) [182], nadolol [183],and palbociclib [183]
Liquorice (Glycyrrhiza) root	P-gp inhibition [184]. CYP3A [185] and CYP2D6 [186] induction Possible increment of toxicity of cardiac glycosides [187]. Diuretics (increased hypokalemia) [188]. Increased insulin sensitivity [189]. Warfarin [50]. MAO-inhibitors [190] Prednisolone [191]. Cyclosporin [192]. Possible interaction with anti-hypertensive drugs [193]
Ilex paraguariensis (mate)	Modulation of CYP2D6 [194] Chemotherapy drugs [195]
Olive and canola oils	None reported

(continued)

Table 14.4 (continued)

Herb	Possible drug-herb interaction (s)
Phyllanthus	Induction of CYP3A and CYP2B1/2 (223) Clopidogrel [196]. Midazolam [197]
Qianggan	None reported
Rosmarinus officinalis	Codeine and paracetamol (synergistic analgesic effects) [198]
Silybum marianum (milk thistle)	Inhibition of cytochrome P450 3A4 [199]. UGT enzyme modulation [175]. Antipsychotic drugs (haloperidol, risperidone, and aripiprazole) [200]
Soy	Induction of CYP3A4 [201] and P-gp [201]. Modulation of UGT enzymes [175]. Interference with OATP2B1 transporter [202]. Tamoxifen [203, 204]. Aromatase inhibitors [205]
Xuezhikang	Inhibition of CYP1A2 and CYP2C19 [206]. Lovastatin [206, 207]

minor effects on the pharmacokinetics of drugs metabolized by CYP enzymes or transported by P-gp [218], some observations report its ability to inhibit the cytochrome P450 3A4 [199] and 2C9 [37] and to modulate UGT enzymes [37, 175]. Interactions with antipsychotic drugs (haloperidol, risperidone, and aripiprazole) are also possible [200].

Of note, herbal products able to interact with drugs, affect hepatic metabolism, and modulate hepatic enzymes can cause liver injury [219, 220] through bioactivation of CYP, oxidative and mitochondrial damage, apoptosis [221], and immune mechanisms [222].

Herb-induced liver injury (HILI), in particular, can develop as acute and chronic hepatobiliary conditions [222]. A recent systematic review of HILI identified 335 hepatotoxic medicinal plants and 296 hepatotoxic ingredients (mainly alkaloids and terpenoids) [223].

Liver toxicity can originate from the potentiation of the toxic effects of drugs, but also from contaminants (i.e., pesticides and heavy metals), adulteration with drugs or synthetic chemicals, or employment of herbs with unknown toxicity [222, 224, 225] and may also depend on individual characteristics such as gender, age, presence of co-morbidities, and gene polymorphisms [223].

Functional Gastrointestinal Disorders (FGIDs)

About one-third of all medicinal plants listed in modern compendia on medicinal herbs are used in patients with FGIDs. Due to the multifactorial origin of FGIDs, these herbs are usually administered in various combinations [226]. This approach can optimize the therapeutic efficacy but can also increase the possibility of herb-drugs interactions. Table 14.5 shows the most popular herbs employed in patients with FGIDs and the reported herb-drug interactions [226, 245]. Peppermint leaf and oil from *Mentha piperita* is frequently used in the treatment of gastrointestinal diseases. Peppermint oil acts by blocking Ca2+ channels and causing the relaxation of

Table 14.5 Most popular herbs employed in patients with functional gastrointestinal disorders and reported herb-drug interactions

Herb	Possible drug interaction(s)
Artichoke (*Cynara scolymus*, Asteraceae)	None reported
Achillea millefolium (common yarrow)	Possible interaction with antidiabetic drugs [227]
Acorus calamus (Calamus)	Interference with CYP450 enzymes [228, 229]. Possible synergistic activity antifungal drugs (fluconazole, clotrimazole, and amphotericin B) [230]. Sodium valproate and carbamazepine [231]
Aesculus hippocastanum	Interference with CYP1A2, CYP2C9, and CYP3A4 enzymes [232]. Anticoagulants and antiplatelet agents [233, 234]
Aloe vera	Altered drug concentration due to inhibition of CYP3A4 and CYP2D6 [62]. P-gp activation [36]. Improved bioavailability of vitamins C and E [63]
Angelica archangelica (Angelica)	None reported
Artemisia absinthium (Absinthe)	CYP2B6 and CYP3A4 induction [75]. Drugs to prevent seizures [76]. Possible interference with warfarin (increased risk of bleeding) [77]
Asafoetida	Inhibitor of CYP2C11 expression [235]. Warfarin [236]
Carum carvi (caraway)	Antitubercular drugs [237]
Chamomile	Cyclosporin [79]
Chelidonium majus (greater celandine)	Inhibition of P-gp, MDR1, and CYP3A4 activity [238]
Cnicus benedictus (St. Benedict's thistle)	None reported
Curcumin	Inhibition of CYP3A4 [80], CYP1A2 [81], and CYP2D6 [82]. Induction of CYP2A6 [81]. Modulation of P-gp [24]. Interactions with camptothecin [83], mechlorethamine [83], paclitaxel [84], doxorubicin [83], cyclophosphamide [83], cyclosporin A [162–165], sulfasalazine [85], methotrexate [86–89], norfloxacin [90], amphotericin B [91], celiprolol and midazolam [92], verapamil [93], tacrolimus [94], acetaminophen [95], ibuprofen [95], and aspirin [95]
Erysimum cheiri (wallflower)	None reported
Foeniculum vulgare	Ciprofloxacin [239]

(continued)

Table 14.5 (continued)

Herb	Possible drug interaction(s)
Gentiana lutea (yellow gentian)	None reported
Ginger	Cyclosporin [21], dabigatran [99], paracetamol [100], and warfarin [101]
Glycyrrhiza glabra (liquorice)	P-gp inhibition [184]. CYP3A [185] and CYP2D6 [186] induction Possible increment of toxicity of cardiac glycosides [187]. Diuretics (increased hypokalemia) [188]. Increased insulin sensitivity [189]. Warfarin [50]. MAO-inhibitors [190] Prednisolone [191]. Cyclosporin [192]. Possible interaction with anti-hypertensive drugs [193]
Iberis amara (bitter candytuft)	None reported
Melissa officinalis (lemon balm)	None reported
Mentha piperita (peppermint)	CYP1A2/2C8/2C9/2C19/2D6 and 3A4 enzymes inhibitor [240–242]. Felodipine [240]. Cyclosporin [243]. 5-fluorouracil [244]
Pimpenella anisum	None reported
Potentilla anserina (common silverweed)	None reported
Schinopsis lorentzii	None reported
Silybum marianum (milk thistle)	Inhibition of cytochrome P450 3A4 [199]. UGT enzyme modulation [175]. Antipsychotic drugs (haloperidol, risperidone, and aripiprazole) [200]

intestinal smooth muscle tissue [246]. This mechanism allows its employment mainly in irritable bowel syndrome (IBS) [247]. As for peppermint oil, a number of other herbs have shown positive outcomes in clinical trials enrolling IBS patients (*Aloe vera*, asafetida, *Pimpinella anisum* oil, the combination of curcumin and *Foeniculum vulgare* oil [11], and the blend of *Schinopsis lorentzii* and *Aesculus hippocastanum*), showing different mechanisms [245, 247]. With few exceptions, all these medicinal herbs show, at least in experimental studies, interactions with several pathways involved in drug absorption, metabolism, and excretion (Table 14.5). In the majority of cases, however, the clinical relevance of such effect is not properly addressed.

Gastro-esophageal Reflux and Esophageal Symptoms

Several herbal products appear in the daily armamentarium to treat gastro-esophageal reflux and other esophageal symptoms (i.e., noncardiac chest pain). The best clinical outcomes exist for Rikkunshito (a traditional Japanese therapy comprising eight herbal extracts) [248, 249], STW5 (a compound of nine herbal extracts) [248], *Ceratonia siliqua*, *Myrtus communis*, *Cydonia oblonga* [249], and *Glycyrrhiza glabra*.

The pharmacodynamic and pharmacokinetic effects of multicomponent herbal products, such as Rikkunshito and STW5, are difficult to assess adequately since specific studies are missing. On the other hand, with the exception of *Glycyrrhiza glabra* (see Table 14.4), clinically relevant herb-drugs interactions have not been reported, until now, for the remaining cited herbs.

Omeprazole (Fig. 14.1), like other prazole molecules, is a widely employed drug for acid-related disorders in the upper gastrointestinal tract (i.e., gastro-esophageal reflux, esophagitis, peptic ulcer disease, and Zollinger–Ellison syndrome). Some herbs, namely St. John's wort, *Ginkgo biloba*, and yin zhi huang, could significantly lower the therapeutic efficacy of omeprazole [250]. This effect is mainly due to a herb-promoted induction of CYP2C19, CYP3A (St. John's wort and yin zhi huang), or CYP2C19 (*Ginkgo biloba*), with a consequent dramatic acceleration of drug elimination [250].

Conclusions

A number of experimental and clinical reports indicate that herbal medicines interact with conventional drugs and that the likelihood of negative effects depends on several variables including polytherapy, genetic polymorphisms, and the presence of mixtures of different herbs. Herb-drug interactions might be frequent, in particular, in patients suffering from chronic gastrointestinal disorders (i.e., IBD and FGIDs) mainly due to the belief they are "natural" and safe to the multifactorial origin of these diseases (requiring different therapeutic strategies) and to frequent dissatisfaction of traditional therapies, in some cases (i.e., FGIDs), still under assessment of clear, efficient, and fully validated guidelines.

Although in the majority of cases, herb-drug interactions have a negligible clinical relevance, the possibility of serious threat to the health of patients cannot be minimized, in particular in the case of possible interactions with antiretroviral, cardiovascular, immunosuppressive, anticoagulant, and anticancer agents.

From this point of view, elderly subjects are at high risk of herb-drug interactions mainly because of the elevated possibility of chronic diseases, polytherapy, and reduced liver and renal function regulating drug clearance.

Healthcare professionals should be properly educated about potential interactions in subjects taking combined treatments (herbs and pharmacologic drugs), in particular in the case of drugs with a narrow therapeutic index. Furthermore, specific clinical trials also exploring pharmacokinetic effects and well-designed translational studies are needed in order to fully evaluate the possibility of herb-drug interactions, at least in the case of the most diffused herbal medicines and in subjects at high risk (children, chronic diseases, and elderly).

References

1. Alissa EM. Medicinal herbs and therapeutic drugs interactions. Ther Drug Monit. 2014;36(4):413–22.
2. Hilsden RJ, Verhoef MJ, Best A, Pocobelli G. Complementary and alternative medicine use by Canadian patients with inflammatory bowel disease: results from a national survey. Am J Gastroenterol. 2003;98(7):1563–8.
3. Langhorst J, Wulfert H, Lauche R, Klose P, Cramer H, Dobos GJ, et al. Systematic review of complementary and alternative medicine treatments in inflammatory bowel diseases. J Crohns Colitis. 2015;9(1):86–106.
4. Joos S. Review on efficacy and health services research studies of complementary and alternative medicine in inflammatory bowel disease. Chin J Integr Med. 2011;17(6):403–9.
5. Triantafyllidi A, Xanthos T, Papalois A, Triantafillidis JK. Herbal and plant therapy in patients with inflammatory bowel disease. Ann Gastroenterol. 2015;28(2):210–20.
6. Liu ZL, Xie LZ, Zhu J, Li GQ, Grant SJ, Liu JP. Herbal medicines for fatty liver diseases. Cochrane Database Syst Rev. 2013;2013(8):CD009059.
7. Shi KQ, Fan YC, Liu WY, Li LF, Chen YP, Zheng MH. Traditional Chinese medicines benefit to nonalcoholic fatty liver disease: a systematic review and meta-analysis. Mol Biol Rep. 2012;39(10):9715–22.
8. Milosevic N, Milanovic M, Abenavoli L, Milic N. Phytotherapy and NAFLD—from goals and challenges to clinical practice. Rev Recent Clin Trials. 2014;9(3):195–203.
9. Loguercio C, Andreone P, Brisc C, Brisc MC, Bugianesi E, Chiaramonte M, et al. Silybin combined with phosphatidylcholine and vitamin E in patients with nonalcoholic fatty liver disease: a randomized controlled trial. Free Radic Biol Med. 2012;52(9):1658–65.
10. Bahrami HR, Hamedi S, Salari R, Noras M. Herbal medicines for the management of irritable bowel syndrome: a systematic review. Electron Physician. 2016;8(8):2719–25.
11. Portincasa P, Bonfrate L, Scribano ML, Kohn A, Caporaso N, Festi D, et al. Curcumin and fennel essential oil improve symptoms and quality of life in patients with irritable bowel syndrome. J Gastrointestin Liver Dis. 2016;25(2):151–7.
12. Patrick L. Gastroesophageal reflux disease (GERD): a review of conventional and alternative treatments. Altern Med Rev. 2011;16(2):116–33.
13. Eardley S, Bishop FL, Prescott P, Cardini F, Brinkhaus B, Santos-Rey K, et al. A systematic literature review of complementary and alternative medicine prevalence in EU. Forsch Komplementmed. 2012;19(Suppl 2):18–28.
14. Dossett ML, Davis RB, Lembo AJ, Yeh GY. Complementary and alternative medicine use by US adults with gastrointestinal conditions: results from the 2012 National Health Interview Survey. Am J Gastroenterol. 2014;109(11):1705–11.
15. Hitl M, Gavaric N, Kladar N, Brkic S, Samojlik I, Dragovic G, et al. Herbal preparations use in prevention and treatment of gastrointestinal and hepatic disorders-data from Vojvodina, Serbia. Complement Ther Med. 2019;43:265–70.
16. Anheyer D, Frawley J, Koch AK, Lauche R, Langhorst J, Dobos G, et al. Herbal medicines for gastrointestinal disorders in children and adolescents: a systematic review. Pediatrics. 2017;139(6).
17. Pike A, Etchegary H, Godwin M, McCrate F, Crellin J, Mathews M, et al. Use of natural health products in children: qualitative analysis of parents' experiences. Can Fam Physician. 2013;59(8):e372–8.
18. Simpson N, Roman K. Complementary medicine use in children: extent and reasons. A population-based study. Br J Gen Pract. 2001;51(472):914–6.
19. Cao F, Liu J, Sha BX, Pan HF. Natural products: experimental efficient agents for inflammatory bowel disease therapy. Curr Pharm Des. 2019;25(46):4893–913.
20. Fugh-Berman A. Herb-drug interactions. Lancet. 2000;355(9198):134–8.
21. Rahman H, Kim M, Leung G, Green JA, Katz S. Drug-herb interactions in the elderly patient with IBD: a growing concern. Curr Treat Options Gastroenterol. 2017;15(4):618–36.

22. Awortwe C, Bruckmueller H, Cascorbi I. Interaction of herbal products with prescribed medications: a systematic review and meta-analysis. Pharmacol Res. 2019;141:397–408.
23. Williamson E, Driver S, Baxter K. Stockley's herbal medicines interactions. London, Chicago: Pharmaceutical Press; 2009.
24. Tarirai C, Viljoen AM, Hamman JH. Herb-drug pharmacokinetic interactions reviewed. Expert Opin Drug Metab Toxicol. 2010;6(12):1515–38.
25. Li Y, Paxton JW. The effects of flavonoids on the ABC transporters: consequences for the pharmacokinetics of substrate drugs. Expert Opin Drug Metab Toxicol. 2013;9(3):267–85.
26. Haefeli WE, Carls A. Drug interactions with phytotherapeutics in oncology. Expert Opin Drug Metab Toxicol. 2014;10(3):359–77.
27. Gerber W, Steyn JD, Kotze AF, Hamman JH. Beneficial pharmacokinetic drug interactions: a tool to improve the bioavailability of poorly permeable drugs. Pharmaceutics. 2018;10(3).
28. Fernandez N, Carriedo D, Sierra M, Diez MJ, Sahagun A, Calle A, et al. Hydrosoluble fiber (Plantago ovata husk) and levodopa II: experimental study of the pharmacokinetic interaction in the presence of carbidopa. Eur Neuropsychopharmacol. 2005;15(5):505–9.
29. Murtaza G, Ullah N, Mukhtar F, Nawazish S, Muneer S, Mariam. Phytotherapeutics: the emerging role of intestinal and hepatocellular transporters in drug interactions with botanical supplements. Molecules. 2017;22(10).
30. Haasbroek A, Willers C, Glyn M, du Plessis L, Hamman J. Intestinal drug absorption enhancement by aloe vera gel and whole leaf extract: in vitro investigations into the mechanisms of action. Pharmaceutics. 2019;11(1).
31. Shi Y, Guo Y, Zhou J, Wu L, Chen L, Sun Y, et al. Herbs-partitioned moxibustion improves intestinal epithelial tight junctions by upregulating A20 expression in a mouse model of Crohn's disease. Biomed Pharmacother. 2019;118:109149.
32. Zhu ML, Liang XL, Zhao LJ, Liao ZG, Zhao GW, Cao YC, et al. Elucidation of the transport mechanism of baicalin and the influence of a Radix Angelicae Dahuricae extract on the absorption of baicalin in a Caco-2 cell monolayer model. J Ethnopharmacol. 2013;150(2):553–9.
33. Kurashima Y, Kiyono H. Mucosal ecological network of epithelium and immune cells for gut homeostasis and tissue healing. Annu Rev Immunol. 2017;35:119–47.
34. Nevo S, Kadouri N, Abramson J. Tuft cells: from the mucosa to the thymus. Immunol Lett. 2019;210:1–9.
35. Turner JR. Intestinal mucosal barrier function in health and disease. Nat Rev Immunol. 2009;9(11):799–809.
36. Yang MS, Yu CP, Huang CY, Chao PL, Lin SP, Hou YC. Aloe activated P-glycoprotein and CYP 3A: a study on the serum kinetics of aloe and its interaction with cyclosporine in rats. Food Funct. 2017;8(1):315–22.
37. Hermann R, von Richter O. Clinical evidence of herbal drugs as perpetrators of pharmacokinetic drug interactions. Planta Med. 2012;78(13):1458–77.
38. Fasinu PS, Manda VK, Dale OR, Egiebor NO, Walker LA, Khan SI. Modulation of cytochrome P450, P-glycoprotein and Pregnane X receptor by selected antimalarial herbs-implication for herb-drug interaction. Molecules. 2017;22(12).
39. Hellum BH, Nilsen OG. In vitro inhibition of CYP3A4 metabolism and P-glycoprotein-mediated transport by trade herbal products. Basic Clin Pharmacol Toxicol. 2008;102(5):466–75.
40. Lamb DC, Waterman MR, Kelly SL, Guengerich FP. Cytochromes P450 and drug discovery. Curr Opin Biotechnol. 2007;18(6):504–12.
41. Langhammer AJ, Nilsen OG. In vitro inhibition of human CYP1A2, CYP2D6, and CYP3A4 by six herbs commonly used in pregnancy. Phytother Res. 2014;28(4):603–10.
42. Yen CC, Liu YT, Lin YJ, Yang YC, Chen CC, Yao HT, et al. Bioavailability of the diterpenoid 14-deoxy-11,12-didehydroandrographolide in rats and up-regulation of hepatic drug-metabolizing enzyme and drug transporter expression. Phytomedicine. 2019;61:152841.
43. Cui Z, Kang H, Tang K, Liu Q, Cao Z, Zhu R. Screening ingredients from herbs against Pregnane X receptor in the study of inductive herb-drug interactions: combining pharmacophore and docking-based rank aggregation. Biomed Res Int. 2015;2015:657159.

44. Staudinger JL, Ding X, Lichti K. Pregnane X receptor and natural products: beyond drug-drug interactions. Expert Opin Drug Metab Toxicol. 2006;2(6):847–57.
45. Xu Y, Zhang Y, Zhou F, Zheng Y, Zhu X. [Human pregnane X receptor-mediated transcriptional regulation of CYP3A4 by extracts of 7 traditional Chinese medicines]. Zhongguo Zhong Yao Za Zhi. 2011;36(11):1524–7.
46. Bartonkova I, Dvorak Z. Essential oils of culinary herbs and spices activate PXR and induce CYP3A4 in human intestinal and hepatic in vitro models. Toxicol Lett. 2018;296:1–9.
47. Kluth D, Banning A, Paur I, Blomhoff R, Brigelius-Flohe R. Modulation of pregnane X receptor- and electrophile responsive element-mediated gene expression by dietary polyphenolic compounds. Free Radic Biol Med. 2007;42(3):315–25.
48. Manda VK, Ibrahim MA, Dale OR, Kumarihamy M, Cutler SJ, Khan IA, et al. Modulation of CYPs, P-gp, and PXR by Eschscholzia californica (California Poppy) and its alkaloids. Planta Med. 2016;82(6):551–8.
49. Feng D, Tang T, Fan R, Luo J, Cui H, Wang Y, et al. Gancao (Glycyrrhizae Radix) provides the main contribution to Shaoyao-Gancao decoction on enhancements of CYP3A4 and MDR1 expression via pregnane X receptor pathway in vitro. BMC Complement Altern Med. 2018;18(1):345.
50. Mu Y, Zhang J, Zhang S, Zhou HH, Toma D, Ren S, et al. Traditional Chinese medicines Wu Wei Zi (Schisandra chinensis Baill) and Gan Cao (Glycyrrhiza uralensis Fisch) activate pregnane X receptor and increase warfarin clearance in rats. J Pharmacol Exp Ther. 2006;316(3):1369–77.
51. Wang YG, Zhou JM, Ma ZC, Li H, Liang QD, Tan HL, et al. Pregnane X receptor mediated-transcription regulation of CYP3A by glycyrrhizin: a possible mechanism for its hepatoprotective property against lithocholic acid-induced injury. Chem Biol Interact. 2012;200(1):11–20.
52. Yu C, Chai X, Yu L, Chen S, Zeng S. Identification of novel pregnane X receptor activators from traditional Chinese medicines. J Ethnopharmacol. 2011;136(1):137–43.
53. Moore LB, Goodwin B, Jones SA, Wisely GB, Serabjit-Singh CJ, Willson TM, et al. St. John's wort induces hepatic drug metabolism through activation of the pregnane X receptor. Proc Natl Acad Sci USA. 2000;97(13):7500–2.
54. Staudinger JL. Clinical applications of small molecule inhibitors of Pregnane X receptor. Mol Cell Endocrinol. 2019;485:61–71.
55. Hogle BC, Guan X, Folan MM, Xie W. PXR as a mediator of herb-drug interaction. J Food Drug Anal. 2018;26(2S):S26–31.
56. Wang J, Huang M, Hu H, Yu L, Zeng S. Pregnane X receptor-mediated transcriptional activation of UDP-glucuronosyltransferase 1A1 by natural constituents from foods and herbs. Food Chem. 2014;164:74–80.
57. Tang JC, Zhang JN, Wu YT, Li ZX. Effect of the water extract and ethanol extract from traditional Chinese medicines Angelica sinensis (Oliv.) Diels, Ligusticum chuanxiong Hort. and Rheum palmatum L. on rat liver cytochrome P450 activity. Phytother Res. 2006;20(12):1046–51.
58. Gao J, Shi Z, Zhu S, Li GQ, Yan R, Yao M. Influences of processed rhubarbs on the activities of four CYP isozymes and the metabolism of saxagliptin in rats based on probe cocktail and pharmacokinetics approaches. J Ethnopharmacol. 2013;145(2):566–72.
59. Yu CP, Lin HJ, Lin SP, Shia CS, Chang PH, Hou YC, et al. Rhubarb decreased the systemic exposure of cyclosporine, a probe substrate of P-glycoprotein and CYP 3A. Xenobiotica. 2016;46(8):677–82.
60. Shia CS, Juang SH, Tsai SY, Lee Chao PD, Hou YC. Interaction of rhubarb and methotrexate in rats: in vivo and ex vivo approaches. Am J Chin Med. 2013;41(6):1427–38.
61. Fabian A, Rutka M, Ferenci T, Bor R, Balint A, Farkas K, et al. The use of complementary and alternative medicine is less frequent in patients with inflammatory bowel disease than in patients with other chronic gastrointestinal disorders. Gastroenterol Res Pract. 2018;2018:9137805.
62. Djuv A, Nilsen OG. Aloe vera juice: IC(5)(0) and dual mechanistic inhibition of CYP3A4 and CYP2D6. Phytother Res. 2012;26(3):445–51.

63. Vinson JA, Al Kharrat H, Andreoli L. Effect of Aloe vera preparations on the human bioavailability of vitamins C and E. Phytomedicine. 2005;12(10):760–5.
64. Pekthong D, Martin H, Abadie C, Bonet A, Heyd B, Mantion G, et al. Differential inhibition of rat and human hepatic cytochrome P450 by Andrographis paniculata extract and andrographolide. J Ethnopharmacol. 2008;115(3):432–40.
65. Ashour ML, Youssef FS, Gad HA, Wink M. Inhibition of cytochrome P450 (CYP3A4) activity by extracts from 57 plants used in traditional Chinese medicine (TCM). Pharmacogn Mag. 2017;13(50):300–8.
66. Ma HY, Sun DX, Cao YF, Ai CZ, Qu YQ, Hu CM, et al. Herb-drug interaction prediction based on the high specific inhibition of andrographolide derivatives towards UDP-glucuronosyltransferase (UGT) 2B7. Toxicol Appl Pharmacol. 2014;277(1):86–94.
67. Chatuphonprasert W, Remsungnen T, Nemoto N, Jarukamjorn K. Different AhR binding sites of diterpenoid ligands from Andrographis paniculata caused differential CYP1A1 induction in primary culture in mouse hepatocytes. Toxicol In Vitro. 2011;25(8):1757–63.
68. Li XP, Zhang CL, Gao P, Gao J, Liu D. Effects of andrographolide on the pharmacokinetics of aminophylline and doxofylline in rats. Drug Res (Stuttg). 2013;63(5):258–62.
69. Thisoda P, Rangkadilok N, Pholphana N, Worasuttayangkurn L, Ruchirawat S, Satayavivad J. Inhibitory effect of Andrographis paniculata extract and its active diterpenoids on platelet aggregation. Eur J Pharmacol. 2006;553(1–3):39–45.
70. Burgos RA, Hidalgo MA, Monsalve J, LaBranche TP, Eyre P, Hancke JL. 14-deoxyandrographolide as a platelet activating factor antagonist in bovine neutrophils. Planta Med. 2005;71(7):604–8.
71. Yoopan N, Thisoda P, Rangkadilok N, Sahasitiwat S, Pholphana N, Ruchirawat S, et al. Cardiovascular effects of 14-deoxy-11,12-didehydroandrographolide and Andrographis paniculata extracts. Planta Med. 2007;73(6):503–11.
72. Suriyo T, Pholphana N, Ungtrakul T, Rangkadilok N, Panomvana D, Thiantanawat A, et al. Clinical parameters following multiple oral dose administration of a standardized Andrographis paniculata capsule in healthy Thai subjects. Planta Med. 2017;83(9):778–89.
73. Balap A, Lohidasan S, Sinnathambi A, Mahadik K. Herb-drug interaction of Andrographis paniculata (Nees) extract and andrographolide on pharmacokinetic and pharmacodynamic of naproxen in rats. J Ethnopharmacol. 2017;195:214–21.
74. Balap A, Lohidasan S, Sinnathambi A, Mahadik K. Pharmacokinetic and Pharmacodynamic interaction of andrographolide and standardized extract of Andrographis paniculata (Nees) with Nabumetone in Wistar rats. Phytother Res. 2017;31(1):75–80.
75. Xing J, Kirby BJ, Whittington D, Wan Y, Goodlett DR. Evaluation of P450 inhibition and induction by artemisinin antimalarials in human liver microsomes and primary human hepatocytes. Drug Metab Dispos. 2012;40(9):1757–64.
76. Skyles AJ, Sweet BV. Alternative therapies. Wormwood. Am J Health Syst Pharm. 2004;61(3):239–42.
77. Acikgoz SK, Acikgoz E. Gastrointestinal bleeding secondary to interaction of Artemisia absinthium with warfarin. Drug Metabol Drug Interact. 2013;28(3):187–9.
78. Kruger P, Kanzer J, Hummel J, Fricker G, Schubert-Zsilavecz M, Abdel-Tawab M. Permeation of Boswellia extract in the Caco-2 model and possible interactions of its constituents KBA and AKBA with OATP1B3 and MRP2. Eur J Pharm Sci. 2009;36(2–3):275–84.
79. Colombo D, Lunardon L, Bellia G. Cyclosporine and herbal supplement interactions. J Toxicol. 2014;2014:145325.
80. Zhang W, Lim LY. Effects of spice constituents on P-glycoprotein-mediated transport and CYP3A4-mediated metabolism in vitro. Drug Metab Dispos. 2008;36(7):1283–90.
81. Chen Y, Liu WH, Chen BL, Fan L, Han Y, Wang G, et al. Plant polyphenol curcumin significantly affects CYP1A2 and CYP2A6 activity in healthy, male Chinese volunteers. Ann Pharmacother. 2010;44(6):1038–45.
82. Al-Jenoobi FI, Al-Thukair AA, Alam MA, Abbas FA, Al-Mohizea AM, Alkharfy KM, et al. Effect of Curcuma longa on CYP2D6- and CYP3A4-mediated metabolism of dex-

tromethorphan in human liver microsomes and healthy human subjects. Eur J Drug Metab Pharmacokinet. 2015;40(1):61–6.

83. Somasundaram S, Edmund NA, Moore DT, Small GW, Shi YY, Orlowski RZ. Dietary curcumin inhibits chemotherapy-induced apoptosis in models of human breast cancer. Cancer Res. 2002;62(13):3868–75.
84. Costa ML, Rodrigues JA, Azevedo J, Vasconcelos V, Eiras E, Campos MG. Hepatotoxicity induced by paclitaxel interaction with turmeric in association with a microcystin from a contaminated dietary supplement. Toxicon. 2018;150:207–11.
85. Kusuhara H, Furuie H, Inano A, Sunagawa A, Yamada S, Wu C, et al. Pharmacokinetic interaction study of sulphasalazine in healthy subjects and the impact of curcumin as an in vivo inhibitor of BCRP. Br J Pharmacol. 2012;166(6):1793–803.
86. Dhanasekaran S, Biswal BK, Sumantran VN, Verma RS. Augmented sensitivity to methotrexate by curcumin induced overexpression of folate receptor in KG-1 cells. Biochimie. 2013;95(8):1567–73.
87. Sankrityayan H, Majumdar AS. Curcumin and folic acid abrogated methotrexate induced vascular endothelial dysfunction. Can J Physiol Pharmacol. 2016;94(1):89–96.
88. Morsy MA, Ibrahim SA, Amin EF, Kamel MY, Rifaai RA, Hassan MK. Curcumin ameliorates methotrexate-induced nephrotoxicity in rats. Adv Pharmacol Sci. 2013;2013:387071.
89. Banji D, Pinnapureddy J, Banji OJ, Saidulu A, Hayath MS. Synergistic activity of curcumin with methotrexate in ameliorating Freund's complete adjuvant induced arthritis with reduced hepatotoxicity in experimental animals. Eur J Pharmacol. 2011;668(1–2):293–8.
90. Pavithra BH, Prakash N, Jayakumar K. Modification of pharmacokinetics of norfloxacin following oral administration of curcumin in rabbits. J Vet Sci. 2009;10(4):293–7.
91. Kudva AK, Manoj MN, Swamy BM, Ramadoss CS. Complexation of amphotericin B and curcumin with serum albumins: solubility and effect on erythrocyte membrane damage. J Exp Pharmacol. 2011;3:1–6.
92. Zhang W, Tan TM, Lim LY. Impact of curcumin-induced changes in P-glycoprotein and CYP3A expression on the pharmacokinetics of peroral celiprolol and midazolam in rats. Drug Metab Dispos. 2007;35(1):110–5.
93. Hou XL, Takahashi K, Tanaka K, Tougou K, Qiu F, Komatsu K, et al. Curcuma drugs and curcumin regulate the expression and function of P-gp in Caco-2 cells in completely opposite ways. Int J Pharm. 2008;358(1–2):224–9.
94. Egashira K, Sasaki H, Higuchi S, Ieiri I. Food-drug interaction of tacrolimus with pomelo, ginger, and turmeric juice in rats. Drug Metab Pharmacokinet. 2012;27(2):242–7.
95. Choi HA, Kim MR, Park KA, Hong J. Interaction of over-the-counter drugs with curcumin: influence on stability and bioactivities in intestinal cells. J Agric Food Chem. 2012;60(42):10578–84.
96. Jalloh MA, Gregory PJ, Hein D, Risoldi Cochrane Z, Rodriguez A. Dietary supplement interactions with antiretrovirals: a systematic review. Int J STD AIDS. 2017;28(1):4–15.
97. Werneke U, Earl J, Seydel C, Horn O, Crichton P, Fannon D. Potential health risks of complementary alternative medicines in cancer patients. Br J Cancer. 2004;90(2):408–13.
98. Miller LG. Herbal medicinals: selected clinical considerations focusing on known or potential drug-herb interactions. Arch Intern Med. 1998;158(20):2200–11.
99. Maadarani O, Bitar Z, Mohsen M. Adding herbal products to direct-acting Oral anticoagulants can be fatal. Eur J Case Rep Intern Med. 2019;6(8):001190.
100. Montserrat-de la Paz S, Garcia-Gimenez MD, Quilez AM, De la Puerta R, Fernandez-Arche A. Ginger rhizome enhances the anti-inflammatory and anti-nociceptive effects of paracetamol in an experimental mouse model of fibromyalgia. Inflammopharmacology. 2018;26(4):1093–101.
101. Leite PM, Martins MAP, Castilho RO. Review on mechanisms and interactions in concomitant use of herbs and warfarin therapy. Biomed Pharmacother. 2016;83:14–21.
102. Parenti C, Arico G, Pennisi M, Venditti A, Scoto GM. Harpagophytum procumbens extract potentiates morphine antinociception in neuropathic rats. Nat Prod Res. 2016;30(11):1248–55.

103. Fernandez N, Lopez C, Diez R, Garcia JJ, Diez MJ, Sahagun A, et al. Drug interactions with the dietary fiber Plantago ovata husk. Expert Opin Drug Metab Toxicol. 2012;8(11):1377–86.
104. Jin C, He X, Zhang F, He L, Chen J, Wang L, et al. Inhibitory mechanisms of celastrol on human liver cytochrome P450 1A2, 2C19, 2D6, 2E1 and 3A4. Xenobiotica. 2015;45(7):571–7.
105. Zhen QS, Ye X, Wei ZJ. Recent progress in research on Tripterygium: a male antifertility plant. Contraception. 1995;51(2):121–9.
106. Fernandez-Banares F, Hinojosa J, Sanchez-Lombrana JL, Navarro E, Martinez-Salmeron JF, Garcia-Puges A, et al. Randomized clinical trial of Plantago ovata seeds (dietary fiber) as compared with mesalamine in maintaining remission in ulcerative colitis. Spanish Group for the Study of Crohn's disease and ulcerative colitis (GETECCU). Am J Gastroenterol. 1999;94(2):427–33.
107. Hanai H, Sugimoto K. Curcumin has bright prospects for the treatment of inflammatory bowel disease. Curr Pharm Des. 2009;15(18):2087–94.
108. Bundy R, Walker AF, Middleton RW, Booth J. Turmeric extract may improve irritable bowel syndrome symptomology in otherwise healthy adults: a pilot study. J Altern Complement Med. 2004;10(6):1015–8.
109. Kumar S, Ahuja V, Sankar MJ, Kumar A, Moss AC. Curcumin for maintenance of remission in ulcerative colitis. Cochrane Database Syst Rev. 2012;10:CD008424.
110. Sebepos-Rogers GM, Rampton DS. Herbs and inflammatory bowel disease. Gastroenterol Clin N Am. 2017;46(4):809–24.
111. Omer B, Krebs S, Omer H, Noor TO. Steroid-sparing effect of wormwood (Artemisia absinthium) in Crohn's disease: a double-blind placebo-controlled study. Phytomedicine. 2007;14(2–3):87–95.
112. Ren J, Tao Q, Wang X, Wang Z, Li J. Efficacy of T2 in active Crohn's disease: a prospective study report. Dig Dis Sci. 2007;52(8):1790–7.
113. Ren J, Wu X, Liao N, Wang G, Fan C, Liu S, et al. Prevention of postoperative recurrence of Crohn's disease: Tripterygium wilfordii polyglycoside versus mesalazine. J Int Med Res. 2013;41(1):176–87.
114. Sun J, Shen X, Dong J, Wang H, Zuo L, Zhao J, et al. Tripterygium wilfordii hook F as maintenance treatment for Crohn's disease. Am J Med Sci. 2015;350(5):345–51.
115. Di Ciaula A, Portincasa P, Maes N, Albert A. Efficacy of bio-optimized extracts of turmeric and essential fennel oil on the quality of life in patients with irritable bowel syndrome. Ann Gastroenterol. 2018;31(6):685–91.
116. Shishodia S, Sethi G, Aggarwal BB. Curcumin: getting back to the roots. Ann N Y Acad Sci. 2005;1056(1):206–17.
117. Lubbad A, Oriowo MA, Khan I. Curcumin attenuates inflammation through inhibition of TLR-4 receptor in experimental colitis. Mol Cell Biochem. 2009;322(1–2):127–35.
118. Billerey-Larmonier C, Uno JK, Larmonier N, Midura AJ, Timmermann B, Ghishan FK, et al. Protective effects of dietary curcumin in mouse model of chemically induced colitis are strain dependent. Inflamm Bowel Dis. 2008;14(6):780–93.
119. Zhang M, Deng CS, Zheng JJ, Xia J. Curcumin regulated shift from Th1 to Th2 in trinitrobenzene sulphonic acid-induced chronic colitis. Acta Pharmacol Sin. 2006;27(8):1071–7.
120. Martelli L, Ragazzi E, di Mario F, Martelli M, Castagliuolo I, Dal Maschio M, et al. A potential role for the vanilloid receptor TRPV1 in the therapeutic effect of curcumin in dinitrobenzene sulphonic acid-induced colitis in mice. Neurogastroenterol Motil. 2007;19(8):668–74.
121. Deguchi Y, Andoh A, Inatomi O, Yagi Y, Bamba S, Araki Y, et al. Curcumin prevents the development of dextran sulfate sodium (DSS)-induced experimental colitis. Dig Dis Sci. 2007;52(11):2993–8.
122. Ukil A, Maity S, Karmakar S, Datta N, Vedasiromoni JR, Das PK. Curcumin, the major component of food flavour turmeric, reduces mucosal injury in trinitrobenzene sulphonic acid-induced colitis. Br J Pharmacol. 2003;139(2):209–18.
123. Sugimoto K, Hanai H, Tozawa K, Aoshi T, Uchijima M, Nagata T, et al. Curcumin prevents and ameliorates trinitrobenzene sulfonic acid-induced colitis in mice. Gastroenterology. 2002;123(6):1912–22.

124. Gupta SC, Patchva S, Aggarwal BB. Therapeutic roles of curcumin: lessons learned from clinical trials. AAPS J. 2013;15(1):195–218.
125. Epstein J, Docena G, MacDonald TT, Sanderson IR. Curcumin suppresses p38 mitogen-activated protein kinase activation, reduces IL-1beta and matrix metalloproteinase-3 and enhances IL-10 in the mucosa of children and adults with inflammatory bowel disease. Br J Nutr. 2010;103(6):824–32.
126. Larmonier CB, Midura-Kiela MT, Ramalingam R, Laubitz D, Janikashvili N, Larmonier N, et al. Modulation of neutrophil motility by curcumin: implications for inflammatory bowel disease. Inflamm Bowel Dis. 2011;17(2):503–15.
127. Jobin C, Bradham CA, Russo MP, Juma B, Narula AS, Brenner DA, et al. Curcumin blocks cytokine-mediated NF-kappa B activation and proinflammatory gene expression by inhibiting inhibitory factor I-kappa B kinase activity. J Immunol. 1999;163(6):3474–83.
128. Volak LP, Hanley MJ, Masse G, Hazarika S, Harmatz JS, Badmaev V, et al. Effect of a herbal extract containing curcumin and piperine on midazolam, flurbiprofen and paracetamol (acetaminophen) pharmacokinetics in healthy volunteers. Br J Clin Pharmacol. 2013;75(2):450–62.
129. Gupta I, Parihar A, Malhotra P, Singh GB, Ludtke R, Safayhi H, et al. Effects of Boswellia serrata gum resin in patients with ulcerative colitis. Eur J Med Res. 1997;2(1):37–43.
130. Gupta I, Parihar A, Malhotra P, Gupta S, Ludtke R, Safayhi H, et al. Effects of gum resin of Boswellia serrata in patients with chronic colitis. Planta Med. 2001;67(5):391–5.
131. Safayhi H, Sailer ER, Ammon HP. Mechanism of 5-lipoxygenase inhibition by acetyl-11-keto-beta-boswellic acid. Mol Pharmacol. 1995;47(6):1212–6.
132. Sailer ER, Subramanian LR, Rall B, Hoernlein RF, Ammon HP, Safayhi H. Acetyl-11-keto-beta-boswellic acid (AKBA): structure requirements for binding and 5-lipoxygenase inhibitory activity. Br J Pharmacol. 1996;117(4):615–8.
133. Dahmen U, Gu YL, Dirsch O, Fan LM, Li J, Shen K, et al. Boswellic acid, a potent antiinflammatory drug, inhibits rejection to the same extent as high dose steroids. Transplant Proc. 2001;33(1–2):539–41.
134. Camarda L, Dayton T, Di Stefano V, Pitonzo R, Schillaci D. Chemical composition and antimicrobial activity of some oleogum resin essential oils from Boswellia spp. (Burseraceae). Ann Chim. 2007;97(9):837–44.
135. Mikhaeil BR, Maatooq GT, Badria FA, Amer MM. Chemistry and immunomodulatory activity of frankincense oil. Z Naturforsch C J Biosci. 2003;58(3–4):230–8.
136. Altmann A, Poeckel D, Fischer L, Schubert-Zsilavecz M, Steinhilber D, Werz O. Coupling of boswellic acid-induced Ca2+ mobilisation and MAPK activation to lipid metabolism and peroxide formation in human leucocytes. Br J Pharmacol. 2004;141(2):223–32.
137. Weber CC, Reising K, Muller WE, Schubert-Zsilavecz M, Abdel-Tawab M. Modulation of Pgp function by boswellic acids. Planta Med. 2006;72(6):507–13.
138. Kokkiripati PK, Bhakshu LM, Marri S, Padmasree K, Row AT, Raghavendra AS, et al. Gum resin of Boswellia serrata inhibited human monocytic (THP-1) cell activation and platelet aggregation. J Ethnopharmacol. 2011;137(1):893–901.
139. Van der Meersch H. Review of the use of artemisinin and its derivatives in the treatment of malaria. J Pharm Belg. 2005;60(1):23–9.
140. Rezaeinodehi A, Khangholi S. Chemical composition of the essential oil of Artemisia absinthium growing wild in Iran. Pak J Biol Sci. 2008;11(6):946–9.
141. Burkhard PR, Burkhardt K, Haenggeli CA, Landis T. Plant-induced seizures: reappearance of an old problem. J Neurol. 1999;246(8):667–70.
142. Li RW, David Lin G, Myers SP, Leach DN. Anti-inflammatory activity of Chinese medicinal vine plants. J Ethnopharmacol. 2003;85(1):61–7.
143. Tao X, Schulze-Koops H, Ma L, Cai J, Mao Y, Lipsky PE. Effects of Tripterygium wilfordii hook F extracts on induction of cyclooxygenase 2 activity and prostaglandin E2 production. Arthritis Rheum. 1998;41(1):130–8.
144. Setty AR, Sigal LH. Herbal medications commonly used in the practice of rheumatology: mechanisms of action, efficacy, and side effects. Semin Arthritis Rheum. 2005;34(6):773–84.

145. Abenavoli L, Izzo AA, Milic N, Cicala C, Santini A, Capasso R. Milk thistle (Silybum marianum): a concise overview on its chemistry, pharmacological, and nutraceutical uses in liver diseases. Phytother Res. 2018;32(11):2202–13.
146. Federico A, Dallio M, Loguercio C. Silymarin/Silybin and chronic liver disease: a marriage of many years. Molecules 2017;22(2).
147. Guo YJ, Zheng SL. Effect of myricetin on cytochrome P450 isoforms CYP1A2, CYP2C9 and CYP3A4 in rats. Pharmazie. 2014;69(4):306–10.
148. Ambroz M, Matouskova P, Skarka A, Zajdlova M, Zakova K, Skalova L. The effects of selected Sesquiterpenes from Myrica rubra essential oil on the efficacy of doxorubicin in sensitive and resistant cancer cell lines. Molecules. 2017;22(6).
149. Singh A, Zhao K, Bell C, Shah AJ. Effect of Berberine on in vitro metabolism of sulfonylureas: a herb-drug interactions study. Rapid Commun Mass Spectrom. 2019:34.
150. Lyu Y, Zhang Y, Yang M, Lin L, Yang X, Cheung SCK, et al. Pharmacokinetic interactions between metformin and berberine in rats: role of oral administration sequences and microbiota. Life Sci. 2019;235:116818.
151. Feng P, Zhao L, Guo F, Zhang B, Fang L, Zhan G, et al. The enhancement of cardiotoxicity that results from inhibiton of CYP 3A4 activity and hERG channel by berberine in combination with statins. Chem Biol Interact. 2018;293:115–23.
152. Li H, Liu L, Xie L, Gan D, Jiang X. Effects of berberine on the pharmacokinetics of losartan and its metabolite EXP3174 in rats and its mechanism. Pharm Biol. 2016;54(12):2886–94.
153. Zhi D, Feng PF, Sun JL, Guo F, Zhang R, Zhao X, et al. The enhancement of cardiac toxicity by concomitant administration of Berberine and macrolides. Eur J Pharm Sci. 2015;76:149–55.
154. Zhou Y, He P, Liu A, Zhang L, Liu Y, Dai R. Drug-drug interactions between ketoconazole and berberine in rats: pharmacokinetic effects benefit pharmacodynamic synergism. Phytother Res. 2012;26(5):772–7.
155. Xin HW, Wu XC, Li Q, Yu AR, Zhong MY, Liu YY. The effects of berberine on the pharmacokinetics of cyclosporin a in healthy volunteers. Methods Find Exp Clin Pharmacol. 2006;28(1):25–9.
156. Chan J, Oshiro T, Thomas S, Higa A, Black S, Todorovic A, et al. Inactivation of CYP2A6 by the dietary Phenylpropanoid trans-Cinnamic aldehyde (Cinnamaldehyde) and estimation of interactions with nicotine and Letrozole. Drug Metab Dispos. 2016;44(4):534–43.
157. Taheri A, Lavasani H, Kasirzadeh S, Sheikholeslami B, Ardakani YH, Rouini MR. Changes in CYP2D enzyme activity following induction of type 2 diabetes, and administration of cinnamon and metformin: an experimental animal study. Xenobiotica. 2018;48(10):984–9.
158. Brancheau D, Patel B, Zughaib M. Do cinnamon supplements cause acute hepatitis? Am J Case Rep. 2015;16:250–4.
159. Mamindla S, Koganti V, Ravouru N, Koganti B. Effect of cinnamomum cassia on the pharmacokinetics and pharmacodynamics of pioglitazone. Curr Clin Pharmacol. 2017;12(1):41–9.
160. Vibes J, Lasserre B, Gleye J, Declume C. Inhibition of thromboxane A2 biosynthesis in vitro by the main components of Crataegus oxyacantha (hawthorn) flower heads. Prostaglandins Leukot Essent Fatty Acids. 1994;50(4):173–5.
161. Dasgupta A, Kidd L, Poindexter BJ, Bick RJ. Interference of hawthorn on serum digoxin measurements by immunoassays and pharmacodynamic interaction with digoxin. Arch Pathol Lab Med. 2010;134(8):1188–92.
162. Yu T, Chen C, Sun Y, Sun H, Li TH, Meng J, et al. ABT-737 sensitizes curcumin-induced anti-melanoma cell activity through facilitating mPTP death pathway. Biochem Biophys Res Commun. 2015;464(1):286–91.
163. Sagiroglu T, Kanter M, Yagci MA, Sezer A, Erboga M. Protective effect of curcumin on cyclosporin A-induced endothelial dysfunction, antioxidant capacity, and oxidative damage. Toxicol Ind Health. 2014;30(4):316–27.
164. Abdel Fattah EA, Hashem HE, Ahmed FA, Ghallab MA, Varga I, Polak S. Prophylactic role of curcumin against cyclosporine-induced nephrotoxicity: histological and immunohistological study. Gen Physiol Biophys. 2010;29(1):85–94.

165. Chueh SC, Lai MK, Liu IS, Teng FC, Chen J. Curcumin enhances the immunosuppressive activity of cyclosporine in rat cardiac allografts and in mixed lymphocyte reactions. Transplant Proc. 2003;35(4):1603–5.
166. Ho BE, Shen DD, McCune JS, Bui T, Risler L, Yang Z, et al. Effects of garlic on cytochromes P450 2C9- and 3A4-mediated drug metabolism in human hepatocytes. Sci Pharm. 2010;78(3):473–81.
167. Foster BC, Foster MS, Vandenhoek S, Krantis A, Budzinski JW, Arnason JT, et al. An in vitro evaluation of human cytochrome P450 3A4 and P-glycoprotein inhibition by garlic. J Pharm Pharm Sci. 2001;4(2):176–84.
168. Hajda J, Rentsch KM, Gubler C, Steinert H, Stieger B, Fattinger K. Garlic extract induces intestinal P-glycoprotein, but exhibits no effect on intestinal and hepatic CYP3A4 in humans. Eur J Pharm Sci. 2010;41(5):729–35.
169. Ang-Lee MK, Moss J, Yuan CS. Herbal medicines and perioperative care. JAMA. 2001;286(2):208–16.
170. Ge B, Zhang Z, Zuo Z. Updates on the clinical evidenced herb-warfarin interactions. Evid Based Complement Alternat Med. 2014;2014:957362.
171. Cloarec N, Solas C, Ladaique A, Tamalet C, Zaegel-Faucher O, Bregigeon S, et al. Subtherapeutic darunavir concentration and garlic consumption; a <<Mediterranean>> drug-food interaction, about 2 cases. Eur J Clin Pharmacol. 2017;73(10):1331–3.
172. Piscitelli SC, Burstein AH, Welden N, Gallicano KD, Falloon J. The effect of garlic supplements on the pharmacokinetics of saquinavir. Clin Infect Dis. 2002;34(2):234–8.
173. Wanwimolruk S, Wong K, Wanwimolruk P. Variable inhibitory effect of different brands of commercial herbal supplements on human cytochrome P-450 CYP3A4. Drug Metabol Drug Interact. 2009;24(1):17–35.
174. Mazzanti G, Menniti-Ippolito F, Moro PA, Cassetti F, Raschetti R, Santuccio C, et al. Hepatotoxicity from green tea: a review of the literature and two unpublished cases. Eur J Clin Pharmacol. 2009;65(4):331–41.
175. Mohamed ME, Frye RF. Effects of herbal supplements on drug glucuronidation. Review of clinical, animal, and in vitro studies. Planta Med. 2011;77(4):311–21.
176. Abdelkawy KS, Abdelaziz RM, Abdelmageed AM, Donia AM, El-Khodary NM. Effects of green tea extract on atorvastatin pharmacokinetics in healthy volunteers. Eur J Drug Metab Pharmacokinet. 2020;45:351.
177. Kiss T, Timar Z, Szabo A, Lukacs A, Velky V, Oszlanczi G, et al. Effect of green tea on the gastrointestinal absorption of amoxicillin in rats. BMC Pharmacol Toxicol. 2019;20(1):54.
178. Golden EB, Lam PY, Kardosh A, Gaffney KJ, Cadenas E, Louie SG, et al. Green tea polyphenols block the anticancer effects of bortezomib and other boronic acid-based proteasome inhibitors. Blood. 2009;113(23):5927–37.
179. Shin SC, Choi JS. Effects of epigallocatechin gallate on the oral bioavailability and pharmacokinetics of tamoxifen and its main metabolite, 4-hydroxytamoxifen, in rats. Anti-Cancer Drugs. 2009;20(7):584–8.
180. Chung JH, Choi DH, Choi JS. Effects of oral epigallocatechin gallate on the oral pharmacokinetics of verapamil in rats. Biopharm Drug Dispos. 2009;30(2):90–3.
181. Lin LC, Wang MN, Tsai TH. Food-drug interaction of (-)-epigallocatechin-3-gallate on the pharmacokinetics of irinotecan and the metabolite SN-38. Chem Biol Interact. 2008;174(3):177–82.
182. Salminen WF, Yang X, Shi Q, Greenhaw J, Davis K, Ali AA. Green tea extract can potentiate acetaminophen-induced hepatotoxicity in mice. Food Chem Toxicol. 2012;50(5):1439–46.
183. Misaka S, Yatabe J, Muller F, Takano K, Kawabe K, Glaeser H, et al. Green tea ingestion greatly reduces plasma concentrations of nadolol in healthy subjects. Clin Pharmacol Ther. 2014;95(4):432–8.
184. Nabekura T, Yamaki T, Ueno K, Kitagawa S. Inhibition of P-glycoprotein and multidrug resistance protein 1 by dietary phytochemicals. Cancer Chemother Pharmacol. 2008;62(5):867–73.

185. Tu JH, He YJ, Chen Y, Fan L, Zhang W, Tan ZR, et al. Effect of glycyrrhizin on the activity of CYP3A enzyme in humans. Eur J Clin Pharmacol. 2010;66(8):805–10.
186. Pandit S, Ponnusankar S, Bandyopadhyay A, Ota S, Mukherjee PK. Exploring the possible metabolism mediated interaction of Glycyrrhiza glabra extract with CYP3A4 and CYP2D6. Phytother Res. 2011;25(10):1429–34.
187. Yorgun H, Aksoy H, Sendur MA, Ates AH, Kaya EB, Aytemir K, et al. Brugada syndrome with aborted sudden cardiac death related to liquorice-induced hypokalemia. Med Princ Pract. 2010;19(6):485–9
188. Yasue H, Itoh T, Mizuno Y, Harada E. Severe hypokalemia, rhabdomyolysis, muscle paralysis, and respiratory impairment in a hypertensive patient taking herbal medicines containing licorice. Intern Med. 2007;46(9):575–8.
189. Eu CH, Lim WY, Ton SH, bin Abdul Kadir K. Glycyrrhizic acid improved lipoprotein lipase expression, insulin sensitivity, serum lipid and lipid deposition in high-fat diet-induced obese rats. Lipids Health Dis. 2010;9:81.
190. Hatano T, Fukuda T, Miyase T, Noro T, Okuda T. Phenolic constituents of licorice. III. Structures of glicoricone and licofuranone, and inhibitory effects of licorice constituents on monoamine oxidase. Chem Pharm Bull (Tokyo). 1991;39(5):1238–43.
191. Chen MF, Shimada F, Kato H, Yano S, Kanaoka M. Effect of oral administration of glycyrrhizin on the pharmacokinetics of prednisolone. Endocrinol Jpn. 1991;38(2):167–74.
192. Hou YC, Lin SP, Chao PD. Liquorice reduced cyclosporine bioavailability by activating P-glycoprotein and CYP 3A. Food Chem. 2012;135(4):2307–12.
193. Wallbach M, Lach N, Stock J, Hiller H, Mavropoulou E, Chavanon ML, et al. Direct assessment of adherence and drug interactions in patients with hypertensive crisis—a cross-sectional study in the Emergency Department. J Clin Hypertens (Greenwich). 2019;21(1):55–63.
194. Feltrin C, Brambila PF, Simoes CMO. Development of Caco-2 cells-based gene reporter assays and evaluation of herb-drug interactions involving CYP3A4 and CYP2D6 gene expression. Chem Biol Interact. 2019;303:79–89.
195. Miranda DD, Arcari DP, Pedrazzoli J Jr, Carvalho Pde O, Cerutti SM, Bastos DH, et al. Protective effects of mate tea (Ilex paraguariensis) on H2O2-induced DNA damage and DNA repair in mice. Mutagenesis. 2008;23(4):261–5.
196. Fatima N, Pingali U, Muralidhar N. Study of pharmacodynamic interaction of Phyllanthus emblica extract with clopidogrel and ecosprin in patients with type II diabetes mellitus. Phytomedicine. 2014;21(5):579–85.
197. Taesotikul T, Nakajima M, Tassaneeyakul W, Yokoi T. Effects of Phyllanthus amarus on the pharmacokinetics of midazolam and cytochrome P450 activities in rats. Xenobiotica. 2012;42(7):641–8.
198. Raskovic A, Milanovic I, Pavlovic N, Milijasevic B, Ubavic M, Mikov M. Analgesic effects of rosemary essential oil and its interactions with codeine and paracetamol in mice. Eur Rev Med Pharmacol Sci. 2015;19(1):165–72.
199. Venkataramanan R, Ramachandran V, Komoroski BJ, Zhang S, Schiff PL, Strom SC. Milk thistle, a herbal supplement, decreases the activity of CYP3A4 and uridine diphosphoglucuronosyl transferase in human hepatocyte cultures. Drug Metab Dispos. 2000;28(11):1270–3.
200. Woron J, Siwek M. Unwanted effects of psychotropic drug interactions with medicinal products and diet supplements containing plant extracts. Psychiatr Pol. 2018;52(6):983–96.
201. Yu CP, Hsieh YW, Lin SP, Chi YC, Hariharan P, Chao PD, et al. Potential modulation on P-glycoprotein and CYP3A by soymilk and miso: in vivo and ex-vivo studies. Food Chem. 2014;149:25–30.
202. Navratilova L, Applova L, Horky P, Mladenka P, Pavek P, Trejtnar F. Interaction of soy isoflavones and their main metabolites with hOATP2B1 transporter. Naunyn Schmiedeberg's Arch Pharmacol. 2018;391(10):1063–71.
203. Ju YH, Doerge DR, Allred KF, Allred CD, Helferich WG. Dietary genistein negates the inhibitory effect of tamoxifen on growth of estrogen-dependent human breast cancer (MCF-7) cells implanted in athymic mice. Cancer Res. 2002;62(9):2474–7.

204. Liu B, Edgerton S, Yang X, Kim A, Ordonez-Ercan D, Mason T, et al. Low-dose dietary phytoestrogen abrogates tamoxifen-associated mammary tumor prevention. Cancer Res. 2005;65(3):879–86.
205. van Duursen MB, Nijmeijer SM, de Morree ES, de Jong PC, van den Berg M. Genistein induces breast cancer-associated aromatase and stimulates estrogen-dependent tumor cell growth in in vitro breast cancer model. Toxicology. 2011;289(2–3):67–73.
206. Chen CH, Uang YS, Wang ST, Yang JC, Lin CJ. Interaction between red yeast rice and CYP450 enzymes/P-glycoprotein and its implication for the clinical pharmacokinetics of lovastatin. Evid Based Complement Alternat Med. 2012;2012:127043.
207. Feng D, Ge C, Tan ZY, Sun JG, Xie Y, Yao L, et al. Isoflavones enhance pharmacokinetic exposure of active lovastatin acid via the upregulation of carboxylesterase in high-fat diet mice after oral administration of Xuezhikang capsules. Acta Pharmacol Sin. 2018;39(11):1804–15.
208. Bagherniya M, Nobili V, Blesso CN, Sahebkar A. Medicinal plants and bioactive natural compounds in the treatment of non-alcoholic fatty liver disease: a clinical review. Pharmacol Res. 2018;130:213–40.
209. Panahi Y, Kianpour P, Mohtashami R, Atkin SL, Butler AE, Jafari R, et al. Efficacy of artichoke leaf extract in non-alcoholic fatty liver disease: a pilot double-blind randomized controlled trial. Phytother Res. 2018;32(7):1382–7.
210. Ben Salem M, Affes H, Ksouda K, Dhouibi R, Sahnoun Z, Hammami S, et al. Pharmacological studies of artichoke leaf extract and their health benefits. Plant Foods Hum Nutr. 2015;70(4):441–53.
211. Ben Salem M, Ksouda K, Dhouibi R, Charfi S, Turki M, Hammami S, et al. LC-MS/MS analysis and hepatoprotective activity of artichoke (Cynara scolymus L.) leaves extract against high fat diet-induced obesity in rats. Biomed Res Int. 2019;2019:4851279.
212. Salekzamani S, Ebrahimi-Mameghani M, Rezazadeh K. The antioxidant activity of artichoke (Cynara scolymus): a systematic review and meta-analysis of animal studies. Phytother Res. 2019;33(1):55–71.
213. Ebrahimi-Mameghani M, Asghari-Jafarabadi M, Rezazadeh K. TCF7L2-rs7903146 polymorphism modulates the effect of artichoke leaf extract supplementation on insulin resistance in metabolic syndrome: a randomized, double-blind, placebo-controlled trial. J Integr Med. 2018;16(5):329–34.
214. Rezazadeh K, Rahmati-Yamchi M, Mohammadnejad L, Ebrahimi-Mameghani M, Delazar A. Effects of artichoke leaf extract supplementation on metabolic parameters in women with metabolic syndrome: influence of TCF7L2-rs7903146 and FTO-rs9939609 polymorphisms. Phytother Res. 2018;32(1):84–93.
215. Grasselli E, Baldini F, Vecchione G, Oliveira PJ, Sardao VA, Voci A, et al. Excess fructose and fatty acids trigger a model of nonalcoholic fatty liver disease progression in vitro: protective effect of the flavonoid silybin. Int J Mol Med. 2019;44(2):705–12.
216. Vecchione G, Grasselli E, Cioffi F, Baldini F, Oliveira PJ, Sardao VA, et al. The Nutraceutic Silybin counteracts excess lipid accumulation and ongoing oxidative stress in an in vitro model of non-alcoholic fatty liver disease progression. Front Nutr. 2017;4:42.
217. Vecchione G, Grasselli E, Voci A, Baldini F, Grattagliano I, Wang DQ, et al. Silybin counteracts lipid excess and oxidative stress in cultured steatotic hepatic cells. World J Gastroenterol. 2016;22(26):6016–26.
218. Soleimani V, Delghandi PS, Moallem SA, Karimi G. Safety and toxicity of silymarin, the major constituent of milk thistle extract: an updated review. Phytother Res. 2019;33(6):1627–38.
219. Lin NH, Yang HW, Su YJ, Chang CW. Herb induced liver injury after using herbal medicine: a systemic review and case-control study. Medicine (Baltimore). 2019;98(13):e14992.
220. Parvez MK, Rishi V. Herb-drug interactions and hepatotoxicity. Curr Drug Metab. 2019;20(4):275–82.
221. Cullen JM. Mechanistic classification of liver injury. Toxicol Pathol. 2005;33(1):6–8.
222. Kaplowitz N. Herb-induced liver injury: a global concern. Chin J Integr Med. 2018;24(9):643–4.

223. He S, Zhang C, Zhou P, Zhang X, Ye T, Wang R, et al. Herb-induced liver injury: phylogenetic relationship, structure-toxicity relationship, and herb-ingredient network analysis. Int J Mol Sci. 2019;20(15).
224. Amadi CN, Orisakwe OE. Herb-induced liver injuries in developing nations: an update. Toxics. 2018;6(2).
225. Lopez-Gil S, Nuno-Lambarri N, Chavez-Tapia N, Uribe M, Barbero-Becerra VJ. Liver toxicity mechanisms of herbs commonly used in Latin America. Drug Metab Rev. 2017;49(3):338 56.
226. Kelber O, Bauer R, Kubelka W. Phytotherapy in functional gastrointestinal disorders. Dig Dis. 2017;35(Suppl 1):36–42.
227. Chavez-Silva F, Ceron-Romero L, Arias-Duran L, Navarrete-Vazquez G, Almanza-Perez J, Roman-Ramos R, et al. Antidiabetic effect of Achillea millefollium through multitarget interactions: alpha-glucosidases inhibition, insulin sensitization and insulin secretagogue activities. J Ethnopharmacol. 2018;212:1–7.
228. Chellian R, Pandy V, Mohamed Z. Pharmacology and toxicology of alpha- and beta-Asarone: a review of preclinical evidence. Phytomedicine. 2017;32:41–58.
229. Pandit S, Mukherjee PK, Ponnusankar S, Venkatesh M, Srikanth N. Metabolism mediated interaction of alpha-asarone and Acorus calamus with CYP3A4 and CYP2D6. Fitoterapia. 2011;82(3):369–74.
230. Kumar SN, Aravind SR, Sreelekha TT, Jacob J, Kumar BS. Asarones from Acorus calamus in combination with azoles and amphotericin B: a novel synergistic combination to compete against human pathogenic Candida species in vitro. Appl Biochem Biotechnol. 2015;175(8):3683–95.
231. Katyal J, Sarangal V, Gupta YK. Interaction of hydroalcoholic extract of Acorus calamus Linn. With sodium valproate and carbamazepine. Indian J Exp Biol. 2012;50(1):51–5.
232. Huang Y, Zheng SL, Zhu HY, Xu ZS, Xu RA. Effects of aescin on cytochrome P450 enzymes in rats. J Ethnopharmacol. 2014;151(1):583–90.
233. Felixsson E, Persson IA, Eriksson AC, Persson K. Horse chestnut extract contracts bovine vessels and affects human platelet aggregation through 5-HT(2A) receptors: an in vitro study. Phytother Res. 2010;24(9):1297–301.
234. McEwen BJ. The influence of herbal medicine on platelet function and coagulation: a narrative review. Semin Thromb Hemost. 2015;41(3):300–14.
235. Korashy HM, Al-Jenoobi FI, Raish M, Ahad A, Al-Mohizea AM, Alam MA, et al. Impact of herbal medicines like Nigella sativa, Trigonella foenum-graecum, and ferula asafoetida, on cytochrome P450 2C11 gene expression in rat liver. Drug Res (Stuttg). 2015;65(7):366–72.
236. Heck AM, DeWitt BA, Lukes AL. Potential interactions between alternative therapies and warfarin. Am J Health Syst Pharm. 2000;57(13):1221–7; quiz 8–30.
237. Sachin BS, Monica P, Sharma SC, Satti NK, Tikoo MK, Tikoo AK, et al. Pharmacokinetic interaction of some antitubercular drugs with caraway: implications in the enhancement of drug bioavailability. Hum Exp Toxicol. 2009;28(4):175–84.
238. El-Readi MZ, Eid S, Ashour ML, Tahrani A, Wink M. Modulation of multidrug resistance in cancer cells by chelidonine and Chelidonium majus alkaloids. Phytomedicine. 2013;20(3–4):282–94.
239. Zhu M, Wong PY, Li RC. Effect of oral administration of fennel (Foeniculum vulgare) on ciprofloxacin absorption and disposition in the rat. J Pharm Pharmacol. 1999;51(12):1391–6.
240. Dresser GK, Wacher V, Wong S, Wong HT, Bailey DG. Evaluation of peppermint oil and ascorbyl palmitate as inhibitors of cytochrome P4503A4 activity in vitro and in vivo. Clin Pharmacol Ther. 2002;72(3):247–55.
241. Unger M, Frank A. Simultaneous determination of the inhibitory potency of herbal extracts on the activity of six major cytochrome P450 enzymes using liquid chromatography/mass spectrometry and automated online extraction. Rapid Commun Mass Spectrom. 2004;18(19):2273–81.
242. Kligler B, Chaudhary S. Peppermint oil. Am Fam Physician. 2007;75(7):1027–30.

243. Wacher VJ, Wong S, Wong HT. Peppermint oil enhances cyclosporine oral bioavailability in rats: comparison with D-alpha-tocopheryl poly(ethylene glycol 1000) succinate (TPGS) and ketoconazole. J Pharm Sci. 2002;91(1):77–90.
244. Abdullah D, Ping QN, Liu GJ. Enhancing effect of essential oils on the penetration of 5-fluorouracil through rat skin. Yao Xue Xue Bao. 1996;31(3):214–21.
245. Fifi AC, Axelrod CH, Chakraborty P, Saps M. Herbs and spices in the treatment of functional gastrointestinal disorders: a review of clinical trials. Nutrients. 2018;10(11).
246. Grigoleit HG, Grigoleit P. Gastrointestinal clinical pharmacology of peppermint oil. Phytomedicine. 2005;12(8):607–11.
247. Hawrelak JA, Wohlmuth H, Pattinson M, Myers SP, Goldenberg JZ, Harnett J, et al. Western herbal medicines in the treatment of irritable bowel syndrome: a systematic review and meta-analysis. Complement Ther Med. 2020;48:102233.
248. Ahuja A, Ahuja NK. Popular remedies for esophageal symptoms: a critical appraisal. Curr Gastroenterol Rep. 2019;21(8):39.
249. Salehi M, Karegar-Borzi H, Karimi M, Rahimi R. Medicinal plants for Management of Gastroesophageal Reflux Disease: a review of animal and human studies. J Altern Complement Med. 2017;23(2):82–95.
250. Li W, Zeng S, Yu LS, Zhou Q. Pharmacokinetic drug interaction profile of omeprazole with adverse consequences and clinical risk management. Ther Clin Risk Manag. 2013;9:259–71.

Food-Drug Interactions 15

Eva Pavić and Valentina Rahelić

Introduction

Most treatments involve the initiation of appropriate pharmacological therapy. It is important to emphasize that appropriate drug dosing must be ensured for their safe and effective use. Drug effects on patients may be inappropriate due to interaction:

1. With another drug (drug-drug interaction)
2. With particular types of food or drink (food-drug interaction)
3. With certain dietary supplements
4. If a patient suffers from other diseases, interactions of drugs with that particular disease

The concept itself is much broader, and it implies the influence of drugs on patient nutritional status. This is why ongoing education about safe and effective drug use is necessary, including the interaction between food and drugs.

When it comes to food-drug interaction, it is important for healthcare professionals to refer patients to what type of food to avoid when taking certain drugs to prevent the inability to use it or to prevent serious health consequences [2, 4].

Food-Drug Interactions and Pharmacologic Aspects

Food can interact with the drug at any time during gastrointestinal absorption, distribution, metabolism and elimination from an organism, while the greatest food effect on the drug itself is during absorption and metabolic reactions [5].

E. Pavić (✉) · V. Rahelić
Department of Nutrition and Dietetics, University Hospital Center Zagreb, Zagreb, Croatia
e-mail: eva.pavic@kbc-zagreb.hr; valentina.rahelic@kbc-zagreb.hr

M. Banić, D. Erceg (eds.), *Drug Interactions in Gastroenterology*, Clinical Gastroenterology, https://doi.org/10.1007/978-3-031-69800-2_15

This is why understanding the very mechanisms of action is necessary to prevent interaction, which is divided into two basic types:

1. Pharmacodynamic interactions
2. Pharmacokinetic interactions [6–8].

Pharmacodynamic Interactions

Pharmacodynamics studies the biochemical and physiological drug effects. The mechanism of action involves drug molecules binding to receptors, enzymes or ion channels, thereby obtaining a physiological response. The response itself can be accelerated or slowed down by other substances' activity.

Pharmacokinetic Interactions

Pharmacokinetics studies the time of drug action including absorption, distribution, biotransformation and excretion from organisms. Absorption involves a number of steps and signifies the drug movement process from its entry into the organism. In this step, food, individual food components and also dietary supplements can affect the process itself, especially in per os administered drugs.

Chemical reactions included in drug and nutrient metabolic reactions can be classified into two groups:

1. First-phase reactions that alter the basic chemical structure of parent molecules
2. Second-phase reactions that result in endogenous substances binding to parent molecule (usually for hydrophilic drugs) or for metabolites as a result of the first-phase reactions (usually for lipophilic drugs)

When the drug leaves systemic circulation, distribution begins. Due to its different chemistry, it is distributed to its target site with the most common transmission method via plasma proteins (e.g., human serum albumin). Drug metabolism takes place in many organs, including the liver which has the most enzymatic systems, digestive system, lungs, kidneys and plasma. The drug is excreted from the organism either in unaltered form, as a metabolite, or as conjugate formed by the reactions of the second phase of metabolism (methylation, acetylation, conjugation with amino acids, sulfoconjugation, glucuronidation or conjugation with glutathione). One of the major enzyme systems that affect drug metabolism is cytochrome P 450 (CYP) enzymes, which act in phase 1 liver detoxification. They can both act as oxidases and peroxidases and catalyze reductive reactions [2, 9–11]. Certain food or active dietary supplement compounds may affect this system, and thus prolong the drug metabolism. As they pass through organisms, drugs become action subjects of enzymatic systems that alter their chemical and biochemical characteristics, most commonly by making lipophilic drugs (more than 70% in practice) become more hydrophilic and, thus more soluble in water, which consequently allows easier excretion by the kidneys. Almost 90% of all oxidative reactions in organisms are catalyzed by CYP enzymes [9].

Certain conditions in kidney tubules can affect drug excretion such as urinary pH change of value, which can lead to the drug returning to the circulatory system. When it comes to dosing and food-drug interaction, it is important to pay attention to individuals who suffer from kidney diseases [2, 10, 11].

Food Ingestion and Drug Interactions

Also, it is important to take into account food type (type of meal), which includes food volume, liquids and solids proportion, osmolality, pH, temperature, calorie content and a number of other components that can influence food or meal outcome.

1. Food volume	Proportional to slowing the gastric emptying
2. Physical properties of gastric contents	Liquids excrete faster than solid foods so the discharge rate is proportional to the size of the solid food that needs to be broken down
3. High-fat food	1. Slows gastric emptying which is proportional to the fatty acids amount in the stomach as well as side chain length 2. Increases lipophilic drug absorption due to improved solubility 3. Decreases hydrophilic drug absorption 4. Increases bile secretion which can interfere with epithelial membranes which increases paracellular drug transport 5. Can stimulate intestinal lymphatic transport for fat-soluble drugs 6. Can inhibit leakage carriers to increase their substrate bioavailability 7. Can lead to diarrhea thereby reducing drug absorption
4. Triglycerides	Unsaturated triglycerides slow gastric emptying more than saturated triglycerides
5. High-protein food	1. Can stimulate the intestinal transport system 2. Can stimulate liver enzyme activity and increase the drug elimination rate 3. Can affect blood-brain barrier 4. Elaborate protein segments can inhibit intestinal amino/peptide transporters which are responsible for some drug absorption
6. Amino acids	Slower gastric emptying which is proportional to the amino acid amount in the stomach
7. Carbohydrate-rich food	1. Have different effects but the primary is delaying gastric emptying 2. Fibers can absorb postprandial bile acid thereby reducing the soluble bile effect 3. Fiber fermentation can reduce metabolism in the intestinal cavity
8. Metals-rich food	Metal ions can form complex compounds with individual drugs
9. Purine-rich food (purine content in food Table 15.1)	Purines can inhibit the intestinal concentrative nucleoside transporter 2 (CNT2) transporter responsible for purine-like drug absorption [11–13]

Table 15.1 Purine content in food [14, 15]

Group 1 (0–15 mg) Low purine content /100 g	Group 2 (40–150 mg) Middle purine content /100 g	Group 3 (150–1000 mg) High purine content /100 g
Potato	Cauliflower, asparagus, broccoli	Offal
Cabbage	Lentil, oat	Bluefish: anchovy, mackerel Anchovies Whitebait
Cucumbers	Beans, peas	
String beans Peas (canned)	Mushrooms	
Tomato	Spinach	
Skim milk	Venison	Mussels, shrimp, etc.
Dairy	Beef	Fish can
Egg	Pork, lamb	Sausages
Rice	Turkey, chicken	Industrial sauces
Polenta	Clams	Meat extract, broth
Cherries, pineapple	Crabs	Yeast
Celery, celery juice, turmeric peanuts, walnuts and almonds, olives	Cod	Alcohol Shitake mushrooms, soy Fructose, fructose glucose syrup

Food composition can affect drug absorption; lipophilic drugs are better absorbed if consumed with fatty food, while on water-soluble drugs, it has no effect. Food can also have a negative effect on drugs made of intramolecular hydrogen bonds with high melting points, which cause them to form poorly soluble crystals, so such drugs are not commonly used as oral agents. As it is noted that numerous environmental factors, physiological environment and health status can affect drug absorption, the simplest and safest administration is orally as most drugs are well absorbed from the digestive system. As described, after ingestion and when entering the bloodstream, it binds most commonly to plasma proteins to reach the site of action. Drugs can be bound to plasma proteins to varying degrees of strength, so those who bind more strongly are more likely to interact with another drug or with a particular nutrient.

For example, cow's milk may reduce the bioavailability of certain drug types due to xanthine oxidase, so it is advised to make 6-h pause between drug intake and milk consumption, Apple juice can inhibit OATP1A2 (organic anion-transporting polypeptide 1A2), while grapefruit juice strongly inhibits CYP3A4 [4, 11]. Table 15.2 shows some significant interactions between fruits, vegetables and drugs.

Table 15.2 Fruit, vegetables and interactions with drugs [16, 17]

Fruit/ vegetables	Molecular goal	Drug interaction
Apple	Inhibits: CYP1A1, OATP	Fexofenadine
Grapefruit	Inhibits: CYP3A4, CYP1A2, MRP2, OATP-B, *P*-glycoprotein	Calcium channel antagonist, central nervous system modulators, HMG-CoA reductase, immunosuppressant, antivirals, phosphodiesterases-5 inhibitor, antihistamines, antiarrhythmics, antibiotics
Grapes	Inhibits: CYP3A4, CYP2E1	Cyclosporine
Mango	Inhibits: CYP1A1, CYP1A2, CYP3A1, CYP2C6, CYP2E1, *P*–glycoprotein	Midazolam, diclofenac, chlorzoxazone, verapamil
Papaya	Inhibits: CYP3A4	/
Sevilla orange	Inhibits: CYP3A4, *P*-glycoprotein, OATP-A, OATP–B	Vinblastine, fexofenadine, glibenclemida, atenolol, ciprofloxacin, cyclosporine, celiprolol, levofloxacin, pravastatin
Tangerine	Stimulates: CYP3A4 Inhibits: *P*-glycoprotein	Nifedipine, digoxin
Broccoli	Inhibits: CYP1A1, CYP2B1/2, CYP3A4, CYP2E1, hGSTA1/2, MRP1, MRP2, BCRP, uridine diphosphate (UDP), glucorosytransterases, sulfotransferases, phenol sulfotransferase (PST) induces: sulfotransferases (SULTs), quinone reductase (QRs), UDP-glucuronosyltransferase (UGT)	/
Carrot	Induces: PST, 7-ethoxycoumarin O-deethylase (ECD) Inhibits: CYP2E1	/
Red pepper	Inhibits: CYP1A2, CYP2A2, CYP3A1, CYP2C11, CYP2B1, CYP2B2, CYP2C6	In vivo and in vitro
Spinach	Possible inhibition: CYP1A2	Heterocyclic aromatic amines
Tomato	Inhibits: CYP1A1, CYP1B1, UGP Increases: CYP2E1, UGT	*Diethyl*nitrosamine, *N*methyl–N--nitrosourea, *1,2-dimethyl*hydrazine

Food-Drug Interactions and Potential Risk Factors

Body composition can significantly affect drug response. If an individual is obese or elderly and has increased fat content compared to a lean part of the body, fat-soluble drugs may accumulate. As a consequence, prolonged excretion and increased toxicity of the drug may occur. Additional risk groups are pregnant women, children, adolescents and malnourished individuals [18–20].

Since the interaction strength between food and drug may vary, interactions can be divided into three groups:

1. *Significant*: can be mediated by food effect on drug absorption degree, more serious with drugs with narrow therapeutic index in which sub and overdose can affect patient, education on drug dosing and timing is crucial.
2. *Moderate*: those that have clinical consequences that can be mitigated if drug dosing and the patient's condition are followed.
3. *Negligible*: those with no clinical implications or with no information about them [3, 21].

Table 15.3 shows some of the food-drug interactions related to particular conditions (allergies, arthritis and pain, asthma, cardiovascular disorders, diabetes, infections, gastrointestinal tract, thyroid preparation and others).

In some cases, the drug is triggered and in others food (food components) (Table 15.4), so that is why it is important to follow recommendations. In the case of individual interactions, as indicated in the table, monitoring and changing diet is in order to prevent interaction development, especially now when every day new drugs and dietary supplements are developing.

Table 15.3 Condition, food-drug interactions [4, 22–24]

Condition	Drug	Interactions food–drug	Recommended drug intake	Possible side effects on nutritional status
Allergies				
	Antihistamine (e.g., diphenhydramine, fexofenadine, loratadine, cetirizine)	Avoid alcohol—increased sedation **Fexofenadine—decreased bioavailability when taken with apple, orange or grapefruit juice*	With water In case of gastrointestinal problems, take with food	
Arthritis and pains				
	Analgesic/antipyretic (e.g., acetaminophen)	Avoid alcohol—increased sedation Caffeine may increase the absorption rate	For rapid relief—take on an empty stomach. If upsets stomach take with food/meal—delays but does not lower absorption	Low levels of vitamin C in platelets
	Corticosteroids (e.g., methylprednisolone, prednisone)	Limit caffeine intake Limit grapefruit or other citrus fruits Avoid alcohol	Take with food or milk to decrease stomach upset	High doses intake can lead to decreased sodium and for supplementation with calcium, vitamins D, K, A, C or protein
	Narcotic analgesics (e.g., codeine with acetaminophen)	Avoid alcohol	Take with food or milk to decrease stomach upset	
	Nonsteroidal anti-inflammatory drugs (NSAIDs) (e.g., aspirin, ibuprofen, naproxen)	Limit caffeine intake Limit/avoid any products that can affect blood coagulation (garlic, ginger, ginkgo, ginseng, horse chestnut) Avoid alcohol	Take with food, water or milk to decrease stomach upset	High doses can lead to an increased need for vitamins C, K and folate **Aspirin—fecal iron loss*

(continued)

Table 15.3 (continued)

Condition	Drug	Interactions food–drug	Recommended drug intake	Possible side effects on nutritional status
Asthma				
	Bronchodilators (e.g., theophylline, albuterol, epinephrine)	Avoid major changes in diet composition (carbohydrates and proteins) Limit caffeine intake from food and drink, chocolate Avoid alcohol **Theophylline—high-fat meals may increase the amount of the drug, while high-carbohydrate meals may decrease it* *Charcoal-broiled meat may decrease the drug effect*	Take with food to decrease stomach upset	*Can leave a bitter aftertaste*
Cardiovascular disorders				
	ACE inhibitors (e.g., captopril, enalapril, lisinopril)	Adequate fluid intake Avoid natural licorice (*Glycyrrhiza glabra*) Avoid salt and calcium **Catropil and moexipril—on an empty stomach 1 h before meal* **Quinapril—high-fat meal decreases absorption*		

	Anticoagulants (e.g., warfarin)	Limit food that is source of vitamin K (vegetables containing vitamin K) because it produces substances that reduce drug effectiveness. The upper limit (UL) for vitamins E and A should not be exceeded, and high doses may prolong clotting time and increase the risk of bleeding Vitamin C is possible for minor interactions *Cooked onions* may increase activity *Charbroiled* may decrease activity *Leafy green vegetables* may develop thromboembolic complications *Cranberry juice* may elevate the international normalized ratio (INR) without bleeding in the elderly High-protein diet raises albumin levels—it may contribute to higher warfarin binding and decrease its effect High-protein and low-carbohydrate diet may contribute to a decreased prothrombin time and international normalized ratio (INR/PT ratio) Avoid alcohol		
	Arrhythmia-specific (e.g., amiodarone, disopyramide)	Grapefruit juice may increase drug availability and absorption		
	Beta-blockers (e.g., atenolol, metoprolol, propranolol, nadolol)	Do not take with orange juice Avoid natural licorice (*Glycyrrhiza glabra*) In accordance with findings, it may be necessary to decrease dietary calcium and sodium—may decrease absorption Avoid alcohol	Take with food 2 h before and 6 h after consuming calcium supplements	

(continued)

Table 15.3 (continued)

Condition	Drug	Interactions food–drug	Recommended drug intake	Possible side effects on nutritional status
	Calcium channel blockers and phenylalkylamine beta blocker	Grapefruit juice may increase drug availability and absorption		
	Cholesterol-lowering (e.g., clofibrate, colestipol, cholestyramine)	Do not take with grapefruit or other citrus fruits Avoid alcohol **Colestipol-cholestyramine—increase intake of high-fiber food and water, avoid grapefruit juice*	Take with food	**Clofibrate—may lead to decreased absorption of A, D, K, B12, folate and iron*
	Diuretics (e.g., furosemide, triamterene)	**Triamterene—avoid large amounts of food that is high in potassium* Avoid natural licorice (*Glycyrrhiza glabra*)	Take on an empty stomach Take with food or milk to decrease stomach upset	Some drugs may cause a loss of magnesium, calcium and potassium so supplements may be needed
	HMG-CoA reductase (statins)	**Atorvastatin, lovastatin, simvastatin—high-fiber foods, at the same time if taken, lowers absorption* *Avoid grapefruit juice* *Avoid alcohol*		
	Nitrates (e.g., isosorbide dinitrate, nitroglycerin)	Avoid alcohol	Take on an empty stomach with water, 1 h before meal or 2 h after	
Infections				
	Antibacterials (e.g., penicillin, amoxicillin, ampicillin)	Avoid guar gum **Penicillin—1 h between drug and fruit juice of other acidic beverage*	Take on an empty stomach with water, 1 h before meal or 2 h later Take with food to decrease stomach upset	Caution with vitamin K supplements

	Antifungals (e.g., fluconazole, ketoconazole, itraconazole)	Avoid alcohol	Take with food to increase absorption Read instructions regarding citrus fruit and grapefruit	
	Cephalosporins (e.g., cefaclor, cefadroxil, cefixime, cefprozil, cephalexin)		Take on an empty stomach 1 h before meal or 2 h later Take with food to decrease stomach upset	
	Macrolides (e.g., azithromycin, clarithromycin)		**Azithromycin—on an empty stomach, 1 h before and 2 h after meal* *Avoid taking with citrus juice and foods, carbonated drinks* Take with food to decrease stomach upset	
	Nitroimidazole (e.g., metronidazole)		Take with food to decrease stomach upset—but food can lower bioavailability Avoid alcohol	
	Tetracyclines (e.g., tetracycline, minocycline)		Take on an empty stomach with 2.5 dL of water Avoid taking with dairy, iron-fortified cereals	Can promote a negative nitrogen balance

(continued)

Table 15.3 (continued)

Condition	Drug	Interactions food–drug	Recommended drug intake	Possible side effects on nutritional status
	Quinolones (e.g., ciprofloxacin, trovafloxacin)		Take on an empty stomach 1 h before meal or 2 h after Take with food to decrease stomach upset not with dairy or calcium-fortified products Do not take with caffeine-containing products—may increase caffeine levels	
Diabetes				
	Insulin and oral diabetic agents	Avoid alcohol—may lead to hypoglycemia or low blood sugar		
Gastrointestinal tract				
	Gastrointestinal stimulants (e.g., cisapride)	Avoid alcohol	Read instructions regarding citrus fruit Grapefruit juice may increase medication availability	
	Histamine blockers (e.g., cimetidine, rupatadine, famotidine, nizatidine)	Avoid alcohol. Caffeine-containing products may irritate the stomach **Cimetidine, rupatadine—with food—increased bioavailability*	Take with or without food with 250 mL water. A bland diet is recommended	Caution with supplements—take 2 h before iron and antacid supplements—decrease iron and B12 absorption
	Laxative (e.g., bisacodyl)	Milk can raise stomach pH	Take on an empty stomach with 250 mL water or juice Stay hydrated	

Thyroid preparation				
	Synthroid	Goitrogenic substances (found in cruciferous vegetables) can interfere with iodine uptake in the thyroid gland	Take on an empty stomach Hypothyroidism induced by goitrogenic food—thorough cooking to inactivate goitrogens in vegetables	Take iron supplements with 4-h pause
	Haloperidol	Avoid alcohol Avoid coffee, tea and fruit juice 1 h before and 2 h after taking	Take with milk or food	Take iron supplements with 4-h pause May lower appetite—weight loss, dry mouth, constipation
Others				
	Benzodiazepines, midazolam, triazolam	Avoid grapefruit juice—may increase availability and absorption		
	Protease inhibitor	Avoid grapefruit juice—may increase availability and absorption		

Table 15.4 Interactions, examples and consequences [3]

Trigger factor—affected object	Consequence	Example
Nutritional status—drug	Treatment failure or drug toxicity	*Obesity*: decreased ertapenem concentration after standard dose administration; acyclovir toxicity after usual dose *Vitamin C deficiency*: prolongs phenobarbital effect
Food or food components—drug	Treatment failure or drug toxicity	*Enteral nutrition*: lowers ciprofloxacin absorption *Food*: can interfere with levodopa and alendronate absorption, but it enhances deferasirox and gabapentin enacarbil absorption *Grapefruit juice*: increases nilotinib bioavailability and simvastatin toxicity
Specific nutrient or other compound in dietary supplements—drug	Treatment failure or drug toxicity	*Daidzein (soy-derived isoflavone)*: increases bioavailability and decreases theophylline clearance *Iron sulfate*: when coadministered with doxycycline lowers its concentration *Vitamin C*: can decrease fluconazole activity *Vitamin D*: decreases atorvastatin concentration
Drug—nutritional status	Impact on nutritional status	*Capecitabine*: can cause hypertriglyceridemia *Low doses of quetiapine*: cause significant weight gain *Sorafenib*: associated with sarcopenia
Drug—specific nutrient	Impact on nutritional status	*Ezetimibe*: lowers vitamin E absorption *Isoniazid*: decreases vitamin B6 status *Carbamazepine*: decreases vitamin D and biotin *Ribavirin and peginterferon-$\alpha 2\beta$*: decreases vitamin B12 status

Potential Interactive Ingredients: Excipients and Food-Drug Interaction

In addition to food-drug interaction, interactions with excipients are also possible. Excipients have many roles, for example, lactose is most commonly used as filler in tablets/pills or capsules, and it is known that a significant amount of lactose can cause digestive disorders in individuals with lactase deficiency.

Individuals with celiac disease have to be sure that the drug does not contain gluten in its composition, and many drugs contain starch (usually originating from wheat, potatoes or corn). That is why it is advised to contact the manufacturer if it is not stated whether the drug contains gluten.

Examples of potential interactive excipients in drugs

1. Albumin	Possible allergic reaction
2. Alcohol (ethanol)	It is recommended that all alcohol and alcohol-containing products should be avoided with certain types of drugs (e.g., disulfiram) to prevent toxicity
3. Aspartame	Non-nutritional sweetener containing phenylalanine in its composition. Individuals with phenylketonuria must be careful because, in significant amounts, it can be toxic to brain tissue
4. Mannitol	Sugar alcohol (from mannitol) used as filler, absorbed more slowly than glucose (releases ½ calories per gram relative to glucose). Soft stools or diarrhea may occur
5. Sorbitol	Sugar alcohol (from sucrose), absorbed more slowly than sucrose as such inhibits the rise in blood glucose levels. Soft stools or diarrhea may also occur
6. Sulfites	Used as antioxidants, including sulfur dioxide, sodium sulfite, sodium and potassium metabisulfite. In individuals with asthma can cause hypersensitivity reactions
7. Tartrazine	Food additives, yellow azo dye. In individuals can cause allergic reactions
8. Vegetable oil	Some types are used as integral parts for parenteral nutrition as non-aqueous substances. Hydrogenated vegetable oil is used as a lubricant in some tablets/pills. Can cause allergic reactions [2]

Certain drugs in their composition can contain excipients that may affect nutritional status as shown in Table 15.5

Table 15.5 Drug examples that contain nutritionally significant excipients [2, 25, 26]

Generic name	US trade name	Excipient	Nutritional significance
Paclitaxel	Taxol	Alcohol (48.7% v/v)	May result in alcohol intoxication in sensitive or low-body-weight individuals
Lansoprazole	Prevacid	Aspartame	Avoid with phenylketonuria (contains 2.5 mg phenylalanine/15 mg tablet)
Clindamycin	Cleocin	Benzyl alcohol 9.45 mg/mL	May lead to fatal "gasping syndrome" in neonates
Duloxetine	Cymbalta	Gelatin	May be avoided by patients with kosher/halal/vegetarian diets
Eszopiclone	Lunesta	Lactose	May cause adverse GI reactions in patients with glucose-galactose malabsorption or hereditary lactase deficiency
Piperacillin/tazobactam	Zosyn	Sodium (65 mg/g piperacillin)	780 mg sodium/day for typical adult dosing

(continued)

Table 15.5 (continued)

Generic name	US trade name	Excipient	Nutritional significance
Gabapentin	Gralise	Soy lecithin	May provoke an allergic reaction
Methylphenidate	Ritalin	Starch	May provoke celiac disease symptoms
Azithromycin	Zithromax	Sucrose (3.87 g/5 mL suspension)	May be significant for patients with diabetes or following ketogenic diets
Niraparib	Zejula	Tartrazine (FD&C yellow no. 5)	May cause allergic reactions, worsening of asthma symptoms

Note: Excipients shown above for US formulations; excipients are brand-specific and may vary *significantly* between formulations and countries. Adapted with permission from www.drugnutritioninteractions.com 2023 by Dean Elbe, PharmD, BCPP

Functional Food

There is a certain food that is considered a functional food because it has beneficial effects in one or more segments. They can have a positive effect on health or can reduce the risk of disease developing.

According to the *International Food Information Council*, functional food is food (or food components) that can ensure more health benefits than a usual diet. The *International Life Sciences Institute of North America* has defined functional food as food that due to the content of physiologically active components provides a health benefit greater than a usual diet. Functional food can be natural food, processed food enriched with bioactive components and also foods that have a reduced proportion of bioactive components.

Some examples are as follows:

1. Carotenoids (β-carotene, α-carotene, lycopene, lutein and astaxanthin) in fruits, vegetables, plant extracts and fortified food: antioxidant and anticancer effect
2. Conjugated linoleic acid in meat and dairy: anticancer effect (breast cancer)
3. Fiber (soluble, insoluble and fructo-oligosaccharides) in cereals, fruits and vegetables: anticancer effect, reduced risk for cardiovascular diseases, immunomodulatory effect, cholesterol-lowering effect, laxative effect and prebiotic effect
4. Glucosinolates and indols in cruciferous vegetables: anticancer effect
5. n-3 fatty acids (linolenic, eicosapentaenoic acid and docosahexaenoic acid) in fatty fish and fortified foods: reduced risk for cardiovascular diseases, triglyceride-lowering effect and improved neurological functions
6. Organosulfur compounds in garlic: immunomodulatory effects, anticancer effect and cholesterol-lowering effect

7. Probiotics (*Lactobacillus, Bifidobacterium*) in dairy products: effect on intestinal microflora and improvement of gastrointestinal health
8. Polyphenols (anthocyanidins, catechins, flavonoids and tannins) in fruits, vegetables, plant extracts and fortified food: antioxidant and anticancer effect and lower risk for cardiovascular diseases
9. Plant sterols and stanols in cereals and fortified foods: cholesterol-lowering effect
10. Soy isoflavones (daidzein and genistein) in soy and soy products: reduction of menopause symptoms, anticancer effects and reduced risk for cardiovascular diseases

Currently, numerous studies are being conducted, based on clinically significant evidence, to establish the safety aspects of functional food, taking into account their acute/chronic toxicity, allergic activity and increased risk for food-drug interaction [27, 28].

Medical Nutrition Therapy

According to the *Academy of Nutrition and Dietetics*, medical nutrition therapy (MNT) is a specific application of the nutrition care process in clinical settings that is focused on the management of diseases it involves in-depth individualized nutrition assessment and duration and frequency of care using the nutrition care process to manage disease [29].

Overall, it is advised to take the patient's anamnesis and food diary that includes intake of over-the-counter (OTC) drugs, dietary supplements, herbal supplements and alcohol. At the same time, anthropometric measurements should be performed, and any body weight change over time, loss of appetite, taste sensation or gastrointestinal problems should be noted.

When it comes to food-drug interaction, medical nutritional therapy itself can be prospective and retrospective.

Prospective medical nutritional therapy takes into account medical nutritional therapy with newly administrated pharmacological therapy. Such medical nutritional therapy should consider not only administered drugs but also dietary supplements and should emphasize pharmacokinetic and pharmacodynamic interactions.

Retrospective medical nutritional therapy considers whether individual patient reactions are related to previously prescribed pharmacological therapy which is regularly taken, where the exact start date of a particular drug and potential patient symptoms may have been critical in determining possible food-drug interaction.

That is one of the reasons why dietitians are important in patient education to ensure adequate diet therapy and educational materials and forewarn possible food-drug interactions [2].

Conclusion

In the twenty-first century, regarding science and technology development and multidisciplinary treatment approaches, it is possible to develop numerous strategies for preventing food-drug interaction.

It is especially important to accent appropriate report preparation, and documentation based on patient monitoring, which forms one of the basis both for the healthcare team and patient education, for the achievement of quality and effective treatment.

As health professionals, our common goal is to determine appropriate pharmacological therapy according to diagnosis with constant and regular patient monitoring. Thereby, the dietitian, as part of a multidisciplinary team, should evaluate, monitor and identify possible food-drug interactions with continuous patient education about appropriate medical nutrition therapy.

References

1. Sjöqvist F, Böttiger Y. Historical perspectives: drug interactions—it all began with cheese. JIM. 2010;268(6):512–5.
2. Mahan LK, Raymond JL. Krause's food & the nutrition care process. 14th ed. Canada: Saunders; 2017.
3. Boullata JI, Hudson LM. Drug–nutrient interactions: a broad view with implications for practice. J Acad Nutr Diet. 2012;112(4):506–17.
4. Bushra R, Aslam N, Yar KA. Food-drug interactions. Oman Med J. 2011;26(2):77–83.
5. Singh BN. Effects of food on clinical pharmacokinetics. Clin Pharmacokinet. 1999;37(3):213–55.
6. O'Shea JP, Holm R, O'Driscoll CM, Griffin BT. Food for thought: formulating away the food effect—a PEARRL review. J Pharm Pharmacol. 2018.
7. Fleisher D, Li C, Zhou Y, Pao LH, Karim A. Drug, meal and formulation interactions influencing drug absorption after oral administration: clinical implications. Clin Pharmacokinet. 1999;36:233–54.
8. Schmidt LE, Dalhoff K. Food-drug interactions. Drugs. 2002;62:1481–502.
9. Rendić S, Medić-Šarić M. Metabolizam lijekova i odabranih ksenobiotika. Zagreb: Medicinska naklada; 2013.
10. McDonnell AM, Dang CH. Basic review of the cytochrome P450 system. J Adv Pract Oncol. 2013;4(4):263–8.
11. Boullata JI, Armenti VT. Handbook of drug-nutrient interactions. 2nd ed. Humana Press; 2010.
12. Deng J, Zhu X, Chen Z, Fan CH, Kwan HS, Wong CH, Shek KY, Zuo Z, Lam TN. A review of food-drug interactions on Oral drug absorption. Drugs. 2017;77:1833–55.
13. McCabe-Sellers B, Frankel EH, Wolfe JJ. Handbook of food-drug interactions. 1st ed. CRC Press; 2003.
14. Jakše B, Jakše B, Pajek M, Pajek J. Uric acid and plant-based nutrition. Nutrients. 2019;11(8):1736.
15. Grahame R, Simmonds HA, Carrey E. Gout—the "at your fingertips". London: Class Publishers; 2003.
16. Ötles S, Senturk A. Food and drug interactions: a general review. Acta Sci Pol Technol Aliment. 2014;13(1):89–102.
17. Fragoso RL, Esparza RJ. Fruit/vegetable-drug interactions: effects on drug metabolizing enzymes and drug transporters. Rijeka: Intech; 2013.

18. Ritschel WA, Kearns GL. Handbook of basic pharmacokinetics including clinical applications. 7th ed. Washington: APhA Publications; 2009.
19. Alonso-Aperte E, Varela-Moreiras G. Drugs-nutrient interactions: a potential problem during adolescence. Eur J Clin Nutr. 2000;54(1):69–74.
20. Custodio JM, Wu CY, Benet LZ. Predicting drug disposition, absorption/elimination/transporter interplay and the role of food on drug absorption. Adv Drug Deliv Rev. 2008;60:717–33.
21. Santos CA, Boullata JI. An approach to evaluating drug-nutrient interactions. Pharmacotherapy. 2005;25(12):1789–800.
22. Bland SE. Drug-food interactions. JPSWI. 1998:28–35.
23. Bellows L, Moore R. Nutrient-drug interactions and food. CSU Extension. 2019:9.
24. Sector of compass group Inc. Manual of clinical nutrition management. 14th ed. Compass Group Morrison Inc; 2013.
25. Pronsky ZM, Crowe JP. Food medication interactions. 17th ed. Penn: Birchrunville; 2012.
26. Elbe D. Drug nutrition interactions. 2023. www.drugnutritioninteractions.com.
27. Gul K, Singh AK, Jabeen R. Nutraceuticals and functional foods: the foods for the future world. Crit Rev Food Sci Nutr. 2016;56:2617–27.
28. Koziolek M, Alcaro S, Augustijns P, et al. The mechanisms of pharmacokinetic food-drug interactions—a perspective from the UNGAP group. Eur J Pharm Sci. 2019;134(5):31–59.
29. Academy of Nutrition and Dietetics. Chicago: MNT Versus Nutrition Education; 2020. https://www.eatrightpro.org/payment/coding-and-billing/mnt-vs-nutrition-education.

How to Avoid Drug Interactions

16

Vesna Bačić Vrca and Ivana Samardžić

Abbreviations

DDI	Drug-drug interactions
BPMH	Best possible medication history best possible medication history
TDM	Therapeutic drug monitoring
OTC	Over-the-counter drugs

Introduction

A drug-drug interaction (DDI) can be defined as the change in the efficacy of a drug due to concomitant or prior administration of another drug. It can also be defined as the occurrence of a pharmacological effect that is not a direct function of two or more concomitantly administered drugs.

DDIs are one of the most common problems related to drug administration. They are also one of the most common causes of adverse drug reactions [1] (see also Chap. 10). DDIs can cause patient harm, complicate the course of the treatment and increase healthcare costs [2]. In addition, DDIs increase the undesirable variability in response to the administered pharmacotherapy. DDIs can cause hospitalization and prolong its duration. DDIs are a preventable cause of morbidity and mortality [3].

Detecting and preventing DDIs is crucial for conducting individualized, optimal and rational pharmacotherapy. DDIs can have the desired synergistic effect in the treatment of certain diseases but can also cause side effects that could lead to

V. Bačić Vrca (✉) · I. Samardžić
Department of Clinical Pharmacy, Dubrava University Hospital, Zagreb, Croatia
e-mail: vesnav@kbd.hr

M. Banić, D. Erceg (eds.), *Drug Interactions in Gastroenterology*, Clinical Gastroenterology, https://doi.org/10.1007/978-3-031-69800-2_16

undesirable treatment outcomes and should therefore be prevented by adequate interventions.

Possible consequences of DDIs are as follows:

- Increase or decrease in a therapeutic effect.
- Prolonged or shortened period necessary to have a therapeutic effect.
- Increased occurrence or intensity of adverse drug reactions.
- Onset of a new adverse drug reaction.
- Intoxication.

Incidence of Interactions

DDIs account for nearly 19% of drug-related adverse effects [4]. Approximately 3–26% of all adverse drug reactions that require hospital admission are caused by DDIs [5]. Estimates about the incidence of DDIs in different settings and countries may vary significantly. Additionally, it is important to emphasize that the results of different DDI studies are not often comparable due to different study designs, methodology and/or patient samples.

An increase in the number of drugs used in pharmacotherapy treatment increases the probability of the onset of DDIs. In general, the incidence of clinically significant DDIs is estimated at 6% in patients taking 2–4 drugs, 50% in those taking five drugs and almost 100% in those taking ten drugs [6]. Sometimes, due to many comorbidities, the administration of multiple drugs is justified. Such therapy is called polytherapy. In particular, polytherapy increases the complexity of therapeutic management and thereby the risk of clinically important DDIs [7]. The prevalence of polytherapy increases with age. However, a patient may also be taking multiple drugs unnecessarily and such therapy is called polypragmasia. An undetected DDI can trigger a cascade in prescribing new drugs, and the patient is at additional risk of new DDIs and side effects.

The incidence of clinically significant DDIs is on the rise, and this number is expected to keep rising for a number of reasons; first, due to increasing drug options and drug consumption. Furthermore, the number of clinically significant DDIs is also expected to rise due to prolonged life expectancy, a rising number of comorbidities and polytherapy.

Clinical drug trials usually do not give real-life data on possible DDIs and their relevance. DDIs are monitored during phase 3 and 4 clinical trials. Drug testing in phase 3 clinical trials generally involves a specific population with particular characteristics of interest and excludes the general population which reduces the chances of occurrence and identification of interactions. Phase 4 clinical trials (the so-called post-marketing surveillance studies) provide more data on DDIs; however, this has also been proven to be insufficient to protect the end-users from serious and life-threatening DDIs. Detecting DDIs is often very difficult. Usually, other potential etiologies of a certain adverse event need to be eliminated first before the event is linked with a DDI. As DDIs mostly occur with an increasing number of drugs where numerous comorbidities exist, it is even more difficult to detect them as they might be presented as an exacerbation of an illness.

Drug withdrawal from the market due to severe DDI can take many years. Some of the drugs that have been withdrawn from the market because of severe DDIs are astemizole, cisapride, mibefradil, tefrenadine and cerivastatin [8]. For example, cerivastatin in combination with gemfibrozil caused severe renal failure and was also found to have a significantly higher risk of developing rhabdomyolysis and fatal outcomes compared to other statins [9, 10].

Patients at Increased Risk

Certain patient groups, such as patients with chronic diseases, patients with renal or hepatic disease, patients with comorbidities, patients undergoing complicated surgical procedures, transplant patients or elderly are at an increased risk of DDIs. Therefore, in order to avoid DDIs, special caution is needed when prescribing pharmacotherapy to this group of patients.

Among the listed patient groups, especially vulnerable to the occurrence of DDIs are certainly the elderly. The share of the elderly is on the rise in total population. This issue was first seen in developed countries and has recently become apparent in developing countries as well [11]. The share of elderly in the population in some countries is over 20%. By 2050, the world population at the age of 60 or over is expected to rise to two billion, which exceeds the figures in 2015 by more than 900 million [12]. The elderly usually take drugs for chronic diseases. Polypharmacy, which is common in elderly patients, increases the risk for DDIs substantially [13]. The most commonly used drug classes in elderly outpatients are analgesics, diuretics, sedatives, hypoglycemics and antihypertensives. The elderly population is especially vulnerable to the occurrence of DDIs due to the changes in physiological functions, which are essential for drug efficacy and metabolism [14]. The most common physiological changes that can affect drug pharmacokinetics are decreased gastric acid secretion, impaired gastrointestinal motility, decreased total absorptive surface area, reduced visceral blood flow, reduced liver and kidney size, reduced hepatic blood flow, decreased glomerular filtration rate, decreased renal tubular filtration, decreased lean body mass, decreased muscle mass, decreased total body water, increased total body fat, decreased concentration of serum albumin, increased alpha 1-acid glycoprotein and various hormonal changes. A greater incidence of DDIs in the elderly can also be attributed to the physiological changes in the body which can affect the pharmacodynamics of drugs, for example, changes in specific receptors and drug target sites. In order to reduce DDIs, the number of drugs used to treat elderly patients must be minimized as possible.

Types of DDIs

In order to avoid DDIs, identifying the right type of interaction is the primary objective that helps us to establish an appropriate intervention. DDIs can be divided into different ways. According to the mechanism of action, DDIs can be classified into two main groups—pharmacokinetic and pharmacodynamic interactions [7]. Furthermore, they can be divided into one-way or two-way interactions. Interactions are also distinguished by the level of clinical significance. Minor drug interactions usually have limited clinical consequences and require no change in therapy or closer monitoring. Clinically significant drug interactions require management and intervention. The interactions may be categorized as potential or already manifest, i.e., actual. In the text below, the types of interactions are briefly described (see more in Chap. 11).

Pharmacokinetic vs. Pharmacodynamic DDIs

In pharmacokinetic interactions, DDIs occur at the level of absorption, distribution, metabolism or elimination of a drug. Pharmacokinetic interactions result in a change in the drug concentration with subsequent toxicity or decreased efficacy. In pharmacodynamic interactions, interference usually occurs at the target sites of drug action. Pharmacodynamic interactions can also be defined as interactions in which drugs influence each other's effects directly [14]. Pharmacodynamic interactions generally involve additive, synergistic or antagonistic effects of drugs acting on the same receptors or physiological system. Pharmacodynamic interactions do not involve changes in the drug concentration in plasma or at the targeted site of action. These types of interactions are probably more common in elderly patients than pharmacokinetic interactions. Pharmacodynamic interactions are more difficult to detect and study than pharmacokinetic interactions [15]. B*ased on the above-mentioned,* it is important to underline that DDIs often involve more than one mechanism. DDIs can change the therapeutic effect of one or both included drugs and be divided into so-called one-way or two-way interactions. The systematic knowledge about pharmacokinetic and pharmacodynamic characteristics of concomitantly administered drugs helps us to understand and prevent DDIs.

Clinically Significant DDI

When identifying a DDI and considering a possible intervention, it is important to differentiate clinically significant from clinically insignificant DDIs. The summary of product characteristics (SPC) is the primary source of information on DDIs for healthcare professionals. Unfortunately, the SPC may be insufficient regarding information about the clinical significance of DDIs. In addition, they are not updated frequently enough compared to the article publications. When identifying potential

DDIs, many other tools can be useful such as interaction databases and DDI screening software. However, it must be emphasized that critical professional interpretation is irreplaceable [16, 17]. A multidisciplinary approach is required when assessing the benefit of a particular drug combination compared to the potential risk of such pharmacotherapy treatment. Screening software can categorize DDIs according to their clinical significance. For example, we differentiate the level of clinical significance which requires closer monitoring of patients and DDIs which require certain modifications of therapy in order to avoid or minimize potential risk of DDIs. Modification may, for example, include the titration of one or both drugs involved in the interaction, the adjustment of dosage regimen or dosing intervals, changing the route of drug administration or selecting another drug from the same class which might be at a more favorable level of interaction. The highest level of interaction includes drugs whose concomitant administration is considered contraindicated and such a combination of drugs should not be further considered as an option in pharmacotherapy treatment.

Potential vs. Actual DDIs

The occurrence of potential DDIs should be differentiated from actual DDIs [18], especially in the context of study results interpretation. There is less available data on the incidence of actual DDIs than potential interactions. Furthermore, when considering the incidence of actual DDIs, studies usually measure only the incidence of interactions that resulted in a side effect, whereas other possible effects, such as decreased drug efficacy, remain undetected or are not considered a consequence of a DDI. It should also be noted that the consequences of actual drug interactions may be attributed to exacerbation of the disease, drug inefficiency or toxicity. Monitoring, documenting and reporting potential or actual clinically significant DDIs are still not at an acceptable level. Specifically designed studies are required in order to monitor the incidence of potential and actual DDIs.

Importance of CYP Enzyme in Avoiding DDI

Drug metabolism is achieved through phase I reactions, phase II reactions or both. The most common phase I reaction is oxidation, which is catalyzed by the CYP system. CYP is a major biotransformation enzyme, which has more than 1000 isoenzymes, five of which (CYP3A4, CYP2D6, CYP2C9, CYP2C19 and CYP1A2) metabolize 90% of all drugs. CYP enzyme system is recognized by regulatory authorities as an important cause of drug interactions [19]. Genetic polymorphism of CYP enzymes plays a significant role in the clinical effects of drugs as well as in the development of DDIs [20]. Even though it is not used routinely, the prediction of the role of CYP polymorphism should be considered for certain drugs as an

Table 16.1 Drugs that act as CYP3A4 substrates, inhibitors or inducers

Substrates	Inhibitors	Inducers
Carbamazepine	Allopurinol	Carbamazepine
Ethosuximide	Amiodarone	Corticosteroids
Felbamate	Cyclosporin	Phenytoin
Phenobarbital	Fluconazole	Omeprazole
Phenytoin	Quinolones	Oxcarbazepine
Tiagabine	Valproic acid	Rifampin

instrument that could contribute to reducing the frequency and clinical significance of DDIs.

The CYP enzymes have been estimated to catalyze almost 75% of all the reactions in the body. Mainly, lipophilic molecules are bound to CYP enzymes. CYP enzyme activity can be induced or inhibited by specific drugs. CYP enzymes are found in the liver and extrahepatic tissues, so drug metabolism can occur in various organs. Nevertheless, the liver is considered the main organ for drug metabolism. CYP enzymes that are *predominantly* expressed in the liver are CYP1A2, CYP2B6, CYP2C, CYP2D6, CYP2E1 and CYP3A. For each of these enzymes, there are certain specifications regarding drug metabolism. For example, CYP2D6 is responsible for the oxidative metabolism of up to 25% of commonly prescribed drugs such as antidepressants, antipsychotics, opioids, antiarrhythmics and tamoxifen [21]. The importance of CYP2C9 polymorphism should be particularly considered when prescribing drugs with a narrow therapeutic range (S-warfarin, phenytoin and tolbutamide) [22]. The CYP2C19 enzyme has a particularly pronounced interethnic variability, whereas CYP3A4 exhibits high interindividual variability in its expression. CYP3A4 is the most abundant enzyme in drug metabolism [23]. To avoid DDIs, it is very important to know substrates, potential inducers and inhibitors of CYP enzymes (see more in Chap. 12).

Some commonly prescribed drugs that are substrates, inhibitors and inducers of CYP3A4 enzymes are shown in Table 16.1.

Importance of Transport Proteins in Avoiding DDI

Transport proteins are involved in drug absorption, distribution and elimination, and they play an important role in the transfer of the drug to the target site of action (see more in Chap. 12). Transport proteins can be divided into influx and efflux proteins as they either contribute to the uptake of the drug in or out of the cell. They are widely distributed throughout the body, but they are particularly expressed in body systems involved in the absorption and elimination of drugs. Like the CYP enzyme system, the activity of transport proteins can also be inhibited or induced by certain drugs which can result in a DDI. In the case of DDI occurrence, the most frequently mentioned transport protein is P-glycoprotein (P-gp).

Table 16.2 Drugs that act as P-gp substrates, inhibitors or inducers

Substrates	Inhibitors	Inducers
Cyclosporine	Amiodarone	Aspirin
Dipyridamole	Atorvastatin	Carbamazepine
Digoxin	Carvedilol	Cyclosporine
Diltiazem	Cyclosporine	Dexamethasone
Losartan	Digoxin	Paclitaxel
Tacrolimus	Spironolactone	Rimfapin

P-gp is one of the members of the ATP-binding cassette (ABC) transporters. It is encoded by the ABCB1 gene (also called the multidrug resistance 1 gene or MDR1 gene). Although the endogenous function of P-gp is not completely understood, the prevailing view is that P-gp acts as a physiological barrier and defense mechanism against harmful xenobiotics. P-gp is expressed on the luminal surface of the intestinal epithelium, kidney proximal tubular epithelium, bile duct hepatocyte membranes, the placenta and the blood-brain barrier [24]. P-gp can extract a wide range of structurally distinct compounds from cells. Hundreds of different substrates, usually hydrophobic, interfere with this ATP-dependent transporter. One of the important features of P-gp is the structural diversity of its substrates. Drugs from different anatomical therapeutic classes are P-gp substrates. Some of the P-gp substrates are anticancer drugs, immunosuppressants, steroid hormones, calcium channel blockers, beta blockers and cardiac glycosides. P-gp is overexpressed in cancer cells and may be responsible for the ineffectiveness of chemotherapy. Various strategies are developed to overcome the difficulties associated with P-gp in optimal drug delivery. Changes in the transporting function of P-gp can cause clinically significant drug interactions. Like enzymes involved in drug metabolism, P-gp substrates can potentially act as inhibitors or inducers of its function. Inhibition of P-gp may result in increased bioavailability of a drug, whereas induction of P-gp decreases its bioavailability. The anatomical localization of P-gp and the fact that it has a broad substrate profile can significantly favor the occurrence and frequency of DDIs. It should be highlighted that many drug interactions involve both P-gp and CYP3A4 because of overlapping substrate specificity between cytochrome P450 (CYP) 3A4 and P-gp [25].

Commonly used drugs that act as P-gp substrates, inducers and inhibitors are listed in Table 16.2.

Targeted DDIs

DDIs are sometimes used intentionally with the goal of achieving a better therapeutic outcome. Such an approach is no exception in, for instance, the treatment of hypertension, diabetes, hyperlipidemia, epilepsy, infection, prevention and treatment of thromboembolic events. In this way, different mechanisms of action are used in order to establish a better control of a disease. However, this pharmacotherapeutic approach may be associated with an increased risk of side effects and must be closely monitored in order to achieve the desired outcomes and minimize the risk of side effects. Monitoring of targeted interactions usually involves increased clinical and/or laboratory monitoring of the patient.

For instance, when using targeted pharmacodynamic interactions between multiple antihypertensives, symptoms and signs of hypotension should be closely monitored. Concomitant use of multiple antidiabetic drugs, especially if the therapy includes insulin, should be used with particular caution with regard to hypoglycemia. Multiple drugs may also be required in the treatment of dyslipidaemia. Special caution should be used when prescribing statins and fibrates, especially gemfibrozil. Taking gemfibrozil with statins is generally considered to be contraindicated, whereas its administration with other fibrates (e.g., fenofibrate) has a lower risk of muscular toxicity. The older generation of antiepileptics (phenytoin, carbamazepine and valproic acid) may interfere with the metabolism of each other in two-way interactions and result in a concentration change of both drugs. The newer generations of antiepileptics do not interfere with each other and are generally considered to be less susceptible to drug interactions. Pharmacodynamic interaction and the synergism of two or more anti-infectives in the treatment of a resistant pathogen can frequently be seen in clinical practice. Interactions of multiple anti-infective drugs are generally manifested in more frequent and more pronounced side effects of anti-infective pharmacotherapy such as nephrotoxicity, ototoxicity, neurotoxicity, QT prolongation and serotonin syndrome. There are certain conditions in which multiple antithrombotic drugs are indicated such as a concomitant acute myocardial infarction and atrial fibrillation. DDIs between antithrombotic agents can lead to a greatly increased risk of bleeding. Careful patient stratification and monitoring can lead to better patient management and outcomes.

Unit Dose Drug Distribution System

The European Association of Hospital Pharmacists and the International Pharmaceutical Federation, in their publications on patient safety, recommend the implementation of the Unit Dose Drug Distribution System (UDDDS) as an evidence-based system for the safety of hospitalized patients. The UDDDS is a system of dispensing a 24-h supply of medication for each hospitalized patient in a hospital ward. UDDDS is a useful instrument to improve prescription practices and avoid DDIs. Hospital pharmacists should make sure that all conditions are fulfilled prior to implementation [26]. By systematically monitoring the prescribed therapy, a pharmacist can be actively involved in the prevention of clinically significant DDIs as well as other medication errors in drug prescriptions. Another benefit of this model is that this significantly increases the chances of timely identification and management of potential clinically significant drug interactions.

Medication Reconciliation

Medication reconciliation is another model that can significantly contribute to the identification and management of potential DDIs. Medication reconciliation identifies and resolves unintentional discrepancies between patients' medication lists across transitions in care [27]. The main purpose of medication reconciliation is to avoid medication errors such as dose omission, therapeutic duplication, errors in drug dosing and dosing intervals as well as DDIs. In order to minimize the errors, it is important to adjust the therapy at each step of healthcare delivery and each transition between different levels of healthcare, i.e., whenever a new or current pharmacotherapy is prescribed or dispensed. Medication reconciliation is the process of comparing the list of medications prescribed by the physician with all the medications the patient actually uses. It can also be defined as a comparison of the best possible medication history (BPMH), with all the prescribed therapy by a physician on patient admission, transfer and discharge. It is a process of identification and reconciliation of any medication discrepancies. A BPMH is a precise list of all the medications a patient uses. Studies have confirmed that medication reconciliation performed by a pharmacist is a very effective strategy in reducing medication errors and has the greatest impact when performed at the point of patient admission or discharge [28]. Medication reconciliation is a complex process for healthcare facilities and requires full integration into hospital systems and processes. Through medication reconciliation, we can not only reduce the incidence of clinically significant DDIs, the number of emergency admissions and hospitalizations but we can also make considerable pharmacoeconomic savings.

Therapeutic Drug Monitoring

Therapeutic drug monitoring (TDM) should also be considered as an instrument for reducing the incidence and clinical significance of DDIs. TDM is a clinical practice that involves measuring drug concentrations in a patient's blood or plasma at a specific time point in order to provide guidelines on the dosage regimen necessary to maintain therapeutic concentrations. TDM is particularly important for drugs that have a narrow therapeutic index, when there is no easy way to measure the outcomes, when a drug has severe side effects, when there are significant interindividual variations in response to the therapy and when specific endogenous and exogenous factors alter the drug exposure. In certain situations, regular monitoring of the drug concentrations in patients might be required for certain immunosuppressive drugs, antibiotics, antifungal drugs, antiviral drugs, cardioactive drugs, anticonvulsants, antipsychotics and antidepressants. However, in practice, therapeutic drug monitoring is underused due to limited resources and sometimes insufficient information on the benefits of this tool.

Standardization of Patient Counseling and Intervention

Standardization is very important in conducting pharmacist interventions regarding drug interactions. Standardized protocols are required, especially for certain drug combinations that have a greater clinical significance and a greater frequency of occurrence. In the absence of standardization, it is difficult to measure the quantity and quality of interventions. Also, it is difficult to achieve content implementation of interventions and measure improvements. Standardization regarding DDIs and pharmacist interventions should be pursued at the national level and beyond. In order to carry out standardization, it is very important to have information on the incidence and significance of potential clinically significant interactions in the prescribed pharmacotherapy. A prerequisite for standardization is developing a special national drug interactions register. Such registers and models would make it easier to identify the most common problems related to DDIs and to provide the best possible interventions. Standardization improves the quality of healthcare as well as decreases the costs of pharmacotherapy. Forming specialized multidisciplinary teams dedicated to leading and overseeing such a process would be valuable to the healthcare system.

Over-the-Counter Drugs

A common and potentially dangerous assumption is that over-the-counter drugs (OTC) are safer than prescription drugs. Prescription drugs are the cause of the majority of drug interactions; however, there are some important over-the-counter drugs that are often overlooked when drug interactions are considered. The use of over-the-counter drugs without consulting a physician or a pharmacist is a particular problem regarding DDIs. Over-the-counter drugs, such as proton pump inhibitors, H2 receptor antagonists, analgesics and various antihistamines, can also significantly interfere with each other or with prescribed pharmacotherapy, which often goes undetected due to its way of dispensing. When it comes to dispensing drugs to outpatients, the optimal model to strive for would be dispensing complete pharmacotherapy in one single pharmacy. This would provide a complete insight into the overall therapy that a patient is taking as well as the potential drug combinations that might interact with each other. Pharmacists are in a unique position to help patients manage certain health conditions [29]. The pharmacist can assist in designing an appropriate medication schedule by suggesting appropriate drug dosing intervals and finding the necessary interventions to avoid and/or reduce the risk of the occurrence of drug interactions.

Clinical Pharmacist

In the age of modern and personalized pharmacotherapy, clinical pharmacy as a specialty has the ability to respond to the growing need to provide quality pharmaceutical care. Many studies have shown that clinical pharmacists can effectively identify and prevent clinically significant drug-related problems [30]. The activities of a clinical pharmacist, acting as a member of a multidisciplinary healthcare team, can influence safe and rational pharmacotherapy at three different levels: before, during and after drug prescription. The pharmacist, by their role and position in the route of medication from prescribing to administration, takes the place of the last professional supervisor who is obliged and able to significantly influence the safe and rational administration of drugs. A clinical pharmacist is specifically educated in pharmacotherapy monitoring. Clinical pharmacist contributes with their clinical skills, unique insight and important medication recommendations to the effective, safe and optimal use of drugs. In addition to the above-mentioned, a clinical pharmacist has a unique opportunity to timely identify potential clinically significant interactions, and in collaboration with the physician and the patient, take timely preventative measures in order to avoid DDIs.

Conclusion

Patient safety should be an imperative to the healthcare system. DDIs are a very important aspect of safe, optimal and rational drug administration. In most cases, through applying proper interventions, DDIs can be prevented or their potential toxicity can be reduced. A systematic knowledge of the pharmacokinetic and pharmacodynamic properties of concurrently prescribed drugs is crucial for predicting and preventing DDIs. In order to avoid DDIs, standardized protocols are required, particularly for specific drug combinations that have a greater clinical significance and a greater frequency of occurrence. By choosing appropriate models, we should improve and develop this aspect of healthcare, especially in the future, when the choice of drugs is ever-growing, and when polytherapy is practically the rule and monotherapy the exception.

References

1. Köhler GI, Bode-Böger SM, Busse R, Hoopmann M, Welte T, Böger RH, et al. Drug-drug interactions in medical patients: effects of in-hospital treatment and relation to multiple drug use. Int J Clin Pharmacol Ther. 2000;38(11):504–13.
2. Arnold RJG, Tang J, Schrecker J, Hild C. Impact of definitive drug-drug interaction testing on medication management and patient care. Drugs Real World Outcomes. 2018;5(4):217–24.
3. Juurlink DN, Mamdani M, Kopp A, Laupacis A, Redelmeier DA. Drug-drug interactions among elderly patients hospitalized for drug toxicity. JAMA. 2003;289(13):1652–8.
4. Reimche L, Forster AJ, van Walraven C. Incidence and contributors to potential drug-drug interactions in hospitalized patients. J Clin Pharmacol. 2011;51(7):1043–50.

5. Ferner RE, Aronson JK. Communicating information about drug safety. BMJ. 2006;333(7559):143–5.
6. Patel PS, Rana DA, Suthar JV, Malhotra SD, Patel VJ. A study of potential adverse drug-drug interactions among prescribed drugs in medicine outpatient department of a tertiary care teaching hospital. J Basic Clin Pharm. 2014;5(2):44–8.
7. Palleria C, Di Paolo A, Giofrè C, Caglioti C, Leuzzi G, Siniscalchi A, et al. Pharmacokinetic drug-drug interaction and their implication in clinical management. J Res Med Sci. 2013;18(7):601–10.
8. Delafuente JC. Understanding and preventing drug interactions in elderly patients. Crit Rev Oncol Hematol. 2003;48(2):133–43.
9. Tornio A, Filppula AMN, M, Backman JT. Clinical studies on drug–drug interactions involving metabolism and transport: methodology, pitfalls, and interpretation. Clin Pharmacol Ther. 2019;105(6):1345–61.
10. Furberg CD, Pitt B. Withdrawal of cerivastatin from the world market. Curr Control Trials Cardiovasc Med. 2001;2(5):205–7.
11. Graham DJ, Staffa JA, Shatin D, Andrade SE, Schech SD, La Grenade L, et al. Incidence of hospitalized rhabdomyolysis in patients treated with lipid-lowering drugs. JAMA. 2004;292(21):2585–90.
12. Brahma DK, Wahlang JB, Marak MD, Ch Sangma M. Adverse drug reactions in the elderly. J Pharmacol Pharmacother. 2013;4(2):91–4.
13. World Health Organization. https://www.who.int/news-room/fact-sheets/detail/ageing-and-health. Accessed 30 Dec 2019.
14. Cascorbi I. Drug interactions-principles, examples and clinical consequences. Dtsch Arztebl Int. 2012;109(33–34):546–56.
15. Mallet L, Spinewine A, Huang A. Prescribing in elderly people 2: the challenge of managing drug interactions in elderly people. Lancet. 2007;370(9582):185–91.
16. Bacic-Vrca V, Marusic S, Erdeljic V, Falamic S, Gojo-Tomic N, Rahelic D, et al. The incidence of potential drug–drug interactions in elderly patients with arterial hypertension. Pharm World Sci. 2010;32(6):815–21.
17. Bacic Vrca V, Becirević-Lacan M, Bozikov V, Birus M. Prescribing medication errors in hospitalised patients: a prospective study. Acta Pharma. 2005;55(2):157–67.
18. Marusic S, Bacic Vrca V, Obreli Neto PR, Franic M, Erdeljic V, Gojo-Tomic N. Actual drug-drug interactions in elderly patients discharged from internal medicine clinic: a prospective observational study. Eur J Clin Pharmacol. 2013;69(9):1717–24.
19. Sychev DA, Ashraf GM, Svistunov AA, Maksimov ML, Tarasov VV, Chubarev VN, et al. The cytochrome P450 isoenzyme and some new opportunities for the prediction of negative drug interaction in vivo. Drug Des Devel Ther. 2018;12:1147–56.
20. Hocum BT, White JR, Heck JW, Thirumaran RK, Moyer N, Newman R, et al. Cytochrome P-450 gene and drug interaction analysis in patients referred for pharmacogenetic testing. Am J Health Syst Pharm. 2016;73(2):61–7.
21. Samer CF, Lorenzini KI, Rollason V, Daali Y, Desmeules JA. Applications of CYP450 testing in the clinical setting. Mol Diagn Ther. 2013;17(3):165–84.
22. Daly AK, Rettie AE, Fowler DM, Miners JO. Pharmacogenomics of CYP2C9: functional and clinical considerations. J Pers Med. 2017;8(1).
23. Konig J, Muller F. Transporters and drug-drug interactions: important determinants of drug disposition and effects. Pharmacol Rev. 2013;65(3):944–66.
24. Tanigawara Y. Role of P-glycoprotein in drug disposition. Ther Drug Monit. 2000;22(1):137–40.
25. Lin JH, Yamazaki M. Role of P-glycoprotein in pharmacokinetics: clinical implications. Clin Pharmacokinet. 2003;42(1):59–98.
26. EAHP. https://statements.eahp.eu/statements/statement-54. Accessed 30 Dec 2019.
27. Kwan JL, Lo L, Sampson M, et al. Medication reconciliation during transitions of care as a patient safety strategy: a systematic review. Ann Intern Med. 2013;158:397–403.

28. Mekonnen AB, McLachlan AJ, Brien JE. Effectiveness of pharmacist-led medication reconciliation programmes on clinical outcomes at hospital transitions: a systematic review and meta-analysis. BMJ Open. 2016;6(2):e010003.
29. Obreli-Neto PR, Marques Dos Reis T, Guidoni CM, Girotto E, Guerra ML, de Oliveira Baldoni A, et al. A systematic review of the effects of continuing education programs on providing clinical community pharmacy services. Am J Pharm Educ. 2016;80(5):88.
30. Viktil KK, Blix HS. The impact of clinical pharmacists on drug-related problems and clinical outcomes. Basic Clin Pharmacol Toxicol. 2008;102(3):275–80.

Part IV

Comorbidity in Digestive Diseases

Influence of Disease on Drug Interaction 17

Marko Luka Bošković and Robert Likić

As our population ages, each day more and more patients live with multiple chronic conditions (MCCs). Because of this, the most frequent medical intervention performed is the writing of a prescription. Poor prescribing is unfortunately a common occurrence as doctors overwhelmingly prescribe medications on a disease-indication basis.

Prescription medications are often added for patients with MCCs without much deliberation, and to their detriment, they are reluctantly removed. This lack of a holistic approach leads to polypharmacy in MCC patients, which has exponential effects on drug interaction. Failing to prescribe efficiently leads to detrimental effects through adverse drug events (ADEs), especially prevalent in patients with MCCs. In order to protect this population, close care must be taken to optimize drug therapy.

Comorbidity vs. Multimorbidity

The distinction of whether a patient with MCCs has a comorbid or multimorbid condition may seem inconsequential. However, it is important because it reflects how different parts of healthcare view and interact with patients who have MCCs [1].

The concept of comorbidity is applied in secondary and tertiary care settings, which have traditionally been structured around diseases or body systems. In these

M. L. Bošković
Dr. Ivan Barbot Neuropsychiatric Hospital, Popovača, Croatia

R. Likić (✉)
School of Medicine, University of Zagreb, Zagreb, Croatia

Division for Clinical Pharmacology and Therapeutics, Department of Internal Medicine, University Hospital Center Zagreb, Zagreb, Croatia
e-mail: robert.likic@mef.hr

M. Banić, D. Erceg (eds.), *Drug Interactions in Gastroenterology*, Clinical Gastroenterology, https://doi.org/10.1007/978-3-031-69800-2_17

settings, patients are viewed as having a central disease that is targeted, with associated comorbid conditions.

The concept of multimorbidity is more applied in a primary care or generalist setting. Here the patient is viewed as having multimorbid conditions that are of equal value, where care can easily change according to patients' priorities. Employing this perspective treats the patient as a whole and instead of a specific disease; aligning more closely to modern concepts of patient-centered care. The patient's experience and priorities, as well as their overall treatment burden, are the primary focus with no condition being prioritized over any other.

For example, a patient with diagnosed chronic kidney disease, type 2 diabetes and hypertension, when seeing their nephrologist is considered by the specialist to have chronic kidney disease, with comorbidities of type 2 diabetes and hypertension. When seeing their endocrinologist and cardiologist, similar subjective perspectives are applied. This form of care leads to multiple silos of healthcare, where drugs are being prescribed for each indication.

In this environment, the burden of treatment can equate to or surpass the therapeutic effect, especially in patients with MCCs. With different non-communicating silos, drugs interact and produce adverse drug events, which continue to be the largest cause of preventable hospitalizations.

Conversely, it can on occasion be appropriate in clinical practice to focus on single conditions, when this is the patients' main priority or source of symptoms. For example, a patient with existing chronic conditions develops severe heart failure which, due to its seriousness, becomes the focus of care, while comorbidities may influence treatment decisions [2, 3].

The comorbid disease model that tertiary health centers follow is closely aligned with biotechnology's approach. Most treatments developed are targeted at treating a specific condition or groups of similar conditions, purposing them for disease-indication use. Moreover, in trial populations, patients with multimorbidity are generally underrepresented [4]. One of the common errors for secondary analyses of these data sets is to assume that the patients with MCCs in the trial are representative of all patients with multimorbidity.

Physicians are left in a difficult position when prescribing patients with MCCs. This is a large reason why adverse drug events continue to be a massive hindrance in healthcare.

Adverse Drug Reactions (ADRs)

An adverse drug reactions (*ADRs*) refers to any injury occurring from a drug (see also Chap. 10). Any potential impact on drug metabolism and circulating concentration can lead to an ADR. ADRs comprise the single largest category of adverse events experienced by hospitalized patients, accounting for 19% of all injuries [5]. The occurrence of ADR is associated with increased hospitalization, increased morbidity and mortality, as well as a higher cost of care [6–8]. In order to decrease adverse drug reactions, vulnerable populations must be identified and treated with special consideration.

Older adults and patients with multimorbidity are at particular risk of developing ADRs due to their multiple chronic conditions and multiple drug therapies. Not only do patients' drugs interact with one another but they also interact with different physiological systems, which in MCC patients are often impaired. Drug-disease interactions are situations where the pharmacotherapy used to treat a disease causes the worsening of another disease. These medications interact with an existing disease and cause an adverse event, most often due to kidney failure [9]. Renal impairment accounts for the vast majority of drug-disease interactions and becomes prominent in geriatric populations as creatinine clearance decreases in the later stages of life. In order to avoid drug-disease interactions, drugs must be prescribed with all other chronic conditions considered.

For patients with stable renal functions, creatinine clearance and kidney function can be estimated according to published formulas; however, one must keep in mind that decreasing muscle mass in older adults leads to lower serum creatinine levels and may not accurately reflect renal function.

Other changes that also require attention in multimorbid patients is the volume of distribution in older adults as body fat increases and muscle mass decreases. A high body fat percentage in older adults leads to large drug storage reservoirs for lipophilic drugs. Combined with the expected decreased renal clearance and potentially decreased liver functionality, this undesirable combination results in prolonged half-lives and a higher plasma concentration; both of which are predisposing factors to drug-disease interactions and adverse drug events.

As ADRs have been shown to be dose-dependent [10, 11], a correct dose must be assigned in order to avoid high circulating concentrations. A general rule that can be followed when prescribing medications to multimorbid patients is the initial dose should be significantly reduced and titrated up to an effective dose, all while following closely for adverse events. Ideally, doses would be adjusted in high-risk patients based on creatinine clearance, CYP enzyme activity, age, weight and body fat percentage; as a common cause of ADR is failure to dose based on these parameters [12]. With the consideration of all of the relevant parameters, serum concentrations are interrupted from accumulating to harmful concentrations. The use of mechanistic models can be used to aid clinical decision-making in avoiding known drug-drug or drug-disease interactions.

Polypharmacy: Less Is More

Polypharmacy is defined simply as the use of five or more medications by a patient [13]. A review in 2010 found that an average American 81-year-old consumes an average of 15 different medications, ranging from 6 to 28 [14]. As patients with MCCs have many different prescribers, the role of comparing the absolute benefit of long-term preventative treatments is usually unfilled [15]. Patients with multimorbidity develop polypharmacy which results in a high treatment burden, potentially outweighing benefits. While polypharmacy most often refers to prescription medication, it is also important to consider the use of over-the-counter drugs and herbal medications.

Multiple drug therapies from non-communicating silos in healthcare oftentimes lead to unpredictable "prescribing cascades." Defined as a new symptom arising as a result of an ADE and being treated improperly with a new drug, resulting in an additional prescription and additional drug-drug interaction [16]. Prescribing cascades are often shown in older adults with multimorbidity, as their multiple-drug therapy offers fertile soil for drug-drug interaction and adverse events.

One of the best-recognized examples of a prescribing cascade relates to the initiation of anti-parkinsonian therapy for symptoms arising from the use of metoclopramide and antipsychotics [17–20]. The now newly added antiparkinsonian drug can lead to new symptoms, including orthostatic hypotension and delirium; causing additional medication to be implemented and perpetuating the cascade. In a case-control study of 3512 Medicaid patients, patients who were prescribed an antipsychotic medication in the preceding 90 days were 5.4 times more likely to be prescribed anti-parkinsonian therapy than patients who had not received an antipsychotic [21]. This is an excellent example that highlights inappropriate prescribing. Failing to review patients' prescriptions as symptoms arise or care settings change predisposes them to the effects of drug cascades.

Changing Care Setting

A survey of American community-dwelling adults showed that five or more medications were used by 36% of the population, while Medicare beneficiaries who had been recently discharged from acute care were prescribed an average of 14 medications [22], one-third of which are medications that could exacerbate geriatric syndromes.

When we examine the spike in the number of medications used from outpatient settings compared to acute in-patient care, one may identify that as patients transition back to their homes, many of the drugs prescribed in acute settings are not discontinued. Among 384 veterans, 44% were found to have at least one unnecessary drug therapy at the time of discharge [23].

Factors that contribute to these unnecessary prescriptions are "routine" medications for hospitalization such as antacids, stool softeners, benzodiazepines and the presence of multiple prescribers. When multiple physicians are contributing to the same drug regimen, often drugs are added freely and reluctantly removed. Efforts must be taken to more efficiently "hand off" patient care from one setting to another. Simple ways to improve setting transitions are keeping accurate medication lists and critically analyzing the drug regimen at each change in the care setting. Installing a check-up on patients' medications commonly called "brown bag checks" provides the opportunity to prevent harm before it is done.

Over-the-Counter and Herbal Medications, the Silent Silo

As the use of natural and herbal medications has been on the rise since 1960 as part of a larger movement toward natural and non-conventional healthcare, drug-herb interactions must be considered alongside the drug-drug interactions of prescription medication (see also Chap. 14).

As patients with MCCs are sometimes driven away from prescription medications due to the increased therapeutic burden, they often turn toward herbal medications. Data from the National Health Interview Survey showed that 17.7% of Americans had used herbal medications in the year prior [24], and increasing data has been showing the potential for herbal medications to cause herb-drug interactions with prescription medication [25]. Many herbal medications and over-the-counter (OTC) drugs are commonly thought to be benign in origin (such as the commonly used fish oils and probiotics). In contrast, other commonly used herbal medications show more dangerous effects. The use of coenzyme Q10 and St. John's wort, commonly used over-the-counter drugs, shows the impact on the expression of liver enzymes, increasing the expression of cytochrome P450 3A4. With the increase in liver enzyme activity, the metabolism of other drugs that use the same metabolic pathway is affected. Warfarin, digoxin, protease inhibitors, oral contraceptives and all other CYP3A4 substrates are affected, leading to a faster metabolism, decreased serum concentration and eventually the failure of therapy [25, 26].

Surveys have shown that the majority of patients who use herbal medications do not disclose this information to their doctors [27]. About 46% of patients taking herbal medication reported that the reason why they did not share this information is that "it wasn't important for the doctor to know," and 57% reported that "the doctor never asked" [28].

The consideration of patient's pharmacokinetics must include all of the medications they are taking. Without considering OTC and herbal medications, physicians are left in the dark regarding P450 activity, and the practice of prescribing becomes more inaccurate.

Another advantage of discussing herbal medications is opening a dialogue about patients' concerns. Many patients take herbal medications to remedy illnesses that cause psychological stress for them. For example, upon questioning the patient regarding herbal medication, they report the use of vitamin E, coenzyme Q10 and garlic, revealing anxiety about myocardial infarction due to family history. Upon measuring cardiovascular risk markers and educating the patient, the unnecessary drugs may be removed, decreasing the potential for drug-herb interaction.

Medication Appropriateness: (Is It Kind, Is It True) Is It Necessary

Medication appropriateness is particularly important in patients with MCCs. When reviewing current medications and prescribing additional medication, remaining life expectancy and goals of care must be considered. For example, if a patient has a short-term life expectancy, prescribing prophylactic medication must be contested. A concept of "time to benefit" in relation to drug prescribing in adults with multiple comorbidities can be used when making therapeutic decisions [29].

Various criteria have been proposed for the appropriateness of drug prescribing. A drug burden index has been modeled, which incorporates drugs with anticholinergic activity and sedative effects, as well as incorporating the total number of medications used and daily dosing.

An increased burden was associated with anticholinergic and sedative drugs [30]. In particular, zolpidem was implicated in 21% of emergency department visits for ADE related to psychiatric medication in people aged 65 or older [31]. High drug burden is related to cognitive decline and increases the risk of falls in residents in long-term care [32]. It is important to consider the appropriateness of anticholinergic drugs and other medications with a high drug burden before prescribing; and if the prescription is warranted, to take careful consideration on the dose prescribed. Alternative drugs with lower anticholinergic activity are available; however, other adverse drug reactions outside of anticholinergic activity must be considered.

Concurrent with the efforts of avoiding burdensome drugs is utilizing appropriate medication. Clinicians may be better at avoiding over-prescribing inappropriate drug therapy than prescribing indicated drug therapy. As an example, one study of older adults found that 50% of patients had not been prescribed a recommended therapy, while only 3% were prescribed medications classified as inappropriate [33]. Another study found that over and underutilization were equally prevalent, where 65% of patients were treated with either over or underutilized medication and both under and overutilization occurred in 42% of patients [34].

Screening tool to alert doctors to the right treatment (START) is a set of 34 validated criteria developed by a consensus of experts in geriatric pharmacotherapy, aimed at identifying potential prescribing omissions in older hospitalized patients [35, 36]. Factors that lead to underutilization include clinicians not being aware of potential benefits, affordability and dose availability.

Preventing Adverse Drug Events

Because chronic illness increases with advancing age, older patients are more likely to have conditions that require multiple drug therapy. The risk of an adverse event due to drug-drug interaction is substantially higher when multiple medications are being prescribed. As an example, the risk of bleeding with warfarin therapy increases with the coadministration of selective and nonselective nonsteroidal anti-inflammatory drugs (NSAID), selective serotonin reuptake inhibitors, omeprazole, lipid-lowering agents, amiodarone and fluorouracil [37]. Optimizing drug therapy by removing ineffective and inappropriate medication and decreasing drug-to-drug interaction is a standard approach to decreasing ADE.

An analysis of a group of Italian patients with a mean age of 78 revealed that the number of drugs being prescribed and the prior history of ADR were the strongest predictors for subsequent ADR. When comparing patients who receive five or fewer medications, the risk was doubled for those prescribed five to seven medications and fourfold for those with eight or more [38]. Each drug that can be removed from a regimen greatly decreases the risk of adverse events.

Inappropriate ordering and inadequate monitoring are the most common errors associated with preventable ADE. Again, the population at highest risk are patients in long-term care settings. Steps such as using computerized decision-making aids and consulting clinical pharmacologists can be taken to avoid inappropriate ordering.

Reviewing drug therapy, especially as patients develop new symptoms, provides an opportunity to correct drug cascades. Periodic reviews or "brown bag checks" are an essential component of medical care for an older patient. During reviews, physicians must review current drug therapy for relevance and effectiveness as well as make sure patients are adherent to their prescriptions. A medication review should consider the patient's status (hepatic and renal function), potential drug-to-drug interaction, symptoms of polypharmacy and goals of care.

Physicians are often reluctant to stop medications, especially if they did not initiate the treatment themselves. Continuing unnecessary medications leads to increased risk for adverse events with limited therapeutic benefit. A common example is digoxin in older adults, often prescribed where indications have not been met.

Unfortunately, there is limited research on how to effectively remove medications from a regimen. It is reasonable to gradually taper off most medication to minimize potential medical withdrawal while monitoring for potential symptoms. Drugs that require tapering include beta-blockers, gabapentin, clonidine, antidepressants, opioids and barbiturates.

As many ADEs are dose-related, tittering a patient's dose to the minimum concentration necessary for therapeutic benefit is necessary to reduce drug-drug interaction. As an example, one case-controlled study in patients over 70 who received thyroid supplementation identified a correlation between the risk of fracture and the dose of levothyroxine [39], indicating the importance of following levels of T4 and adjusting the dose accordingly.

Considering non-pharmacologic treatment is generally overlooked. Although many patients are reluctant to abandon sedentary lifestyles, any treatment that may be non-pharmacologic is high-value.

Maintaining mobility and cognitive ability is key to maintaining the quality of life in older adults. Avoiding high-risk drugs and continual assessment of drug regimens provides opportunities for simple inspections and corrections. Although many medications may be necessary for older patients' multimorbidity, small corrections along the way may be decisive in adding life to their years and years to their life.

References

1. Dumbreck S, Flynn A, Nairn M, Wilson M, Treweek S, Mercer SW, et al. Drug-disease and drug-drug interactions: systematic examination of recommendations in 12 UK national clinical guidelines BMJ. 2015:350.

2. Boyd CM, Darer J, Boult C, et al. Clinical practice guidelines and quality of care for older patients with multiple comorbid diseases: implications for pay for performance. JAMA. 2005;294:716–24.
3. Fortin M, Soubhi H, Hudon C, et al. Multimorbidity's many challenges. BMJ. 2007;334:1016–7.
4. Hanlon P, Hannigan L, Rodriguez-Perez J, et al. Representation of people with comorbidity and multimorbidity in clinical trials of novel drug therapies: an individual-level participant data analysis. BMC Med. 2019;17:201.
5. Leape LL, Brennan TA, Laird N, et al. The nature of adverse events in hospitalized patients. Results of the Harvard Medical Practice Study II. N Engl J Med. 1991;324:377.
6. Classen DC, Pestotnik SL, Evans RS, et al. Adverse drug events in hospitalized patients. Excess length of stay, extra costs, and attributable mortality. JAMA. 1997;277:301.
7. Phillips DP, Christenfeld N, Glynn LM. Increase in US medication-error deaths between 1983 and 1993. Lancet. 1998;351:643.
8. Fanikos J, Cina JL, Baroletti S, et al. Adverse drug events in hospitalized cardiac patients. Am J Cardiol. 2007;100:1465.
9. Guthrie B. Better guidelines for better care: accounting for multimorbidity in clinical guidelines—structured examination of exemplar guidelines and health economic modelling. Health Serv Delivery Res. 2017;5:1.
10. Ray WA, Griffin MR, Schaffner W, et al. Psychotropic drug use and the risk of hip fracture. N Engl J Med. 1987;316:363.
11. Tamblyn R, Abrahamowicz M, du Berger R, et al. A 5-year prospective assessment of the risk associated with individual benzodiazepines and doses in new elderly users. J Am Geriatr Soc. 2005;53:233.
12. Breton G, Froissart M, Janus N, et al. Inappropriate drug use and mortality in community-dwelling elderly with impaired kidney function—the Three-City population-based study. Nephrol Dial Transplant. 2011;26:2852.
13. Ferner RE, Aronson JK. Communicating information about drug safety. BMJ. 2006;3(33):143.
14. Rochon PA, Gurwitz JH. Optimising drug treatment for elderly people: the prescribing cascade. BMJ. 2007;315(7115):1096–9.
15. Harrison C, Fortin M, van den Akker M, Mair F, Calderon-Larranaga A, Boland F, et al. Comorbidity versus multimorbidity: why it matters. J Multimorb Comorb. 2021;11:2633556521993993.
16. Eisenberg DM, Davis RB, Ettner SL, et al. Trends in alternative medicine use in the United States, 1990-1997: results of a follow-up national survey. JAMA. 1998;280:1569.
17. Rochon PA, Gurwitz JH. Optimising drug treatment for elderly people: the prescribing cascade. BMJ. 1997;315:1096.
18. Avorn J, Bohn RL, Mogun H, et al. Neuroleptic drug exposure and treatment of parkinsonism in the elderly: a case-control study. Am J Med. 1995;99:48.
19. Rochon PA, Stukel TA, Sykora K, et al. Atypical antipsychotics and parkinsonism. Arch Intern Med. 2005;165:1882.
20. Stephen PJ, Williamson J. Drug-induced parkinsonism in the elderly. Lancet. 1984;2:1082.
21. Avorn J, Gurwitz JH, Bohn RL, et al. Increased incidence of levodopa therapy following metoclopramide use. JAMA. 1995;274:1780.
22. Saraf AA, Petersen AW, Simmons SF, et al. Medications associated with geriatric syndromes and their prevalence in older hospitalized adults discharged to skilled nursing facilities. J Hosp Med. 2016;11:694.
23. Hajjar ER, Hanlon JT, Sloane RJ, et al. Unnecessary drug use in frail older people at hospital discharge. J Am Geriatr Soc. 2005;53:1518.
24. Clarke TC, Black LI, Stussman BJ, et al. Trends in the use of complementary health approaches among adults: United States, 2002-2012 Natl Health Stat Rep. 2015:1.
25. Catalano KRN. Update on the National Patient Safety Goals—Changes for 2005. AORN J. 2005;81:335.
26. Gardiner P, Sadikova E, Filippelli AC, et al. Medical reconciliation of dietary supplements: don't ask, don't tell. Patient Educ Couns. 2015;98:512.

27. Ashar BH, Rowland-Seymour A. Advising patients who use dietary supplements. Am J Med. 2008;121:91.
28. Ang-Lee MK, Moss J, Yuan CS. Herbal medicines and perioperative care. JAMA. 2001;286:208.
29. Holmes HM, Min LC, Yee M, et al. Rationalizing prescribing for older patients with multimorbidity: considering time to benefit. Drugs Aging. 2013;30:655.
30. Carrière I, Fourrier-Reglat A, Dartigues JF, et al. Drugs with anticholinergic properties, cognitive decline, and dementia in an elderly general population: the 3-city study. Arch Intern Med. 2009;169:1317.
31. Hampton LM, Daubresse M, Chang HY, et al. Emergency department visits by adults for psychiatric medication adverse events. JAMA Psychiatry. 2014;71:1006.
32. Gray SL, Anderson ML, Dublin S, et al. Cumulative use of strong anticholinergics and incident dementia: a prospective cohort study. JAMA Intern Med. 2015;175:401.
33. Higashi T, Shekelle PG, Solomon DH, et al. The quality of pharmacologic care for vulnerable older patients. Ann Intern Med. 2004;140:714.
34. Steinman MA, Landefeld CS, Rosenthal GE, et al. Polypharmacy and prescribing quality in older people. J Am Geriatr Soc. 2006;54:1516.
35. O'Mahony D, O'Sullivan D, Byrne S, et al. STOPP/START criteria for potentially inappropriate prescribing in older people: version 2. Age Ageing. 2015;44:213.
36. Onder G, Petrovic M, Tangiisuran B, et al. Development and validation of a score to assess risk of adverse drug reactions among in-hospital patients 65 years or older: the GerontoNet ADR risk score. Arch Intern Med. 2010;170:1142.
37. Holbrook AM, Pereira JA, Labiris R, et al. Systematic overview of warfarin and its drug and food interactions. Arch Intern Med. 2005;165:1095.
38. Turner MR, Camacho X, Fischer HD, et al. Levothyroxine dose and risk of fractures in older adults: nested case-control study. BMJ. 2011;342:d2238.
39. Zhu J, Weingart S. Prevention of adverse drug events in hospitals. UpToDate. https://www.uptodate.com/contents/prevention-of-adverse-drug-events-in-hospitals.

Functional Status of GI Mucosa and Oral Drug Absorption

18

Srećko Marušić, Ivana Marinović, and Ivana Samardžić

Abbreviations

ATP	Adenosine triphosphate
ATPase	Adenosine triphosphatase
ABC transporters	ATP-binding cassette transporters
BCRP/ABCG2	Breast cancer resistance protein
CYP450	Cytochrome P450
DPP4	Dipeptidyl peptidase-4
ECL cells	Enterochromaffin-like cells
GIP	Gastric inhibitory polypeptide
GLP-1	Glucagon-like peptide-1
H_2	Histamine
IEC	Intestinal epithelial cells
MRP2	Multidrug resistance-associated protein 2
OATP2B1	Organic anion-transporting polypeptide 2B1
PEPT1	Proton-coupled oligopeptides transporters
P-gp	P-glycoprotein
PLA2	Phospholipase A2
PPIs	Proton pump inhibitors
TFF3	Protease-resistant trefoil factor
SLC	Solute carriers
SULT	Sulfotransferase
UGT	Uridine diphospho-glucuronosyltransferase

S. Marušić (✉)
Department of Endocrinology, Dubrava University Hospital, Zagreb, Croatia

School of Medicine, University of Zagreb, Zagreb, Croatia

I. Marinović · I. Samardžić
Department of Endocrinology, Dubrava University Hospital, Zagreb, Croatia

M. Banić, D. Erceg (eds.), *Drug Interactions in Gastroenterology*, Clinical Gastroenterology, https://doi.org/10.1007/978-3-031-69800-2_18

Introduction

The main function of the GI system is to isolate and prepare the essential nutrients for use at the cellular level. In addition, the GI system has a defensive role, because it protects against unwanted substances and microorganisms while eliminating the excess of unnecessary substances from the body. The GI system comprises its main pillar, the digestive tube, the digestive organs and a number of accessories smaller and larger glands [1].

The wall surrounding the lumen of the digestive tract is made up of four layers: mucous membrane, submucosa, muscular layer and serosa. The mucosa is made up of the covering epithelium, the lamina propria and the muscularis mucosa. The lamina propria is made of loose connective tissue rich in blood and lymphatic vessels, smooth muscle cells, glands and lymphatic tissue. The lamina propria provides support and nutrition to the epithelium [2]. The muscularis of the mucosa are usually built of a thin internal (circular) and outer (longitudinal) layer of smooth muscle cells which separate the mucosa from the submucosa. The mucosa is also called the mucous membrane.

Accessory glands are located along the whole digestive system, producing mucus, specific enzymes and hormones important for nutrient digestion and absorption. Specific complex glands, the pancreas and the liver, are also in synergy with the GI system: they empty their contents into the GI system, thus contributing to normal digestion and absorption. GI glands secrete substances depending on different stimuli. Some of these stimuli are mechanical, hormonal, chemical or nervous.

A whole range of GI hormones and intestinal peptides are synthesized and released from the GI tract. Their functions have only been extensively investigated to a lesser extent. GI hormones are synthesized in the specialized cells of the GI mucosa called enteroendocrine cells. Enteroendocrine cells constitute the largest endocrine organ in the body and play a crucial role in controlling the secretion and motility of the GI system, food intake regulation, postprandial glucose levels and metabolism [3]. The targets of digestive hormones are also located outside the digestive system. The efforts have been invested in understanding precisely their role as a target for the development of new drugs.

The GI tract immune system is a complex system of immune cells and their interactions with the intestinal milieu. It is built of immunocompetent cells, such as neutrophils, monocytes, macrophages and lymphocytes, but also cells whose role in immune responses and immunomodulatory processes is still being discovered, such as epithelial and dendritic cells. The GI mucosa is in constant contact with a number of exogenous antigens that induce an immune response. However, the mucosa provides homeostasis using the mucosal immune system and commensal bacteria [4]. The role of the GI mucosa is to establish tolerance to own tissue antigens, food antigens, inhalation antigens and normal microbial flora (GI microbiota) but also to destroy and eliminate pathogens. In a healthy organism, these processes are balanced.

The absorption of a drug from the gut into the bloodstream involves the disintegration of the solid dosage form, the dissolution of the active pharmaceutical ingredient and its transport across the gut wall [1].

In order to understand the process of drug absorption, it is crucial to understand the functional differentiation of the mucosa along the GI system. Absorption is an integrated process, determined by the functional characteristics of the mucous membranes of certain GI regions and the drug.

GI Mucosa

The GI mucosa lays the surface of the GI tract, playing a functional role in the digestion, absorption, excretion and body protection. The epithelial monolayer of the mucosa is very important in regulating the passage of nutrients and drugs by various transport mechanisms. The layer of epithelial cells supports the extracellular matrix, which comprises lamina, collagen and proteoglycans. Together they form a solid barrier to the immune system, which is also the barrier that limits drug absorption. A mucosal barrier function disorder affects the development and course of a variety of GI diseases such as reflux esophagitis, inflammatory bowel disease, functional GI disorders and cancers. Functional differentiation of the GI mucosa differs depending on the tissues of the oesophagus, stomach and small and large intestines, leading to characteristics specific to a particular GI region [1].

The GI mucosa is covered by a layer of mucus whose composition varies depending on the main function of each part of the GI tract. Mucus is a thick protective secretion that lubricates the GI tract. In other words, mucus protects cells along the GI tract from mechanical and chemical damage caused by food, acidity and damage from digestive system enzymes. The GI mucus consists mainly of water (95%), electrolytes, lipids and glycoproteins [5].

The first mucous glands of the GI tract are found already in the oral cavity. Saliva counts as a digestive juice and its average secretion amounts to 1 L/day. Saliva contains serous and mucous secretions. Serous secretions contain ptyalin, an enzyme important for the digestion of starch, while mucosal secretions contain the enzyme mucin, which is responsible for lubrication and protection. Saliva has a digestive and protective function. Oesophageal secretions are mainly mucus, which has a crucial role in protecting the oesophagus from food damage and facilitating the passage of food through the oesophagus to the stomach. The mucus also protects the oesophagus from gastric acid. A certain amount of acid from the stomach can enter the oesophagus, primarily its lower part. In this respect, mucus also has a protective function for the oesophagus.

Gastric Mucosa

Gastric mucosa comprises different types of cells. In addition to highly epithelial cells, there are other types of cells in various gastric glands such as mucoid cells, zymogenic cells, G cells (also called gastrin cells), D (delta) cells, parietal (oxyntic cells) and enterochromaffin-like cells (ECL cells).

Mucoid cells which are responsible for the secretion of gastric mucus are found in all gastric glands. Zymogenic cells secrete pepsinogen, and G cells secrete gastrin. D cells secrete somatostatin which contributes to the regulation of gastric acid secretion. Parietal cells produce hydrogen ions important for the synthesis of gastric acid. The additional role of parietal cells is to synthesise glycoproteins, the so-called intrinsic factors that are essential for the absorption of vitamin B12 [6]. ECL cells that secrete histamine and thus participate in the synthesis of acid are found in the vicinity of parietal cells. They represent up to 50% of enteroendocrine cells in oxyntic mucosa. Enteroendocrine cells are the largest endocrine organ that regulates the secretion, motility and metabolism of the digestive system.

In addition to the mucous-secreting glands, the acid-secreting gastric glands (fundic or oxyntic glands) and pyloric glands are also located in the stomach. The fundic glands are predominantly located in the stomach fundus and body, while the pyloric glands are located in the antrum of the stomach. The fundic glands secrete hydrochloric acid, pepsinogen, intrinsic factor and mucus. The pyloric glands secrete mainly mucus and the hormone gastrin. They are similar to fundic glands; however, in their structure, mucosal cells are dominant with significantly fewer peptic and parietal cells.

Parietal cells secrete hydrochloric acid by means of the so-called proton pump of the stomach, hydrogen potassium adenosine triphosphatase (ATPase), also known as H^+/K^+ ATPase. The acidity of such content can be very low, as low as 0.8. However, when mixed with other gastric contents, the pH is still slightly higher and is generally 1–3.5. Regulation of gastric acid secretion is mediated by the action of the hormones histamine, gastrin and somatostatin.

Gastrin is the major hormonal factor for gastric acid secretion. It is a linear polypeptide, represented in various forms. It is derived from preprogastrin (consisting of 101 amino acids), which is cleaved into gastrins of different lengths. The most common is the so-called "big gastrin" consisting of 34 amino acids. Gastrin bioactivity is preserved in five amino acid sequences called "pentagastrin," located at the five C-terminal of all members of the gastrin family, regardless of the total size of the gastrin peptide. The hormone gastrin is secreted as a response to the low acidity of gastric contents when food enters the stomach. Also, some food proteins specifically stimulate gastric activity and cause gastrin secretion into the bloodstream. By blood, gastrin is transferred to the ECL cells whose primary role is the secretion of histamine. Histamine then stimulates the parietal cells to secrete hydrochloric acid [7]. Also, it has been found that gastrin participates in regulation of the intestinal mucosa growth and intestinal epithelial cell (IEC) proliferation.

Prostaglandins, hormone-like substances, have a protective effect on the GI mucosa and have a certain inhibitory effect on the excretion of hydrochloric acid [8]. The secretion of hydrochloric acid can also be modified by certain drugs. Proton pump inhibitors (PPIs) inhibit the acid secretion in parietal cells by binding to $H^+/$

K+ ATPase (the proton pump). These are drugs used in a variety of indications which in their etiology have impaired secretion of gastric acid and are used in different doses and regimens. For example, they have a significant role in the pharmacotherapy treatment for eradication of *Helicobacter pylori*. In addition to the mentioned PPIs, reduced gastric acid secretion can be achieved with the use of histamine (H_2) receptor antagonists [9].

Gastric mucosa secretes up to 1.5 L of gastric juice per day. Gastric secretion can be functionally divided into three phases: cephalic, gastric and intestinal. The cephalic phase precedes the arrival of food in the stomach and accounts for about 30% of the secretion. The major part of secretion (about 60% of total gastric acid secretion) occurs during the gastric phase when food arrives in the stomach [10]. Gastric juice is a variable mixture of water, hydrochloric acid, electrolytes (sodium, potassium, calcium, phosphate, sulphate and bicarbonate) and organic matter (mucus, pepsin and protein). This juice is highly acidic due to its hydrochloric acid content and is also rich in enzymes. An important ingredient in gastric juice is the digestive enzyme pepsin. The peptic and mucous cells of the gastric glands secrete several different types of pepsinogens, but their function is basically the same. Once excreted, pepsinogen must be converted to pepsin in order to be active. Pepsin plays an important role in protein degradation. In general, proteins are only absorbed when broken down into basic units—amino acids. The secretion and activity of pepsinogens depend on the current presence and the amount of acid in the stomach and are also triggered by the stimulation of peptic cells by acetylcholine. The optimum pH for pepsinogen activity is 1.5–2. If the pH is higher, the proteolytic activity weakens, and it is absent above pH 5 [11, 12]. Patients with a reduced amount of gastric acid are also commonly found to have reduced amounts of pepsinogen.

Pepsin affects only the partial degradation of proteins. More precisely, it just starts this process. Proteins, peptones and polypeptides are broken down by protein pepsin, while most of the digestion is then taken up by pancreatic enzymes, mainly in the upper intestine. The last phase is the breakdown of proteins into amino acids. Enterocytes, located in the small intestine, play the main role in the last phase. They catalyse the process by secreting specific peptidases, the most important of which are aminopolypeptidases and dipeptidases.

The intrinsic factor is secreted together with hydrochloric acid from parietal cells. It is a protein that helps the organism absorb vitamin B12 from the ileum. The intrinsic factor deficiency can be acquired during life, or it can be hereditary. Vitamin B12 deficiency is associated with the development of pernicious anaemia [13]. Vitamin B12 is essential for the maturation process of red blood cells. Intrinsic factor deficiency can be observed in diseases that destroy parietal cells. For example, it is not uncommon for the elderly to develop this kind of deficiency due to atrophic gastritis which can then lead to pernicious anaemia. Also, the proper function of certain cells in the central and peripheral nervous systems is thought to be related to the intrinsic factor.

Small Intestine Mucosa

The small intestine is the main organ of the digestive tract. With 2–3 cm in diameter and 4–6 m in length, the small intestine is the longest part of the digestive tract. The major functional segments of the small intestine are the duodenum, jejunum and ileum. The basic functions of the small intestine are the mixing and transport of intraluminal contents and the production of enzymes and other ingredients necessary for digestion and absorption. Most processes in the small intestine dissolve carbohydrates, proteins and fats and reduce them to simpler organic compounds. The entire intestinal mucosa is arranged into numerous villi of about 1 mm in length, protruding into the lumen of the small intestine and increasing the absorption surface. Simple tubular glands, intestinal glands or the crypts of Lieberkühn open into the lumen at the bases of the villi.

The intestinal mucosa also contains a number of functional cells: enterocytes, enteroendocrine cells, goblet cells and Paneth cells. Columnar epithelial cells (enterocytes) are the predominant cell type in the villous epithelium, and their primary function is to absorb digested nutrients. Columnar epithelial cells (enterocytes) also help maintain the integrity of the physical and chemical mucosal barrier. Tight junctions composed of claudins, zone occludens (ZO), members of the occludin family and junctional adhesion molecules (JAM) seal the intercellular space of the intestinal epithelium. Different expression of claudins determines barrier properties. Tight junctions are expressed differentially along the GI tract. Barrier is relatively leaky in small intestinal tissue, while gastric and colonic mucosa are of intermediate tightness [1]. Intestinal epithelial cells derive from the pluripotent intestinal epithelial stem cells located in the intestinal crypts. Some other epithelial and non-epithelial cell types have been found at the mucosal surface including M cells, tuft cells and intraepithelial lymphocytes.

Paneth cells are key effectors in the gut mucosal defence system. The granules of Paneth cells contain high concentrations of various antimicrobial proteins, including α-defensin, lysozyme, C-type lectins and phospholipase A2 (PLA2) that together guard the intestinal crypt stem cells against bacterial invasion and create a highly hygienic local environment [14]. Paneth cells protect from physical and chemical stress, and also they have a bactericidal effect [2].

Peyer's patches are aggregated lymphoid follicles in the small intestine submucosa, and they also contain lymph nodes. About 50% of lymphocytes B in these nodes synthesize immunoglobulin IgA, the so-called "secretory IgA." Its basic function is the local protection of the mucous membranes against viruses and bacteria. This is achieved through binding with microorganisms, which prevents them from penetrating the mucous membrane and entering into the body. Epithelial cells of the intestinal mucosa play an essential role in the transfer of antigens from the intestines to lymphatic structures. The M cells (or microfold cells) are particularly specialized for antigen sampling that form pocket-like structures on the basolateral cell membrane. In the process called endocytosis, these cells absorb antigens from the mucosal surface and transport them trapped in vesicles into the pockets containing T and B lymphocytes and macrophages.

The main role of goblet cells is to secrete mucus in order to protect the intestinal mucosa. Two main goblet cell products are mucin-type MUC2 and the small, protease-resistant trefoil factor (TFF3) [15].

Intestinal mucus is secreted by the Brunner's glands. The mucus contains a large number of hydrogencarbonate ions that neutralize hydrochloric acid coming from the stomach. Large amounts of hydrogencarbonate ions also come with the secretions from the liver and pancreas, which flow into the duodenum. Intestinal juice is slightly alkaline (7.5–8) and is generally reabsorbed by intestinal villi. Enterocytes, especially those in the region of the intestinal villi, contain a large number of different types of enzymes (peptidases, lipases, saccharases, lactases and maltases). During nutrient absorption through the intestinal surface, nutrients are broken down into smaller units, which the body can absorb. Each small intestine region can absorb and digest a variety of nutrients, including carbohydrates, proteins, fats, water and vitamins, minerals and fat-soluble micronutrients [16].

GI hormones undergo synthesis in specified cells of the GI mucosa known as enteroendocrine cells. Numerous subpopulations of these cells can be distinguished: G cells, I cells, S cells, K cells, Mo cells, L cells and D cells, whose primary function is the secretion of gastrin, cholecystokinin, secretions, gastric inhibitory polypeptide (GIP), motilin, glucagon-like peptide-1 (GLP-1) and somatostatin. Interestingly enough, many subpopulations of enteroendocrine cells are capable of secreting more hormones, but hormonal gene expression is controlled by location in the GI tract [17]. In enteroendocrine cells, hormones are found in specific granules that are secreted after specific food stimulation in the process of exocytosis [3]. GI hormone release is linked to G protein-coupled receptors in response to changes in luminal content. GI hormones have a number of different effects: contraction and release of smooth muscles, digestive enzymes secretion, fluid and electrolytes secretion, effect on GI tract tissue growth and regulation of secretion of other GI peptides. The GI hormones are classified as endocrine, paracrine or neurocrine, based on the method by which the molecule gets delivered to its target cells.

In the context of the development of new drugs, particular attention should be paid to incretin hormones. GLP-1 and GIP are two main incretin hormones. They are secreted in response to food intake and stimulate a decrease in blood glucose levels by increasing pancreatic insulin secretion. Secretive incretin response to insulin (the so-called incretin effect) accounts for at least 50% of the total insulin secreted after peroral glucose intake [18]. Therefore, by definition, incretins are insulinotropic hormones, i.e. they induce insulin secretion. It has also been shown that they stimulate beta-cell proliferation and inhibit apoptosis. The final result is an increase in total beta-cell mass [19]. Their half-life is very short, between 2 and 5 min, which limits their effect on glucose homeostasis. Both incretins are rapidly deactivated by an enzyme called dipeptidyl peptidase-4 (DPP4), which is widespread in the body. Drugs that act on the incretin system include dipeptyl peptidase-4 inhibitors and incretin mimetics (incretin receptor agonists) that prolong and enhance endogenous incretin action. DPP4 enzyme inhibitors inhibit the breakdown of endogenous incretins and extend their life span to 12–24 h.

Incretin receptor agonists have shown therapeutic benefits for patients with type 2 diabetes, primarily because they improve insulin secretion regardless of blood glucose level. GIP also plays an important role in gastric emptying and inducing satiety in diabetic patients and overweight patients. With the use of molecular modification, the lifespan of synthetic analogues was significantly prolonged, as well as their effect on glucoregulation and other metabolic effects.

Colonic Mucosa

The organization of colonic function is determined by the roles of the luminal bacterial flora, the function of various types of mucosal epithelial cells, immunocompetent cells and neuromusculature. The epithelial barrier is composed of specialized cells with diverse functions that emerge from stem cells at the crypt base. The majority of epithelial cells are absorptive colonocytes interspersed with specialized epithelial lineages, including secretory goblet and enteroendocrine cells.

The primary function of the colon is the absorption and transport of water and electrolytes. In average adult humans, the colon absorbs about 1.5 L of fluid per day. In certain bacterial infections, parts of the colon may become more irritated, which can result in increased excretion of water and electrolytes. Diarrhoea occurs when excretion exceeds absorption processes [20]. Colonic mucosa is lined with numerous crypts of Lieberkühn, but unlike the small intestine, it has no intestinal villi. Epithelial cells contain almost no enzymes at all. They are mostly mucous cells that secrete only mucous. In the colon, mucus also has a protective function. In addition to the aforementioned, colonic mucus is important for propelling faecal matter. Colonic epithelial cells exist in symbiosis with commensal microflora: the two-layer structure of the colonic mucus with an inner zone devoid of bacteria and an upper zone that is colonized by bacteria and varies in thickness as the mucin is digested [21]. They coordinate the absorptive and immunology process.

Absorption

Peroral drug administration is the most common and desirable route of administration because it is inexpensive, convenient and safer for patients [22]. Intravenous administration is a method by which the entire dose of the drug is injected directly into the systemic circulation and is available for further distribution to all the tissues in the body. On the other hand, the passage of orally administrated drugs through the GI tract is influenced by a number of physiological factors and characteristics of the drug itself. Oral drug bioavailability is also often limited by first-pass hepatic and intestinal drug extraction, which requires higher doses compared to the intravenous route of administration. After absorption through the gastric or intestinal epithelium, drugs are carried through the portal vein into the bloodstream. After passing through the liver, certain drugs are actively secreted from hepatocytes into the bile and then transported to the gut, where they can be reabsorbed again. This process is referred to as enterohepatic cycling. In order to improve absorption and therapeutic success rate, the pharmaceutical industry is making great efforts in drug design.

Bioavailability is a fraction of a drug dose that reaches, in an unchanged form, the systemic circulation. More specifically, it is the amount of drug that reaches the target site of action. However, plasma drug concentrations are more commonly used because the amount of the unchanged drug is difficult or impossible to measure at the exact target site of action. Plasma concentration generally correlates well with the concentration at the target site of action.

Bioavailability is a key pharmacokinetic parameter described by the following equation:

$$F = F_{\text{abs}} \times (1 - E_{\text{G}}) \times (1 - E_{\text{H}})$$

where F is the bioavailability, and E_{G} and E_{H} are the fractions extracted in the gut wall and liver, respectively. The fraction of the dose that is absorbed (F_{abs}) and its absorption rate are largely determined by a large number of different biopharmaceutical factors.

In order to achieve a sufficiently high systemic bioavailability, most drug products require pharmaceutical development to produce a plasma concentration-time profile that provides the optimal pharmacodynamic response with minimized side effects. This is especially important for modified-release products. In general, oral products with poor bioavailability (F below 25%–35%) are recognized as having more intra- and interindividual variability in plasma exposure [23].

Drug-Related Factors Affecting Drug Absorption

Drug absorption is also determined by the physicochemical properties of the drug. The drug has to be dissolved first in order to be absorbed. Solid drug formulations should be properly dissolved to achieve proper absorption. A drug formulation comprises an active substance and often a number of excipients incorporated into one integrated complex. With proper drug formulation, the existing properties of the active substance should be adjusted in order to produce adequate absorption. Drug-related factors affecting drug absorption are drug structure, solubility (lipophilicity and hydrophilicity), molecular polarity, molecule size, pharmaceutical form and excipient type.

The hydrophilic and hydrophobic properties of a drug strongly affect its solubility and absorption. Drugs that are polar or hydrophilic usually do not easily pass through the cell membranes of the gut wall. The hydrophobic property of the drug can be expressed by the partition coefficient P or its logarithm logP.

$$P_{\text{noctanol/w}} = C_{\text{n-octanol}} / C_{\text{Water}}$$

A partition coefficient $P_{\text{n-octanol/w}}$ is the ratio of the concentration of a substance in n-octanol ($C_{\text{n-octanol}}$) to the concentration in water (C_{water}). The solubility of a drug in n-octanol is similar to that in biofilm; therefore, n-octanol may be used to simulate the lipid barrier of the digestive tract. LogP measures the relative distribution of non-ionized molecules between n-octanol and water [24]. Generally, the hydrophilic/lipophilic properties of a drug can be altered by changing the substituent on the molecule. For example, the hydrophilicity of too many polar drugs can be reduced by removing or masking the polar functional groups. This strategy has proven successful in modifying molecules derived from natural sources (alkaloids or endogenous peptides). Following that, the binding of the lipophilic molecule to the active drug may contribute to better bioavailability. Lipophilic carriers can also be useful in reducing the metabolic changes of the first passage through the liver. Prodrugs have proven to be useful in the temporary masking of functional groups which are important for binding to the active site but which, at the same time, reduce drug absorption. It is also possible to design a drug that utilizes transport proteins in the cell membrane, which will allow it to reach the target site of action more easily.

Most drugs are weak organic acids or bases, and they exist in non-ionized and ionized forms in an aqueous environment. The non-ionized form is usually lipid-soluble (lipophilic) and rapidly passes through the cell membranes. The ionized form has low lipid-solubility (but high water-solubility, i.e. hydrophilicity) and high electrical resistance and, therefore, cannot easily penetrate the cell membranes. The proportion of the present non-ionized form (and thus the ability of the drug to pass into the membrane) is determined by the pH of the medium and the pKa of the drug (acid dissociation constant). pKa is the pH at which the concentrations of ionized and non-ionized forms are equal.

The Henderson-Hasselbalch equation is used to calculate the ratio of the ionized and non-ionized fraction of the weak acid or the weak base, the pKa of these molecules and the pH of the medium:

$$\log(\text{ionized fraction} / \text{non} - \text{ionized fraction}) = \text{pKa} - \text{pH}.$$

Acidic drugs are less ionized in an acidic medium and more easily absorbed in the stomach. Basic drugs that are ionized in an acidic medium will be poorly absorbed in the stomach. By increasing the pH to neutral in the small or large intestine, the absorption of basic drugs increases as well. If the drugs are broken down at acidic pH, capsule formulation can protect the active substance until the drug reaches the small intestine.

Physiological Factors in the GI Tract Affecting Drug Absorption

A number of physiological factors in the GI tract affect the absorption of the drug, for example, GI transit time, the presence of food in the GI tract, specificity of surface area, regional pH, enzymatic activity, colonic microflora, age and certain diseases.

Transit Time and Absorptive Surface

The retention of the drug in the stomach is very variable and it depends, among other things, on the dosage form and the presence of food in the stomach. It usually ranges from 5 min to 2 h. The stomach has a relatively large surface of the epithelium, but the absorption from the stomach is generally weak, primarily because it lacks the typical membrane with intestinal villi and the epithelial cells are interconnected by tight junctions. The mucous layer of the stomach and shorter retention of food are the limiting factors for absorption. Food intake especially affects absorption from the stomach, which is less visible in other parts of the GI system. Food can change the pH, blood flow and GI tract secretion. Furthermore, food can complex drugs and compete with drugs for absorption.

The largest part of drug absorption takes place in the small intestine, given it has the maximum absorption area of 60 m^2 in both the jejunum and ileum. In this way, the small intestine maximizes absorption. It is also considered to be the most permeable part of the GIT, given its tight junctions [1]. The drug is retained in the small intestine for 3–4 h. Drug retention in the small intestine is especially important for controlled-release drugs, drugs that dissolve in the intestinal medium, drugs that are solely absorbed in the intestines, drugs that require specific GI tract transporters and drugs that have a weak absorption in the colon.

In the colon, the surface area is much smaller and totals around 0.25 m^2 as there are no villi. Transit time in the colon also depends on a number of factors and can range from 2 to 48 h. The tight junctions between the epithelial cells of the colon are much tighter than those in the small intestine. Most of the absorption in the colon occurs in its proximal half, while its distal part is mostly used for the storage of faecal matter. The mucus is a thin and discontinuous layer in the small intestine that facilitates the absorption of a larger range of molecular nutrients, as opposed to the thick two-layer system in the colon (range: 20–52.5 μm) [25, 26].

pH

The pH is variable along the GI tract, the lowest being in the stomach which is acidic due to the secretion of hydrochloric acid by parietal cells. Gastric pH values in the fasted state range from 1 to 3.5, while in the fed state they can range from 3 to 7. The pH gradually increases in the small intestine ranging from 6 to about 7.4 in the terminal ileum. The pH drops to 5.7 in the caecum, but gradually increases again, reaching pH 6.7 in the rectum. The pH can cause drug degradation. For example, erythromycin and proton pump inhibitors degrade rapidly at acidic pH values and, therefore, have to be formulated as enteric capsules. In that way, they are protected from the aggressive environments of the stomach and delivered into the intestinal region [27, 28]. Antacids and foods can increase the pH of the GIT, which consequently enhances the absorption of basic drugs while having an adverse effect on the absorption of acidic drugs. The negative interference with the absorption degree can be avoided by temporarily separating the two drugs.

Intestinal Metabolism

Intestinal metabolism limits the bioavailability of a drug. Therefore, predicting the quality and quantity of intestinal metabolism plays a significant role in drug design. Intestinal metabolism can occur in the gut lumen and enterocytes. Different types of chemical reactions (such as hydrolysis, reduction, acetylation and deacetylation) are also mediated by enzymes of commensal microflora, which can be significant but overlooked [29]. Luminal enzymes can modify the chemical structure of a drug and affect its activity in two ways. Certain drugs are subject to enzymatic inactivation in the GI lumen, while some other drugs are activated, i.e. transformed by the luminal enzymes into their active form.

Various types of cytochromes P450 (CYP450), uridine diphosphoglucuronosyltransferase (UGT) and sulfotransferase (SULT) are considered to be the most important drug-metabolizing enzymes in human enterocytes.

The CYP3A enzyme should be particularly emphasized because it is often included in the human intestinal metabolism. CYP3A is predominantly localized in functionally mature enterocytes. The total mass of CYP3A in the entire small intestine from isolated enterocytes is estimated to be less than 1% of liver enzymes. However, the intestine significantly contributes to or even equates to the liver CYP3A in the total metabolism of the first passage of some drugs (e.g. cyclosporine and verapamil). Extensive presystemic intestinal metabolism is probably the consequence of positioning of the intestine with respect to the liver; a higher drug concentration in the intestines, prolonged drug transit time, and the fact that, unlike hepatic metabolism, the presystemic metabolism is not limited by plasma protein binding or blood perfusion rate but by enterocyte permeability [22].

Age

Physiological changes that occur with aging also alter the absorption of the drug. It should be noted that, in the treatment of children, for example, the absorption is much slower in infants than in older children. In older children, absorption correlates with their age. Specific structural and functional changes in the GI system that can affect absorption occur in the elderly, for example, a decrease in gastric secretion, an increase in gastric pH, the gastric emptying is slowed down, the total resorptive surface becomes smaller and the motility of the intestines is slowed down.

Diseases

Various diseases are likely to influence absorption in the GI system and hence the bioavailability of drugs (see also Chap. 17). Diseases such as cystic fibrosis, AIDS and Parkinson's disease can cause changes in the gut microbiome [30]. Lower pH and increased secretin secretion are often seen in patients with AIDS. A lower pH is also present in inflammatory bowel diseases (ulcerative colitis and Chron's disease), while significantly reduced secretion of gastric acid can be found in diabetes, thereby increasing the pH. Gastroparesis can be present in early and advanced Parkinson's disease. Weaker intercellular connections are found in celiac disease, which increases intestinal permeability. Due to pathological changes in the intestinal mucosa caused by cystic fibrosis, the transition time through the small intestine is prolonged.

Types of Drug Absorption

The GI membrane separates the lumen of the stomach and intestines from the systemic circulation. The membrane is composed of a bimolecular bilayer of lipids and proteins inserted into the membrane or attached to one of the surfaces of the membrane. Many membrane proteins and glycolipids often have oligosaccharide chains exposed to the extracellular environment. The bimolecular lipid layer is impermeable to most water-soluble molecules because they are not soluble in the hydrophobic core of the bilayer. The permeability coefficient is the measure of the ability to diffuse a molecule through the membrane barrier. In the case of small molecules, the permeability coefficient of the lipid bilayer mostly correlates with their solubility in non-polar solvents. For example, steroids can pass more easily through the lipid bilayer than electrolytes. Non-lipid-soluble molecules pass the lipid bilayer using proteins inserted into the bilayer that form channels for ion and small molecule transport and serve as carriers for larger molecules.

There are two main ways of drug passage through the GIT membrane, and these are the transcellular and paracellular pathways. The paracellular pathway refers to the passage of a drug between the cells. This way of transport may be important for small hydrophilic charged molecules (logP < 0). Transcellular transport can be divided into several categories:

- Passive diffusion.
- Facilitated passive diffusion.
- Active transport.
- Pinocytosis.

Passive Diffusion

Drugs diffuse across the cell membrane from areas of high concentration (e.g. from the GI fluid) to those with lower concentrations (e.g. into the blood). Most drugs are absorbed by the passive diffusion process. The diffusion rate is directly proportional to the concentration gradient, but it also depends on the solubility of lipids in the molecule, the size, the degree of ionization and the absorption surface. Because the cell membrane is lipid, generally the lipid-soluble drugs diffuse at the fastest rate. In addition to that, small molecules diffuse faster through cell membranes than larger ones. The small intestine, especially the duodenum, has the largest absorption surface, and passive diffusion is most pronounced in that area.

Fick's laws of diffusion describe the passive diffusion:

$$\begin{aligned}&\text{Molecule flux}\left(\text{number of molecules per unit time}\right)\\&=\left(C_1-C_2\right)\times\left(\text{surface}\times\text{permeability coefficient / thickness}\right)\end{aligned}$$

where C_1 represents a higher concentration, C_2 represents a lower concentration, the surface refers to the surface through which the diffusion occurs, the permeability coefficient is a measure of drug molecules' mobility in the medium in which the diffusion takes place and the thickness represents the length of the diffusion pathway [31]. In the case of diffusion in the lipoid medium, the partition coefficient of oil/water is a major factor affecting the movement of the molecules, because this coefficient determines how easily the drug enters the lipid membranes from the aqueous medium, thus creating a concentration gradient between the membrane and the bloodstream.

Facilitated Diffusion

Certain low-solubility molecules in lipids (e.g. glucose) penetrate the membranes faster than expected. This is due to the fact that specific transporters are involved in the process. Consequently, facilitated diffusion represents the passive transport of solute from the region of the higher concentration into the region of the lower concentration, mediated by a specific protein carrier. The carrier molecule in the membrane is reversibly combined with the substrate molecule outside of the cell membrane, and the carrier-substrate complex diffuses rapidly through the membrane, releasing the substrate on the inner surface. In this process, the protein carrier appears in two basic conformations. Substrate binding induces a conformational change in the carrier, which consequently enables the release of the solute. Following that, the empty carrier returns to its previous conformation. Consequently, only the transport of substrates of relatively specific molecular configuration occurs through the membrane, and the carrier availability limits the process. This process is completely reversible and the net flow across the membrane depends on the concentration gradient. The process does not require energy consumption, and it cannot occur against a concentration gradient.

The rate at which solute enters a cell by process of facilitated diffusion is determined by the concentration gradient across the membrane, the amount of carrier available (this is a key control step), the solute-carrier interaction affinity and the rate of conformational change.

Active Transport

Active transport is a selective process that consumes energy and acts against a concentration gradient. The energy source can be the adenosine triphosphate (ATP) hydrolysis process or the concentration gradient of sodium or electrical potential. The process appears to be limited to drugs that are structurally similar to endogenous substrates (for example, ions, vitamins, sugars and amino acids). These drugs are absorbed at specific sites of the small intestine. It is estimated that up to 400 different types of transporters are located in the small intestine.

The transport system is similar to the enzyme action because it has a specific binding site for the solute, the carrier can be saturated with the substrate, which has a maximum transport rate and there is a substrate-binding constant for the carrier—K_m (Michaelis-Menten constant) as well as a structurally similar competitive inhibitor which stops the transport. K_m can also be interpreted as the affinity of the compound to the enzyme or transporter. Therefore, transport system kinetics are different from passive diffusion kinetics. The rate of movement in passive diffusion is directly proportional to the concentration of solute, while in the transport process involving carriers, the rate of movement is limited by the availability of carriers. The transport system kinetics obey the rules of the Michaelis-Menten kinetics, in which the concentration at half the maximum velocity (V_{max}) of the transport is equal to the binding constant (K_m) of solute for the carrier [31].

Pinocytosis

Pinocytosis is a form of endocytosis. The cell membrane invaginates, takes in the surrounding fluid and particles and closes once again, thus forming a specific pinocytotic vesicle, which consequently separates from the membrane and enters the cytoplasm. Depending on the size of the invaded particle, pinocytosis is further segregated into micropinocytosis and macropinocytosis. Micropinocytosis occurs in almost all cells, while macropinocytosis occurs only in certain cells. The vesicles produced by pinocytosis are much smaller than those generated by phagocytosis. This process requires energy consumption. In drug transport, this pathway is considered to be of secondary importance.

Transporters and Absorption

Transporters have a major function in intestinal absorption, and they are becoming increasingly important in the field of drug design. Transport proteins are located on the apical and basolateral membranes of enterocytes. We can divide them into influx and efflux transporters, depending on whether they deliver the drug to the cell or pump it out of the cell. Furthermore, the two major superfamilies of transporters are the solute carriers (SLC) and the ATP-binding cassette transporters (ABC transporters). The SLC superfamily mainly includes the influx transporters; among them, the most studied are the proton-coupled oligopeptides transporters (PEPT1) and organic anion transporting polypeptide 2B1 (OATP2B1). The ABC transporters mainly include the efflux transporters; among them, the most described are the P-glycoprotein (P-gp), breast cancer resistance protein (BCRP/ABCG2) and multidrug resistance-associated protein 2 (MRP2) [32].

Influx protein PEPT1 mediates the transport of dipeptides and tripeptides and utilizes a proton gradient as a driving force to concentrate intracellular oligopeptides. It can recognize 400 different peptides and 8000 different tripeptides and also has the potential to transport a variety of drugs, including β-lactam antibiotics, angiotensin-converting enzyme inhibitors and anticancer drugs.

From the OATP2B1 substrate, we will single out some of the more commonly used drugs such as certain statins, glibenclamide and fexofenadine.

ABC transporters are a group of proteins belonging to one of the oldest and biggest families of proteins. ABC transporters are ubiquitous integral membrane proteins that enable the transport of different substrates through the membrane. They obtain the energy for this process through hydrolysis of the ATP transporters [33]. P-gp is one of the best-described and most studied transporters encoded by the multidrug resistance gene, MDR1/ABCB1. P-gp is located in the apical membrane of the entire intestinal system, from the duodenum to the rectum, with the highest expression in the small intestine enterocytes. P-gp has an important function in the removal of toxic substances from the body. Many drugs are substrates of P-gp and can alter its activity. Altered P-gp activity can lead to pharmacokinetic drug interactions as a result of its induction and/or inhibition [34]. For example, systemic exposure to orally administered digoxin (P-gp substrate) decreases with coadministration of rifampicin (P-gp inducer), whereas the administration of P-gp inhibitors, such as quinidine, verapamil and clarithromycin with digoxin, leads to a significant increase in digoxin concentration in the plasma [35, 36].

The fact that certain drugs are substrates of both P-gp and CYP3A4 enzymes can be particularly important for their absorption. By interfering with their action, such drugs return to the GI lumen via the efflux transport protein P-gp and are reexposed to metabolism through the CYP3A4 enzyme [37]. The low bioavailability of certain drugs can be explained through the synergism of P-gp and CYP3A4, which can complicate the pharmacotherapy treatment, especially with regard to drugs with narrow therapeutic indexes, such as cyclosporine and tacrolimus.

Conclusion

Peroral absorption is the preferred route of drug administration; however, it is determined by the complex interference between the physiological characteristics of the GI mucosa and the specific drug characteristics. The properties of the GI mucosa differ throughout the GI tract and largely determine the design of drugs. In the process of peroral drug absorption, there are many other factors and mechanisms whose detailed function and possibility of use for better drug absorption are yet to be studied. The advancements in this area bring a new perspective on drug design and the achievement of better pharmacotherapeutic outcomes.

References

1. Vertzoni M, Augustijns P, Grimm M, Koziolek M, Lemmens G, Parrott N, et al. Impact of regional differences along the gastrointestinal tract of healthy adults on oral drug absorption: an UNGAP review. Eur J Pharm Sci. 2019;134:153–75.
2. Van Eyken P, Fanni D, Gerosa C, Ambu R. The Normal biopsy: mucosa and submucosa. In: Geboes K, Nemolato S, Leo M, Faa G, editors. Colitis. Cham: Springer; 2014. p. 1–16.
3. Latorre R, Sternini C, De Giorgio R, Greenwood-Van Meerveld B. Enteroendocrine cells: a review of their role in brain-gut communication. Neurogastroenterol Motil. 2016;28(5):620–30.
4. Tokuhara D, Kurashima Y, Kamioka M, Nakayama T, Ernst P, Kiyono H. A comprehensive understanding of the gut mucosal immune system in allergic inflammation. Allergol Int. 2019;68(1):17–25.
5. Boegh M, Nielsen HM. Mucus as a barrier to drug delivery—understanding and mimicking the barrier properties. Basic Clin Pharmacol Toxicol. 2015;116(3):179–86.
6. Willet SG, Mills JC. Stomach organ and cell lineage differentiation: from embryogenesis to adult homeostasis. Cell Mol Gastroenterol Hepatol. 2016;2(5):546–59.

7. Schubert ML, Rehfeld JF. Gastric peptides-gastrin and somatostatin. Compr Physiol. 2019;10(1):197–228.
8. Wallace JL. Prostaglandins, NSAIDs, and gastric mucosal protection: why doesn't the stomach digest itself? Physiol Rev. 2008;88(4):1547–65.
9. Sachs G, Shin JM, Hunt R. Novel approaches to inhibition of gastric acid secretion. Curr Gastroenterol Rep. 2010;12(6):437–47.
10. Phan J, Benhammou JN, Pisegna JR. Gastric Hypersecretory states: investigation and management. Curr Treat Options Gastroenterol. 2015;13(4):386–97.
11. O'Connor A, O'Moráin C. Digestive function of the stomach. Dig Dis. 2014;32(3):186–91.
12. Petersen KU. Pepsin and its importance for functional dyspepsia: relic, regulator or remedy? Dig Dis. 2018;36(2):98–105.
13. Annibalc B, Lahner E, Fave GD. Diagnosis and management of pernicious anemia. Curr Gastroenterol Rep. 2011;13(6):518–24.
14. Gassler N. Paneth cells in intestinal physiology and pathophysiology. World J Gastrointest Pathophysiol. 2017;8(4):150–60.
15. Aihara E, Engevik KA, Montrose MH. Trefoil factor peptides and gastrointestinal function. Annu Rev Physiol. 2017;79:357–80.
16. Volk N, Lacy B. Anatomy and physiology of the small bowel. Gastrointest Endosc Clin N Am. 2017;27(1):1–13.
17. Sinagoga KL, McCauley HA, Múnera JO, Reynolds NA, Enriquez JR, Watson C, et al. Deriving functional human enteroendocrine cells from pluripotent stem cells. Development. 2018;145(19).
18. Kim W, Egan JM. The role of incretins in glucose homeostasis and diabetes treatment. Pharmacol Rev. 2008;60(4):470–512.
19. Drucker DJ. The biology of incretin hormones. Cell Metab. 2006;3(3):153–65.
20. Milla PJ. Advances in understanding colonic function. J Pediatr Gastroenterol Nutr. 2009;48(2):S43–5.
21. Johansson ME, Phillipson M, Petersson J, Velcich A, Holm L, Hansson GC. The inner of the two Muc2 mucin-dependent mucus layers in colon is devoid of bacteria. Proc Natl Acad Sci. 2008;105(39):15064–9.
22. Peters SA, Jones CR, Ungell AL, Hatley OJ. Predicting drug extraction in the human gut wall: assessing contributions from drug metabolizing enzymes and transporter proteins using preclinical models. Clin Pharmacokinet. 2016;55(6):673–96.
23. Hellriegel ET, Bjornsson TD, Hauck WW. Interpatient variability in bioavailability is related to the extent of absorption: implications for bioavailability and bioequivalence studies. Clin Pharmacol Ther. 1996;60(6):601–7.
24. Bannan CC, Calabró G, Kyu DY, Mobley DL. Calculating partition coefficients of small molecules in octanol/water and cyclohexane/water. J Chem Theory Comput. 2016;12(8):4015–24.
25. Bajka BH, Rigby NM, Cross KL, Macierzanka A, Mackie AR. The influence of small intestinal mucus structure on particle transport ex vivo. Colloids Surf B Biointerfaces. 2015;135:73–80.
26. Strugala V, Dettmar PW, Pearson JP. Thickness and continuity of the adherent colonic mucus barrier in active and quiescent ulcerative colitis and Crohn's disease. Int J Clin Pract. 2008;62(5):762–9.
27. Fukui E, Miyamura N, Uemura K, Kobayashi M. Preparation of enteric-coated timed-release press-coated tablets and evaluation of their function by in vitro and in vivo tests for colon targeting. Int J Pharm. 2000;204(1–2):7–15.
28. Ogwal S, Xide TU. Bioavailability and stability of erythromycin delayed release tablets. Afr Health Sci. 2001;1(2):90–6.
29. Swanson HI. Drug metabolism by the host and gut microbiota: a partnership or rivalry? Drug Metab Dispos. 2015;43(10):1499–504.
30. Hatton GB, Madla CM, Rabbie SC, Basit AW. Gut reaction: impact of systemic diseases on gastrointestinal physiology and drug absorption. Drug Discov Today. 2019;24(2):417–27.
31. Lin L, Wong H. Predicting Oral drug absorption: mini review on physiologically-based pharmacokinetic models. Pharmaceutics. 2017;9(4):41.

32. Estudante M, Morais JG, Soveral G, Benet LZ. Intestinal drug transporters: an overview. Adv Drug Deliv Rev. 2013;65(10):1340–56.
33. Rees DC, Johnson E, Lewinson O. ABC transporters: the power to change. Nat Rev Mol Cell Biol. 2009;10(3):218–27.
34. König J, Müller F, Fromm MF. Transporters and drug-drug interactions: important determinants of drug disposition and effects. Pharmacol Rev. 2013;65(3):944–66.
35. Igel S, Drescher S, Mürdter T, Hofmann U, Heinkele G, Tegude H, et al. Increased absorption of digoxin from the human jejunum due to inhibition of intestinal transporter-mediated efflux. Clin Pharmacokinet. 2007;46(9):777–85.
36. Wessler JD, Grip LT, Mendell J, Giugliano RP. The P-glycoprotein transport system and cardiovascular drugs. J Am Coll Cardiol. 2013;61(25):2495–502.
37. Benet LZ. The drug transporter-metabolism alliance: uncovering and defining the interplay. Mol Pharm. 2009;6(6):1631–43.

Infections

19

Rok Čivljak and Marta Perović Mihanović

Introduction

The gastrointestinal tract is often involved in infectious diseases, either primarily in gastrointestinal infections or secondarily in infectious diseases of other organ systems, as well as systemic infections. On the other hand, the most common symptoms of gastrointestinal infections, such as nausea, vomiting, diarrhea, and abdominal pain, are not only present in infectious diseases but also in some noninfectious diseases, thereby complicating the assessment of patients with gastrointestinal symptoms. For example, nausea and vomiting could be symptoms of migraine, increased intracranial pressure, central nervous system infection, myocardial infarction and heart failure, pregnancy, endocrine and metabolic disorders, medications, toxic etiologies, and other extraintestinal disorders [1]. Vomiting is frequently seen as a general symptom of many infectious diseases, although it can also indicate psychiatric diseases, labyrinthine disorders, and many noninfectious organic gastrointestinal disorders. Diarrhea can be a consequence of oncological treatment (chemotherapy, radiation), hyperthyroidism, or a side effect of many medications, often antimicrobial, as well as noninfectious bowel diseases, such as mesenteric thrombosis, IBD, and others [2]. In this chapter, we present the most common gastrointestinal infections, the impact of infections on the gastrointestinal tract, and possible interactions among the drugs most frequently used in the treatment of gastrointestinal infections.

R. Čivljak (✉)
Dr. Fran Mihaljević, University Hospital for Infectious Diseases, Zagreb, Croatia

School of Medicine, University of Zagreb, Zagreb, Croatia
e-mail: rok.civljak@bfm.hr

M. Perović Mihanović
Dr. Fran Mihaljević, University Hospital for Infectious Diseases, Zagreb, Croatia
e-mail: mperovic@bfm.hr

M. Banić, D. Erceg (eds.), *Drug Interactions in Gastroenterology*, Clinical Gastroenterology, https://doi.org/10.1007/978-3-031-69800-2_19

Acute Infectious Diarrhea and Other Foodborne Illnesses

Various infectious agents affect the gastrointestinal tract, whether by damaging the anatomic barriers, altering the intestinal microbiota, or even stimulating the production of circulating humoral factors. The most widespread condition in this group is acute infectious diarrhea, caused by various bacteria, viruses, or parasites. The frequency of the individual pathogens, severity of the clinical profiles, and consequences are different in children and in adults, as well in patients in resource-rich and resource-limited settings. For example, gastrointestinal infections are one of the most common causes of morbidity and mortality in children under 5 years of age in the underdeveloped countries of the world but an extremely rare cause of mortality in adults living in developed countries [3].

The characteristics of the host are essential for assessing the severity of infection and prognosis. Bacterial diarrhea in developed countries rarely results in fatal outcomes, although high morbidity is seen among elderly patients, children in children's collectives, travelers visiting developing countries, and men who have sex with men (MSM). We can expect a more severe clinical profile among elderly patients, patients with resected stomachs, patients receiving anti-ulcer therapy, immunodeficient patients, splenectomized patients, those with chronic diseases (diabetes, liver cirrhosis, kidney damage, IBD, malignancies, hemoglobinopathies, AIDS) and organ transplant recipients [4].

Among the classical bacterial gastrointestinal infections, the most common are caused by nontyphoidal *Salmonella*. A person becomes infected by ingesting raw or undercooked food of animal origin. In addition to the amount consumed, the severity of the clinical condition also depends on underlying chronic gastrointestinal diseases, which are primarily gastric hyperacidity, the use of antacids to neutralize stomach acid, intestinal hypermotility, and cancers of the digestive tract [5]. *Salmonella* also affects the small and large intestines and causes diarrhea not only by invading the epithelial cells, but also by producing enterotoxins. The disease is manifested by an elevated temperature; profuse, watery, greenish diarrhea stool; abdominal cramps, nausea, and vomiting. In 1–4% of the cases, the disease is complicated by bacteremia, resulting in distant septic foci (in the gastrointestinal (GI) tract, cholangitis, cholecystitis, and peritonitis), more often seen in the elderly and immunocompromised patients.

Campylobacteriosis can also involve the small and large intestines, and is manifested by watery, bloody diarrhea, rarely accompanied by bacteremia. Today, infections caused by *Shigella*, which create the typical clinical profile of dysenteric syndrome, are increasingly rare.

In the United States, the most common bacterial pathogens in children are *Salmonella enterica* (42%), *Campylobacter* (28%), *Shigella* (21%), *Yersinia* (5%), and *E. coli* O157 (3%) [6].

Bloody diarrhea is a diagnostic challenge because it can be of either infectious or noninfectious origin. Clinical symptoms, such as fever, diarrhea, and vomiting, raise suspicions that the disease is caused by invasive pathogens. In the United

States, *Salmonella*, *Campylobacter*, *C. difficile*, *Shigella,* and Shiga toxin-producing *E. coli* are among the most common causes of infectious bloody diarrhea.

Viral diarrhea is most common among children. In addition to the infectious dose, the severity of the clinical profile is affected by the general physical condition, nutritional status, and/or the presence of congenital immunodeficiency [7].

Parasitic infestations do not usually cause acute diarrhea but are clinically manifested by chronic diarrhea, which can lead to malabsorption. In some infections (e.g., pinworm), a large number of parasites in the intestinal lumen can cause ileus, intussusception, volvulus, bowel perforation, cholangitis, biliary obstruction, appendicitis, or pancreatitis. Studies have also shown that parasitic infections increase the risk of postinfectious chronic gastrointestinal disorders [8].

In immunocompromised patients, diarrheal disease nearly always has a prolonged or relapsing course and can be caused by various bacteria, viruses, parasites, or fungi [9]. The patients most affected are those with impaired cellular immunity, for example, those with advanced AIDS. In addition to the usual pathogens, in such patients, it is necessary to consider *E. coli, Cryptosporidia, microsporidia, Cystoisospora belli, cytomegalovirus*, and *Mycobacterium avium* complex infections [10].

With respect to foodborne diseases, the most common foodborne pathogens are *Campylobacter* spp., *Escherichia coli* O157, *Listeria monocytogenes*, and nontyphoidal *Salmonella* [11]. Elderly adults are also more likely to die of enteric infections. Several age-related factors may contribute to their increased susceptibility: weakened immune system, changes to the gastrointestinal tract, higher prevalence of other conditions, and the frequent use of antacids and immunosuppressive drugs [12].

Following the introduction of the rotavirus vaccine, noroviruses have become the leading cause of viral diarrheal diseases in the United States [13]. Although noroviruses are responsible for a large number of cases, *Salmonella* is responsible for a larger number of hospitalizations, cases with severe clinical profiles and more frequent fatal outcomes [14].

According to the Infectious Disease Society of America (IDSA) Guidelines, the isolation of the etiological pathogen is not necessary in uncomplicated cases of acute diarrhea or other foodborne illnesses; immunocompetent patients; or patients with traveler's diarrhea, unlike those cases characterized by bloody diarrhea, fever, abdominal pain, or the clinical profile of sepsis. In these last cases, the pathogen must be identified by culture or molecular techniques [15].

Infectious diarrhea is treated with symptomatic and antimicrobial therapy. Rehydration is the basis for the treatment of any type of infectious diarrhea. Fluid is compensated for perorally in mild cases, if the patient tolerates peroral intake. It is usually sufficient to administer an oral rehydration solution (ORS), which is officially recommended by the WHO and UNICEF for the treatment of diarrhea in children in third world countries [16]. In the case of vomiting or severe dehydration, rehydration is achieved parenterally. In addition to rehydration, a dietary regime and balanced caloric intake are important, as well as the administration of probiotics to restore equilibrium to the intestinal microflora. Since most diarrhea is of viral etiology and self-limiting, symptomatic treatment alone is usually sufficient. In the treatment of infectious diarrhea, it is important to avoid antimotility drugs, which would slow bacterial excretion, increase the frequency of bacteremia and invasive forms of the disease, and prolong the carrier state. Cases of severe clinical profiles and even fatal outcomes caused by *C. difficile* and *C. perfringens toxins have been recorded in patients receiving loperamide* [17].

When deciding upon the administration of antimicrobial drugs for the treatment of diarrhea, it is necessary to follow the guidelines strictly. Such treatment is indicated when the clinical presentation is moderately severe or severe, according to the antibiogram of the isolated causative agent. The use of an antibiotic to shorten the duration of some types of diarrhea and prevent complications is justified. However, it must be borne in mind that the unjustified prescribing of antibiotics leads to increased bacterial resistance, dysbiosis of the intestinal microflora, *C. difficile* overgrowth, and post-antimicrobial diarrhea, while in some cases antibiotics can also prolong the carrier state. Shortening the duration of the symptoms of the disease and preventing complications are known to occur in shigellosis, Enterotoxigenic Escherichia coli (ETEC) infections, and *V. cholerae* [18]. On the other hand, antibiotic treatment has not been shown to be effective against campylobacter infections, does not lead to a significant reduction in the duration of the disease, and is only justified for patients expected to develop complications (the elderly, immunosuppressed individuals and pregnant women) [19]. In diarrhea caused by nontyphoid salmonella, antibiotics can prolong the carrier state without significantly shortening the duration of the disease or preventing the development of complications. The administration of antibiotics must strictly follow the indications: patients over 50 years of age, infants younger than 3 months of age, patients with chronic intestinal diseases, hemoglobinopathies, pregnant patients with endovascular and valvular defects, patients with artificial valves, and immunosuppressed patients. It is generally thought that antimicrobial treatment of diarrhea should be avoided in children, primarily due to the risk of developing hemolytic-uremic syndrome in children with diarrhea caused by the Shiga toxin *E. coli* [20].

The risk of complications and fatal outcomes during the course of infectious diarrhea is the highest in the extreme age groups, infants and the elderly, as well as in immunosuppressed patients. Complications are most often related to invasive strains of the pathogen entering the bloodstream, that is, bacteremia leading to the formation of septic foci, although pathogens can also promote the development of autoimmune diseases, such as Guillain-Barré syndrome.

In infants, the most common complication is purulent meningitis, while adult patients are susceptible to foreign body endovascular infections, mycotic aneurisms, and the formation of extraintestinal foci (intra-abdominal abscesses, liver and spleen abscesses, cholangitis, cholecystitis, pyelonephritis, arthritis, meningitis, and arteritis). Immunocompromised patients are particularly at risk for developing invasive forms of the disease, bacteremia, fulminant meningitis, intestinal perforation, and fatal outcomes [21].

Clostridioides Difficile-Associated Disease (CDAD)

In addition to the classical bacterial pathogens, in the last two decades, owing to the increasing overuse and misuse of antibiotics, *Clostridioides difficile* has become one of the most frequent causes of diarrhea. Nearly all antibiotics can cause antibiotic-associated diarrhea resulting from the germination of *C. difficile* spores on disrupted intestinal microbiota [22]. The disease is manifested by slimy, bloody, watery stools; dehydration, meteorism and abdominal pain, with or without generalized symptoms or fever. *C. difficile* produces two exotoxins (A and B), which damage the mucous membrane of the colon to produce pseudomembranes. In extremely severe and clinically unrecognized cases, the disease may progress to the development of toxic megacolon and bowel perforation. Particularly severe forms of the disease are encountered in elderly patients and nursing home residents [23].

All antibiotics can contribute to the onset of CDAD. It is estimated that approximately 20% of the patients develop recurrent episodes of CDAD after the successful treatment of a first episode. Recurrent infections can be caused by the germination of bacteria from residual spores in the intestinal mucosa or reinfection with a new bacterial strain. Recurrences mainly occur among elderly patients, patients receiving immunosuppressive therapy, patients hospitalized for a long period of time, and patients using proton pump inhibitors or H2 receptor blockers [24, 25].

The first step in treating CDAD is to terminate the antibiotic treatment that triggered the infection, when possible. Depending on the severity of the infection, treatment may include antibiotics, fecal microbiota transplantation, probiotics, and even surgery.

It is thought that native host-gut microbiota may mediate in the creation of a type of defense from colonization by *C. difficile* spores [26]. The interaction between *C. difficile* and the intestinal microbiota is complex and still not completely understood, although it is known with certainty that the colonization of the intestinal tract by spores alters the structure of the host microflora. One of the mechanisms that leads to clostridial overgrowth in the intestines is the antibiotic-induced increase in the secretion of bile salts, which contributes to spore germination in the intestinal lumen [27].

Stool samples from patients who have developed CDAD following antimicrobial treatment show reduced microbial biological diversity. There is even less such diversity in patients who have experienced repeated episodes of CDAD in comparison to healthy subjects and those who have completed successful treatment [28]. Some animal models have shown that the use of clindamycin leads to the loss of lactobacilli and mucosal overgrowth by species from the *Enterobacteriaceae* family. This is why over 95% of fecal microbiota transplants have successful outcomes [26].

The Risk of Chronic Gastrointestinal Disorders Following Acute Infection

Several studies have linked bacterial intestinal infections to an increased risk of chronic gastrointestinal disorders, including IBD and gastroesophageal reflux disease (GERD) [29–31].

Various bacterial pathogens (*Campylobacter, Shigella, Salmonella*, and *E. coli* O157:H7) are associated with the emergence of postinfectious enteropathy, although which and to what extent are not known. Viral gastroenteritis is a more frequent cause of transient enteropathy than bacterial pathogens [32].

Although the etiology and pathogenesis of IBD are still not well understood, many clinical and observational studies have highlighted the role of the intestinal microbiota at the onset of the disease [33]. One study has demonstrated that the incidence of colonization with *C. difficile* is 7% higher among patients with IBD, compared to the healthy population [34].

A broad range of infectious agents, such as *Salmonella, Shigella, Campylobacter, B. cereus, Staph. aureus, C. perfringens, E. coli*, etc., can damage the wall of the small intestine and lead to malabsorption [35].

Bacterial proliferation in the small intestine can occur due to changes in the intestinal anatomy or gastrointestinal motility, as well as the decreased secretion of gastric acid. It is encountered most frequently in elderly patients with gastric hypoacidity who take several types of medication, some of which can have the side effect of intestinal hypomotility.

The most common bacterial infection that leads to mucosal overgrowth in the small intestine and consequent malabsorption is Whipple's disease (intestinal lipodystrophy), a relapsing chronic disease caused by the actinomycete *Tropheryma whipplei*. Another bacterial causative agent is *Mycobacterium avium*-intracellular complex, an opportunistic pathogen in immunocompromised patients, especially those with AIDS. In an immunocompetent host, the infection does not lead to the development of disease, while in the immunocompromised, the disease is manifested by chronic diarrhea, abdominal pain, and weight loss [36].

Fungi are an important cause of gastrointestinal infections in patients with weakened immunity: transplant patients, AIDS patients, and patients with various congenital immunodeficiencies. The most common fungi involved are *Histoplasma capsulatum* and *Cryptococcus neoformans*.

The most important and most common protozoan infestation responsible for malabsorption is giardiasis. Studies have demonstrated that patients with hypogammaglobulinemia, agammaglobulinemia, IgA-deficiency, and achlorhydria are at the highest risk, while humoral deficiency is not a significant factor in the development of infection. In immunocompromised patients, the infection is manifested by long-term diarrhea, malabsorption, and weight loss, while in adult patients it is most commonly asymptomatic or self-limiting, with mild clinical symptoms. The protozoa responsible for malabsorption in immunocompromised patients are *Cryptosporidium parvum, Cyclospora cayetanensis, Isospora belli, Microsporidium, cryptosporidia*, and *microsporidia* [37].

The most important helminths responsible for malabsorption are *Ancylostoma duodenale* and *Strongyloides stercoralis*. Both lead to the development of chronic bloody diarrhea, resulting in sideropenic anemia, characterized by eosinophilia in the blood and the formation of eosinophilic infiltrates in the small intestinal mucosa.

In the differential diagnosis of immunosuppressed patients with AIDS or IBD, cytomegalovirus infection *should be the first viral pathogen considered. The clinical symptoms are diarrhea, elevated temperature, abdominal pain, and weight loss.* Several studies have shown that intestinal malabsorption can persist after recovery from infectious diseases [38].

Gastrointestinal Involvement in Chronic Infectious Diseases

Some chronic infectious diseases can also cause severe gastrointestinal involvement. One of the most common predisposing factors for liver cirrhosis is infection with hepatitis B (HBV) and hepatitis C (HCV) viruses. Hepatitis B can be manifested as acute hepatitis, nonprogressive chronic hepatitis, progressive chronic disease with transition to cirrhosis, the fulminant necrotizing form or the asymptomatic form. Hepatitis C transitions to the chronic form of the disease more often (85%) than hepatitis B, with 20% of the patients developing liver cirrhosis. Fibrosis underlies the pathogenesis of hepatocellular carcinoma [39].

Several gastrointestinal clinical conditions are symptomatic in HIV-infected patients, mostly resulting from secondary infections. One of them is thrush, a fungal infection of the oral cavity caused by *Candida* spp., which presents as white layers on the soft palate or gingiva [40]. Another disease is oral hairy leukoplakia, caused by the Epstein-Barr virus, usually an asymptomatic lesion on the lateral borders of the tongue [41]. Besides AIDS, it can also be associated with other immunosuppressed conditions. Aphthous ulcerations of the oropharynx, which present with painful swallowing, are clinically common among HIV-infected patients, although their etiology remains unknown. Besides the oral cavity, candidiasis may also involve the esophagus, as well as the small and large bowels.

Esophagitis may be caused by *Candida spp*, cytomegalovirus, herpes simplex virus, Kaposi sarcoma, or lymphoma. Patients may complain of difficulty in swallowing, retrosternal burning, and weight loss. Cytomegalovirus usually causes large deep ulcers, whereas Herpes simplex virus (HSV) presents with multiple small shallow ulcers. Enterocolitis is common among HIV-infected patients. Infections may attack the small or large bowel. Small bowel infection usually presents with periumbilical cramps, extensive watery diarrhea and weight loss, while large bowel infection presents with lower abdominal pain, cramps, and tenesmus.

The differential diagnosis of enterocolitis includes bacterial, protozoal, and viral pathogens. The most common bacterial etiological factors are *Campylobacter*, *Salmonella* spp., and *Shigella* spp. Among parasites, there are *Cryptosporidium parvum*, *Microsporidia,* and *Cystospora belli*. The most commonly isolated pathogens are Cytomegalovirus (CMV) (viruses) and *Histoplasma capsulatum* (fungi). Shigellosis is often sexually transmitted among the MSM population [42]. Generally, bacterial enterocolitis among the HIV-infected population has a prolonged course, often complicated with bacteremia, and may be recurrent [43].

The MSM population frequently presents with symptoms of proctitis, resulting from a sexually transmitted infection, such as *C. trachomatis*, *N. gonorrhoeae*, or *T. pallidum,* and are also at great risk for HPV, anal dysplasia, and anal cancer. Therefore, cancer screening is recommended [44].

Among HIV-infected individuals with chronic enterocolitis, known as HIV-associated enteropathy, the etiological pathogen cannot be determined in some cases. The pathology is not fully understood but HIV seems to be directly involved in the depletion of gut-associated CD4 cells [45].

HIV accelerates both HBV and HCV progression. HIV infection has a strong influence on the course of HBV infection. Patients coinfected with both viruses are at a greater risk of developing chronic HBV infection than those with HBV infection alone [46]. Patients with HBV and HIV coinfection are more likely to develop liver cirrhosis or hepatocellular carcinoma and die of liver disease than patients with only HBV infection [47].

When HIV-infected intravenous drug users are coinfected with HCV, due to shared routes of acquisition, their prognosis becomes more severe. Chronic HCV coinfection may lead to liver fibrosis, cirrhosis, end-stage liver disease, hepatocellular carcinoma, and death [48].

Campylobacteriosis is a risk factor for the development of chronic gastrointestinal disorders, such as IBD and celiac disease [49].

C. albicans is a ubiquitous microorganism. An opportunistic pathogen, it is commonly found in the gastrointestinal tract of immunocompetent persons and poses no danger [50]. However, the use of broad-spectrum antibiotics leads to the dysbiosis of the intestinal microbial environment, stimulates the reproduction of yeasts, and increases colonization in immunocompromised patients, which can cause invasive diseases [51].

Infections and Malignancies of the Gastrointestinal Tract

It has been known for decades that some pathogens of infectious diseases, that is, viruses, bacteria, and parasites, are linked to the onset of certain malignant diseases, including those of the gastrointestinal tract. Worldwide, infections are generally etiologically linked to approximately 15%–20% of all carcinomas, although the percentages are higher in underdeveloped countries. However, many patients with such infections never develop malignant diseases, indicating that additional factors are necessary for malignancies to occur [52].

Worldwide, an estimated 1.9 million cancer cases, representing 17.8% of all human cancers, were attributable to infectious agents in 2002. Most of this burden was related to viral infections (12.1%) (the human papilloma viruses (5.2%), the hepatitis B and C viruses (4.9%), the Epstein-Barr virus (1%), the human immunodeficiency virus [HIV] together with the human herpes virus 8 (0.9%), with 5.6%

related to infection with the bacterium *Helicobacter pylori*, and a very small proportion (about 0.1%) to parasitic infections). The percentage of infections attributable to cancer is higher in developing countries (26.3%) than in developed countries (7.7%), reflecting a higher prevalence of infection with the major causative agents (hepatitis viruses, HPV, *H. pylori*, and HIV) [53].

A 2020 study by the Pan-Cancer Analysis of Whole Genomes (PCAWG) Consortium found that 16% of cancers were associated with viruses, such as the Epstein-Barr virus (EBV), hepatitis B virus (HBV), and human papillomaviruses (HPV, e.g., HPV16 or HPV18). For HBV, viral integration was associated with local variations in genomic copy numbers [54].

These cancers might be easily prevented through vaccination (e.g., papillomavirus vaccines), diagnosed with simple blood tests and treated with less-toxic antiviral compounds [55].

Some of the infections of the gastrointestinal tract associated with the occurrence of gastrointestinal cancer are as follows:

- *Helicobacter pylori* is the main cause of chronic gastritis and gastric ulcer, and it also plays a role in the development of adenocarcinoma and gastric lymphoma [56].
- *Streptococcus gallolyticus* (formerly known as *Streptococcus bovis*) is associated with the development of colorectal cancer and adenoma in 25–80% of cases [57], although the mechanism is still insufficiently understood. In every case of bacteremia caused by these bacteria, colon cancer should be suspected and confirmed/excluded by a diagnostic workup.
- Hepatitis B and C viruses cause infections that can lead to the development of hepatocellular carcinoma when left untreated. In Europe, 60–70% of the cases of hepatocellular carcinoma are associated with HCV infection, and 10–15% are associated with HBV infection [58].
- *Salmonella typhi* can cause chronic infections associated with gallbladder carcinoma [59] and cholangiocellular carcinoma [60].
- *S. mansoni* is associated with adenocarcinoma of the colon [61].
- Several trematode parasites are known to be epidemiologically linked with malignancy in humans, such as the liver flukes *Clonorchis sinensis* and *Opisthorchis viverrini,* which are known predisposing factors for the development of cholangiocarcinoma [62].

Patients with cirrhosis of the liver have impaired cellular immunity, suffer from protein malnutrition and vitamin deficiencies, and are prone to develop sepsis and spontaneous bacterial peritonitis. The cytotoxic drugs used in the treatment of patients with carcinoma directly suppress the bone marrow and also impair cellular and humoral immunity. Given that they act on cells that multiply rapidly, they damage the epithelium of the gastrointestinal system and increase the risk of colonization by various Gram-positive and Gram-negative pathogens and fungi. Radiation therapy also damages the epithelium of the gastrointestinal mucosa [63].

Transplantation and Infection

Despite all the advances in health care, patients with solid organ transplants are still most likely to contract and die from bacterial infections [64]. This usually involves infections caused by multidrug resistant (MDR) Gram-negative pathogens *(Klebsiella pneumoniae, Acinetobacter baumannii, Pseudomonas aeruginosa, Escherichia coli), which may present clinically as sepsis, urinary tract infections, pneumonia, or surgical wound infections* [65]. The likelihood of acquiring an infection increases with the length of hospitalization and whether the patient has received immunosuppressive therapy and/or broad-spectrum antibiotics [66].

Infections with human polyomaviruses, small nonenveloped DNA viruses that asymptomatically infect about 80% of healthy adults, are associated with human disease, particularly in immunocompromised individuals, such as organ transplant recipients, including those of the gastrointestinal tract (particularly liver transplant recipients). The BK virus (BKV) is associated with tubulointerstitial nephritis, ureteral stenosis, and graft dysfunction in kidney transplant and nonkidney solid organ transplant patients, as well as hemorrhagic cystitis in hematopoietic stem cell transplant patients, whereas the JC virus (JCV) is associated with a fatal brain disease known as progressive multifocal leukoencephalopathy. The majority of the episodes of polyomavirus DNAemia in transplant patients are subclinical, although, in some cases, BKV DNAemia is associated with kidney rejection, while JCV DNAemia is accompanied by nonspecific symptoms. These observations were most common in kidney and/or pancreas transplant patients (26%), although they were also noted, to a lesser extent, in liver transplant patients (4%). The effect of BKV and JCV viremia on transplant outcomes is less clear, especially in Solid organ transplant (SOT) patients at high risk of contracting the CMV disease [67].

A systematic review by Umbro et al. showed that BKV viruria and/or viremia in liver transplantation is less prevalent than in kidney or heart transplantation, except when renal dysfunction is present. In general, viruric and viremic liver transplant patients have elevated levels of serum creatinine. Therefore, renal dysfunction in liver transplantation may be an additional causative factor in immunologic dysfunction, which could render patients more susceptible to BKV infection [68]. Another study on the effects of polyomavirus infection in hematopoietic stem cell transplant recipients by Hu et al. [69] showed that CMV infection was found to be an independent risk factor for JCV infection (OR: 8.528), while transplants with mismatched human leukocyte antigens (proteins on human cells) (HLA) are more susceptible to BKV infection (OR: 12,000). The liver function of JCV-infected subjects was worse than that of uninfected subjects, leading to the conclusion that JCV infections should be considered in cases of unexplained liver function deterioration, especially those with CMV-JC coinfection. Therefore, further studies are needed to assess the long-term clinical relevance of polyomavirus infection in liver transplant recipients.

Drug Interactions in the Treatment of Gastrointestinal Infections

Broad-spectrum antibiotics often cause dysbiosis of the intestinal microflora, which can lead to malabsorption syndrome. When antacids and antimotility drugs are administered in combination with antibiotics, chelates or complexes often form, which either prevent or retard antibiotic absorption. Moreover, antimotility drugs contribute to the prolonged retention of drugs in the stomach lumen, where antibiotics are inactivated by gastric acid. In such cases, the drugs should not be administered at the same time but rather at intervals of at least 2 h apart. Such clinically significant interactions occur between tetracyclines and quinolones. Antacids form insoluble complexes with tetracyclines, thereby reducing antibiotic absorption by over 90%. In combination with tetracyclines such as ciprofloxacin and ofloxacin, absorption is reduced by 50–90% [70].

Antimotility drugs, such as loperamide, demonstrate a synergistic effect with antibiotics in the treatment of mild forms of traveler's diarrhea [71]. However, this group of drugs should be avoided in patients with fever and abdominal cramps due to the risk of developing toxic megacolon or intestinal perforation [72].

The eradication of *H. pylori* infection is an example of the synergistic action of antibiotics and proton pump inhibitors. *H. pylori* infections are most commonly asymptomatic, although in a minority of symptomatic cases they can be manifested by dyspepsia caused by increased gastric acid secretion from ulcers. The objective of combined antimicrobial therapy is to eradicate bacteria, while the simultaneous administration of proton pump inhibitors reduces the secretion of gastric acid by the gastric parietal cells, which accelerates the eradication of the causative agent [73].

A recent study conducted in Europe among patients with liver cirrhosis showed a significant increase in the incidence of multidrug-resistant (MDR) bacteria [74]. This particularly applies to ciprofloxacin resistance, present in over 40% of these patients, which is of importance to the extent that ciprofloxacin is the antibiotic of choice in the prophylaxis of spontaneous bacterial peritonitis, which may lead to the development of life-threatening intraperitoneal infections [75].

Beta-lactam antibiotics are among the most commonly prescribed antibiotics. In the treatment of many infectious syndromes, they are often combined with other antibiotics, primarily aminoglycosides and macrolides. However, the combination of antimicrobial drugs often does not contribute to their effectiveness, increasing the risk of side effects and adverse reactions while encouraging the development of resistance. It is conceivable that treatment with two antibiotics to prevent resistance among typical bacterial pathogens would amount to a pyrrhic victory, reducing resistance at the site of infection in the short term but resulting in selection for resistance in the microbiome and environment to two antibiotics rather than one, triggering the loss of efficacy for both drugs in the long run. Therefore, combined administration is rarely justified, especially in environments where the incidence of antimicrobial resistance is low [76].

Amoxicillin affects the pharmacokinetic profile of the aspirin-active metabolite salicylic acid by slowing the metabolic activity of aspirin through the intestinal flora. The interaction between amoxicillin and aspirin mediated by the intestinal flora may affect the efficacy of aspirin and cause more significant adverse effects [77].

Cephalosporins are generally considered to be among the safest antibiotics but can cause certain side effects, particularly in the gastrointestinal tract, especially when used in combination with other drugs. A rare side effect of ceftriaxone treatment is the occurrence of pseudolithiasis, the precipitation of the calcium salts of the ceftriaxone in the gall bladder, which usually does not cause symptoms, except rare incidences of nausea and epigastric pain, which can quickly be verified ultrasonically. Resorption usually occurs spontaneously after treatment is discontinued. This symptom usually occurs in the pediatric population, with the use of higher doses of ceftriaxone per unit of body weight [78]. However, less commonly this phenomenon can also be found in adult patients [79].

Caution should be exercised when coadministering cephalosporins and vitamin K, as the effect of the vitamin K can be enhanced by cephalosporins. When cephalosporins are given in combination with aminoglycosides, they may weaken the effect by reducing the serum concentration of the aminoglycosides. The use of cephalospirins can also lead to a reduction in the therapeutic effect of probiotics of the order *Lactobacillus* [80].

Coadministration of various drugs can influence the severity of aminoglycoside-induced nephrotoxicity. While vancomycin and teicoplanin amplify experimental aminoglycoside-induced nephrotoxicity, extended-spectrum penicillins reduce the risk of kidney injury. Animal experiments with an aminoglycoside plus cephalothin, cefazolin, or cefamandole indicated either no effect or an attenuation of nephrotoxicity in comparison with an aminoglycoside plus placebo [81].

Macrolide antibiotics often cause gastrointestinal side effects, while azithromycin may induce the prolongation of the QT interval. Therefore, caution is needed when prescribing this drug to elderly patients and those with bradycardia, hypokalemia, and heart disease [82]. Azithromycin may increase the effect of statins on rhabdomyolysis and increase the concentration of tacrolimus. Caution is required with patients on anticoagulant therapy because azithromycin can also increase the serum concentration of vitamin K antagonists [83].

Quinolones are also frequently used in the treatment of gastrointestinal infections, especially ciprofloxacin. Therefore, it should be borne in mind that ciprofloxacin inhibits the group of cytochrome P450 monooxygenase enzymes, which otherwise participate in the metabolism of many drugs and toxins. It has been demonstrated that ciprofloxacin diminishes the elimination of theophylline and methylxanthine substrates, so these drugs should be avoided in combination with ciprofloxacin. If treatment with ciprofloxacin is essential, the doses of these drugs should be reduced and their plasma levels monitored [84]. Nonsteroidal anti-inflammatory drugs can enhance central nervous system stimulation caused by fluoroquinolones through the displacement of the neurotransmitter gamma-aminobutyric acid from the receptor sites, thereby lowering the seizure threshold [85].

Treatment with metronidazole can cause a disulfiram reaction. Drugs containing alcohol, parenteral cotrimoxazole and cough syrups can also lead to disulfiram reactions when coadministered with metronidazole. Treatment with metronidazole and disulfiram can result in acute psychosis or confusion [86]. Cases of sudden death have also been reported in patients treated with metronidazole in combination with ethanol [87]. In psychiatric patients, caution is needed because metronidazole can cause lithium retention, which increases its toxicity [88]. In cardiology, it has been shown that the administration of metronidazole in combination with drugs that prolong the QT interval cause polymorphic ventricular tachycardia, known as *torsades de pointes*. This occurred in a patient treated with a combination of metronidazole and amiodarone [89]. In a study on solid organ transplant recipients with *C. difficile* infections, treatment with metronidazole led to increased serum concentrations of tacrolimus [90].

The nephrotoxicity and ototoxicity of vancomycin has long been recognized. Treatment with some drug combinations can increase these undesirable side effects, such as the administration of a combination of parenteral vancomycin and aminoglycosides, which can increase the nephrotoxicity of the aminoglycosides [91]. Concomitant treatment with nonsteroidal anti-inflammatory drugs and parenteral vancomycin can raise the serum concentration of vancomycin, as does combination treatment with vancomycin and piperacillin [92]. With the peroral administration of vancomycin, there is generally no resorption from the intestinal lumen so the drug does not usually enter the systemic circulation. Nevertheless, this can still happen in cases of IBD or pseudomembranous colitis caused by *C. difficile.* Peroral administration of vancomycin can reduce the therapeutic effect of *Lactobacillus.*

Trimethoprim therapy can enhance the hyperkalemic effect of coprescribed angiotensin-converting enzyme inhibitors or angiotensin receptor blockers [93]. The chemoprophylaxis or treatment of *Pneumocystis* infection with trimethoprim in HIV-infected patients can increase the serum concentrations of lamivudine and zidovudine [94], as well as metformin, and thus potentiate the hypoglycemic effect in patients with diabetes [95]. Treatment with sulfonamides in patients on vitamin K antagonist therapy can potentiate the anticoagulant effect of vitamin K, so a 10 or 20% reduction in the dose of vitamin K antagonist should be considered before administering sulfonamides [96].

The antiviral drugs used in the treatment of chronic infection with the hepatitis C virus can interact with other drugs and, therefore, should be prescribed with caution. Such interactions can lead to the development of severe side effects, a lack of clinical response, or viral resistance. Badri et al. investigated interactions between a combination of antiviral drugs for the treatment of chronic hepatitis C infection (ombitasvir/paritaprevir/ritonavir) and 11 different types of medications, including statins (pravastatin, rosuvastatin) and a proton pump inhibitor (omeprazole). The study showed that when the combination of antiviral drugs is administered with a statin, a lower dose of the statin is required, whereas a higher dose of omeprazole may be required when administered with the combination of antiviral drugs. It is not necessary to adjust the dose of the antiviral drug in either of these two instances [97]. It has been demonstrated that various highly active antiretroviral therapies (HAART), which suppress HIV viremia, alter the intestinal microflora in various ways, especially drugs from the group of protease inhibitors [98]. However, the mechanism is still unknown. Further research would be required in order to determine the optimal approach to the treatment of disorders of the intestinal mucosa.

Cytomegalovirus infection is an important cause of morbidity and mortality among patients with solid organ transplants [99]. In this group of patients, infection can occur when the virus is reactivated, for example, due to the administration of immunosuppressive therapy or exogenously, for example, via the transplanted organ. Symptomatic CMV infection usually occurs during the first 3 months after transplantation in patients who have not received antiviral prophylaxis. Although the virus can affect almost all organs, it usually affects the gastrointestinal and respiratory tracts. In the gastrointestinal tract, it usually causes hepatitis but the virus can also affect other parts, creating a clinical picture of esophagitis, gastritis, enteritis, or colitis. Infections most often occur in CMV-negative recipients who received organs from seropositive donors [100]. Antiviral prophylaxis with valganciclovir is usually administered for 3–6 months, although preemptive therapy has recently been shown to be superior in reducing the incidence of CMV infection over a 12-month period [101].

Ganciclovir and valganciclovir, alone or in combination with other drugs, are known to cause myelosuppression, particularly leucopenia. Ganciclovir has many overlapping toxic side effects with other drugs used in transplant medicine, cytoreductive chemotherapy, and immunosuppression therapy. The nephrotoxicity of other drugs administered with ganciclovir (e.g., cyclosporine or amphotericin B) can reduce the excretion of ganciclovir and thereby increase the risk of myelosuppression. Caution should also be exercised in the simultaneous administration of ganciclovir and co-trimoxazole due to potentially serious myelosuppression and nephrotoxicity. The combination of ganciclovir and imipenem increases the risk of epileptic seizures [102]. When introducing ganciclovir into therapy, urea and creatinine levels must be monitored at least once a week, since the dose must be adjusted if kidney failure occurs [103].

The first drug to be discovered for the treatment of malaria was quinine, followed by improved synthesized forms, chloroquine and hydroxychloroquine. In recent years, it has been shown that antimalarial drugs also possess certain immunomodulatory properties. Thus, they have found certain applications in the treatment of various autoimmune diseases (arthritis, *Sjögren's syndrome,* systemic lupus erythematosus [SLE], rheumatoid arthritis [RA]), cardiovascular and oncological diseases, but also metabolic diseases. Thus, the administration of hydroxychloroquine to patients suffering from SLE, RA, and diabetes has been shown to lower glycemic levels [104].

In the treatment of echinococcosis, conservative or surgical treatment is used, depending on the size and site of the cyst, the viability of the *Echinococcus* and the potential for cyst rupture and the dissemination of the protoscolex. In inoperable cases, the treatment options are albendazole, mebendazole, and praziquantel. In the search for new drugs, it has been shown that *E. multilocularis,* metacestodes, and malignant tumors have some similarities: the capacity for continuous cell growth, the ability to moderate the immune response, the secretion of proteolytic enzymes in order to reach the target organ, the stimulation of angiogenesis, and the potential for metastasis [105]. These similarities have aroused suspicions that antiproliferative drugs could also affect the metacestode *Echinococcus*, and many antiparasitic drugs, such as artemisinin, mefloquine, and the derivative *nitazoxanide have antiproliferative activity* [106]. One of the first antiproliferative drugs in the treatment of alveolar *Echinococcus* was doxorubicin, but its use was soon abandoned due to its toxicity [107].

Probiotics help re-establish intestinal microflora disrupted by illness and, among other things, antimicrobial therapy, and are considered safe for immunocompetent patients. However, the benefits from administering them to immunocompromised patients are dubious. Some types, for example, *Saccharomyces* and lactobacilli, are associated with the development of infections in immunocompromised patients and, therefore, the clinician should weigh the potential risks and benefits [108].

References

1. Quigley EMM, Hasler WL, Parkman HP. AGA technical review on nausea and vomiting. Gastroenterology. 2001;120:263.
2. Getto L, Zeserson E, Breyer M. Vomiting, diarrhea, constipation, and gastroenteritis. Emerg Med Clin North Am. 2011;29:211, viii.
3. Liu L, Johnson HL, Cousens S, Perin J, Scott S, et al. Global, regional, and national causes of child mortality: an updated systematic analysis for 2010 with time trends since 2000. Lancet. 2012;379:2151–61.
4. Haessler S, Granowitz EV. Norovirus gastroenteritis in immunocompromised patients. N Engl J Med. 2013;368:971.
5. Guerrant RL, Van Gilder T, Steiner TS, Thielman NM, Slutsker L, Tauxe RV, et al. Practice guidelines for the management of infectious diarrhea. Clin Infect Dis. 2001;32:331–51.
6. Esposito DH, Holman RC, Haberling DL, et al. Baseline estimates of diarrhea-associated mortality among United States children before rotavirus vaccine introduction. Pediatr Infect Dis J. 2011;30:942–7.
7. Stuempfig ND, Seroy J. Viral gastroenteritis. In: StatPearls. Treasure Island, FL: StatPearls Publishing; 2020. p. 2020.
8. Blitz J, Riddle MS, Porter CK. The risk of chronic gastrointestinal disorders following acute infection with intestinal parasites. Front Microbiol. 2018;9:17.
9. Krones E, Högenauer C. Diarrhea in the immunocompromised patient. Gastroenterol Clin N Am. 2012;41:677–701.
10. Stark D, Barratt JL, van Hal S, Marriott D, Harkness J, Ellis JT. Clinical significance of enteric protozoa in the immunosuppressed human population. Clin Microbiol Rev. 2009;22:634–50.
11. Scallan E, Crim SM, Runkle A, et al. Bacterial enteric infections among older adults in the United States: foodborne diseases active surveillance network, 1996–2012. Foodborne Pathog Dis. 2015;12:492–9.
12. Lund BM, O'Brien SJ. The occurrence and prevention of foodborne disease in vulnerable people. Foodborne Pathog Dis. 2011;8:961–73.
13. Payne DC, Vinjé J, Szilagyi PG, et al. Norovirus and medically attended gastroenteritis in U.S. children. N Engl J Med. 2013;368:1121–30.
14. Crump JA, Sjölund-Karlsson M, Gordon MA, Parry CM. Epidemiology, clinical presentation, laboratory diagnosis, antimicrobial resistance, and antimicrobial Management of Invasive Salmonella Infections. Clin Microbiol Rev. 2015;28:901–37.
15. Shane AL, Mody RK, Crump JA, et al. 2017 Infectious Diseases Society of America clinical practice guidelines for the diagnosis and management of infectious diarrhea. Clin Infect Dis. 2017;65:e45–80.

16. UNICEF. The State of the World's Children 2019. Children, food and nutrition: growing well in a changing world. New York: UNICEF. p. 2019.
17. Koo HL, Koo DC, Musher DM, DuPont HL. Antimotility agents for the treatment of *Clostridium difficile* diarrhea and colitis. Clin Infect Dis. 2009;48:598–605.
18. Christopher PR, David KV, John SM, Sankarapandian V. Antibiotic therapy for *Shigella* dysentery. Cochrane Database Syst Rev 2010;2010:CD006784.
19. Ternhag A, Asikainen T, Giesecke J, Ekdahl K. A metaanalysis on the effects of antibiotic treatment on duration of symptoms caused by infection with *Campylobacter* species. Clin Infect Dis. 2007;44:696–700.
20. Bianchi L, Gaiani F, Vincenzi F, et al. Hemolytic uremic syndrome: differential diagnosis with the onset of inflammatory bowel diseases. Acta Biomed. 2018;89:153–7.
21. Dhanoa A, Fatt QK. Non-typhoidal Salmonella bacteraemia: epidemiology, clinical characteristics and its' association with severe immunosuppression. Ann Clin Microbiol Antimicrob. 2009;8:15.
22. Abt MC, McKenney PT, Pamer EG. Clostridium difficile colitis: pathogenesis and host defence. Nat Rev Microbiol. 2016;14:609–20.
23. Desai J, Elnaggar M, Hanfy AA, Doshi R. Toxic megacolon: background, pathophysiology, management challenges and solutions. Clin Exp Gastroenterol. 2020;13:203–10.
24. Loo VG, Bourgault AM, Poirier L, Lamothe F, Michaud S, Turgeon N. Host and pathogen factors for Clostridium difficile infection and colonization. N Engl J Med. 2011;365:1693–703.
25. Barletta JF, El-Ibiary SY, Davis LE, Nguyen B, Raney CR. Proton pump inhibitors and the risk for hospital-acquired Clostridium difficile infection. Mayo Clin Proc. 2013;88:1085–90.
26. Britton RA, Young VB. Role of the intestinal microbiota in resistance to colonization *by Clostridium difficile*. Gastroenterology. 2014;146:1547–53.
27. Howerton A, Ramirez N, Abel-Santos E. Mapping interactions between germinants and Clostridium difficile spores. J Bacteriol. 2011;193:274–82.
28. Chang JY, Antonopoulos DA, Kalra A, et al. Decreased diversity of the fecal microbiome in recurrent Clostridium difficile-associated diarrhea. J Infect Dis. 2008;197:435–8.
29. Connor BA, Riddle MS. Post-infectious sequelae of travelers' diarrhea. J Travel Med. 2013;20:303–12.
30. Hanevik K, Wensaas KA, Rortveit G, Eide GE, Morch K, Langeland N. Irritable bowel syndrome and chronic fatigue 6 years after *giardia* infection: a controlled prospective cohort study. Clin Infect Dis. 2014;59:1394–400.
31. Futagami S, Itoh T, Sakamoto C. Systematic review with metaanalysis: post-infectious functional dyspepsia. Aliment Pharmacol Ther. 2015;41:177–88.
32. Marshall JK, Thabane M, Borgaonkar MR, James C. Postinfectious irritable bowel syndrome after a food-borne outbreak of acute gastroenteritis attributed to a viral pathogen. Clin Gastroenterol Hepatol. 2007;5:457–60.
33. Jostins L, Ripke S, Weersma RK, et al. Host-microbe interactions have shaped the genetic architecture of inflammatory bowel disease. Nature. 2012;491:119–24.
34. Clayton EM, Rea MC, Shanahan F, et al. The vexed relationship between *Clostridium difficile* and inflammatory bowel disease: an assessment of carriage in an outpatient setting among patients in remission. Am J Gastroenterol. 2009;104:1162–9.
35. Ensari A. The malabsorption syndrome and its causes and consequences. Pathobiol Human Disease. 2014:1266–1287.
36. Giezendanner S, Wirth HP, Zala G, Weber R, Flury R, Meyenberger C. Klinische Manifestationen und Verlauf der Zytomegalievirus-Kolitis bei Aids-Patienten [Clinical manifestations and course of cytomegalovirus colitis in AIDS patients]. Schweiz Med Wochenschr. 1995;125:2417–22. German.
37. Nsagha DS, Njunda AL, Assob NJC, et al. Intestinal parasitic infections in relation to CD4(+) T cell counts and diarrhea in HIV/AIDS patients with or without antiretroviral therapy in Cameroon. BMC Infect Dis. 2016;16:9.

38. Woodward J, Gkrania-Klotsas E, Kumararatne D. Chronic norovirus infection and common variable immunodeficiency. Clin Exp Immunol. 2017;188:363–70.
39. Li H, Yan L, Shi Y, Lv D, Shang J, Bai L, Tang H. Hepatitis B virus infection: overview. Adv Exp Med Biol. 2020;1179:1–16.
40. Mohamed AA, Lu XL, Mounmin FA. Diagnosis and treatment of esophageal candidiasis: current updates. Can J Gastroenterol Hepatol. 2019;2019:3585136.
41. Lauritano D, Moreo G, Oberti L, et al. Oral manifestations in HIV-positive children: a systematic review. Pathogens. 2020;9:E88.
42. Aragón TJ, Vugia DJ, Shallow S, Samuel MC, Reingold A, Angulo FJ, Bradford WZ. Case-control study of shigellosis in San Francisco: the role of sexual transmission and HIV infection. Clin Infect Dis. 2007;44(3):327–34.
43. Huppmann AR, Orenstein JM. Opportunistic disorders of the gastrointestinal tract in the age of highly active antiretroviral therapy. Hum Pathol. 2010;41:1777–87.
44. Piketty C, Selinger-Leneman H, Grabar S, et al. Marked increase in the incidence of invasive anal cancer among HIV-infected patients despite treatment with combination antiretroviral therapy. AIDS. 2008;22:1203–11.
45. Kotler DP. HIV infection and the gastrointestinal tract. AIDS. 2005;19:107–17.
46. Kellerman SE, Hanson DL, McNaghten AD, Fleming PL. Prevalence of chronic hepatitis B and incidence of acute hepatitis B infection in human immunodeficiency virus-infected subjects. J Infect Dis. 2003;188:571–7.
47. Dharel N, Sterling RK. Hepatitis B virus-HIV coinfection: forgotten but not gone. Gastroenterol Hepatol. 2014;10:780–8.
48. Limketkai BN, Mehta SH, Sutcliffe CG, Higgins YM, Torbenson MS, Brinkley SC, et al. Relationship of liver disease stage and antiviral therapy with liver-related events and death in adults Coinfected with HIV/HCV. JAMA. 2012;308:370–8.
49. Riddle MS, Gutierrez RL, Verdu EF, Porter CK. The chronic gastrointestinal consequences associated with campylobacter. Curr Gastroenterol Rep. 2012;14:395–405.
50. Gutierrez D, Weinstock A, Antharam VC, et al. Antibiotic-induced gut metabolome and microbiome alterations increase the susceptibility to Candida albicans colonization in the gastrointestinal tract. FEMS Microbiol Ecol. 2020:96:
51. Sahni V, Agarwal SK, Singh NP, et al. Candidemia—an under-recognized nosocomial infection in Indian hospitals. J Assoc Physicians India. 2005;53:607–11.
52. Bouvard V, Baan R, Straif K, Grosse Y, Secretan B, El Ghissassi F, et al. A review of human carcinogens—part B: biological agents. WHO International Agency for Research on Cancer Monograph Working Group. Lancet Oncol. 2009;10:321–2.
53. Parkin DM. The global health burden of infection—associated cancers in the year 2002. Int J Cancer. 2006;118:3030–44.
54. Zapatka M, Borozan I, Brewer DS, Iskar M, Grundhoff A, Alawi M, et al. The landscape of viral associations in human cancers. Nat Genet. 2020;52:320–30.
55. Roden RBS, Stern PL. Opportunities and challenges for human papillomavirus vaccination in cancer. Nat Rev Cancer. 2018;18:240–54.
56. Parsonnet J, Friedman GD, Vandersteen DP, Chang Y, Vogelman JH, Orentreich N, Sibley RK. Helicobacter pylori infection and the risk of gastric carcinoma. N Engl J Med. 1991;325:1127–31.
57. Abdulamir AS, Hafidh RR, Abu BF. The association of Streptococcus bovis/gallolyticus with colorectal tumors: the nature and the underlying mechanisms of its etiological role. J Exp Clin Cancer Res. 2011;30:11.
58. Trichopoulos D, Bamia C, Lagiou P, et al. Hepatocellular carcinoma risk factors and disease burden in a European cohort: a nested case-control study. J Natl Cancer Inst. 2011;103:1686–95.
59. Kumar S, Kumar S, Kumar S. Infection as a risk factor for gallbladder cancer. J Surg Oncol. 2006;93:633–9.
60. Robbins S, Chuang VP, Hersh T. The development of hepatobiliary cancer in a carrier of *Salmonella typhus*. Am J Gastroenterol. 1988;83:675–8.

61. Madbouly KM, Senagore AJ, Mukerjee A, Hussien AM, Shehata MA, Navine P, Delaney CP, Fazio VW. Colorectal cancer in a population with endemic Schistosoma mansoni: is this an at-risk population? Int J Color Dis. 2007;22:175–81.
62. Kim YI. Liver carcinoma and liver fluke infection. Arzneimittelforschung. 1984;34:1121–6.
63. Lu L, Li W, Chen L, Su Q, Wang Y, Guo Z, Lu Y, Liu B, Qin S. Radiation-induced intestinal damage: latest molecular and clinical developments. Future Oncol. 2019;15:4105–18.
64. Wadström J, Ericzon B-G, Halloran PF, et al. Advancing transplantation: new questions, new possibilities in kidney and liver transplantation. Transplantation. 2017;101:S1–S42.
65. Ferrarese A, Zanetto A, Becchetti C, et al. Management of bacterial infection in the liver transplant candidate. World J Hepatol. 2018;10:222–30.
66. Shafiekhani M, Mirjalili M, Vazin A. Prevalence, risk factors and treatment of the most common gram-negative bacterial infections in liver transplant recipients: a review. Infect Drug Resist. 2019;12:3485–95.
67. Razonable RR, Brown RA, Humar A, Covington E, Alecock E, Paya CV. A longitudinal molecular surveillance study of human polyomavirus viremia in heart, kidney, liver, and pancreas transplant patients. J Infect Dis. 2005;192:1349–54.
68. Umbro I, Tinti F, Muiesan P, Mitterhofer AP. Different behaviour of BK-virus infection in liver transplant recipients. World J Gastroenterol. 2016;22:1532–40.
69. Hu J, Li S, Yang M, Xu L, Zhang X, Zhao H, et al. Incidence, risk factors and the effect of polyomavirus infection in hematopoietic stem cell transplant recipients. J Int Med Res. 2017;45:762–70.
70. Gugler R, Allgayer H. Effects of antacids on the clinical pharmacokinetics of drugs. An update. Clin Pharmacokinet. 1990;18:210–9.
71. Lääveri T, Sterne J, Rombo L, Kantele A. Systematic review of loperamide: no proof of antibiotics being superior to loperamide in treatment of mild/moderate travellers' diarrhoea. Travel Med Infect Dis. 2016;14(4):299–312. https://doi.org/10.1016/j.tmaid.2016.06.006. Epub 2016 Jun 27
72. Barrett J, Brown M. Travellers' diarrhoea. BMJ. 2016;353:i1937.
73. de Brito BB, da Silva FAF, Soares AS, Pereira VA, Santos MLC, Sampaio MM, Neves PHM, de Melo FF. Pathogenesis and clinical management of helicobacter pylori gastric infection. World J Gastroenterol. 2019;25(37):5578–89.
74. Piano S, Singh V, Caraceni P, Maiwall R, Alessandria C, Fernandez J, et al. Epidemiology and effects of bacterial infections in patients with cirrhosis worldwide. Gastroenterology. 2019;156:1368–1380.e10.
75. Patel VC, Williams R. Antimicrobial resistance in chronic liver disease. Hepatol Int. 2020;14:24–34.
76. Leibovici L, Paul M. Aminoglycoside/beta-lactam combinations in clinical practice. J Antimicrob Chemother. 2007;60:911–2.
77. Zhang J, Sun Y, Wang R, Zhang J. Gut microbiota-mediated drug-drug interaction between amoxicillin and aspirin. Sci Rep. 2019;9:16194.
78. Schaad UB, Tschäeppeler H, Lentze MJ. Transient formation of precipitations in the gallbladder associated with ceftriaxone therapy. Pediatr Infect Dis. 1986;5:708–10.
79. Yamabe A, Irisawa A, Wakabayashi H, Tsunoda T, Tominaga K. Ceftriaxone-associated pseudolithiasis in the gallbladder and bile duct of an elderly patient. Intern Med. 2020;59:2725–8.
80. Turnidge JD. The pharmacodynamics of beta-lactams. Clin Infect Dis. 1998;27:10–22.
81. Leggett JE. Aminoglycosides. In: Bennett JE, Dolin R, Blaser MJ, editors. Mandell, Douglas, and Bennett's principles and practice of infectious diseases. 9th ed. Philadelphia, PA: Elsevier; 2020. p. 305–17.
82. Hancox JC, Hasnain M, Vieweg WV, Crouse EL, Baranchuk A. Azithromycin, cardiovascular risks, QTc interval prolongation, torsade de pointes, and regulatory issues: a narrative review based on the study of case reports. Ther Adv Infect Dis. 2013;1:155–65.
83. Shaeer KM, Chahine EB, Varghese Gupta S, Cho JC. Macrolide allergic reactions. Pharmacy (Basel). 2019;7:135.

84. Stahlmann R, Schwabe R. Safety profile of grepafloxacin compared with other fluoroquinolones. J Antimicrob Chemother. 1997;40 Suppl A:83–92.
85. Hori S, Shimada S. Effects of quinolones on the central nervous system. In: Hooper DC, Wolfson JS, editors. Quinolone antimicrobial agents. 2nd ed. Washington, DC: American Society for Microbiology; 1993. p. 513.
86. Lau AH, Lam NP, Piscitelli SC, Wilkes L, Danziger LH. Clinical pharmacokinetics of metronidazole and other nitroimidazole anti-infectives. Clin Pharmacokinet. 1992;23:328–64.
87. Williams CS, Woodcock KR. Do ethanol and metronidazole interact to produce a disulfiram-like reaction? Ann Pharmacother. 2000;34:255–7.
88. Teicher MH, Altesman RI, Cole JO, Schatzberg AF. Possible nephrotoxic interaction of lithium and metronidazole. JAMA. 1987;257:3365–6.
89. Kounas SP, Letsas KP, Sideris A, Efraimidis M, Kardaras F. QT interval prolongation and torsades de pointes due to a coadministration of metronidazole and amiodarone. Pacing Clin Electrophysiol. 2005;28:472–3.
90. Early CR, Park JM, Dorsch MP, Pogue KT, Hanigan SM. Effect of metronidazole use on tacrolimus concentrations in transplant patients treated for Clostridium difficile. Transpl Infect Dis. 2016;18:714–20.
91. Gan IM, van Dissel JT, Beekhuis H, Swart W, van Meurs JC. Intravitreal vancomycin and gentamicin concentrations in patients with postoperative endophthalmitis. Br J Ophthalmol. 2001;85:1289–93.
92. Reardon J, Lau TT, Ensom MH. Vancomycin loading doses: a systematic review. Ann Pharmacother. 2015;49:557–65.
93. Antoniou T, Gomes T, Juurlink DN, Loutfy MR, Glazier RH, Mamdani MM. Trimethoprim-sulfamethoxazole-induced hyperkalemia in patients receiving inhibitors of the renin-angiotensin system: a population-based study. Arch Intern Med. 2010;170:1045–9.
94. Thomas CF, Limper AH. Treatment and prevention of pneumocystis pneumonia in HIV-infected patients. Post TW editor. UpToDate. Waltham, MA: UpToDate Inc. http://www.uptodate.com. Accessed 9 Dec 2019.
95. Strevel EL, Kuper A, Gold WL. Severe and protracted hypoglycaemia associated with co-trimoxazole use. Lancet Infect Dis. 2006;6:178–82.
96. Sulfamethoxazole-Trimethoprim. In: LiverTox: clinical and research information on drug-induced liver injury. Bethesda, MD: National Institute of Diabetes and Digestive anf Kidney Diseases; 2017b.
97. Badri PS, Dutta S, Wang H, et al. Drug interactions with the direct-acting antiviral combination of ombitasvir and paritaprevir-ritonavir. Antimicrob Agents Chemother. 2015;60:105–14.
98. Pinto-Cardoso S, Klatt NR, Reyes-Terán G. Impact of antiretroviral drugs on the microbiome: unknown answers to important questions. Curr Opin HIV AIDS. 2018;13:53–60.
99. Fayek SA, Mantipisitkul W, Rasetto F, Munivenkatappa R, Barth RN, Philosophe B. Valganciclovir is an effective prophylaxis for cytomegalovirus disease in liver transplant recipients. HPB (Oxford). 2010;12:657–63.
100. Griffiths P, Lumley S. Cytomegalovirus. Curr Opin Infect Dis. 2014;27:554–9.
101. Singh N, Winston DJ, Razonable RR, Lyon GM, Silveira FP, Wagener MM, Stevens-Ayers T, Edmison B, Boeckh M, Limaye AP. Effect of preemptive therapy vs antiviral prophylaxis on cytomegalovirus disease in seronegative liver transplant recipients with seropositive donors: a randomized clinical trial. JAMA. 2020;323:1378–87.
102. Genentech, Inc. Cytovene-IV (ganciclovir sodium for injection). 2010. http://www.gene.com/gene/products/information/cytovene/pdf/pi.pdf. Accessed 23 July 2012.
103. Tice AD, Rehm SJ, Dalovisio JR, Bradley JS, Martinelli LP, Graham DR, Gainer RB, Kunkel MJ, Yancey RW, Williams DN, IDSA. Practice guidelines for outpatient parenteral antimicrobial therapy. IDSA guidelines. Clin Infect Dis. 2004;38(12):1651–72.
104. Penn SK, Kao AH, Schott LL, et al. Hydroxychloroquine and glycemia in women with rheumatoid arthritis and systemic lupus erythematosus. J Rheumatol. 2010;37:1136–42.
105. Hemphill A, Stadelmann B, Rufener R, et al. Treatment of echinococcosis: albendazole and mebendazole—what else? Parasite. 2014;21:70.

106. Müller J, Sidler D, Nachbur U, Wastling J, Brunner T, Hemphill A. Thiazolides inhibit growth and induce glutathione-S-transferase Pi (GSTP1)-dependent cell death in human colon cancer cells. Int J Cancer. 2008;123:1797–806.
107. Liance M, Nemati F, Bories C, Couvreur P. Experience with doxorubicin-bound polyisohexyl-cyanoacrylate nanoparticles on murine alveolar echinococcosis of the liver. Int J Parasitol. 1993;23:427–9.
108. Riddle MS, DuPont HL, Connor BA. ACG clinical guideline: diagnosis, treatment, and prevention of acute diarrhea infections in adults. Am J Gastroenterol. 2016;111:602–22.

Cardiorespiratory Disorders 20

Mario Udovičić, Danijela Grizelj, and Hrvoje Falak

Introduction

The prevalence of cardiovascular and respiratory disorders in the general population is relatively high and it is thus not unusual to encounter digestive disease patients with cardiovascular or respiratory comorbidities.

There is a whole set of common risk factors for developing both cardiovascular and digestive disease [1]. All those disorders influence each other in a bidirectional manner through several mechanisms. These include altered hemodynamics, systemic inflammation, bacterial overgrowth, and interactions and adverse effects of medications. It is therefore uneasy to separate the two systems.

Very often, modern therapeutic protocols impose polypharmacy in the management of cardiovascular and respiratory diseases that can cause upper gastrointestinal symptoms. Not unusual is also overlapping of similar symptoms, such as epigastric pain and aginan pecotris. In this review, we present a few common cardiovascular and respiratory comorbidities frequently encountered in patients with digestive diseases, and their repercussions in the digestive system.

Atrial Fibrillation

Atrial fibrillation (AF) is the most common cardiac arrhythmia worldwide and is associated with significant morbidity and mortality [2].

AF is defined as supraventricular tachyarrhythmia, documented by surface Electrocardiograph (ECG), with uncoordinated atrial electrical activation and consequently ineffective atrial contraction. Electrocardiographic characteristics of AF

M. Udovičić (✉) · D. Grizelj · H. Falak
Division of Cardiovascular Diseases, Department of Internal Medicine, Dubrava University Hospital, Zagreb, Croatia

M. Banić, D. Erceg (eds.), *Drug Interactions in Gastroenterology*, Clinical Gastroenterology, https://doi.org/10.1007/978-3-031-69800-2_20

include: irregular R-R intervals (when atrioventricular conduction is not impaired), absence of distinct repeating P waves, and irregular atrial activations [3]. The central characteristic of AF is very rapid and uncoordinated electrical atrial activity with the absence of effective atrial contraction. This increases the risk of blood coagulation and thrombosis, particularly in the left atrial appendage. The resulting rapid and irregular ventricular contractions reduce its performance, aggravating existing heart failure or even precipitating de novo heart failure [4].

AF is classified as first diagnosed (not diagnosed before, irrespective of its duration), paroxysmal if it terminates spontaneously or with intervention within 7 days of onset, persistent if it is continuously sustained for >7 days, long-standing persistent if it is present continuously for >1 year when decided to adopt a rhythm control strategy, or as permanent arrhythmia—it is accepted by the patient and physician, and no further attempts to restore/maintain sinus rhythm will be undertaken [3].

Its prevalence is around 1–2% in the adult European population [5], rising from less than 0.5% among less than 40 year olds up to 15% for patients aged >80 years. Men are more likely affected than women; the lifetime risk for people over 40 years is at around 25% [6]. The risk of AF rises with the severity of a preexisting structural heart disease.

The pathophysiology of AF is complex [7]. A number of risk factors have been associated with AF and are broadly cardiovascular and noncardiovascular. The common cardiovascular conditions predisposing AF include hypertension, heart failure, valvular disease, ischemic and rheumatic heart disease, while noncardiovascular risk factors include smoking, obesity, diabetes mellitus, chronic kidney disease, hyperthyroidism, sepsis, chest infection, and obstructive sleep apnea [8].

Diseases of the liver and gastrointestinal tract also contribute to AF risk through various mechanisms, while vice versa the treatment for AF predisposes gastrointestinal and liver diseases [2].

Gastrointestinal (GI) disorders share several common risk factors with AF [9] such as stress, smoking, alcohol, obesity, hypertension diabetes mellitus, as well as inflammation [2, 10].

Chronic and acute inflammatory states have been shown to play an important role in the pathogenesis and promotion of persistence of AF. Neurohormonal mechanisms and autonomic imbalance are also associated with AF, with episodes caused by excitement, stimulants, vagal stimulation, or medications such as digitalis, and overactive thyroid function [2].

AF is associated with a series of serious complications and increased morbidity and more admissions to hospital. Complications include a near fivefold excess risk of stroke [11], a two- to threefold increased risk of heart failure [12], an increased risk of premature dementia [13], and finally with a nearly twofold increased risk of mortality [12] compared to those who do not have AF.

Therapy starts with primary AF prevention by treating cardiovascular risk-factors. Also various comorbidities, including lifestyle factors, have to be addressed and modified. Stroke prevention is primarily achieved by oral anticoagulation therapy (OAC) by vitamin K antagonists and direct oral anticoagulants (DOACs). A stroke risk stratification model CHA2DS2-VA (Congestive heart failure, Hypertension, Age ≥75 years (2 points), Diabetes mellitus, prior Stroke/transient ischaemic attack/arterial thromboembolism (2 points), Vascular disease, Age 65–74 years) is used for patients with nonvalvular AF (NVAF). Current guidelines recommend using oral anticoagulation for CHA2DS2-VA ≥2. The few absolute contraindications to OAC include active serious bleeding, severe thrombocytopenia, or severe anemia under investigation, and a recent high-risk bleeding event such as intracranial hemorrhage (ICH). Nondrug options may be considered in cases such as left appendage occluder.

The rhythm control strategy is the concept to restore and maintain sinus rhythm. It comprises of several treatment approaches, such as cardioversion, antiarrhythmic medication, and catheter ablation. Rate control is another important part of AF management, if rhythm control strategy is abandoned, and may often be sufficient to improve symptoms by controlling the heart rate. The optimal heart-rate target in AF patients is unclear, and very little robust evidence exists. Modalities are antiarrhythmic drugs and ablation of the atrioventricular node and pacemaker implantation, if the former fails.

Gastrointestinal Bleeding

Patients with AF and CHA_2DS_2-VA scores greater than one require oral anticoagulation. Treatment options consist either of warfarin or DOACs: dabigatran, rivaroxaban, edoxaban, and apixaban.

Among these patients, GI bleeding remains one of the most common complications of anticoagulant therapy for AF [2]. Very often patients on anticoagulation with major gastrointestinal bleeding (MGIB) have an underlying gastrointestinal malignancy. One study found that 1 in 12 MGIB events was associated with occult cancer [14].

While MGIB rates are more variable in the published literature for dabigatran and rivaroxaban, overall, DOACs have a similar or lower MGIB rate compared to warfarin [15].

Although studies directly comparing the DOACs are not available, existing real-world data and multiple meta-analyzes of GI bleeding suggest that apixaban may have fewer MGIB occurrences compared to dabigatran and rivaroxaban and should be considered as the preferred treatment for patients at an increased risk of bleeding [2, 16, 17].

Anticoagulation and Liver Injury

Patients with AF on treatment with OAC are also at risk for acute liver injury (ALI). All DOACs undergo varying degrees of hepatic metabolism, with much lower hepatic metabolism for dabigatran [18]. Therefore, the risk of liver injury was the lowest for those treated with dabigatran, intermediate for patients on rivaroxaban, and highest for those treated with warfarin [17]. Vitamin K antagonists (VKAs) have been in use for decades, but ALI has been seldom reported. Rare cases of DOAC-induced ALI have been reported with dabigatran [19], rivaroxaban [20], and apixaban [21].

Risk factors for ALI hospitalization included underlying hepatobiliary disease, failty, history of alcohol-use disorder, cancer, anemia, kidney disease, and heart failure [2, 18].

However, the results of a recent large cohort study based on the French health care database do not suggest an increased risk of ALI in DOAC patients with NVAF compared to VKA patients in the first year after treatment initiation, irrespective of a history of liver disease [18].

Patients with chronic liver disease often have abnormalities in coagulation characterized by clinical bleeding and decreased levels of most procoagulant factors [22]. However, this is accompanied by decreases in the levels of anticoagulants as antithrombin and protein C. Accumulating evidence contradicts the notion that patients with liver disease are "auto-anticoagulated" and protected against stroke and systemic thromboembolism associated with AF [22].

As the patients with liver disease have largely been excluded from trials of OACs, and all currently approved OACs undergo metabolism in the liver to at least some degree, hepatic dysfunction may cause increased bleeding. Thus, the optimal anticoagulation regimen for patients with AF who have liver dysfunction remains unclear [23].

Amiodarone Effects on Liver

Amiodarone is a very potent antiarrhythmic agent used in the treatment of ventricular and atrial arrhythmias, including AF.

Its use is associated with several serious adverse effects, which also encompass liver dysfunction. The mechanism of liver injury includes decrease in δ-oxidation of fatty acid levels, increase of lipid peroxidation, increased reactive oxygen species generation, and lipogenesis. Up to 30% of patients taking the drug have an asymptomatic acute elevation of liver enzyme levels after intravenous infusion [24].

Symptomatic and more aggressive conditions such as hepatitis, extensive hepatocellular necrosis, Reye syndrome-like illness, cholestatic hepatitis, liver failure, and cirrhosis from amiodarone have also been reported, but are fortunately rare (0–3% of amiodarone users). The risk increases with prolonged use and high doses.

With prolonged use, amiodarone is concentrated in the liver and its hepatic levels can be 100 to 500 times higher than serum levels. Chronic liver injury caused by amiodarone is a function of its cumulative dose. Amiodarone hepatotoxicity takes time to settle and may sometimes present itself even after amiodarone has been discontinued [24, 25].

Mesenteric Ischemia

In patients with AF, one of the fatal consequences may be mesenteric ischemia, which is mostly due to a thromboembolic event originating from the left atrium and appendage, rather than in situ formation [26]. The chance of mesenteric ischemia is higher with increasing CHA_2DS_2-VASc scores [4], main risk factors being a previous stroke, age over 75 years, arterial hypertension, and structural heart disease [27], while women are particularly at risk [28].

Heart Failure

Heart failure is not a single pathological diagnosis, but a complex clinical syndrome consisting of cardinal symptoms and signs caused by a failure to meet the systemic demands of circulation that results from a functional or structural heart disorder impairing ventricular filling or ejection of blood to the systemic circulation [29, 30].

In Western countries, coronary artery disease (CAD) and hypertension are the most common etiologies of HF, but cardiomyopathies, valvular heart disease, arrhythmias, congenital heart disease, and other causes are also prevalent [29].

The overall prevalence of HF is estimated at 1–2% of adults in developed countries [29], but this refers only to the diagnosed cases of HF, and the true prevalence being higher. It rises to ≥10% among people older than 70 years, while among those over 65 years of age presenting to primary care with breathlessness on exertion, one in six will have unrecognized HF. Despite multiple effective therapies, HF patients still have a poor long-term prognosis, and therefore HF represents one of the major challenges for health care systems [31, 32].

HF is a complex multifactorial systemic disorder resulting in a systemic inflammation state affecting a whole range of organ systems: renal, cerebral, musculoskeletal, immune, and digestive systems.

Mechanisms of gastrointestinal and hepatic dysfunction in HF are still not entirely understood, but their presence is associated with increased morbidity and mortality [33]. This involvement of the digestive system in HF results in a bidirectional relationship that has been called the cardiointestinal syndrome [34].

The clinical presentation of digestive symptoms in HF varies depending on the onset and duration of HF (acute or chronic), etiology, (also possibly shared etiologies such as alcohol abuse), and medications used with liver and or cardiac side effects.

The splanchnic venous system holds a large number of α-1 and α-2 receptors and is thus responsive to the sympathetic nervous system. Therefore, it has a much higher compliance than the peripheral venous system and is a relatively greater venous reservoir [35]. In HF, the activation of the sympathetic nervous system leads to a decrease in the capacitance of splanchnic veins and a shift of fluid out of the splanchnic veins, thereby increasing the effective circulating volume and the preload without increasing total body volume [36].

The symptoms of abdominal discomfort, nausea, constipation, and diarrhea in advanced HF patients are attributed also to these changes [33].

Chronic Liver Congestion

HF may directly lead to increased central venous pressure due to prolonged right heart failure or indirectly by elevated left ventricular filling pressures and secondary pulmonary hypertension. The elevated central venous pressure is transmitted with minimal attenuation to the hepatic sinusoidal bed as a consequence of a lack of hepatic venous valves, creating hepatic venous sinus congestion and decreasing oxygen diffusion to hepatocytes [37].

This backward failure is seen in right or biventricular congestive heart failure, valvular disease, severe pulmonary hypertension, cor pulmonale, pericardial diseases, and constrictive pericarditis, causing chronic venous outflow obstruction and hepatic venous congestion called "congestive hepatopathy" [37].

The resulting hepatic congestion may result in nausea, bloating, right upper quadrant pain, jaundice (imitating biliary disease or hepatitis), hepatomegaly, abnormal liver enzyme levels, high protein ascites, and prolongation of the prothrombin time [38]. Sometimes congestion is severe enough to produce diarrhea, malabsorption, proteinlosing enteropathy anorexia, and even cardiac cachexia [39, 40].

Low flow states in HF may cause a reduction of intestinal blood flow in those patients, resulting in intestinal motor dysfunction, abdominal discomfort as well as increased juxtamucosal bacterial growth [41]. Chronic hypoxemia and prolonged congestion may further result in hepatic fibrosis, and if left untreated, even progress to cardiac cirrhosis [42].

Acute Liver Injury

In contrast to chronic congestion, acute cardiogenic liver injury (ACLI), known as "ischemic hepatitis" or "shock liver," is described as hepatocytic injury with a sudden onset, that occurs in critically ill patients with multiple underlying comorbid conditions, most frequently cardiovascular disease [43]. The pathogenesis of ischemic hepatitis seems to originate from a "two-hit" mechanism when the liver at risk for hepatic injury, due to right-sided heart failure with resultant passive hepatic venous congestion, is subsequently exposed to systemic hypoperfusion and ischemia [44]. Underlying cardiac disease is typical if not mandatory.

It is characterized by a rapid and profound rise of serum aminotransferases and lactate dehydrogenase levels in 1–3 days after the hemodynamic insult, which tend to normalize within 7–10 days in the absence of any further insult. Alkaline phosphatase and bilirubin levels typically remain minimally affected, while jaundice is rare, except in most severe cases.

There is no specific management option besides correction of the underlying cause of hemodynamic disturbance, which is most often directed at the cardiovascular system, and which typically results in a complete and rapid resolution of liver abnormalities. [43]. The use of diuretics, inotropes, or vasodilators was reported to be associated with favorable outcomes [45].

The mortality rate is high and the prognosis of the patient depends largely on the underlying cause of hypotension. Unfavorable outcomes are mostly associated with comorbidities, while the likelihood of the development of acute liver failure due to ischemic hepatitis is controversial [43].

Cardiac Cachexia in Heart Failure

Cachexia is caused by an imbalance between catabolic and anabolic mechanisms [46]. It is defined as unintentional weight loss, with or without skeletal muscle wasting, of at least 5% of baseline weight during the previous year [47]. Cachexia is a well-known problem in patients with chronic end-stage HF, and while it is estimated that cardiac cachexia (CC) is overtly present in about 10–15% of HF patients [48], up to 50% of patients with HF may be malnourished using broader definitions [49]. Very often, a precise distinction between the terms malnutrition and cachexia is not made, and while they may be phenotypically similar, and often overlap and coexist, they have different origins [50]. The foundation for the definition is the presence or absence of inflammation [51]. Nutrition risk in the absence of an inflammatory condition is classified as starvation-related malnutrition (intake-driven), while the presence of either chronic or acute inflammation results in chronic or acute disease-related malnutrition (disease-driven), which is traditionally designated as cachexia. Since loss of appetite is often coupled with inflammation, starvation malnutrition frequently coexists with cachexia, which hinders to determine the relative contributions of each in a specific patient [50].

The pathophysiology of CC in HF is complex and multifactorial due to a combination of factors. The mechanisms by which HF promotes cachexia include direct consequences of HF itself and mechanisms common to other chronic disease states [50].

First of all, patients with HF have dyspnea, and work of breathing leads to the consumption of a significant amount of energy, contributing to loss of weight and fatigue.

Likewise, HF is characterized by activation of the renin-angiotensin-aldosterone system and the adrenergic nervous system, raising the levels of noradrenaline and cortisol. This leads to increasing insulin resistance promoting a cellular catabolic state and peripheral vasoconstriction [50].

As already mentioned, HF is a systemic response characterized by inflammatory activation. This may initially be beneficial by inducing short term cytoprotective responses, but over time it becomes maladaptive. The central role is here attributed to tumor necrosis factor (TNF)–α, originally called cachexin. Its long-term activation leads to a direct myocardial depressant effect, induces myocardial apoptosis and reduces peripheral blood flow causing exercise intolerance, cellular damage, and inflammation.

Additionally, there is a reduced food intake, which may be caused by several factors: low sodium, tasteless diets prescribed to the patient; depression and chronic fatigue; systemic proinflammatory state; abnormal increase in leptin and adiponectin levels; early satiety due to hepatomegaly with gastric compression. Also several drug side effects can contribute to the decreased intake of nutrients, such as reduction of intestinal motility due to zinc and potassium depletion caused by diuretics; or digitalis induced anorexia and vomiting [52].

Splanchnic congestion, bowel wall hypoperfusion, edema, and collagen accumulation in the intestinal mucosa lead to the thickening of the gastrointestinal wall, and to an increase of the distance between the capillaries and the enterocytes, thus causing intestinal malabsorption [53].

Additionally, there is an increasing concentration of the intestinal bacterial flora and higher adhesion of the biofilm to the sigmoid mucosa. Increased mucosal permeability and impaired intestinal barrier function due to underperfusion lead to bacterial translocation of lipopolysaccharides derived from enteric Gram-negative bacteria resulting in the stimulation of the production of TNF-α, again aggravating the state of systemic inflammation [52, 53].

The resulting metabolic imbalance favors catabolism with eventual wasting of all tissue compartments: skeletal muscle, fat, and, later, bone [54]. Insufficient protein and energy delivery also causes immunologic dysfunction and impairs the maintenance of integrity of protective barriers causing frequent infections. Muscle weakness further exacerbates the poor exercise tolerance from decreased cardiac output. Cardiac cachexia is common among patients with HF and is a strong predictor of poor prognosis and has been associated with a poor quality of life, increased mortality rates, and a high readmission rate.

The management options include a multidisciplinary approach consisting of exercise, active screening of patients with HF for malnutrition, individualized nutritional counseling, and diets to ensure that sufficient calories and essential micronutrients are consumed. However, the best intervention appears to be optimization of HF therapy [50].

Aortic Stenosis

Aortic stenosis (AS) is the most common primary acquired valvular disease in the Western world with rising prevalence as a consequence of the ageing population [55].

The classic triad of symptoms (angina pectoris, HF, and syncope) associated with severe symptomatic aortic stenosis is well known, but AS has been linked to manifestations in other systems, including increased incidence of GI bleeding.

The connection between aortic stenosis and intestinal angiodysplasia has been contentious, as both are common in the elderly, but evidence that aortic stenosis is the cause of the coagulopathy appears much stronger than the supposition of a casual connection [56]. It is referred to as Heyde syndrome—a triad consisting of aortic stenosis, acquired coagulopathy—von Willebrand syndrome type 2A (vWS-2A) and sideropenic aaemia due to bleeding from GI angiodysplasia or from an idiopathic site. The exact prevalence and frequency of aortic stenosis in patients with bleeding GI angiodysplasia remains controversial [57].

The most convincing pathological mechanism is the acquired degradation and deficiency of von Willebrand factor (vWF) causing vWS-2A. It is presumed that it is the high shear stress due to valvular or large vessel stenosis, which elevates the von Willebrand factor–cleaving metalloprotease activity, and leads to the proteolysis of high molecular weight multimers of the von Willebrand factor, leading to degradation or clearance of vWF. The severity of vWF deficit is directly proportional to the severity of the aortic stenosis, the percentage of high molecular weight multimers being negatively correlated to the mean transvalvular pressure gradient [58].

Although AS is the most common cardiovascular etiology for vWS-2A, other possible causes are also reported: hypertrophic cardiomyopathy (with left ventricular outflow tract obstruction), dysfunctional prosthetic valves, ventricular septal defect, persistent ductus arteriosus, and left ventricular support systems [59]. An aortic peak pressure gradient of at least 50 mmHg or more seems to be required for Heyde syndrome to develop in AS [60]. The usually concomitant antithrombotic or anticoagulation therapy prescribed in this patient group may exacerbate the bleeding.

Endoscopic cautery, angiographic embolization, and intestinal resection are possible short-term therapies. However, in almost all reported cases of Heyde syndrome, definite termination of bleeding has been accomplished by aortic valve replacement. Gastrointestinal bleeding ceased in 95% of cases, compared to only 5% in cases controlled by laparotomy with or without bowel resection [61].

An issue at hand is also the choice of the valve prosthesis, and although anticoagulation is preferably avoided in an elderly patient with intestinal bleeding due to Heyde syndrome, bleeding has been reported to cease promptly following valve replacement in these patients, notwithstanding the type of the prosthesis or subsequent use of oral anticoagulation [62, 63]. In conclusion, Heyde syndrome should be considered in all patients with severe aortic stenosis and sideropenic anemia due to gastrointestinal bleeding.

Cardiovascular Disease

Cardiovascular diseases (CVD), including coronary artery disease (CAD), cerebrovascular disease, and peripheral arterial disease are the leading cause of death globally, with an estimated 17.9 million people dying from CVDs in 2019, or 32% of all global deaths. Of these deaths, 85% were due to heart attack and stroke. Individuals at risk of cardiovascular diseases often have elevated blood pressure, are overweight, or obese [64].

Epigastric pain or heart burn as the initial symptom of angina or infarction can mimic GI disease and sometimes be notoriously difficult to distinguish from noncardiac disorders [65]. Organs derived from the embryonic foregut can all produce pain in the midline epigastric region. Epigastric discomfort therefore has a large differential that involves both severe and benign disorders [66].

After the diagnosis of CAD has been established, treatment options include cardiac revascularization (percutaneous or surgical) and medication, which again may affect the digestive system.

The use of smooth muscle relaxants (calcium channel antagonists, nitroglycerin) is widespread, which improves coronary blood flow but also relaxes the lower esophageal sphincter (LES), thereby promoting gastroesophageal reflux disease [40], which may contribute to the increasing incidence of esophageal adenocarcinoma. Assuming a causal relation, about 10% of the esophageal adenocarcinomas occurring in the population may be attributable to intake of lower esophageal sphincter (LES)-relaxing drugs [67].

Statins inhibit HMG-CoA reductase in the liver depleting intracellular cholesterol and in turn inducing the production of LDL receptors. Generally, they are contraindicated in patients with active liver disease. However, there is also a concern that statins might worsen hepatic function in patients with chronic liver disease. The use of statins has often been associated with being asymptomatic and usually the transient elevation of serum aminotransferase levels occurs in the first 12 months of therapy [68]. The rise is greater than three times the upper limit of normal (ULN) in about 1% of patients. But, as it is not correlated with histopathological changes or liver synthetic dysfunction, it therefore does not constitute a liver injury [69]. The available data suggest that the statin treatment of patients with elevated transaminases levels up to three times the ULN appears safe and does not lead to severe liver disease [70].

Clinically significant, statin-induced, severe liver injury is an extremely rare event, reported in $\approx$1 in 100,000 individuals treated with statins [71].

Statins also appear safe in people with nonalcoholic fatty liver disease (NAFLD), with appropriate monitoring. However, despite some encouraging results in several small studies, there is still no definite evidence that statin therapy reduces the progression of liver disease, and statins should not be used for this indication [70]. Data on safety in people with advanced or decompensated liver disease are insufficient, and statin treatment is therefore generally discouraged in this setting.

Platelet activation and aggregation play a significant role in the pathogenesis of arterial thrombosis and are directly correlated with ischemic events. Low dose acetylsalicylic acid (ASA) (<325 mg) is the cornerstone of the secondary prevention of myocardial infarction, and it is also used for primary prevention among patients with an increased risk of cardiovascular events or among patients with diabetes mellitus, although these indications appear more controversial [72].

The association of ASA with GI adverse effects (ranging from peptic ulcer to fatal bleeding or perforation) is well-known and established [73].

Patients who undergo percutaneous coronary intervention (PCI) require dual antiplatelet therapy (DAPT) for at least 3 months (exceptionally 1 month) after elective PCI in stable coronary disease or for at least 6 months after PCI in acute coronary syndrome, in order to prevent stent thrombosis and other cardiovascular events [74].

DAPT consists of ASA and a P2Y12 antagonist (such as clopidogrel, prasugrel, or ticagrelor) that separately inhibit the cyclooxygenase-1 (COX-1) and the adenosine diphosphate-dependent pathways. Together, they confer greater protection against platelet activation and stent thrombosis than either antagonist alone [75]. However, DAPT also doubles the risk of gastrointestinal (GI) bleeding compared with single antiplatelet therapy (SAPT) [76].

Proton pump inhibitors (PPIs) decrease the risk of gastroduodenal ulcers and upper GI bleeding in patients taking aspirin alone or in combination with clopidogrel, and despite some concerns due to shared metabolic pathways involving hepatic P450 of PPIs and clopidogrel, no definitive evidence supporting a clinically important drug-drug interaction was found. Therefore, patients on clopidogrel should be given PPI as an adjunct if they have a history or additional risk factors for upper GI bleeding [77].

Chronic Obstructive Pulmonary Disease

Chronic obstructive pulmonary disease (COPD) is defined by The Global Initiative for Chronic Obstructive Lung Disease as a common, preventable, and treatable disease that is characterized by persistent respiratory symptoms and airflow limitation that is due to airway and/or alveolar abnormalities usually caused by significant exposure to noxious particles or gases [78]. Approximately 10% of individuals aged 40 years or older have COPD, although the prevalence varies between countries and increases with age and it is the third leading cause of death worldwide [79]. Three major subtypes have been distinguished in earlier definitions with partial overlapping: emphysema, chronic bronchitis, and chronic obstructive asthma [80].

The clinical course is often marked by acute exacerbations [81], which increase the risk of morbidity and mortality of COPD [82] and lead to worsening of lung function and declining quality of life [83].

COPD is understood to be a condition that has an impact on other organs, the so-called systemic effects [84, 85]. It is associated with significant concomitant chronic diseases, which increase its morbidity and mortality. COPD can directly lead to or accelerate co-morbidities through hypoxia, dyspnea, polycythemia, pulmonary hypertension, and decreased activity [86].

Regarding the digestive system, COPD is associated with gastroesophageal reflux disease (GERD), peptic ulcer disease, weight loss, and obesity as well as cachexia.

Chronic Obstructive Pulmonary Disease and Gastroesophageal Reflux Disease

The prevalence of GERD in COPD ranges widely from 17 to 78%, due to different diagnostic approaches, but is generally higher than in healthy control patients (18%) [87]. Using the 24-h pH monitoring, 62% of patients with severe COPD (FEV1 range 20–49%) had GERD in contrast to only 19% of controls [88].

GERD is also implicated in COPD exacerbations, and a bidirectional relationship is assumed between GERD and respiratory disorders, especially with asthma.

Asthma induces mechanistic and physiological changes, which can also lead to GERD. Anti-asthmatic medications such as β-2-adrenergic receptor agonists or theophylline are proposed to relax smooth muscles including the lower esophageal sphincter (LES) [89]. Another supposed mechanism is the obstructive pattern of asthma that leads to increased negative intrathoracic pleural pressure and increased diaphragmatic pressure, which favor the regurgitation of gastric content across the LES due to the pressure difference [90].

Conversely, GERD can induce asthma by two proposed mechanisms. Reflux theory stipulates that direct retrograde reflux into the esophagus with subsequent aspiration into the lungs causes chronic inflammation, which can lead to impaired gas exchange and airway obstruction [91]. The theory is the reflex theory, which states that direct acidification to the lower esophagus and subsequent microaspiration in the respiratory tract lead to airway hyperresponsiveness and overactive bronchial smooth muscles [31] via stimulation of acid-sensitive receptors in the distal esophagus of the shared the vagus nerve.

Peptic Ulcer Bleeding

Patients with COPD are also at a higher risk of developing recurrent peptic ulcer bleeding (PUB) [92, 93]. COPD is an independent risk factor for peptic ulcers and nonvariceal ulcer bleeding as has been shown in several studies and observed in subgroup analyses involving stratification by age, sex, the use of ulcerogenic drugs, *H. pylori* status, and comorbidities [92]. As COPD is a systemic inflammation state, the patients are also subjected to chronic hypoxia and oxidative stress producing reactive oxygen species [94] that may damage gastric or small intestinal mucosa [95].

They also have other smoking-related chronic diseases, such as hypertension, coronary artery disease, or heart failure, and use therefore more anti-platelet agents, that increase ulcer bleeding risk [96].

Furthermore, COPD patients often use steroids for controlling lung inflammation. The mechanism by which corticosteroids induce GI bleeding or perforation has not been fully established, but corticosteroids may cause tissue repair, thus leading to delayed wound healing. [97, 98].

Cigarette smokers have a higher risk of developing poorly healing peptic ulcer disease [99].

Therefore, it is reasonable to consider administering gastroprotective medication in patients with COPD [92].

Conclusion

Cardiac and respiratory diseases are the leading cause of death worldwide and have a high prevalence and incidence in the general population.

Although at first glance, it seems that the digestive system on the one hand and cardiac or respiratory systems on the other hand do not have much in common, there is a plethora of evidence of links between those systems, documenting an intricate interplay between them, both in health and disease, and share an elaborate bi- or multidirectional relationship.

References

1. Sbeit W, Kadah A, Mahamid M, Mari A, Khoury T. The interplay between gastrointestinal and cardiovascular diseases: a narrative review focusing on the clinical perspective. Eur J Gastroenterol Hepatol. 2021;32(2):132–9.
2. Long MT, Ko D, Arnold LM, Trinquart L, Sherer JA, Keppel SS, et al. Gastrointestinal and liver diseases and atrial fibrillation: a review of the literature. Ther Adv Gastroenterol. 2019;12:1756284819832237.
3. Hindricks G, Potpara T, Dagres N, Arbelo E, Bax JJ, Blomström-Lundqvist C, et al. 2020 ESC guidelines for the diagnosis and management of atrial fibrillation developed in collaboration with the European Association for Cardio-Thoracic Surgery (EACTS): the task force for the diagnosis and management of atrial fibrillation of the European Society of Cardiology (ESC) developed with the special contribution of the European Heart Rhythm Association (EHRA) of the ESC. Eur Heart J. 2020;42(5):373–498.
4. Lip GY, Nieuwlaat R, Pisters R, Lane DA, Crijns HJ. Refining clinical risk stratification for predicting stroke and thromboembolism in atrial fibrillation using a novel risk factor-based approach: the euro heart survey on atrial fibrillation. Chest. 2010;137(2):263–72.
5. Wilke T, Groth A, Mueller S, Pfannkuche M, Verheyen F, Linder R, et al. Incidence and prevalence of atrial fibrillation: an analysis based on 8.3 million patients. Europace. 2013;15(4):486–93.
6. Lip GY, Fauchier L, Freedman SB, Van Gelder I, Natale A, Gianni C, et al. Atrial fibrillation. Nat Rev Dis Primers. 2016;2:16016.
7. Omran H, Gutleben KJ, Molatta S, Fischbach T, Wellmann B, Horstkotte D, et al. Second generation cryoballoon ablation for persistent atrial fibrillation: an updated meta-analysis. Clin Res Cardiol. 2018;107(2):182–92.
8. Ball J, Carrington MJ, McMurray JJ, Stewart S. Atrial fibrillation: profile and burden of an evolving epidemic in the 21st century. Int J Cardiol. 2013;167(5):1807–24.
9. Tetta C, Moula AI, Matteucci F, Parise O, Maesen B, Johnson D, et al. Association between atrial fibrillation and Helicobacter pylori. Clin Res Cardiol. 2019;108(7):730–40.
10. Gesualdo M, Scicchitano P, Carbonara S, Ricci G, Principi M, Ierardi E, et al. The association between cardiac and gastrointestinal disorders: causal or casual link? J Cardiovasc Med (Hagerstown). 2016;17(5):330–8.
11. Wolf PA, Abbott RD, Kannel WB. Atrial fibrillation as an independent risk factor for stroke: the Framingham study. Stroke. 1991;22(8):983–8.
12. Wang TJ, Larson MG, Levy D, Vasan RS, Leip EP, Wolf PA, et al. Temporal relations of atrial fibrillation and congestive heart failure and their joint influence on mortality: the Framingham heart study. Circulation. 2003;107(23):2920–5.
13. Kalantarian S, Stern TA, Mansour M, Ruskin JN. Cognitive impairment associated with atrial fibrillation: a meta-analysis. Ann Intern Med. 2013;158(5 Pt 1):338–46.
14. Flack KF, Desai J, Kolb JM, Chatterjee P, Wallentin LC, Ezekowitz M, et al. Major gastrointestinal bleeding often is caused by occult malignancy in patients receiving warfarin or dabigatran to prevent stroke and systemic embolism from atrial fibrillation. Clin Gastroenterol Hepatol. 2017;15(5):682–90.
15. Cangemi DJ, Krill T, Weideman R, Cipher DJ, Spechler SJ, Feagins LA. A comparison of the rate of gastrointestinal bleeding in patients taking non-vitamin K antagonist Oral anticoagulants or warfarin. Am J Gastroenterol. 2017;112(5):734–9.

16. Miller CS, Dorreen A, Martel M, Huynh T, Barkun AN. Risk of gastrointestinal bleeding in patients taking non-vitamin K antagonist oral anticoagulants: a systematic review and meta-analysis. Clin Gastroenterol Hepatol. 2017;15(11):1674–83 e3.
17. Abraham NS, Noseworthy PA, Yao X, Sangaralingham LR, Shah ND. Gastrointestinal safety of direct oral anticoagulants: a large population-based study. Gastroenterology. 2017;152(5):1014–22 e1.
18. Maura G, Bardou M, Billionnet C, Weill A, Drouin J, Neumann A. Oral anticoagulants and risk of acute liver injury in patients with nonvalvular atrial fibrillation: a propensity-weighted nationwide cohort study. Sci Rep. 2020;10(1):11624.
19. Rochwerg B, Xenodemetropoulos T, Crowther M, Spyropoulos A. Dabigatran-induced acute hepatitis. Clin Appl Thromb Hemost. 2012;18(5):549–50.
20. Licata A, Puccia F, Lombardo V, Serruto A, Minissale MG, Morreale I, et al. Rivaroxaban-induced hepatotoxicity: review of the literature and report of new cases. Eur J Gastroenterol Hepatol. 2018;30(2):226–32.
21. Cordeanu M, Lambert A, Gaertner S, Nouri S, Mirea C, Alt-Tebacher M, et al. Apixaban-induced hepatotoxicity. Int J Cardiol. 2016;204:4–5.
22. Tripodi A, Mannucci PM. The coagulopathy of chronic liver disease. N Engl J Med. 2011;365(2):147–56.
23. Qamar A, Vaduganathan M, Greenberger NJ, Giugliano RP. Oral anticoagulation in patients with liver disease. J Am Coll Cardiol. 2018;71(19):2162–75.
24. Patel V, Sanyal AJ. Drug-induced steatohepatitis. Clin Liver Dis. 2013;17(4):533–46. vii
25. Chang CC, Petrelli M, Tomashefski JF Jr, McCullough AJ. Severe intrahepatic cholestasis caused by amiodarone toxicity after withdrawal of the drug: a case report and review of the literature. Arch Pathol Lab Med. 1999;123(3):251–6.
26. Halperin JL, Hart RG. Atrial fibrillation and stroke: new ideas, persisting dilemmas. Stroke. 1988;19(8):937–41.
27. Hughes M, Lip GY, Guideline Development Group NCGfMoAFiP, Secondary Care NIfH, Clinical E. Stroke and thromboembolism in atrial fibrillation: a systematic review of stroke risk factors, risk stratification schema and cost effectiveness data. Thromb Haemost. 2008;99(2):295–304.
28. Bekwelem W, Connolly SJ, Halperin JL, Adabag S, Duval S, Chrolavicius S, et al. Extracranial systemic embolic events in patients with Nonvalvular atrial fibrillation: incidence, risk factors, and outcomes. Circulation. 2015;132(9):796–803.
29. McDonagh TA, Metra M, Adamo M, Gardner RS, Baumbach A, Bohm M, et al. Corrigendum to: 2021 ESC guidelines for the diagnosis and treatment of acute and chronic heart failure: developed by the task force for the diagnosis and treatment of acute and chronic heart failure of the European Society of Cardiology (ESC) with the special contribution of the Heart Failure Association (HFA) of the ESC. Eur Heart J. 2021;42(48):4901.
30. Malik A, Brito D, Vaqar S, Chhabra L, Doerr C. Congestive heart failure (nursing). StatPearls; 2021.
31. Platz E, Jhund PS, Claggett BL, Pfeffer MA, Swedberg K, Granger CB, et al. Prevalence and prognostic importance of precipitating factors leading to heart failure hospitalization: recurrent hospitalizations and mortality. Eur J Heart Fail. 2018;20(2):295–303.
32. Lena A, Ebner N, Anker MS. Cardiac cachexia. Eur Heart J Suppl. 2019;21(Supplement_L):L24–L7.
33. Sundaram V, Fang JC. Gastrointestinal and liver issues in heart failure. Circulation. 2016;133(17):1696–703.
34. Sandek A, Rauchhaus M, Anker SD, Von Haehling S. The emerging role of the gut in chronic heart failure. Curr Opin Clin Nutr Metab Care. 2008;11(5):632–9.
35. Gelman S, Warner DS, Warner MA. Venous function and central venous pressure: a physiologic story. J Am Soc Anesthesiol. 2008;108(4):735–48.
36. Anker SD, Von Haehling S. Inflammatory mediators in chronic heart failure: an overview. Heart. 2004;90(4):464–70.

37. Pabolu S, Dudekula A, Pitchumoni CS. Gastrointestinal manifestations of non-GI disorders. In: Pitchumoni CS, Dharmarajan TS, editors. Geriatric gastroenterology. Cham: Springer International Publishing; 2021. p. 2117–66.
38. Kubo SH, Walter BA, John DHA, Clark M, Cody RJ. Liver function abnormalities in chronic heart failure: influence of systemic hemodynamics. Arch Intern Med. 1987;147(7):1227–30.
39. King D, Smith ML, Chapman TJ, Stockdale HR, Lye M. Fat malabsorption in elderly patients with cardiac cachexia. Age Ageing. 1996;25(2):144–9.
40. Israeli E, Bernstein CN. Gastrointentinal manifestations of systemic diseases. Yamada's textbook of gastroenterology; 2015. pp. 2399–439.
41. Sandek A, Swidsinski A, Schroedl W, Watson A, Valentova M, Herrmann R, et al. Intestinal blood flow in patients with chronic heart failure: a link with bacterial growth, gastrointestinal symptoms, and cachexia. J Am Coll Cardiol. 2014;64(11):1092–102.
42. Rodriguez Ziccardi M, Pendela VS, Singhal M. Cardiac cirrhosis. In: StatPearls. Treasure Island, FL: StatPearls Publishing LLC; 2022.
43. Lightsey JM, Rockey DC. Current concepts in ischemic hepatitis. Curr Opin Gastroenterol. 2017;33(3):158–63.
44. Seeto RK, Fenn B, Rockey DC. Ischemic hepatitis: clinical presentation and pathogenesis. Am J Med. 2000;109(2):109–13.
45. Denis C, De Kerguennec C, Bernuau J, Beauvais F, Cohen SA. Acute hypoxic hepatitis ('liver shock'): still a frequently overlooked cardiological diagnosis. Eur J Heart Fail. 2004;6(5):561–5.
46. von Haehling S. Muscle wasting and sarcopenia in heart failure: a brief overview of the current literature. ESC Heart Failure. 2018;5(6):1074.
47. Evans WJ, Morley JE, Argilés J, Bales C, Baracos V, Guttridge D, et al. Cachexia: a new definition. Clin Nutr. 2008;27(6):793–9.
48. von Haehling S, Anker MS, Anker SD. Prevalence and clinical impact of cachexia in chronic illness in Europe, USA, and Japan: facts and numbers update 2016. Wiley Online Library; 2016. p. 507–9.
49. Grossniklaus DA, O'Brien MC, Clark PC, Dunbar SB. Nutrient intake in heart failure patients. J Cardiovasc Nurs. 2008;23(4):357–63.
50. Rahman A, Jafry S, Jeejeebhoy K, Nagpal AD, Pisani B, Agarwala R. Malnutrition and cachexia in heart failure. JPEN J Parenter Enteral Nutr. 2016;40(4):475–86.
51. White JV, Guenter P, Jensen G, Malone A, Schofield M, Academy of N, et al. Consensus statement of the Academy of Nutrition and Dietetics/American Society for Parenteral and Enteral Nutrition: characteristics recommended for the identification and documentation of adult malnutrition (undernutrition). J Acad Nutr Diet. 2012;112(5):730–8.
52. André TR, Santos AL, Neto IG. Cardiac cachexia syndrome. Cardiology. 2017.
53. Valentova M, von Haehling S, Bauditz J, Doehner W, Ebner N, Bekfani T, et al. Intestinal congestion and right ventricular dysfunction: a link with appetite loss, inflammation, and cachexia in chronic heart failure. Eur Heart J. 2016;37(21):1684–91.
54. Loncar G, Fulster S, von Haehling S, Popovic V. Metabolism and the heart: an overview of muscle, fat, and bone metabolism in heart failure. Int J Cardiol. 2013;162(2):77–85.
55. Vahanian A, Beyersdorf F, Praz F, Milojevic M, Baldus S, Bauersachs J, et al. 2021 ESC/EACTS guidelines for the management of valvular heart disease: developed by the task force for the management of valvular heart disease of the European Society of Cardiology (ESC) and the European Association for Cardio-Thoracic Surgery (EACTS). Eur Heart J. 2021;43(7):561–632.
56. Massyn MW, Khan SA. Heyde syndrome: a common diagnosis in older patients with severe aortic stenosis. Age Ageing. 2009;38(3):267–70.
57. Warkentin TE, Moore JC, Anand SS, Lonn EM, Morgan DG. Gastrointestinal bleeding, angiodysplasia, cardiovascular disease, and acquired von Willebrand syndrome. Transfus Med Rev. 2003;17(4):272–86.
58. Vincentelli A, Susen S, Le Tourneau T, Six I, Fabre O, Juthier F, et al. Acquired von Willebrand syndrome in aortic stenosis. N Engl J Med. 2003;349(4):343–9.

59. Hudzik B, Wilczek K, Gasior M. Heyde syndrome: gastrointestinal bleeding and aortic stenosis. CMAJ. 2016;188(2):135–8.
60. Tsuji A, Tanabe M, Onishi K, Kitamura T, Okinaka T, Ito M, et al. Intravascular hemolysis in aortic stenosis. Intern Med. 2004;43(10):935–8.
61. Scheffer SM, Leatherman LL. Resolution of Heyde's syndrome of aortic stenosis and gastrointestinal bleeding after aortic valve replacement. Ann Thorac Surg. 1986;42(4):477–80.
62. Mishra PK, Kovac J, de Caestecker J, Fancourt G, Logtens E, Spyt T. Intestinal angiodysplasia and aortic valve stenosis: let's not close the book on this association. Eur J Cardiothorac Surg. 2009;35(4):628–34.
63. Abi-Akar R, El-Rassi I, Karam N, Jassar Y, Slim R, Jebara V. Treatment of Heyde's syndrome by aortic valve replacement. Curr Cardiol Rev. 2011;7(1):47–9.
64. World Health Organization. Cardiovascular diseases (CVDs). 2021. https://www.who.int/news-room/fact-sheets/detail/cardiovascular-diseases-(cvds).
65. Robinson P, Perkins JC Jr. Approach to patients with epigastric pain. Emerg Med Clin North Am. 2016;34(2):191–210.
66. Williams JF, Sontag SJ, Schnell T, Leya J. Non-cardiac chest pain: the long-term natural history and comparison with gastroesophageal reflux disease. Am J Gastroenterol. 2009;104(9):2145–52.
67. Lagergren J, Bergström R, Adami HO, Nyrén O. Association between medications that relax the lower esophageal sphincter and risk for esophageal adenocarcinoma. Ann Intern Med. 2000;133(3):165–75.
68. Jose J. Statins and its hepatic effects: newer data, implications, and changing recommendations. J Pharm Bioallied Sci. 2016;8(1):23–8.
69. Calderon RM, Cubeddu LX, Goldberg RB, Schiff ER. Statins in the treatment of dyslipidemia in the presence of elevated liver aminotransferase levels: a therapeutic dilemma. Mayo Clin Proc. 2010;85(4):349–56.
70. Newman CB, Preiss D, Tobert JA, Jacobson TA, Page RL 2nd, Goldstein LB, et al. Statin safety and associated adverse events: a scientific statement from the American Heart Association. Arterioscler Thromb Vasc Biol. 2019;39(2):e38–81.
71. Bjornsson E, Jacobsen EI, Kalaitzakis E. Hepatotoxicity associated with statins: reports of idiosyncratic liver injury post-marketing. J Hepatol. 2012;56(2):374–80.
72. Zheng SL, Roddick AJ. Association of Aspirin use for primary prevention with cardiovascular events and bleeding events: a systematic review and meta-analysis. JAMA. 2019;321(3):277–87.
73. Farrell B, Godwin J, Richards S, Warlow C. The United Kingdom transient ischaemic attack (UK-TIA) aspirin trial: final results. J Neurol Neurosurg Psychiatry. 1991;54(12):1044–54.
74. Neumann F-J, Sousa-Uva M, Ahlsson A, Alfonso F, Banning AP, Benedetto U, et al. 2018 ESC/EACTS Guidelines on myocardial revascularization. Eur Heart J. 2018;40(2):87–165.
75. Bittl JA, Laine L. Gastrointestinal injury caused by aspirin or clopidogrel monotherapy versus dual antiplatelet therapy. J Am Coll Cardiol. 2022;79(2):129–31.
76. Investigators. Effects of clopidogrel added to aspirin in patients with recent lacunar stroke. N Engl J Med. 2012;367(9):817–25.
77. Levine GN, Bates ER, Blankenship JC, Bailey SR, Bittl JA, Cercek B, et al. 2011 ACCF/AHA/SCAI guideline for percutaneous coronary intervention: executive summary: a report of the American College of Cardiology Foundation/American Heart Association task force on practice guidelines and the Society for Cardiovascular Angiography and Interventions. Circulation. 2011;124(23):2574–609.
78. Singh D, Agusti A, Anzueto A, Barnes PJ, Bourbeau J, Celli BR, et al. Global strategy for the diagnosis, management, and prevention of chronic obstructive lung disease: the GOLD science committee report 2019. Eur Respir J. 2019;53(5):1900164.
79. Organization WH. The top 10 causes of death. 2021.
80. Han M, Dransfield MT, Martinez FJ. Chronic obstructive pulmonary disease: definition, clinical manifestations, diagnosis, and staging. Uptodate. 2018:14.

81. Seemungal TA, Donaldson GC, Paul EA, Bestall JC, Jeffries DJ, Wedzicha JA. Effect of exacerbation on quality of life in patients with chronic obstructive pulmonary disease. Am J Respir Crit Care Med. 1998;157(5):1418–22.
82. Vos T, Flaxman AD, Naghavi M, Lozano R, Michaud C, Ezzati M, et al. Years lived with disability (YLDs) for 1160 sequelae of 289 diseases and injuries 1990–2010: a systematic analysis for the global burden of disease study 2010. Lancet. 2012;380(9859):2163–96.
83. Seemungal TA, Donaldson GC, Bhowmik A, Jeffries DJ, Wedzicha JA. Time course and recovery of exacerbations in patients with chronic obstructive pulmonary disease. Am J Respir Crit Care Med. 2000;161(5):1608–13.
84. MacNee W. Systemic inflammatory biomarkers and co-morbidities of chronic obstructive pulmonary disease. Ann Med. 2013;45(3):291–300.
85. Choudhury G, Rabinovich R, MacNee W. Comorbidities and systemic effects of chronic obstructive pulmonary disease. Clin Chest Med. 2014;35(1):101–30.
86. Charbek E, Espiritu JR, Nayak R, Morley JE. Editorial: frailty, comorbidity, and COPD. J Nutr Health Aging. 2018;22(8):876–9.
87. Lee AL, Goldstein RS. Gastroesophageal reflux disease in COPD: links and risks. Int J Chron Obstruct Pulmon Dis. 2015;10:1935–49.
88. Casanova C, Baudet J, del Valle Velasco M, Martin J, Aguirre-Jaime A, de Torres JP, et al. Increased gastro-oesophageal reflux disease in patients with severe COPD. Eur Respir J. 2004;23(6):841–5.
89. Naik RD, Vaezi MF. Extra-esophageal gastroesophageal reflux disease and asthma: understanding this interplay. Expert Rev Gastroenterol Hepatol. 2015;9(7):969–82.
90. Bor S, Kitapcioglu G, Solak ZA, Ertilav M, Erdinc M. Prevalence of gastroesophageal reflux disease in patients with asthma and chronic obstructive pulmonary disease. J Gastroenterol Hepatol. 2010;25(2):309–13.
91. Jack CI, Calverley PM, Donnelly RJ, Tran J, Russell G, Hind CR, et al. Simultaneous tracheal and oesophageal pH measurements in asthmatic patients with gastro-oesophageal reflux. Thorax. 1995;50(2):201–4.
92. Huang KW, Kuan YC, Chi NF, Huang YH, Luo JC, Chien LN. Chronic obstructive pulmonary disease is associated with increased recurrent peptic ulcer bleeding risk. Eur J Intern Med. 2017;37:75–82.
93. Huang KW, Luo JC, Leu HB, Lin HC, Lee FY, Chan WL, et al. Chronic obstructive pulmonary disease: an independent risk factor for peptic ulcer bleeding: a nationwide population-based study. Aliment Pharmacol Ther. 2012;35(7):796–802.
94. Islam M, Sultana M, Hoque M. Prevalence of peptic ulcer disease in patients with chronic obstructive pulmonary disease in a teaching hospital. TAJ: J Teachers Assoc. 2018;30:36.
95. Magnussen H, Watz H. Systemic inflammation in chronic obstructive pulmonary disease and asthma: relation with comorbidities. Proc Am Thorac Soc. 2009;6(8):648–51.
96. Moermans C, Heinen V, Nguyen M, Henket M, Sele J, Manise M, et al. Local and systemic cellular inflammation and cytokine release in chronic obstructive pulmonary disease. Cytokine. 2011;56(2):298–304.
97. Garrow D, Delegge MH. Risk factors for gastrointestinal ulcer disease in the US population. Dig Dis Sci. 2010;55(1):66–72.
98. Narum S, Westergren T, Klemp M. Corticosteroids and risk of gastrointestinal bleeding: a systematic review and meta-analysis. BMJ Open. 2014;4(5):e004587.
99. Maity P, Biswas K, Roy S, Banerjee RK, Bandyopadhyay U. Smoking and the pathogenesis of gastroduodenal ulcer—recent mechanistic update. Mol Cell Biochem. 2003;253(1–2):329–38.

21 Renal Insufficiency

Ivica Horvatić and Ivan Durlen

Abbreviations

ADAMTS13	A disintegrin and metalloproteinase with a thrombospondin type 1 motif, member 13
AKI	Acute kidney injury
ANA	Antinuclear antibodies
ANCA	Antineutrophil cytoplasmic autoantibodies
ATI	Acute tubular injury
CKD	Chronic kidney disease
COX-2	Cyclooxygenase 2
CYP	Cytochrome P
EGPA	Eosinophilic granulomatosis with polyangiitis
EXTRIP	Extracorporeal Treatments in Poisoning
FSGS	Focal segmental glomerulosclerosis
GFR	Glomerular filtration rate
eGFR	Estimated glomerular filtration rate
GPA	Granulomatosis with polyangiitis
HIV	Human immunodeficiency virus
HUS	Hemolytic-uremic syndrome
IBD	Inflammatory bowel disease
KDIGO	Kidney Disease Improving Global Outcomes

I. Horvatić (✉)
School of Medicine, University of Zagreb, Zagreb, Croatia

Faculty of Pharmacy and Biochemistry, University of Zagreb, Zagreb, Croatia

Department of Nephrology and Dialysis, Dubrava University Hospital, Zagreb, Croatia

I. Durlen
Department of Nephrology and Dialysis, Dubrava University Hospital, Zagreb, Croatia

M. Banić, D. Erceg (eds.), *Drug Interactions in Gastroenterology*, Clinical Gastroenterology, https://doi.org/10.1007/978-3-031-69800-2_21

MCD	Minimal change disease
MPA	Microscopic polyangiitis
NSAIDs	Non-steroidal anti-inflammatory drugs
PPIs	Proton pump inhibitors
RLV	Renal limited vasculitis
RRT	Renal replacement therapy
SCr	Serum creatinine
TMA	Thrombotic microangiopathy
TTP	Thrombotic thrombocytopenic purpura

Introduction

Renal insufficiency and renal disorders are often connected to gastrointestinal (GI) disease in the same patient. There is increased awareness that primarily GI disorders and their therapy are affecting the kidney and possibly causing kidney disease through hemodynamic, toxic, metabolic, immunologic, and infective mechanisms. On the other hand, primarily renal disorders and their therapy also can cause GI disease. Renal disorders are considerably affecting the pharmacokinetics and pharmacodynamics of the majority of drugs that are used in gastroenterology [1, 2]. Recently one other connection between kidney and GI systems, namely through gut microbiota, and the so-called gut-kidney axis has been found. Changes in gut microbiota have considerable effects on kidney function, and renal insufficiency causes gut dysbiosis [3].

Renal insufficiency is a syndrome, which is characterized by the reduction or loss of the majority of kidney functions. First and foremost, this refers to the reduction in the glomerular filtration rate (GFR). This is then categorized as acute kidney injury (AKI) or as chronic kidney disease (CKD), which are new terms that replaced older terms and syndromes of acute and chronic renal insufficiency.

Also, reduction or loss of other kidney functions are considered renal insufficiency. Glomerular diseases are presented with hematuria and/or proteinuria, tubulointerstitial diseases manifest as electrolyte and acid/base disorders, as well as decreased urine concentrating ability and nephrocalcinosis or nephrolithiasis.

Acute Kidney Injury (AKI)

AKI is a syndrome characterized by a rapid loss of kidney excretory function (decreased GFR) and diagnosed by the rapid accumulation of nitrogenous waste products (urea, creatinine) and/or decreased urine output. The definition was introduced in 2012 by The Kidney Disease Improving Global Outcomes (KDIGO) as a replacement for various different definitions used before and today is broadly accepted [4, 5]. According to this, AKI is defined as an increase in serum creatinine (SCr) levels by $\geq$26.5 μmol/L within 48 h or increase in SCr levels to $\geq$1.5 times baseline, which is known or presumed to have occurred within the prior 7 days or urine volume $<$ 0.5 mL/kg/h for 6 h.

The incidence of AKI varies from 295 cases per million people per year (dialysis requiring AKI) to 5000 cases per million people per year (nondialysis-requiring AKI) [6]. The prevalence is reported from 1 to 9% in hospitalized patients [4] and rises to more than 60% in intensive care unit admissions [7].

Traditionally, causes of AKI are divided into three categories: prerenal, intrinsic renal, and postrenal (Table 21.1).

Prerenal AKI is a consequence of hemodynamic changes in renal circulation resulting in renal hypoperfusion that do not cause significant injury to renal intrinsic cells (the most susceptible to ischemic changes are tubular epithelial cells). Hypovolemia (due to GI, renal, skin, respiratory, or other fluid loss) is the most common cause. Also, hypotension due to other causes (sepsis, heart failure, low intravascular volume in liver failure, or nephrotic syndrome) and drugs that alter renal hemodynamics, causing imbalance between vasoconstriction and vasodilation, can lead to this type of AKI.

Table 21.1 Causes of acute kidney injury (AKI)

Prerenal	True volume depletion		GI fluid loss—bleeding, vomiting, diarrhea Renal fluid loss—diuretics, osmotic diuresis Bleeding, burns, sweating, crush injuries
	Hypotension		Cardiogenic shock, septic shock
	Edematous states		Heart failure—cardiorenal syndrome Hepatic failure—hepatorenal syndrome Nephrotic syndrome
	Selective renal ischemia		Renal thromboembolism Renal artery stenosis
	Drugs affecting glomerular hemodynamics		NSAIDs, Angiotensin-converting enzyme (ACE) inhibitors, angiotensin II antagonists, calcineurin inhibitors
Intrinsic renal	Acute tubular injury	Renal ischemia	As prerenal just prolonged
		Sepsis	Microbes
		Nephrotoxins	Vancomycin, aminoglycosides, hemoglobin, myoglobin, cisplatin, radiocontrast agents, pentamidine, foscarnet, cidofovir, tenofovir, mannitol, hydroxyethyl starch, synthetic cannabinoids, snake poison, mushrooms, ethylene glycol, oxalates
	Glomerulonephritis		IgA nephropathy, lupus nephritis, infection-related glomerulonephritis, C3 glomerulopathy
	Tubulointerstitial nephritis		Acute allergic tubulointerstitial nephritis
	Small-vessel vasculitis		ANCA vasculitis
	Thrombotic microangiopathy		Hemolytic-uremic syndrome, thrombotic thrombocytopenic purpura, disseminated intravascular coagulation, malignant hypertension
Postrenal	Obstruction within the urinary tract		Lithiasis, stenoses, tumors
	Obstruction outside the urinary tract		Retroperitoneal fibrosis, tumors, gynccologic disease/ prostate hypertrophy

Intrinsic renal injury as a cause of AKI is most commonly due to acute tubular injury (ATI). It is characterized by structural damage to renal tubular epithelial cells ranging from mild damage (loss of epithelial brush-border) to severe (acute tubular necrosis). The causes of ATI can be ischemic or toxic. Ischemic ATI is a result of prolonged hemodynamic changes and ischemia (factors that cause prerenal AKI but last longer and are more severe), but also systemic inflammation and sepsis cause this type of AKI. Toxic ATI is a result of various drugs (antibiotics, chemotherapeutics), heme pigments, toxins (alcohols, snake or mushroom toxins, radiocontrast agents), as well as bacterial toxins and cytokines in sepsis.

Other causes of intrinsic renal AKI are glomerular diseases (acute or rapid-progressive glomerulonephritis), tubulointerstitial diseases (acute allergic tubulointerstitial nephritis), and vascular disorders (small- and middle-size vessel vasculitis, thrombotic microangiopathy). Postrenal causes of AKI include diseases that cause obstruction within or outside the urinary tract (Table 21.1).

Chronic Kidney Disease (CKD)

CKD is a syndrome, formerly known as chronic renal insufficiency, and currently defined by KDIGO guidelines, as decreased excretory kidney function (GFR < 60 mL/min/1.73 m^2) or findings of markers of kidney damage (proteinuria or hematuria or known parenchymal kidney disease) or both of at least 3 months duration [8]. The most common causes are diabetes mellitus and hypertension in high- and middle-income countries, followed by glomerular diseases [9]. Prevalence varies by ethnicity and socioeconomic factors, methods used to determine GFR and markers of kidney damage, ranging from less than 5% to more than 20%, and in high-income countries, like USA and Australia, being around 11% [9]. GFR is usually determined by estimation (estimated GFR, eGFR), using several equations, most commonly Chronic Kidney Disease Epidemiology Collaboration (CKD-EPI) and Modification of Diet in Renal Disease study (MDRD) equation [10, 11].

Glomerular, Tubulointerstitial, and Vascular Renal Disease

Glomerular and microvascular renal disorders present themselves with proteinuria and/or hematuria with or without reduced GFR. Several clinical syndromes are found: asymptomatic proteinuria and/or hematuria (proteinuria <3.5 g/24 h/1.73m^2 and/or hematuria, with normal GFR and without hypertension), nephrotic syndrome (proteinuria >3.5 g/24 h/1.73m^2, hypoalbuminemia, hyperlipidemia, pro-coagulative state) and nephritic syndrome (hematuria and reduced GFR and azotemia). Nephritic syndrome can further be divided, depending on the duration of azotemia, into acute (azotemia develops within a few days), rapidly progressive (azotemia progresses within few weeks), and chronic (duration of azotemia at least 3 months, without progression). Renal biopsy is needed for the diagnosis. Glomerular diseases are caused by immunological disorders (deposition of circulating immune complexes in glomeruli or in situ formation of immune complexes, circulating permeability factors, disorders of complement regulation), deposition of nonimmunogenic molecules or mechanical factors like hyperfiltration. The most common primary glomerular diseases are IgA nephropathy, focal segmental glomerulosclerosis (FSGS), membranous nephropathy, and C3 glomerulonephritis. The most common secondary glomerular disorders are secondary FSGS (due to hyperfiltration or following other glomerular diseases), diabetic nephropathy, infection-related glomerulonephritis, and lupus nephritis [12, 13].

Microvascular renal disorders include small-vessel vasculitis and thrombotic microangiopathy (TMA). Small-vessel vasculitis is mostly caused by antineutrophil cytoplasmic autoantibodies (ANCA). ANCA-associated vasculitis is characterized by the inflammation of predominantly small-sized vessels and the presence of circulating ANCA. It is classified into four clinical subtypes: granulomatosis with polyangiitis (GPA), microscopic polyangiitis (MPA), eosinophilic GPA (EGPA), and renal limited vasculitis (RLV) [14]. The GPA, MPA, and EGPA are systemic diseases that can affect every organ system, but most commonly affect the respiratory tract and kidneys. The GI system could also be affected; most often, it is the intestinal tract that is affected. Also, autoimmune hepatobiliary diseases are in some cases associated with ANCA. ANCA-associated vasculitis presents most often with rapidly progressive nephritic syndrome. Other causes of small-vessel vasculitis include immune complex diseases like cryoglobulinemic vasculitis (associated with hepatitis C) and IgA vasculitis (Henoch-Schoenlein purpura). TMA is characterized by thrombocytopenia, microangiopathic hemolytic anemia (the presence of schistocytes, elevated serum bilirubin levels, LDH, lowered haptoglobin levels), and organ injury. Clinical presentation can vary depending on organs affected, but two best described syndromes are hemolytic-uremic syndrome (HUS), characterized by acute kidney injury, and thrombotic thrombocytopenic purpura (TTP), characterized predominantly with neurologic symptoms and AKI. TMA is classified into infection-associated TMA (*shiga*-toxin producing *E.coli*, *Streptococcus pneumoniae*, HIV), primary hereditary TMA (ADAMTS13 deficiency-causing mutations, complement alternative pathway factors, or regulators mutations), primary acquired TMA (autoantibodies to ADAMTS13 or complement alternative pathway factors or regulators) and secondary TMA (malignant hypertension, pregnancy-associated TMA, malignancy-associated TMA, TMA with glomerular diseases, TMA after bone marrow transplantation, drug-induced TMA) [15].

The most common glomerular and microvascular renal disorders with their typical clinical presentations are listed in Table 21.2.

Tubulointerstitial disease is characterized by varying degrees of reduced GFR, subnephrotic range proteinuria, and electrolyte disorders (sodium, potassium, calcium, magnesium), acid-base disorders, and reduced urine concentrating ability. Acute tubulointerstitial allergic nephritis is caused by various commonly used drugs [16] and is characterized by AKI with some systemic allergic manifestations (rash, eosinophilia). Chronic tubulointerstitial disorders include chronic tubulointerstitial nephritis in systemic autoimmune disease (sarcoidosis, Sjogren syndrome), analgesic nephropathy, or uricemic nephropathy [16]. Chronic tubulointerstitial disorders

Table 21.2 The most common glomerular and microvascular renal disorders with their typical clinical presentation

Clinical presentation	Disorder
Asymptomatic proteinuria and/or hematuria	IgA nephropathy, hereditary nephritis, hypertensive nephropathy, diabetic nephropathy, secondary focal segmental glomerulosclerosis, lupus nephritis
Nephrotic syndrome	Membranous nephropathy, primary focal segmental glomerulosclerosis, minimal change disease, amyloidosis, diabetic nephropathy
Acute nephritic syndrome	Poststreptococcal or other infection-related glomerulonephritis, C3 glomerulopathy, cryoglobulinemic glomerulonephritis/vasculitis
Rapidly progressive nephritic syndrome	ANCA-associated vasculitis, IgA vasculitis, lupus nephritis
Chronic nephritic syndrome	IgA nephropathy, hereditary nephritis, C3 glomerulopathy
Acute kidney injury	Thrombotic microangiopathy

can be accompanied with nephrocalcinosis and nephrolithiasis due to a defect in calcium transport in renal tubules.

Basic Principles of Pharmacokinetics and Pharmacodynamics in Renal Disorders

Pharmacokinetics and pharmacodynamics of many drugs are altered in kidney disease, depending on the disease and the drug. Pharmacokinetics reflects processes of absorption, distribution, metabolism, and excretion, all of which could be altered in patients with kidney disease. The changes in those processes dictate adjustments in the dosing regimen of drugs to achieve an optimal therapeutic effect. Guidelines for adjustments of the dosing regimen in varying stages of kidney disease (AKI or CKD) are provided by the manufacturer and should always be considered before administering the drug. The basic pharmacokinetic parameters that are altered in patients with kidney disease are clearance and distribution volume [1, 2]. The distribution volume is usually increased in the setting of AKI (except prerenal causes), CKD, and glomerular disease with nephrotic syndrome. This requires an increase in the dose of medications to achieve maximal concentration. On the other hand, renal clearance is the result of GFR, active secretion, and passive reabsorption in renal tubules. In various kidney diseases usually all those processes are altered. Decreased GFR does not necessarily mean that the dose of the drug should be reduced, because the tubular secretion may be preserved [1, 2, 17–20]. When considering tubular reabsorption and secretion, one should also take into account the impact of coprescribed drugs due to potential inhibition or stimulation of renal tubular transporters. Also, kidney disease often decreases the non-renal clearance of drugs. Some possible mechanisms for that include the inhibition of enzymes and transporters by circulating uremic toxins, changes in protein expression, and binding and alteration of drug blood transport [21–27].

The minimal change in kidney function that necessitates change in dosage is not well-defined, but there is a principle that dose adjustment is not required if the pharmacokinetic parameter changes by less than 30% [1, 28], but some authors think that decrease in kidney function is likely to be clinically significant, if drug clearance decreases by more than 50% [1, 28]. The extent to which drugs or their metabolites are excreted by the kidney is an important determinant in dose adjustment. In general, dose adjustment is unlikely to be required when less than 30% of the drug is excreted by the kidneys [29, 30]. Dose adjustment may be required for selected drugs with pharmacokinetics that change significantly in kidney disease, and also if there is a high risk of drug accumulation and severe and/or irreversible toxicity (narrow therapeutic range) [1].

Criteria for potential clinically significant decrease in kidney function due to either AKI or CKD were proposed by the Extracorporeal Treatments in Poisoning (EXTRIP) group [28, 31]:

- eGFR <45 mL/min/1.73 m^2
- Stage 2 or 3 AKI
- In adults without a baseline plasma creatinine, plasma creatinine >176 μmol/L in adults, or >132 μmol/L in the elderly or those with low muscle mass
- Plasma creatinine levels greater than two times the upper limit of normal for age and weight in children without a baseline plasma creatinine concentration
- The presence of oligo/anuria

Pharmacodynamics reflects on the processes of drug action, and it is rarely considered when calculating the optimal dose in patients with kidney disease [2]. Pharmacodynamics is primarily determined by pharmacokinetics, but other factors that also determine pharmacodynamics of drugs include: [1] factors that act primarily by affecting drug concentration (drug dose, receptor number, organ response, counter-regulating or competing factors at the receptor); [2] pathological processes (aging, AKI or CKD, decreased number and sensitivity of the receptors, decreased receptor binding, and signal transduction); [3] competition of other drugs for similar receptors (synergistic or antagonistic effects, drugs toxicity) [2]. In pharmacodynamics, the reversible effects (receptor-mediated and saturable) and irreversible effects (direct and proportional to rising concentrations; target an on-off mechanism or an active cell, bacteria, cancer cell, or immune cell) can be distinguished.

When designing a dosing regimen, it is important to consider the therapeutic target, the initial dose, the maintenance dose, the dosing frequency, and the timing of dosage adjustment. Although these data in patients with renal impairment should be obtained from published pharmacokinetic and pharmacodynamic data, they are often difficult to ascertain because during drug development, only a small number of patients with CKD, and especially with AKI, are included.

In CKD, drug absorption is highly variable. It may decrease due to gut wall edema, but some studies found an increase in absorption because of gut wall impairment [28, 32]. Also, the decreased activity of hepatic transporters and cytochrome-P 450 (CYP) enzymes during the first-pass of drugs may increase bioavailability. The volume of distribution is often not significantly increased, because there are increasing factors on one side (fluid retention and hypoalbuminemia) and decreasing factors on the other side (sarcopenia, especially in advanced CKD). Renal drug clearance is proportionally decreased to GFR, but this depends also on the renal compartment where the damage is located. When tubules are relatively intact, tubular elimination of drugs can increase renal drug clearance, compared to glomerular disease accompanied with significant tubulointerstitial damage. Extrarenal drug clearance is thought to be decreased in CKD due to decreased activity of CYP enzymes, but this is often poorly quantified. Some guidelines may apply to dosing regimens in patients with CKD: a loading dose may be required in some patients, for example, for hydrophilic drugs that require a rapid onset of action like antibiotics; in most patients, when kidney excretion is decreased by more than 50%, a proportional decrease in the amount or frequency of the maintenance dose is required; this is especially the case for drugs predominantly secreted in proximal tubules in patients with tubulointerstitial disease regardless of the GFR [28].

In AKI, the situation regarding the dosing regimen is much more complicated, because of numerous changes in physiology, organ function, and volume status that occur very quickly within a few hours and affect the pharmacokinetics and pharmacodynamics of drugs. Also, AKI is defined with SCr concentration or urine output, and not with changes in GFR. Changes in SCr often lag behind those of GFR [33] and therapy-like intravenous fluids decrease SCr concentration understating the severity of AKI. The absorption of drugs in AKI is not well-quantified, but may decrease [28]. The volume of distribution of drugs remains not significantly changed or may increase [28]. Renal clearance is decreased and is rapidly changing. The data on extrarenal drug clearance in AKI are mostly lacking. Changes in bowel, hepatic, and kidney perfusion may alter drug absorption and distribution also. Recommendations for initial, loading, and maintenance dose in AKI are often difficult to make. Here, more often than in CKD, therapeutic drug monitoring is used to assist dosage adjustments. Drug concentrations are measured in the patient and if concentration is outside the desired therapeutic range, the dosing regimen is adjusted accordingly. This should especially be applied to anti-infective drugs or drugs with a narrow therapeutic range.

Principles of Drug Dosing with Renal Replacement Therapy (RRT)

RRT replaces the non-endocrine, blood-filtering function of the kidneys. Techniques include dialysis (hemodialysis (diffusion), peritoneal dialysis), hemofiltration (convection), and hemodiafiltration (diffusion and convection) and could be done intermittently (3–4 h every other day) or continuously. Drug clearance by RRT depends on the modality of RRT and is also additive to endogenous clearance, so all should be accounted for in determining the appropriate dosing regimen. Unfortunately, the data concerning the RRT effect on drug clearance is often highly variable or not available—differences in dialysis regimen in trials and in local practice (blood and dialysate flow, filter type, and size) [28]. Most important parameters that increase drug elimination during conventional hemodialysis are low molecular weight (under 500 daltons), small distribution volume, and less than 90% protein binding. Increasing blood flow and dialysate rate increases elimination. Using high-flux dialysis (larger pores) results in better elimination of molecules with higher molecular weight. Regarding the timing of the dose, with intermittent hemodialysis, we should administer the drugs after the treatment. One possible exception is prescribing of aminoglycosides to patients with ESRD (end-stage renal disease) on intermittent hemodialysis, where a large dose can be administered immediately before dialysis to optimize the concentration profile [28]. Continuous methods are applied for a longer period of time and have a lower hourly clearance than intermittent dialysis; however, because of the prolonged duration, the method removes a significant amount of the drug. The data about drug clearance in continuous RRT is scarce, and it is mostly limited to antibiotics. Therapeutic drug monitoring confirms that desired drug concentrations are achieved and should be used routinely in RRT patients, especially on anti-infectives [28]. The additional effect on the drug clearance of peritoneal dialysis is probably low [28]. Some common medications used in gastroenterology and their doses in RRT patients are listed in Table 21.3.

Renal Disorders Following Primary GI Disease

Renal disorders can be a direct or indirect consequence of primary GI disease as well as caused by various drugs used in the treatment of gastrointestinal disease. Several mechanisms can be involved in the pathogenesis of such renal disorders: hemodynamic, toxic, infective, immunological, or metabolic. Renal disorders include all disorders mentioned before: acute kidney injury, chronic kidney disease, glomerular, tubulointerstitial, and vascular disorders, as well as nephrolithiasis. Renal biopsy is needed in the majority of cases for the diagnosis of those disorders. In Table 21.4, the most common renal disorders following GI diseases are listed [34–38].

Drug-Induced Renal Disorders

There is a frequent association between drugs and different types of kidney disorders, acute as well as chronic. Drugs can cause glomerular, tubular, and vascular kidney disorders, consequently leading to AKI and/or CKD. The incidence is difficult to determine, but it can be as high as 18% [16]. Most episodes of drug-induced renal disorders are reversible, especially when discovered early, but can sometimes lead to CKD.

Glomerular Disorders Induced by Drugs

They can be classified into two pathogenic types: as a result of direct injury to glomerular cells and as a result of immune-mediated injury. Direct glomerular cell injury can involve podocytes resulting in Minimal Change Disease (MCD) or Focal

Table 21.3 Common medications used in gastroenterology and their doses in RRT patients

Drug	Hemodialysis	CAPD	CRRT
Amoxicillin	q24h, dose post HD	250 mg q8h	As normal GFR
Azathioprine	As normal	50%	75%
Cefazolin	0.5–1.0 g post HD	0.5 g q12h	q12h
Cefepime	1.0 g post HD	q24–48h	Not recommended
Ceftriaxone	As normal GFR, post HD	As normal GFR	As normal GFR
Cholestyramine	As normal GFR	As normal GFR	As normal GFR
Cimetidine	25%	25%	50%
Ciprofloxacin	250 mg q12h	250 mg q8h	200 mg iv q12h
Dexamethasone	As normal GFR	As normal GFR	As normal GFR
Diazepam	As normal GFR	As normal GFR	As normal GFR
Fluconazole	50%	50%	As normal GFR
Imipenem	25%	25%	50%
Lamivudine	25 mg qd	25 mg qd	50–150 mg qd
Lansoprazole	As normal GFR	As normal GFR	As normal GFR
Levofloxacin	25–50%	25–50%	50%
Methylprednisolone	As normal GFR	As normal GFR	As normal GFR
Metoclopramide	50%	50%	50–75%
Metronidazole	As normal GFR	100% q12h	As normal GFR
Mycophenolate mofetil	50–100%	50–100%	As normal GFR
Omeprazole	As normal GFR	As normal GFR	As normal GFR
Penicillamine	125–250 mg thrice weekly post HD	Avoid	Avoid
Propofol	As normal GFR	As normal GFR	As normal GFR
Ranitidine	50%	50%	100%
Ribavirin	50%	50%	100%
Tacrolimus	As normal GFR	As normal GFR	As normal GFR
Vancomycin	500 mg q48–96h	500 mg q48–96h	500 mg q12–48h

Segmental Glomerular Sclerosis (FSGS) with nephrotic syndrome, endothelial cells resulting in thrombotic microangiopathy, or mesangial cells leading to mesangial nodular sclerosis [39, 40] (Table 21.5). Immune-mediated glomerular injury is usually caused by the induction of autoantibodies (most common are ANCA leading to ANCA-associated vasculitis and ANA leading to drug-induced lupus) or by the

Table 21.4 The most common renal disorders associated with primarily GI disease

Renal disorder		GI disease	Mechanisms
Acute kidney injury		Infective or autoimmune bowel disease (gastroenterocolitis)	Ischemic (hemodynamic)—vomiting, diarrhea
		Peptic ulcers, esophagogastric varices, angiodysplasia, tumors	Ischemic (hemodynamic)—bleeding
		Liver cirrhosis	Ischemic (hemodynamic)—neurohumoral disbalance—hepatorenal syndrome
		Drugs (see Table 21.7)	Toxic, ischemic
Glomerular disorders	IgA nephropathy	Chronic liver disease, pancreatic neoplasms, inflammatory bowel disease (IBD), hepatitis C	Immunologic—immune complex-mediated
	Membranous nephropathy	GI neoplasms Hepatitis B, rectal abscesses, IBD	Immunologic—immune complex-mediated
	Focal segmental glomerulosclerosis	Hepatitis C and B	Direct injury to podocytes
	Minimal change disease	Colon or pancreatic carcinomas, IBD	Immunologic—immune complex-mediated
	Membrano proliferative glomerulonephritis	Hepatitis C and B Visceral abscesses, IBD, hepatitis B	Cryoglobulinemia Immunologic—immune complex-mediated
	AA amyloidosis	IBD, chronic inflammatory diseases	Serum amyloid A deposition
	Anti-glomerular basement membrane glomerulonephritis	IBD	Immunologic—immune complex-mediated
Vascular disorders	ANCA-associated vasculitis	Drugs (see Table 21.6)	Immunologic
	Thrombotic microangiopathy	Drugs (see Table 21.5)	Immunologic, direct endothelial injury
	Polyarteritis nodosa	Hepatitis B and C	Immunologic—immune complex-mediated
Tubulo-interstitial disorders	Acute tubulointerstitial nephritis	Various drugs (see Table 21.7)	Immunologic—allergic
	Chronic tubulointerstitial nephritis	IBD	Immunologic
	Nephrolithiasis	IBD	Metabolic—calcium oxalate, uric acid
Chronic kidney disease		Nonalcoholic fatty liver disease	Metabolic

Table 21.5 The most common drugs inducing glomerular disorders by direct injury

	Podocyte injury	Endothelial injury
Pathological changes	Minimal change disease/ focal segmental glomerulosclerosis	Thrombotic microangiopathy
Drugs	IFN-⟨ and -®, bisphosphonates—pamidronate, NSAIDs, COX-2 inhibitors, lithium, anabolic steroids, sirolimus	Antiangiogenic agents (bevacizumab, aflibercept, Tyr-kinase inhibitors), chemotherapeutics (mitomycin-C, gemcitabine, cisplatin/carboplatin, cytarabine, bleomycin, daunorubicin, hydroxyurea), IFN-⟨ and -®, calcineurin inhibitors, antimicrobial agents (valacyclovir, penicillins, metronidazole, tetracycline, sulfisoxazole, albendazole), NSAIDs, quinine

Table 21.6 The most common drugs inducing glomerular disorders by immune-mediated injury

	ANCA-associated vasculitis	Drug-induced lupus	Membranous nephropathy
Pathological changes	Crescentic glomerulonephritis	Proliferative glomerulonephritis	Diffuse thickening of glomerular basement membranes
Drugs	Allopurinol, sulfasalazine, penicillamine, minocycline, propylthiouracil, levamisole	TNF-⟨ inhibitors, procainamide, hydralazine, quinidine	Gold salts, penicillamine, mercury, NSAIDs, COX-2 inhibitors

Table 21.7 The most common drugs inducing tubulointerstitial disorders

	Acute tubular injury (necrosis)		Acute tubulointerstitial nephritis
Mechanism	Ischemic	Toxic	Allergic
Drugs	NSAIDs, diuretic, ACE inhibitors, calcineurin inhibitors, radiocontrast agents, vasodilators	Radiocontrast agents, aminoglycosides, amphotericin B, quinolones, pentamidine, tetracycline, cisplatin, mithramycin, foscarnet, ifosfamide, cidofovir, adefovir, tenofovir, mannitol, hydroxyethyl starch	NSAIDs, COX-2 inhibitors, PPIs, antimicrobial agents (penicillins, methicillin, ampicillin, rifampin, cephalosporins, ciprofloxacin, clarithromycin, sulphonamides), thiazides, allopurinol, cytosine arabinoside, furosemide

formation of immune complexes in situ in glomeruli (membranous nephropathy) [41] (Table 21.6).

Tubulointerstitial Disorders Induced by Drugs

There are several mechanisms causing drug-induced tubulointerstitial injury. First, there is acute tubular injury (necrosis), which can be either ischemic (by the reduction of renal perfusion) or toxic (by direct injury to tubular epithelial cells) [16] (Table 21.7). Some ubiquitously used drugs (often over-the-counter) can cause this type of injury like non-steroidal anti-inflammatory drugs (NSAIDs). By blocking the production of vasodilatory prostaglandin, they can cause renal ischemia, especially in patients with reduced intravascular volume. All classes of NSAIDs have been associated with this type of injury including acetic acid derivatives (diclofenac, sulindac, and tolmetin), enolic acid derivatives (piroxicam), and propionic acid derivatives (ketoprofen, fenoprofen, and ibuprofen), as well as cyclooxygenase-2 (COX-2) inhibitors (etodolac and celecoxib) [16]. This should prompt awareness and vigilance when using this drug group. Also, there is a frequent use of radiocontrast agents in modern medicine, and those can cause acute tubular necrosis by both types of mechanisms. Preventive measures should be carried out before diagnostic procedures using radiocontrast agents (hydration of patients, withdrawal of drugs that reduce renal perfusion), as well as a close follow-up of renal function parameters after the procedure. Allergic acute tubulointerstitial nephritis is the second most common drug-induced renal disorder [16]. Pathogenesis involves the binding of medications to renal tubular antigens, mimicking renal tubular antigens, or the induction of an immune reaction following deposition in the interstitium [16]. It is associated with some general symptoms like fever, rash, arthralgias, as well as eosinophilia, AKI, leukocyturia, eosinophiluria, hematuria, and mild proteinuria. Literally every drug can cause this type of disorder, but the most common causes are again NSAIDs, as well as some common drugs used in gastroenterology like proton pump inhibitors (PPIs), mesalazine, and antibiotics [16, 42] (Table 21.7). Diagnosis usually requires renal biopsy, and treatment includes withdrawal of the suspected drug and glucocorticoids during 3–6 months [16].

Other Renal Disorders Induced by Drugs

Other types of renal disorders induced by drugs include: cholesterol emboli (with anticoagulants—heparin, warfarin, alteplase), chronic interstitial nephritis (analgesic nephropathy—phenacetin, NSAIDs, acetaminophen, aspirin; mesalazine; lithium; cidofovir; acyclovir, PPIs), formation of crystals or stones (acyclovir, methotrexate, triamterene, ganciclovir, antibiotics) [16]. Antibiotics have been recently associated with an increased risk of stone formation, and the proposed mechanism includes disturbances in gut and urinary microbiome, leading to metabolic disorders, especially in oxalate metabolism and consequently to calcium oxalate stone formation [43, 44]. The highest risk was found for sulphonamides, cephalosporins, and fluoroquinolones. Also, worth mentioning, some drugs can cause pseudo-elevation in SCr levels by the competitive tubular secretion of creatinine or interference with laboratory determination (trimethoprim, cimetidine, triamterene, probenecid, spironolactone, ascorbic acid, cefoxitin, cephalothin, flucytosine, methyldopa), as well as pseudo-elevation in blood urea nitrogen levels (glucocorticoids, tetracycline) [16].

GI Disorders Following Primary Renal Disorders

GI Manifestations in AKI and CKD

GI manifestations of acute kidney injury and chronic kidney disease are very common, probably much more than reported and acknowledged. Especially in patients with ESRD (end-stage renal disease) on dialysis, it is estimated that about 80% of patients have some type of GI manifestation [45]. Mostly these symptoms are due to uremia, and symptoms can vary regarding the degree of uremia. Nonspecific symptoms (nausea, vomiting, anorexia, uremic fetor, hiccups, diarrhea, irritable bowel syndrome) are most common, around 60% [46]. These nonspecific symptoms usually disappear on starting renal replacement therapy. Malnutrition is very common in CKD patients because of low food intake (anorexia, but often connected to dietary restrictions of low protein diet), lower intestinal absorption, and chronic inflammation. The most acute potential complication of AKI or CKD is GI hemorrhage, occurring in up to 36.8% of patients and is associated with a significantly increased risk of hospitalization and death. Causes of GI bleeding are impaired platelet function (uremia), use of heparin (dialysis), and higher incidence of ulcers [47, 48]. The prophylactic use of proton-pump inhibitors is beneficial. Regarding the upper digestive tract, CKD manifestations could be hyperpigmentation of the lips, stomatitis, gingivitis, esophagitis, gastroparesis (uremia, autonomic neuropathy), gastritis (increased gastrin serum levels), peptic ulcers (*H. Pylori*, NSAIDs). Angiodysplasia is a frequent cause of GI bleeding, especially in dialysis patients. Regarding the lower digestive tract, constipation is common (could be induced by phosphate binder therapy). Diverticular disease has the same incidence in CKD as in the general population but CKD patients are at higher risk for acute diverticulitis and complications [49]. Due to uremia and fluid overload in AKI and CKD mucosal and submucosal edema could occur causing colitis. Drug absorption could be impaired because of intestinal mucosal edema, so higher doses of oral medication or parenteral use could be necessary. Colon perforation has a higher incidence in patients on hemodialysis as well as peritoneal dialysis (necrosis due to pressure) [46]. Intestinal ischemia and ischemic colitis (vasculitis, amyloidosis) are less common complications of CKD and its treatment. There appears to be a higher incidence of cholelithiasis in CKD patients [50], and bile reflux is found in 19% of patients on hemodialysis, which contributes to gastric erosions [46]. It remains unclear whether acute pancreatitis (AP) is more prevalent in patients with CKD, but it is certain that CKD patients with AP have higher mortality and add substantial burden to the health care system [51]. CKD patients mostly have elevated levels of pancreatic enzymes continuously (since they are partially excreted by the kidneys), without signs of acute pancreatitis. The most common cause of AP in CKD patients, in contrast to the general population, is hypercalcemia. Liver manifestations of AKI and CKD could mostly be due to fluid overload, drug-induced or viral. Hepatitis B and hepatitis C virus infections are the most common and serious causes of liver damage in CKD patients. Ascites could occur due to volume overload and low albumin concentration, especially in ESRD patients.

GI Manifestations in AKI and CKD Treatment

The common GI manifestations related to the technique of peritoneal dialysis include reflux esophagitis, hernias, bowel erosion by catheter pressure, peritonitis, and pancreatitis. Complications related to hemodialysis include nausea, vomiting, intestinal ischemia due to hypotension, GI bleeding (uremia/heparin), pancreatitis. In contrast, patients after renal transplantation mostly develop opportunistic infections (CMV, candida, and herpes) and drug-related toxicity in the colon (MMF—mycophenolate mofetil-related colitis). Dialysis patients are at a higher risk for *Clostridium difficile*-associated diarrhea [52].

GI Manifestations in Glomerular Disease

GI manifestations in glomerular disease differ regarding the underlying cause and presentation of glomerular disease. With nephrotic syndrome, intestinal edema is most common; in some cases, it leads to intussusception (can also be caused by peristalsis incoordination) [53]. Thromboembolism is a major complication in nephrotic syndrome, but although not so common in the GI tract, mesenteric ischemia could occur [54]. Most other manifestations are connected to uremia and fluid overload and were discussed earlier. Pancreatitis could occur due to hypertriglyceridemia.

GI Manifestations in Tubular Disease

GI manifestations in tubular disease patients happen due to uremia, acid-base and electrolyte imbalance (especially hyperkalemia and acidosis), hyperphosphatemia, hypocalcemia, and fluid overload. Most of the manifestations were discussed earlier.

GI Manifestations in Renal Vascular Disease

Mesenteric ischemia and ischemic colitis are the most common GI manifestations of systemic vasculitis. Much rarer complications are ischemic hepatitis and acute pancreatitis. A rare condition presenting with hematuria and abdominal pain, commonly forgotten, is the nutcracker syndrome—compression of the left renal vein by abdominal aorta and superior mesenteric artery.

GI Manifestations Connected to Medication Therapy of Renal Disease

Almost all medications stated in this chapter could cause general side-effects like nausea, dyspepsia, diarrhea, constipation, abdominal pain, dry mouth, and so these will not be noted later. The most common drugs used in nephrology are antihypertensive drugs. ACE inhibitors are probably the most widely used antihypertensive drug (also lowering proteinuria levels) that could also cause pancreatitis, and less commonly but severe, intestinal angioedema or hepatitis (cytotoxic or cholestatic). With angiotensin receptor blockers we should stress the possibility of olmesartan causing enteropathy (chronic diarrhea and weight loss), and as a group they could cause hepatic failure. Calcium channel blockers, with other most common side effects, could cause gastritis, pancreatitis, hepatitis, and gingival hyperplasia. The most common side-effect of moxonidine is mouth dryness. Another group of medications commonly used in nephrology is diuretics. Furosemide and torsemide could cause hypokalemia and paralytic ileus (furosemide), liver failure, and encephalopathy and acute pancreatitis. Indapamide could cause hepatitis, hepatic encephalopathy, and acute pancreatitis. Spironolactone could cause gastric ulcer and bleeding and hepatitis. Eplerenone could cause cholecystitis and is contraindicated with severe hepatic failure. Glucocorticoids, most commonly used in glomerular disease patients, increase the risk of gastritis, gastric ulcers, and GI bleeding, rarely visceral perforation or hepatic steatosis [55]. The combined use of glucocorticoids and NSAIDs significantly increases the risk of GI side-effects, especially bleeding. The most common GI manifestations of cyclophosphamide and cyclosporine are nausea, vomiting and appetite loss, but diarrhea, mouth sores, and liver failure could occur. GI adverse events associated with MMF (mycophenolate mofetil) are frequent, and in 40–50% of cases lead to dose reduction or withdrawal, most commonly diarrhea [56]. In patients treated with rituximab, new-onset abdominal pain should prompt an investigation for acute abdomen—bowel obstruction, GI perforation should be excluded [57, 58]. All of these drugs affecting the immune system could increase the chance of GI infections.

Of medications used in dialysis patients, phosphate binders have most common GI manifestations. Sevelamer is commonly associated with vomiting, nausea, diarrhea, constipation, and in some cases, fecal impaction and bleeding [59]. Patients on hemodialysis have a higher risk for GI bleeding because of the need for anticoagulation during hemodialysis procedures.

References

1. Lea-Henry TN, Carland JE, Stocker SL, Sevastos J, Roberts DM. Clinical pharmacokinetics in kidney disease: fundamental principles. Clin J Am Soc Nephrol. 2018;13:1085–95.
2. Keller F, Hann A. Clinical pharmacodynamics: principles of drug response and alterations in kidney disease. Clin J Am Soc Nephrol. 2018;13:1413–20.
3. Lehto M, Groop PH. The gut-kidney Axis: putative interconnections between gastrointestinal and renal disorders. Front Endocrinol (Lausanne). 2018;9:553.
4. Bellomo R, Kellum JA, Ronco C. Acute kidney injury. Lancet. 2012;380:756–66.
5. The Kidney Disease Improving Global Outcomes (KDIGO) Working Group. Definition and classification of acute kidney injury. Kidney Int. 2012;Suppl 2:19–36.
6. Hsu CY, McCullough CE, Fan D, Ordonez JD, Cherow GM, Go AS. Community-based incidence of acute renal failure. Kidney Int. 2007;72:208–12.

7. Liangos O, Wald R, O'Bell JW, Price L, Pereira BJ, Jaber BL. Epidemiology and outcomes of acute renal failure in hospitalized patients: a national survey. Clin J Am Soc Nephrol. 2006;1:43–51.
8. Kidney Disease: Improving Global Outcomes (KDIGO) CKD Work Group. KDIGO 2012 clinical practice guideline for the evaluation and management of chronic kidney disease. Kidney Int Suppl. 2013:1–150.
9. Webster AC, Nagler EV, Morton RL, Masson P. Chronic kidney disease. Lancet. 2017;389:1238–52.
10. Levey AS, Bosch JP, Lewis JB, Greene T, Rogers N, Roth D. A more accurate method to estimate glomerular filtration rate from serum creatinine: a new prediction equation. Modification of Diet in Renal Disease Study Group. Ann Intern Med. 1999;130:461–70.
11. Levey AS, Stevens LA, Schmid CH, Zhang YL, Castro AF III, Feldman HI, Kusek JW, Eggers P, Van LF, Greene T, Coresh J. A new equation to estimate glomerular filtration rate. Ann Intern Med. 2009;150:604–12.
12. Floege J, Amann K. Primary glomerulonephritides. Lancet. 2016;387:2036–48.
13. KDIGO Glomerulonephritis Work Group. KDIGO clinical practice guideline for Glomerulonephritis. Kidney Int Suppl. 2012;2:139–274.
14. Jennette JC, Falk RJ, Bacon PA, Basu N, Cid MC, Ferrario F, et al. 2012 revised international chapel hill consensus conference nomenclature of vasculitides. Arthritis Rheum. 2013;65:1–11.
15. Brocklebank V, Wood KM, Kavanagh D. Thrombotic Microangiopathy and the kidney. Clin J Am Soc Nephrol. 2018;13:300–17.
16. Choudhury D, Ahmed Z. Drug-associated renal dysfunction and injury. Nat Clin Pract Nephrol. 2006;2:80–91.
17. Joy MS, Frye RF, Nolin TD, Roberts BV, La MK, Wang J, et al. In vivo alterations in drug metabolism and transport pathways in patients with chronic kidney diseases. Pharmacotherapy. 2014;34:114–22.
18. Putt TL, Duffull SB, Schollum JB, Walker RJ. GFR may not accurately predict aspects of proximal tubule drug handling. Eur J Clin Pharmacol. 2014;70:1221–6.
19. Roberts DM. The relevance of drug clearance to antibiotic dosing in critically ill patients. Curr Pharm Biotechnol. 2011;12:2002–14.
20. McIntyre CW, Owen PJ. Prescribing drugs in kidney disease. In: Brenner BM, editor. Brenner & Rector's the kidney. Philadelphia: Saunders Elsevier; 2008. p. 1930–56.
21. Greenblatt DJ. Hepatic clearance of drugs in patients with renal insufficiency. Clin Pharmacol Drug Dev. 2013;2:295–7.
22. Nolin TD, Appiah K, Kendrick SA, Le P, McMonagle E, Himmelfarb J. Hemodialysis acutely improves hepatic CYP3A4 metabolic activity. J Am Soc Nephrol. 2006;17:2363–7.
23. Nolin TD, Frye RF, Le P, Sadr H, Naud J, Leblond FA, et al. ESRD impairs nonrenal clearance of fexofenadine but not midazolam. J Am Soc Nephrol. 2009;20:2269–76.
24. Volpe DA, Tobin GA, Tavakkoli F, Dowling TC, Light PD, Parker RJ. Effect of uremic serum and uremic toxins on drug metabolism in human microsomes. Regul Toxicol Pharmacol. 2014;68:297–303.
25. Sun H, Frassetto L, Benet LZ. Effects of renal failure on drug transport and metabolism. Pharmacol Ther. 2006;109:1–11.
26. De Martin S, Orlando R, Bertoli M, Pegoraro P, Palatini P. Differential effect of chronic renal failure on the pharmacokinetics of lidocaine in patients receiving and not receiving hemodialysis. Clin Pharmacol Ther. 2006;80:597–606.
27. Yeung CK, Shen DD, Thummel KE, Himmelfarb J. Effects of chronic kidney disease and uremia on hepatic drug metabolism and transport. Kidney Int. 2014;85:522–8.
28. Roberts DM, Sevastos J, Carland JE, Stocker SL, Lea-Henry TN. Clinical pharmacokinetics in kidney disease: application to rational Design of Dosing Regimens. Clin J Am Soc Nephrol. 2018;13:1254–63.
29. FDA. Pharmacokinetics in patients with impaired renal function—study design, data analysis, and impact on dosing and labeling. 2010. https://www.fda.gov/downloads/drugs/guidancecomplianceregulatoryinformation/guidances/ucm204959.pdf. Accessed 24 Nov 2019.

30. Khanal A, Castelino RL, Peterson GM, Jose MD. Dose adjustment guidelines for medications in patients with renal impairment: how consistent are drug information sources? Intern Med J. 2014;44:77–85.
31. Lavergne V, Nolin TD, Hoffman RS, Roberts D, Gosselin S, Goldfarb DS, et al. The EXTRIP (EXtracorporeal TReatments in poisoning) workgroup: guideline methodology. Clin Toxicol (Phila). 2012;50:403–13.
32. Velenosi TJ, Urquhart BL. Pharmacokinetic considerations in chronic kidney disease and patients requiring dialysis. Expert Opin Drug Metab Toxicol. 2014;10:1131–43.
33. Chiou WL, Hsu FH. Pharmacokinetics of creatinine in man and its implications in the monitoring of renal function and in dosage regimen modifications in patients with renal insufficiency. J Clin Pharmacol. 1975;15:427–34.
34. Angeletti A, Cantarelli C, Cravedi P. HCV-associated nephropathies in the era of direct acting antiviral agents. Front Med (Lausanne). 2019;6:20.
35. Kupin WL. Viral-associated GN: hepatitis B and other viral infections. Clin J Am Soc Nephrol. 2017;12:1529–33.
36. Kupin WL. Viral-associated GN: hepatitis C and HIV. Clin J Am Soc Nephrol. 2017;12:1337–42.
37. Ambruzs JM, Larsen CP. Renal manifestations of inflammatory bowel disease. Rheum Dis Clin N Am. 2018;44:699–714.
38. Rosato V, Masarone M, Dallio M, Federico A, Aglitti A, Persico M. NAFLD and extra-hepatic comorbidities: current evidence on a multi-organ metabolic syndrome. Int J Environ Res Public Health. 2019;16:E3415.
39. Markowitz GS, Bomback AS, Perazella MA. Drug-induced glomerular disease: direct cellular injury. Clin J Am Soc Nephrol. 2015;10:1291–9.
40. Radhakrishnan J, Perazella MA. Drug-induced glomerular disease: attention required! Clin J Am Soc Nephrol. 2015;10:1287–90.
41. Hogan JJ, Markowitz GS, Radhakrishnan J. Drug-induced glomerular disease: immune-mediated injury. Clin J Am Soc Nephrol. 2015;10:1300–10.
42. Al-Aly Z, Maddukuri G, Xie Y. Proton pump inhibitors and the kidney: implications of current evidence for clinical practice and when and how to deprescribe. Am J Kidney Dis. 2019;75(4):497–507.
43. Ferraro PM, Curhan GC, Gambaro G, Taylort EN. Antibiotic use and risk of incident kidney stones in female nurses. Am J Kidney Dis. 2019:74.
44. Tasian G, Miller A, Lange D. Antibiotics and kidney stones: perturbation of the gut-kidney Axis. Am J Kidney Dis. 2019;74:724–6.
45. Cano AE, Neil AK, Kang JY, Barnabas A, Eastwood JB, Nelson SR, Hartley I, Maxwell D. Gastrointestinal symptoms in patients with end-stage renal disease undergoing treatment by hemodialysis or peritoneal dialysis. Am J Gastroenterol. 2007;102(9):1990–7.
46. Santacoloma Osorio M, Camilo Giraldo G. Gastrointestinal manifestations of chronic kidney disease. Rev Colomb Nefrol. 2017;4(1);17–26.
47. Fiaccadori E, Maggiore U, Clima B, Melfa L, Rotelli C, Borghetti A. Incidence, risk factors, and prognosis of gastrointestinal hemorrhage complicating acute renal failure. Kidney Int. 2001;59(4);1510–9.
48. Thomas R, Panackal C, John M, Joshi H, Mathai S, Kattickaran J, Iqbal M. Gastrointestinal complications in patients with chronic kidney disease—a 5-year retrospective study from a tertiary referral center. Ren Fail. 2013;35(1):49–55.
49. Chang SS1, Huang N, Hu HY. Patients with end-stage renal disease were at an increased risk of hospitalization for acute diverticulitis. Medicine (Baltimore). 2016;95(39): 4881.
50. Kazama JJ, Kazama S, Koda R, et al. The risk of gallbladder stone formation is increased in patients with predialysis chronic kidney disease but not those undergoing chronic hemodialysis therapy. Nephron Clin Pract. 2009;111:167–72.
51. Kroner PT, Mareth K, Raimondo M, et al. Acute Pancreatitis in Advanced Chronic Kidney Disease and Kidney Transplant Recipients: Results of a US Nationwide Analysis. Mayo Clin Proc Innov Qual Outcomes. 2019;3(2):160–8.

52. Eui Oh S, Lee SM, Lee YK, et al. Clostridium difficile-associated diarrhea in dialysis patients. Kidney Res Clin Pract. 2013;32(1):27–31.
53. Ete T, Mondal S, Sinha D, et al. Small bowel intussusception in an adult with nephrotic syndrome. Indian J Nephrol. 2014;24(2):136–7.
54. Park BS, Park S, Jin K, et al. Nephrotic syndrome complicated with portal, splenic, and superior mesenteric vein thrombosis. Kidney Res Clin Pract. 2014;33(3):161–4.
55. Piper JM, Ray WA, Daugherty JR, Griffin MR. Corticosteroid use and peptic ulcer disease: role of nonsteroidal anti-inflammatory drugs. Ann Intern Med. 1991;114(9):735–40.
56. Bunnapradist S, Ambühl PM. Impact of gastrointestinal-related side effects on mycophenolate mofetil dosing and potential therapeutic strategies. Clin Transplant. 2008;22(6):815–21.
57. Cornejo A, Bohnenblust M, Harris C, Abrahamian GA. Intestinal perforation associated with rituximab therapy for post-transplant lymphoproliferative disorder after liver transplantation. Cancer Chemother Pharmacol. 2009;64:857–60.
58. Kasi PM, et al. Clinical review: Serious adverse events associated with the use of rituximab - a critical care perspective. Crit Care. 2012;16:231.
59. Yuste C, Mérida E, Hernández E, et al. Gastrointestinal complications induced by sevelamer crystals. Clin Kidney J. 2017;10(4):539–44.

Hepatic Insufficiency 22

Ivana Mikolašević, Tajana Filipec Kanižaj, Viktor Domislović, and Duško Kardum

Introduction

The safety of drugs is a frequent concern in patient management. This is also the case in cirrhotic patients which represent the challenging population of patients to manage. Currently, there are no guidelines for medical management of liver cirrhosis patients [1–3]. Over the last decade, there has been an increase in liver cirrhosis and global annual mortality to over one million. The most frequent etiology of liver cirrhosis in Europe are chronic hepatitis B (HBV) and C (HCV) virus infections, chronic alcohol consumption and liver disease because of metabolic syndrome named nonalcoholic fatty liver disease (NAFLD) [1–3]. Regardless of etiology, the pathophysiology from acute inflammation to fibrosis and cirrhosis is similar. Namely, hepatic tissue injury triggers an inflammatory response, which if persistent, progresses to fibrosis. An early stage of liver fibrosis is usually without obvious symptoms, in contrast to advanced fibrosis or cirrhosis which causes significant loss of hepatocyte function, tissue scarring, formation of regenerative nodules, etc.

I. Mikolašević (✉)
Department of Gastroenterology, University Hospital Center Rijeka, Rijeka, Croatia

School of Medicine, University of Rijeka, Rijeka, Croatia

T. Filipec Kanižaj
Department of Gastroenterology, Merkur University Hospital, Zagreb, Croatia

V. Domislović
Department of Gastroenterology and Hepatology, University Hospital Center Zagreb, Zagreb, Croatia

D. Kardum
University of North, Varaždin, Croatia

Department of Gastroenterology, Merkur University Hospital, Zagreb, Croatia

Faculty of Medicine, J.J. Strossmayer University of Osijek, Osijek, Croatia

M. Banić, D. Erceg (eds.), *Drug Interactions in Gastroenterology*, Clinical Gastroenterology, https://doi.org/10.1007/978-3-031-69800-2_22

These processes result in increased portal vein pressure and clinical manifestations and complications of portal hypertension [2–8]. Liver cirrhosis is defined as compensated if complications are absent, and if progression occurs, complications such as bleeding or hepatic encephalopathy (HE) can be life-threatening.

Child-Pugh score assesses chronic liver disease (CLD) using five components: existence of ascites and encephalopathy, bilirubin levels, prothrombin time and albumin levels. Hence, the Child-Pugh (CP) score assesses chronic hepatic injury as follows: 5–6 is mild hepatic damage and is usually classified as CP grade A, 7–9 moderate hepatic damage classified as grade B and 10–15 is severe hepatic damage (grade C) [1, 9]. Additionally, the model for end-stage liver Disease (MELD) is also a classification system for liver disease severity, which is calculated using bilirubin, the parameter of kidney function (i.e., creatinine), international normalized ratio (INR) and finally the cause of CLD. This score system can predict 3-month mortality in patients on the waiting list for liver transplantation. Hence, it is now used in priority allocation for patients expecting liver transplantation. These classifications are not specific and sensitive enough to quantitate drug metabolism by the liver; therefore, pharmacological adjustment based on these equations is not in regular or frequent use [1, 10]. However, according to data, adjustment of drug dosage in patients with liver disease should be considered according to the Child-Pugh score. European Medicines Agency (EMA) and the Food and Drug Administration (FDA) require kinetic studies in CLD patients for new drug authorization and dose adjustment [11, 12]. This information, which is provided in the summary of product characteristics (SPC), can be very helpful. However, most of the clinical studies include patients with Child-Pug A (good hepatic function), therefore recommendations on drug dose adjustments in Child-Pugh class C (advanced liver dysfunction) cannot be given. In contrast to renal insufficiency, no specific guidelines or algorithms in order to adjust the dose of specific drugs exist in CLD patients. There is an increasing interest in updating current SPC information [1].

Currently, an exact and established method for assessing liver failure which would be in good correlation with liver drug clearance does not exist. The semi-quantitative Child-Pugh score is inappropriate due to imprecision and lack of ability to quantify exact liver capacity for drug metabolization. The Child-Pugh score is associated with complication development and survival in cirrhotic patients. Furthermore, when calculating the Child-Pugh score some of the components are prone to subjectivity, such as evaluation of ascites and encephalopathy.

Increasing dysfunction of hepatocytes is affecting both metabolic and synthetic liver function. This includes endogenous and exogenous substances such as bilirubin, plasma proteins or various medications. Thus, decreased ability to excrete toxic products may result in increased levels of neurotoxins which can precipitate the development of HE. Hypoalbuminemia along with portal hypertension can lead to ascites. Portal hypertension has well-known complications such as gastric or esophageal varices as a result of portosystemic collaterals. Cirrhosis and its complications can lead to alterations in pharmacokinetic (PK) as well as alterations in pharmacodynamic (PD) characteristics of the drug which can be clinically highly significant [2–9].

The liver is one of the central organs which has an important role in drug absorption, but also in drug distribution and elimination. The liver affects PK and PD not just through the process of biotransformation but also through processes of blood flow through the liver, the binding capacity of plasma proteins, excretion of drugs throughout the biliary system, all of which can be highly significant. Portosystemic collaterals may reduce drug elimination through diminished first-pass effect, while decreased blood flow through the liver may reduce high extraction drugs (flow-limited drugs). These facts point out the importance of dose adjustment in CLD patients. Also, there are some other considerations that could have a significant influence on drug metabolism such as renal function. Thus, in CLD patients, we have to evaluate renal clearance as well as the presence or absence of kidney dysfunction associated with liver cirrhosis (i.e., hepatorenal syndrome). Thus, kinetic changes in CLD patients can occur due to the following mechanisms [1–12]: (i) necrosis of hepatocytes, (ii) portosystemic collaterals and development of shunts, (iii) decrease in levels of proteins that bind drugs, changes in (iv) distribution volume, (v) drug metabolism (vi) elimination, (vii) pharmacodynamics, association with (viii) renal failure and occurrence of (ix) interactions between drugs.

Drugs administered to CLD patients, such as those with liver cirrhosis, should be dose-adjusted. Currently, there has not been any biomarker identified that would reflect hepatic function and that would be used in daily clinical practice. However, drugs that have high extraction in the liver have higher bioavailability in cirrhotic patients, which is the result of reduced hepatic clearance. Such drugs, if administered orally, should be initially dose adjusted according to extraction in the liver. In addition, the dose for maintaining should also be in line with available kinetic studies in liver cirrhosis. It is important to note that CLD does not affect bioavailability for low hepatic extraction drugs, but hepatic clearance may be impaired, thus the maintenance regimen should be adjusted, i.e., they should be reduced. Accordingly, the first dose should be administered in the lower range of normal for drugs with an intermediate liver extraction. On the other hand, reduction of maintenance doses is highly recommended in the case of drugs with a high liver extraction. Some drugs may be predominantly excreted via the biliary tract; therefore, cholestasis may affect their levels. Antineoplastic medications often have dose adjustment recommendations in biliary obstruction or cholestatic liver lesions, but this is not the case for most of the drugs that are eliminated via the biliary system. Therefore, dose adjustment in this situation is difficult but should be made along with the expected toxicity and pharmacological effect. Along with kinetic changes, dynamics can also be altered in drugs such as opiates, benzodiazepines, NSAIDs and diuretics. Side effects might occur; therefore, one should bear in mind that dose adjustment recommendations are general and should not be substituted for clinical monitoring, which should always have an advantage over recommendations [1–14]. Finally, drug level and adverse event monitoring should be frequently performed if possible.

Pharmacokinetic Changes

Pathophysiology of changes and influence on PK parameters are shown in Table 22.1 [10–13]. Consequently, drug levels might be lowered, or the exposure to the drugs might be considerably high, depending on the drug and patient's features.

Patient Characteristics

Patient characteristics might have a significant influence on drug PK, such as cirrhosis severity, underlying liver disease severity, nutritional status, genetic polymorphisms, etc. [6, 7, 14–27].

Table 22.1 Pathophysiological changes and pharmacokinetic parameters in liver cirrhosis patients

Changes in pathophysiology	Changes in pharmacokinetics
Absorption	
– Gastropathy due to portal hypertension – Impairment of gastrointestinal motility – Delay of gastric emptying – Increased intestinal permeability	– Decreased absorption – Alteration of drug absorption
– Reduced intrinsic clearance – Altered liver blood flow	– Lowered first-pass effect – Increased bioavailability – Diminished pro-drug metabolism
Distribution	
– Hypoproteinemia—impaired liver synthesis	– Larger fraction of unbound drug to proteins
– Endogenous substance accumulation (e.g., bilirubin), plasma protein displaced binding site	– Enlarged distribution volume
– Retention of fluid	
Metabolism	
Impaired hepatic architecture (e.g., hepatocellular necrosis and formation of nodules)	– Reduced intrinsic clearance – Enzyme sensitivity on these changes varies among different enzymes (e.g., CYP2C19 is sensitive and CYP2D6 is affected in later stages) – Stereoselectivity change of liver drug metabolism
Decreased liver blood flow	Delay in drug clearance
Elimination	
Biliary obstruction Reduced expression of protein transporter	Reduction in biliary excretion Disrupted enterohepatic recycling
Renal impairment (advanced stage of cirrhosis)	Reduced renal elimination

(a) *Influence of liver cirrhosis severity*

Increased liver cirrhosis severity or CLD progression decreases the activity of enzymes included in metabolism, which can consequently lead to changes in PK [7, 15]. This often results in higher exposure to medicines due to increased drug plasma levels [6, 16–27]. In addition, renal function can also decline with increasing severity of cirrhosis. In pharmacokinetic studies, the use of CLD scoring systems such as CP classification is warranted in the categorization of patients regarding liver dysfunction severity, and this is the reason why product labels may contain Child-Pugh-based recommendations [7, 19, 20].

(b) *Influence of liver cirrhosis etiology*

The etiology of cirrhosis, i.e., underlying CLD could have an influence on the changes in PK and their extent via alteration of drug metabolizing enzymatic activity. For example, whether the CLD is the result of the cholestatic or hepatocellular liver lesion can result in different CYP-enzyme expression [7, 21]. Prasad et al. showed the abundance of most enzymes that are involved in metabolism (decreased 25–50% compared to healthy individuals), in those that were transplanted due to alcoholic cirrhosis versus HCV etiology. At the time of transplantation, their CP score was C [22]. For example, a different pathophysiological mechanism is that the cirrhotic liver of alcoholic etiology decreased alcohodehydrogenase type 1A, 1B as well as UGT1A4 in comparison to the cirrhotic liver of HCV etiology [7, 22].

Breimer et al. showed that subjects with cirrhotic liver of alcoholic etiology had the lowest clearance of antipyrine which has low EH, while there was overlap in subjects with other CLDs [14]. In another study, patients with cirrhosis had decreased clearance, while there was no difference between the cirrhosis groups based on the etiology [23]. Also, it is important to point out jaundice as a confounding factor which is probably a reflection of the severity of hepatic impairment. In conclusion, different types of liver disease may differently affect and alter plasma drug levels; however, clinical implications still need to be determined [7].

(c) *Other characteristics of liver cirrhosis patients*

Regarding genetic polymorphisms, current data are scarce. Ohnishi and colleagues compared cirrhosis patients and healthy controls in regard to CYP2C19 activity using the omeprazole hydroxylation index and found that poor metabolizers (PM) genotype had similar enzyme activity in comparison to cirrhotic patients with CYP2C19 homozygous and heterozygous genotype [7, 28]. Also, data have shown that pantoprazole exposure in Child-Pugh cirrhosis B and C (unknown genotype) was comparable to healthy subjects of CYP2C19 PM (7,30). Furthermore, the CYP2D6 genotype (188C > T) has been shown as a predictor for propranolol response in cirrhotic patients, although without a control group [29].

Medication Characteristics

(a) *Pharmacokinetics*

The influence of changes in pathophysiology in liver cirrhosis patients on PK is presented in Table 22.1. There is a frequent use of a well-stirred model in explaining the influence of drug plasma level changes [7, 13–15, 30].

According to this model, three components influence hepatic drug clearance: (i) liver blood flow, (ii) intrahepatic clearance (drug metabolism in hepatocytes) and (iii) unbound fraction of the drug. The hepatic extraction ratio (EH) drug fraction is removed from the circulation with a single hepatic passage. According to the well-stirred model, drugs are divided by EH into EH that is higher than 0.7 (high), EH: 0.3–0.7 (intermediate) and EH that is lower than 0.3 (low) extraction [7, 13–15]. For high EH drugs, liver blood flow is the limiting factor, hence, these drugs are "flow-limited." First-pass metabolism in these drugs is high when administered orally if taken from healthy individuals [7, 31]. On the other side, portosystemic shunts may have a significant influence. For example, naltrexone has a bioavailability of 5–40% in healthy subjects, while in patients with compensated and decompensated liver cirrhosis, its bioavailability is much higher [7, 31]. Low EH medicines are less efficiently cleared from the blood by the liver, and their clearance is mostly intrinsic and depends on the free fraction. Examples of drugs with low EH are proton pump inhibitors (PPIs), lansoprazole and pantoprazole [32]. Also, there has been a CYP2C19 activity decrease in cirrhotic patients, which results in larger exposure to drugs. Thus, intermediate EH drugs such as paroxetine are influenced by all three components (liver blood flow, status of liver metabolism activity and unbound drug fraction) [7, 33]. Gonzales et al. reported pharmacokinetic studies that explain the association of drug properties with PK changes in cirrhotic patients [7, 27]. Drugs with higher EH ratios and moderate-to-severe liver dysfunction had elevated drug exposure, with uncertain clinical meaning since some of the low EH medicines had increased exposure. The negative PK predictor for impairment was high elimination through the kidney, which could also be affected in liver cirrhosis, thus, this result should be interpreted with caution [7, 15, 27].

(b) *Administration route*

All administration routes that are related to the first-pass effect may affect all administration routes, especially drugs with high EH. Hence, oral and parenteral administration routes differ. Isradipine and nifedipine, which have intermediate EH, had higher bioavailability. Namely, the bioavailability of oral isradipine was 17% and 37% in healthy subjects and subjects with cirrhosis, respectively [34]. In addition, nifedipine bioavailability was 50% in healthy, while it was 90% in liver cirrhosis patients [35]. Furthermore, when oral naltrexone is administered in patients with liver cirrhosis, exposure is a fivefold to tenfold increase depending on the liver compensation status [31]. This was not the case after intramuscular injection of naltrexone where there was no PK difference comparing mild and moderate cirrhosis with healthy subjects [36]. Data on rectal administration and its influence on bioavailability are lacking [7].

Pharmacodynamic Changes

In pathological situations such as liver cirrhosis, penetration of the drug to the target site may be impaired. This may result in lower or higher response to medications; thus, it could lead to diminished effect or potential toxicity [7].

Alteration in Toxicological Effects

There is an increased risk of toxicological effects of drugs in cirrhotic patients. An overview of side effects in CLD patients has been published [7, 37].

Neurotoxicity

Some of the medicines could be neurotoxic in cirrhotic patients and may precipitate HE. This has been shown in five percent of 913 HE cases with relation to benzodiazepines, 4% to opioids and one percent to hypnotics [38]. In addition, it seems that benzodiazepine use is a significant risk factor in developing HE by fivefold, if the therapy is used for 3–10 days [7, 39]. It is important to mention some of the pathophysiological mechanisms for neurotoxicity such as increased blood-brain barrier (BBB) permeability, increased brain receptor affinity or density and increased levels of neurotoxins in circulation. Increased BBB permeability has been shown with the presence of medications and metabolites in cerebrospinal fluid (CSF) of patients with HE, which are shown to be in healthy controls [7, 40]. For example, higher levels of cimetidine in CFS have been reported [7, 41]. The exact pathophysiological mechanism of the increase in BBB permeability has not been fully explained. It has been hypothesized that increased bilirubin exposure might lead to downregulation or occupation of efflux pumps such as P-glycoprotein and multi-drug resistance protein 1 [7, 40]. Also, sedation with benzodiazepines was more excessive in cirrhotic patients compared to controls [7, 42, 43]. On the other hand, benzodiazepine CSF levels were not higher than those in controls [44]. Additionally, deceased patients with HE had a higher density of "peripheral-type" benzodiazepine receptors, and the upregulation may be enhanced by inflammation [45, 46]. Moreover, the pathogenesis of HE can be also linked to increased neurosteroid synthesis that can occur in this setting, which may modulate the gamma-aminobutyric acid receptor system [46]. Another possible mechanism for neurotoxicity is an increase in known neurotoxic agents such as ammonia, lactate and manganese [47]. For example, HE can occur in acetazolamide, which decreases ammonia excretion, which results in increased levels of ammonia in the blood, which consequently crosses BBB at high levels [48, 49]. Overall, medication neurotoxicity in liver cirrhosis may be multifactorial; therefore, further research is warranted [7].

Alteration of Pharmacological Effect

There are data regarding some of the more frequent therapies such as diuretics, beta-blocker therapy, therapy with muscle relaxants and inhibitors of the renin-angiotensin-aldosterone system. Decreased response to diuretics has been hypothesized to be the consequence of the reduction in diuretic potential of the kidney [7, 49–52]. Also, a less pronounced effect of beta-blocker metipranolol was noted in cirrhotic patients, possibly due to the downregulation of beta-adrenergic receptors [7, 53]. However, some of the data report dose-dependent propranolol response which does not differ from healthy controls after control for alterations in PK [54]. Furthermore, response to muscle relaxants may also differ in cirrhotic patients, but these were in correlation with the parameters of PK. Also, data suggest that the proportion of angiotensin-converting enzyme (ACE) inhibition in cirrhosis was like healthy subjects, while, on the other hand, decreased activation of enalapril was reported with a similar effect on values of the blood pressure to the healthy subjects [7, 55–57].

Impairment of Renal Function

Data that investigated the use of nonsteroidal anti-inflammatory (NSAIDs) medications [58] reported that there is a decrease in glomerular filtration rate in about a third of liver cirrhosis patients following NSAID administration. Another paper reported renal impairment in around half of patients with liver cirrhosis using ibuprofen [59]. According to this paper, liver cirrhosis patients can develop renal impairment caused by ibuprofen (50% of patients reported) [58, 59]. RAAS inhibitors may also contribute to a decrease in renal function in patients with decompensated cirrhosis [60]. Pathophysiologic mechanisms have been proposed, especially since the association of renal hemodynamics and cirrhosis-associated hemodynamics have been well-described [61]. Liver cirrhosis is connected with impaired hemodynamics with development of the portal hypertension and splanchnic vasodilatation that leads to RAAS system activation (vasodilatation of afferent with prostaglandins and vasoconstriction of efferent arterioles with AT-II), which is a mechanism to preserve renal function [62]. This interference with RAAS inhibitors and NSAIDs which inhibit AT-II and prostaglandin synthesis might cause acute renal failure [7, 61]. An additional mechanism is the direct toxic effect on renal tubules, such as with aminoglycosides [61, 63].

Immunological Effects

Liver cirrhosis is a state of systemic impairment of multiple organs, and thus liver cirrhosis can often lead to immune dysfunction which can be precipitated using immunosuppressive therapy [64]. Patients with liver cirrhosis using interferon-α have an increased prevalence of infections [65, 66]. Furthermore, earlier data had suggested that the use of PPIs can lead to a higher risk of spontaneous bacterial peritonitis and other infections in liver cirrhosis patients, possibly due to pH changes and consequently bacterial colonization, overgrowth and translocation [18, 67].

Hematological Effects

Alterations in hematological parameters such as thrombocytopenia, erithrocytopenia or impaired coagulation status are often present in liver cirrhosis due to various pathophysiological mechanisms such as hypersplenism, decreased synthesis of thrombopoietin, erythropoietin and coagulation factors [7, 68, 69]. One study reported a decreased ability to increase thrombopoietin as a compensatory mechanism [70]. Furthermore, data suggest that the risk of cytopenia (i.e., hematological toxicity) is higher in liver cirrhosis patients using azathioprine than in those without cirrhosis [71, 72]. Also, since the metabolism of azathioprine is related to the liver, changes in PK could also occur [73]. Similarly, interferon-α may cause thrombocytopenia and leukopenia [74]. In a randomized study with 60 patients treated with interferon-α because of viral infection, there were more cases of neutropenia or thrombocytopenia in the cirrhosis group (22% vs. 5%) [75]. Similarly, results were reported in another study [76]. Also, ribavirin-induced hemolytic anemia may occur, which has been shown in HCV patients with lower baseline platelet levels which had a greater drop in hemoglobin levels [77]. It is expected that patients with liver cirrhosis have impaired laboratory parameters, which might precipitate hematological toxicity of the applied drug, especially if such drug has known and potential hematological adverse effects. Another concern is coagulation impairment and misbalance of procoagulants and anticoagulants, which represents a large challenge when considering anticoagulant therapy [7, 78].

Hepatotoxicity

According to data, patients with CLD have a more severe form of drug-induced liver injury (DILI) in comparison to patients without CLD [7, 79, 80] with higher mortality (16% vs. 5.2%). The exact causality of liver injury (DILI or progression of CLD) is sometimes difficult to determine [7]. For example, drugs such as obeticholic acid or some antiviral HCV treatment have been associated with additional liver injury [81, 82]. In addition, regarding virus clearance, there is a possibility that a paradoxical response of the liver to virus clearance is involved [83]. Regarding obeticholic acid, the FDA issued a warning due to several incidents that resulted lethally in CP B and C liver cirrhosis, but this was most likely due to inadequate dosing (once daily instead of once weekly) [7, 83, 84].

Specific Medications in Liver Cirrhosis

Next, we will mention the use of some specific group of drugs in patients with cirrhosis.

Use of Antibiotics in Liver Cirrhosis Patients

Patients with liver cirrhosis have increased bacteriemia due to impaired function of the reticular endothelial system and hepatic destruction, therefore frequently requiring antibiotic therapy for either therapeutic or prophylactic purposes [85, 86]. In cirrhosis, prolonged half-life has been reported for tetracycline, isoniazid and rifampin, and excretion by the liver has been reported for macrolide antibiotics such as erythromycin, azithromycin, chloramphenicol and lincomycin [85]. Metronidazole and antifungal drugs such as itraconazole, ketoconazole, fluconazole and miconazole, as well as nitrofurantoin pyrazinamide should be used with caution. Additionally, in the case of the use of beta-lactams, we have to keep in mind that it can be connected with leucopenia. Aminoglycosides are connected with a higher risk of renal injury, while vancomycin can be related to increased toxicity in liver failure patients [85]. Drug prescribing information should always be investigated when using medications in special circumstances. For example, rifampicin+isoniazid-based antituberculosis therapy (ATT) has higher hepatotoxicity and higher mortality when used in patients with cirrhosis, and only in CP A, may be used as in the general population, with strict monitoring. Pyrazinamide should be avoided. In liver cirrhosis patients with CP score C, drugs such as quinolone, ethambutol and one second-line agent may be used for 12–18 months [13, 85–88]. Ketoconazole and miconazole can be used, but it is recommended to monitor their concentrations. The dose for metronidazole should be reduced by half in severe cirrhosis or with renal failure in combination. According to the literature, there is no data regarding the safe use of nitrofurantoin, chloramphenicol and pyrazinamide, and they could have potentially toxic effects, so their administration in CLD is not recommended [85, 87] (Table 22.2).

Cardiovascular Drug Therapy

Cardiovascular drug therapy and its interactions with liver cirrhosis are especially important. Patients with non-alcoholic cirrhosis related to steatosis have an increased incidence of metabolic syndrome components and associated risk factors. Labetalol, methyldopa, captopril, amiodarone and ticlopidine can be hepatotoxic; therefore, caution is needed. Alpha-blockers, ACE inhibitors, angiotensin II receptor antagonists and other drugs used in cardiovascular diseases have been reviewed regarding the need for dose adjustment [81, 89]. Statins have a good safety profile, and according to the current data, the development of liver lesions in patients on statin therapy and placebo is similar. On the other hand, idiosyncratic DILI is rare but can be potentially fatal. However, it seems that statins are safe in patients with CLD, for example, for the treatment of dyslipidemia in NAFLD and in compensated patients with chronic HBV or HCV infection [85, 90, 91].

Other Medications

In this part, we will briefly report the use of some medications such as those that are used in anesthesia as well as those that are used for pain treatment and also anticonvulsants. For example, a single dose of midazolam has been shown to have minimal

Table 22.2 List of drugs that are causing hepatotoxicity [89]

Fulminant hepatic failure
– Ketoconazole
– Trovafloxacin
– Sulfonamides
– Trimethoprim-sulfamethoxazole
Cholestatic injury
– Nitrofurantoin, Trimethoprim-sulfamethoxazole
– Penicillin G, cloxacillin, oxacillin
– Cephalosporins
– Erythromycin
– Floxacillin
– Clarithromycin
– 5-Fluorocytosine
– Trovafloxacin
– Griseofulvin
– Thiabendazole
Hepatocellular injury
– Penicillin G
– Amoxicillin
– Clindamycin
– Chloramphenicol
– Trimethoprim-sulfamethoxazole
– Trovafloxacin
– Oxacillin
– Itraconazole
– Ketoconazole
– Amphotericin

impact in patients with CP A, but there is a need for caution in liver cirrhosis patients with CP B and C scores. Accordingly, flumazenil is safe to use when there is a need to reverse the benzodiazepine effect. Similarly, the use of fentanyl in liver cirrhosis is quite safe due to almost normal elimination. Accordingly, the toxic effects of opioids can be treated with naloxone. In liver cirrhosis patients who have a need for sedation due to endoscopic procedures, the use of propofol is a good option due to its short half-life. One should bear in mind the potential adverse effects (hypotension, tachycardia, hypoventilation and QT prolongation) [85, 92–94]. On the other hand, there are some concerns regarding general anesthesia in patients with cirrhosis because it can be connected with the reduction of the hepatic blood flow that may lead to decompensation of liver cirrhosis. Safe agents are isoflurane and desflurane which are not metabolized in the liver. On the other hand, some agents such as halothane and volatile agents should be avoided. Furthermore, a combination of drugs may be beneficial since it may reduce the need for other anesthetic agents [85, 87].

Regarding pain management, there is great concern when using NSAIDs since they can lead to some serious complications. For example, the use of NSAIDs can be connected with bleeding from the gastrointestinal system, as well as with renal impairment connected with cirrhosis such as hepatorenal syndrome, and finally, their use can be related to HE and increased mortality. Thus, NSAIDs should be avoided. On the other hand, opioid analgesic drugs could precipitate encephalopathy and should also be used with caution [95, 96]. Analgesic choices should be made on an individual level taking into account the risk of adverse events and potential benefits [87, 97].

Regarding the use of anticonvulsants in liver cirrhosis patients, drugs such as phenytoin, carbamazepine and valproate can be used in cirrhosis patients with caution because they can cause hepatotoxicity. Lamotrigine and topiramate also need dose adjustment. Furthermore, antidepressants such as paroxetine and fluoxetine require dose adjustment [85, 87]. Finally, an antiemetic drug that is widely used (i.e., metoclopramide) requires significant dose reduction in cirrhotic patients.

Conclusion

Liver cirrhosis as well as other stages of CLD are multi-systemic diseases that are often associated with other comorbidities, and the liver has often a central role in drug metabolism and immunologic response. Therefore, the management of this specific group of patients is complicated. When considering influence on the drug PK both patient and drug characteristics must be taken into account. Also, alterations in pharmacological or toxicological response are possible due to pathophysiological changes in liver cirrhosis.

References

1. Periáñez-Párraga L, Martínez-López I, Ventayol-Bosch P, Puigventós-Latorre F, Delgado-Sánchez O. Drug dosage recommendations in patients with chronic liver disease. Rev Esp Enferm Dig. 2012;104:165–84.
2. Weersink RA, Bouma M, Burger DM, et al. Evidence-based recommendations to improve the safe use of drugs in patients with liver cirrhosis. Drug Saf. 2018;41:603–13.
3. Lewis JH, Stine JG. Review article: prescribing medications in patients with cirrhosis—a practical guide. Aliment Pharmacol Ther. 2013;37:1132–56.
4. Asrani SK, Devarbhavi H, Eaton J, et al. Burden of liver diseases in the world. J Hepatol. 2018;70:151–71.
5. Tsochatzis EA, Bosch J, Burroughs AK. Liver cirrhosis. Lancet. 2014;383(9930):1749–61.
6. Ge PS, Runyon BA, Campion EW. Treatment of patients with cirrhosis. N Engl J Med. 2016;375:767–77.
7. Weersink RA, Burger DM, Hayward KL, Taxis K, Drenth JPH, Borgsteede SD. Safe use of medication in patients with cirrhosis: pharmacokinetic and pharmacodynamic considerations. Expert Opin Drug Metab Toxicol. 2020;16:45–57.
8. Poordad FF. Presentation and complications associated with cirrhosis of the liver. Curr Med Res Opin. 2015;31:925–37.
9. Pugh RN, Murray-Lyon IM, Dawson JL, Pietroni MC, Williams R. Transection of the oesophagus for bleeding oesophageal varices. Br J Surg. 1973;60:646–9.
10. Cholongitas E, Marelli L, Shusang V, Senzolo M, Rolles K, Patch D, et al. A systematic review of the performance of the model for endstage liver disease (MELD) in the setting of liver transplantation. Liver Transpl. 2006;12:1049–61.

11. Guidance for industry: pharmacokinetics in patients with impaired hepatic function: study design, data analysis, and impact on dosing and labelling. U.S. Department of Health and Human Services, Food and Drug Administration, Center for Drug Evaluation and Research and Center for Biologics Evaluation and Research FDA, 2003. Availabe at http://www.fda.gov/cber/gdlns/imphep.pdf
12. Guideline on the evaluation of the pharmacokinetics of medicinal products in patients with impaired hepatic function. Committee for medicinal products for human use. EMA (CPMP/EWP/2339/02), 2005. Available at http://www.emea.europa.eu/pdfs/human/ewp/23390.
13. Delcò F, Tchambaz L, Schlienger R, Drewe J, Krähenbühl S. Dose adjustment in patients with liver disease. Drug Saf. 2005;28:529–45.
14. Breimer D. Pharmacokinetics in liver disease. Pharm Weekbl [Sci]. 1987;9(2):79–84.
15. Verbeeck RK. Pharmacokinetics and dosage adjustment in patients with hepatic dysfunction. Eur J Clin Pharmacol. 2008;64(12):1147–61.
16. Nasser AF, Heidbreder C, Liu Y, et al. Pharmacokinetics of sublingual buprenorphine and naloxone in subjects with mild to severe hepatic impairment (Child-Pugh classes A, B, and C), in hepatitis C virus-seropositive subjects, and in healthy volunteers. Clin Pharmacokinet. 2015;54(8):837–49.
17. Albarmawi A, Czock D, Gauss A, et al. CYP3A activity in severe liver cirrhosis correlates with Child-Pugh and model for end-stage liver disease (MELD) scores. Br J Clin Pharmacol. 2014;77(1):160–9.
18. Orlando R, Piccoli P, De Martin S, et al. Cytochrome P450 1A2 is a major determinant of lidocaine metabolism in vivo: effects of liver function. Clin Pharmacol Ther. 2004;75(1):80–8.
19. Food and Drug Administration. Guidance for industry: pharmacokinetics in patients with impaired hepatic function: study design, data analysis, and impact on dosing and labeling. Rockville 2003. [cited 2020 Nov 25]. Available from: https://www.fda.gov/media/71311/download.
20. European Medicines Agency. Guideline on the evaluation of the pharmacokinetics of medicinal products in patients with impaired hepatic function. London. 2005. [cited 2020 Nov 25]. Available from: https://www.ema.europa.eu/en/documents/scientific-guideline/guideline-evaluation-pharmacokinetics-medicinal-productspatients-impaired-hepatic-function_en.pdf.
21. Hasler JA, Estabrook R, Murray M, et al. Human cytochromes P450. Mol Asp Med. 1999;20(1–2):55–65.
22. Prasad B, Bhatt DK, Johnson K, et al. Abundance of phase 1 and 2 drug-metabolizing enzymes in alcoholic and hepatitis C cirrhotic livers: a quantitative targeted proteomics study. Drug Metab Dispos. 2018;46(7):943–52.
23. Gilmore IT, Thompson RP. Kinetics of 14C-glycocholic acid clearance in normal man and in patients with liver disease. Gut. 1978;19(12):1110–5.
24. Chalasani N, Gorski JC, Patel NH, et al. Hepatic and intestinal cytochrome P450 3A activity in cirrhosis: effects of transjugular intrahepatic portosystemic shunts. Hepatology. 2001;34(6):1103–8.
25. De Winter S, Verelst S, Wauters J, et al. Pharmacokinetic changes after placement of a transjugular intrahepatic portosystemic shunt. Eur J Clin Pharmacol. 2014;70(3):377.
26. Spriet I, Meyfroidt G, Maleux G, et al. The impact of a transjugular intrahepatic portosystemic shunt on the pharmacokinetics of caspofungin in a critically ill patient. Pharmacology. 2012;90(5–6):247–50.
27. Gonzalez M, Goracci L, Cruciani G, et al. Some considerations on the predictions of pharmacokinetic alterations in subjects with liver disease. Expert Opin Drug Metab Toxicol. 2014;10(10):1397–408.
28. Ohnishi A, Murakami S, Akizuki S, et al. In vivo metabolic activity of CYP2C19 and CYP3A in relation to CYP2C19 genetic polymorphism in chronic liver disease. J Clin Pharmacol. 2005;45(11):1221–9.
29. Ferron GM, Preston RA, Noveck RJ, et al. Pharmacokinetics of pantoprazole in patients with moderate and severe hepatic dysfunction. Clin Ther. 2001;23(8):1180–92.

30. Palatini P, De Martin S. Pharmacokinetic drug interactions in liver disease: an update. World J Gastroenterol. 2016;22:1260–78.
31. Bertolotti M, Ferrari A, Vitale G, et al. Effect of liver cirrhosis on the systemic availability of naltrexone in humans. J Hepatol. 1997;27(3):505–11.
32. Weersink RA, Bouma M, Burger DM, et al. Safe use of proton pump inhibitors in patients with cirrhosis. Br J Clin Pharmacol. 2018;84:1806–20.
33. Dalhoff K, Almdal TP, Bjerrum K, et al. Pharmacokinetics of paroxetine in patients with cirrhosis. Eur J Clin Pharmacol. 1991;41(4):351–4.
34. Cotting J, Reichen J, Kutz K, et al. Pharmacokinetics of isradipine in patients with chronic liver disease. Eur J Clin Pharmacol. 1990;38(6):599–603.
35. Kleinbloesem C, Van Harten J, Wilson J, et al. Nifedipine: kinetics and hemodynamic effects in patients with liver cirrhosis after intravenous and oral administration. Clin Pharmacol Ther. 1986;40(1):21–8.
36. Turncliff RZ, Dunbar JL, Dong Q, et al. Pharmacokinetics of long acting naltrexone in subjects with mild to moderate hepatic impairment. J Clin Pharmacol. 2005;45(11):1259–67.
37. Croxen F. Undesirable side effects. In: North-Lewis P, editor. Drugs and the liver: a guide to drug handling in liver dysfunction. London: Pharmaceutical Press; 2008. p. 135–43.
38. Bajaj JS, O'Leary JG, Tandon P, et al. Targets to improve quality of care for patients with hepatic encephalopathy: data from a multi-centre cohort. Aliment Pharmacol Ther. 2019;49:1518–27.
39. Grønbæk L, Watson H, Vilstrup H, et al. Benzodiazepines and risk for hepatic encephalopathy in patients with cirrhosis and ascites. United Eur Gastroenterol J. 2018;6(3):407–12.
40. Weiss N, Saint Hilaire PB, Colsch B, et al. Cerebrospinal fluid metabolomics highlights dysregulation of energy metabolism in overt hepatic encephalopathy. J Hepatol. 2016;65(6):1120–30.
41. Schentag JJ, Cerra FB, Calleri GM, et al. Age, disease, and cimetidine disposition in healthy subjects and chronically ill patients. Clin Pharmacol Ther. 1981;29(6):737–43.
42. Bakti G, Fisch HU, Karlaganis G, et al. Mechanism of the excessive sedative response of cirrhotics to benzodiazepines: model experiments with triazolam. Hepatology. 1987;7(4):629–38.
43. Jochemsen R, Joeres RP, Wesselman JG, et al. Pharmacokinetics of oral brotizolam in patients with liver cirrhosis. Br J Clin Pharmacol. 1983;16(Suppl 2):322S.
44. Perney P, Butterworth RF, Mousseau DD, et al. Plasma and CSF benzodiazepine receptor ligand concentrations in cirrhotic patients with hepatic encephalopathy: relationship to severity of encephalopathy and to pharmaceutical benzodiazepine intake. Metab Brain Dis. 1998;13(3):201–10.
45. Lavoie J, Layrargues GP, Butterworth RF. Increased densities of peripheral-type benzodiazepine receptors in brain autopsy samples from cirrhotic patients with hepatic encephalopathy. Hepatology. 1990;11(5):874–8.
46. Prakash R, Mullen KD. Mechanisms, diagnosis and management of hepatic encephalopathy. Nat Rev Gastroenterol Hepatol. 2010;7(9):515–25.
47. Butterworth RF. The liver-brain axis in liver failure: neuroinflammation and encephalopathy. Nat Rev Gastroenterol Hepatol. 2013;10(9):522–8.
48. Margo CE. Acetazolamide and advanced liver disease. Am J Ophthalmol. 1986;101(5):611.
49. Wijdicks EFM, Longo DL. Hepatic encephalopathy. N Engl J Med. 2016;375(17):1660–70.
50. Gentilini P, La Villa G, Marra F, et al. Pharmacokinetics and pharmacodynamics torasemide and furosemide in patients with diuretic resistant ascites. J Hepatol. 1996;25(4):481–90.
51. Schwartz S, Brater DC, Pound D, et al. Bioavailability, pharmacokinetics, and pharmacodynamics of torsemide in patients with cirrhosis. Clin Pharmacol Ther. 1993;54(1):90–7.
52. Villeneuve JP, Verbeeck RK, Wilkinson GR, et al. Furosemide kinetics and dynamics in patients with cirrhosis. Clin Pharmacol Ther. 1986;40(1):14–20.
53. Janků I, Perlik F, Tkaczykova M, et al. Disposition kinetics and concentration-effect relationship of metipranolol in patients with cirrhosis and healthy subjects. Eur J Clin Pharmacol. 1992;42(3):337–40.
54. Taegtmeyer AB, Haschke M, Tchambaz L, et al. A study of the relationship between serum bile acids and propranolol pharmacokinetics and pharmacodynamics in patients with liver cirrhosis and in healthy controls. PLoS One. 2014;9(6):e97885.

55. Baba T, Murabayashi S, Tomiyama T, et al. The pharmacokinetics of enalapril in patients with compensated liver cirrhosis. Br J Clin Pharmacol. 1990;29(6):766–9.
56. Thiollet M, Funck-Brentano C, Grange J, et al. The pharmacokinetics of perindopril in patients with liver cirrhosis. Br J Clin Pharmacol. 1992;33(3):326–8.
57. Ohnishi A, Tsuboi Y, Ishizaki T, et al. Kinetics and dynamics of enalapril in patients with liver cirrhosis. Clin Pharmacol Ther. 1989;45(6):657–65.
58. Clària J, Kent JD, López-Parra M, et al. Effects of celecoxib and naproxen on renal function in nonazotemic patients with cirrhosis and ascites. Hepatology. 2005;41(3):579–87.
59. Laffi G, Daskalopoulos G, Kronborg I, et al. Effects of sulindac and ibuprofen in patients with cirrhosis and ascites: an explanation for the renal-sparing effect of sulindac. Gastroenterology. 1986;90(1):182–7.
60. Tandon P, Abraldes JG, Berzigotti A, et al. Renin–angiotensin–aldosterone inhibitors in the reduction of portal pressure: a systematic review and meta-analysis. J Hepatol. 2010;53(2):273–82.
61. Salerno F, Badalamenti S. Drug-induced renal failure in cirrhosis. In: Ginès P, Arroyo V, Rodés J, editors. Ascites and renal dysfunction in liver disease. Oxford: Blackwell Publishing Ltd; 2005. p. 372–82.
62. Bernardi M, Domenicali M. The renin-angiotensin-aldosterone system in cirrhosis. In: Ginès P, Arroyo V, Rodés J, editors. Ascites and renal dysfunction in liver disease. Oxford: Blackwell Publishing Ltd.; 2005. p. 41–53.
63. Hampel H, Bynum GD, Zamora E, et al. Risk factors for the development of renal dysfunction in hospitalized patients with cirrhosis. Am J Gastroenterol. 2001;96(7):2206–10.
64. Bunchorntavakul C, Chamroonkul N, Chavalitdhamrong D. Bacterial infections in cirrhosis: a critical review and practical guidance. World J Hepatol. 2016;8(6):307–21.
65. Perrillo RR, Tamburro C, Regenstein F. Low-dose, titratable interferon alfa in decompensated liver disease caused by chronic infection with hepatitis B virus. Gastroenterology. 1995;109(3):908–16.
66. Hoofnagle JHJ, Di Bisceglie AM, Waggoner JG. Interferon alfa for patients with clinically apparent cirrhosis due to chronic hepatitis B. Gastroenterology. 1993;104(4):1116–21.
67. Bajaj JS, Zadvornova Y, Heuman DM, et al. Association of proton pump inhibitor therapy with spontaneous bacterial peritonitis in cirrhotic patients with ascites. Am J Gastroenterol. 2009;104(5):1130–4.
68. Mitchell O, Feldman DM, Diakow M, et al. The pathophysiology of thrombocytopenia in chronic liver disease. Hepat Med. 2016;8:39–50.
69. Marks PW. Hematologic manifestations of liver disease. Semin Hematol. 2013;50(3):216–21.
70. Peck-Radosavljevic M, Wichlas M, Pidlich J, et al. Blunted thrombopoietin response to interferon alfa–induced thrombocytopenia during treatment for hepatitis C. Hepatology. 1998;28(5):1424–9.
71. Heneghan MA, Allan ML, Bornstein JD, et al. Utility of thiopurine methyltransferase genotyping and phenotyping, and measurement of azathioprine metabolites in the management of patients with autoimmune hepatitis. J Hepatol. 2006;45(4):584–91.
72. Czaja AJ, Carpenter HA. Thiopurine methyltransferase deficiency and azathioprine intolerance in autoimmune hepatitis. Dig Dis Sci. 2006;51(5):968–75.
73. Aspen Pharma Trading Limited. Summary of product characteristics imuran 25 mg: medicines evaluation board; [cited 2020 Nov 28]. Available from: https://www.geneesmiddeleninformatiebank.nl/smpc/h05565_smpc.pdf.
74. Pardo M, Marriott E, Moliner MC, et al. Risks and benefits of interferon-α in the treatment of hepatitis. Drug Saf. 1995;13(5):304–16.
75. Causse X, Godinot H, Chevallier M, et al. Comparison of 1 or 3 MU of interferon alfa-2b and placebo in patients with chronic non-A, non-B hepatitis. Gastroenterology. 1991;101(2):497–502.
76. Rakela J, Wood JR, Czaja AJ, et al. Long-term versus short-term treatment with recombinant interferon alfa-2a in patients with chronic hepatitis B: a prospective, randomized treatment trial. Mayo Clin Proc. 1990;65(10):1330–5.

77. Van Vlierberghe H, Delanghe JR, De Vos M, et al. Factors influencing ribavirin-induced hemolysis. J Hepatol. 2001;34(6):911–6.
78. Lisman T, Kamphuisen PW, Northup PG, et al. Established and new generation antithrombotic drugs in patients with cirrhosis–possibilities and caveats. J Hepatol. 2013;59(2):358–66.
79. Gupta NK, Lewis JH. The use of potentially hepatotoxic drugs in patients with liver disease. Aliment Pharmacol Ther. 2008;28(9):1021–41.
80. Chalasani N, Bonkovsky HL, Fontana R, et al. Features and outcomes of 899 patients with drug-induced liver injury: the DILIN prospective study. Gastroenterology. 2015;148(7):1352.
81. Food and Drug Administration. FDA warns about serious liver injury with ocaliva (obeticholic acid) for rare chronic liver disease. 2017.[cited 2020 Now 27]. Available from: https://www.fda.gov/media/107517/download.
82. Food and Drug Administration. FDA drug safety communication: FDA warns of serious liver injury risk with hepatitis C treatments viekira pak and technivie. 2015. [cited 2020 Now 27]. Available from: https://www.fda.gov/media/94262/download.
83. Health NIo. Drug record—viekira pak: dasabur, ombitasvir, paritraprevir and ritonavir. [cited 2020 Now 27]. Available from: https://livertox.nih.gov/ViekiraPak.htm.
84. Intercept statement regarding ocaliva® (obeticholic acid) safety and dosing in Primary Biliary Cholangitis (PBC) patients. New York: Globe Newswire; 2017; Sept. 25, [4]. Available from: http://ir.interceptpharma.com/static-files/8013669f-4f8c-4543-90eb-8b479682a1e8
85. Amarapurkar DN. Prescribing medications in patients with decompensated liver cirrhosis. Int J Hepatol. 2011;2011:519526.
86. Rolando N, Philpott-Howard J, Williams R. Bacterial and fungal infection in acute liver failure. Semin Liver Dis. 1996;16:389–402.
87. Lewis JH. The rational use of potentially hepatotoxic medications in patients with underlying liver disease. Expert Opin Drug Saf. 2002;1(2):159–72.
88. Sonika U, Kar P. Tuberculosis and liver disease: management issues. Trop Gastroenterol. 2012;33(2):102–6.
89. Sokol SI, Cheng A, Frishman WH, Kaza CS. Cardiovascular drug therapy in patients with hepatic diseases and patients with congestive heart failure. J Clin Pharmacol. 2000;40(1):11–30.
90. Vuppalanchi R, Chalasani N. Statins for hyperlipidemia in patients with chronic liver disease: are they safe? Clin Gastroenterol Hepatol. 2006;4(7):838–9.
91. Kalaitzakis E, Björnsson ES. Use of statins in patients with liver disease. Minerva Gastroenterol Dietol. 2014;60(1):15–24.
92. Rodighiero V. Effects of liver disease on pharmacokinetics. An update. Clin Pharmacokinet. 1999;37:399–431.
93. Bamji N, Cohen LB. Endoscopic sedation of patients with chronic liver disease. Clin Liver Dis. 2010;14:185–94.
94. Chandok N, Watt KD. Pain management in the cirrhotic patient: the clinical challenge. Mayo Clin Proc. 2010;85:451–8.
95. Rossi S, Assis DN, Awsare M, et al. Use of over-the-counter analgesics in patients with chronic liver disease: physicians' recommendations. Drug Saf. 2008;31(3):261–70.
96. Khalid SK, Lane J, Navarro V, Garcia-Tsao G. Use of over-the-counter analgesics is not associated with acute decompensation in patients with cirrhosis. Clin Gastroenterol Hepatol. 2009;7(9):994–9.
97. Tegeder I, Lötsch J, Geisslinger G. Pharmacokinetics of opioids in liver disease. Clin Pharmacokinet. 1999;37(1):17–40.

23 Comorbidity and Comedication in Irritable Bowel Syndrome Patients

Žarko Babić

Introduction

Irritable Bowel Syndrome

Irritable bowel syndrome (IBS) is one of the most common causes of sickness in gastroenterology and internal medicine [1]. IBS is a functional gastrointestinal disorder (FIGD), recently renamed neuro-gastroenterological and motility disorder. The first definition, diagnostic, and therapeutic procedure are stated according to the Rome I consensus (criteria), which we have developed to the Rome IV consensus [2–5].

The Rome IV consensus distinguishes five groups of bowel disorders in group C, and they are irritable bowel syndrome, functional constipation, functional diarrhea, functional abdominal pain, functional abdominal bloating/distension, unspecified functional bowel disorder, and opioid-induced constipation [2–7].

The diagnostic criteria for Rome IV consensus IBS are recurrent abdominal pain, occurring on average, at least 1 day per week in the last 3 months and are associated with two or more of the following: related to defecation, associated with a change in frequency of stool, and associated with a change in form (appearance) of stool. The criteria should be fulfilled for the last 3 months with symptoms onset at least 6 months prior to diagnosis [6, 7]. The constipation and dyspepsia are differentiated according to Rome criteria and are treated per se.

Patients with IBS suffer from chronic abdominal pain, cramping, distension, and flatulating (SIC-P), mostly in the lower abdomen, with a characteristic disturbed bowel pattern, which can be constipation (SIC-C), diarrhea (SIC-D), or alternating

Ž. Babić (✉)
Department of Interventional Gastroenterology, Dubrava University Hospital, Zagreb, Croatia
e-mail: zarko.babic@zg.t-com.hr

M. Banić, D. Erceg (eds.), *Drug Interactions in Gastroenterology*, Clinical Gastroenterology, https://doi.org/10.1007/978-3-031-69800-2_23

constipation and diarrhea (SIC-M), and at the end the unclassified form (IBS-U). The patient can change the form of the disease and the intensity of the disease [6, 7]. Prevalence rates for IBS in studies around the world are from 2% to 25%. In Western countries, it is generally in the range of 10–20% for adults who have completed diagnostic criteria for IBS [6]. Most of these patients are women up to 70% [6, 7].

Comorbidity in IBS

Comorbidity is the presence of one or more additional conditions co-occurring with a primary condition [7]. The term can indicate a condition existing simultaneously, but independently with another condition or a related medical condition [7].

Whitehead et al. found that 50% of IBS patients have at least one co-morbid somatic complaint. He found also that many IBS patients have motility disorder. We have known for a while for overlap of IBS and FIGD, functional dyspepsia (FD), etc. [8].

Comorbid or extraintestinal symptoms occur frequently with irritable bowel syndrome and account for up to three-fourths of excess healthcare visits [8]. Comorbidity with other functional gastrointestinal disorders is high. The reason for this is the sharing of pathophysiological mechanisms [8].

There are a lot of comorbidity functional syndromes and common other symptoms such as other functional GI disorders (e.g., various forms of functional constipation, gastroparesis, intestinal pseudo-obstruction, etc.), fibromyalgia, chronic fatigue syndrome, multiple chemical sensitivity syndrome, post-traumatic stress disorder, chronic pelvic pain, psychological comorbidity (somatization disorder, depression, anxiety, and panic disorder), interstitial cystitis and dysuria, migraine and tension headaches, temperomandibular joint disorder, sexual-related disorders, dyspareunia, exacerbation of IBS during menstrual period, decreased libido, sleeping problems, muscle pain, fatigue, headache, dizziness, palpitations, back pain, shortness of breath, dry mouth, etc. [8–11].

IBS and Other FGID

The patient has often more than gastrointestinal functional (motility) disorder. The most common overlap is with functional dyspepsia, so Ford et al. found that it is 15–42% [10, 12].

Riedel et al. found that patients suffering from IBS have a twofold increase in intestinal and extraintestinal comorbidity rates and have impaired quality of life [6, 9]. The prevalence of IBS eightfold increased in patients with dyspepsia. Based on Rome III criteria, Wang's study has found that 24.8% of functional dyspepsia (FD) patients and 31.5% of IBS patients also had the diagnostic criteria of the other disorder [11, 13]. We have also been known for the overlap among IBSs, FD, and gastroesophageal reflux disease (GERD) for a long time, with the overlapping of IBS and FD over 80% in this study [14]. During the time the IBS patients developed FD, 22% of patients changed their symptom profile from FD to IBS, mostly female patients [8]. The overlap of IBS and GERD is significantly greater (19–25%) than the incidence of individual prevalence [8]. Overlapping patients showed higher levels of anxiety compared with patients who had only one FGID, had higher symptom ratings of GERD, and had lower quality of life [8, 15]. The visceral hyperalgesia can explain the high prevalence of overlapping [8].

IBS and Other Gastrointestinal Diseases

IBS and inflammatory bowel disease (IBD) are in some individuals difficult to distinguish because symptoms can be very similar to each other, due to sharing pathophysiological mechanisms [8]. Some forms of IBS have similar, not only clinical manifestations but also similar endoscopy and pathohistological findings. Further diagnostic procedures can distinguish that doubt (e.g., fecal calprotectin, follow-up of IBS patient, etc.)

A similar condition is in exocrine pancreatic insufficiency (EPI), where the EPI is detected in 6% of patients who fulfilled Rome II criteria for IBS, but further diagnostic procedures can distinguish that doubt [16]. Similar inflammatory processes are probably the reason for that [8, 16].

Lactose intolerance can cause confusion in the IBS diagnosis and sometimes can share the symptoms with IBS-D, also causing inflammatory processes in the intestine [8].

IBS and Other Extraintestinal Disorders

Non-gastrointestinal disorders are extraintestinal disorders such as fibromyalgia syndrome (FMS), chronic fatigue syndrome (CFS), chronic pelvic pain (CPP), sexual dysfunction (SXD), and sleep disturbances (SLD) [8].

Somatic Disorders

The prevalence of IBS in patients with FMS ranges from 30% to 35% but in some studies up to 70% [8].

FMS is considered a disorder of somatic hypersensitivity, while IBS is considered a disorder of visceral hypersensitivity [12, 13]. Both groups of patients, IBS and FMS, had more severe disorders such as global feeling of well-being, sleep disturbances, relation of stress to symptoms, physician visits, concerns about illness, and psychological distress, than those with IBS only [8, 12, 13].

The prevalence of CFS is about 0.4% in the general population, up to 70% in FMS and 14–92% in IBS patients [8, 17], and the overlapping with the abovementioned syndromes is significantly higher [8].

CPP has a prevalence of 14% in IBS patients and 29–79% in women IBS patients. Unfortunately, 47% of women patients undergoing laparoscopy have had CPP, at least had IBS, but some of them have without any pathological finding, and all of that we have known for a lot of time [18, 19].

SXD is increased in IBS patients such as reduced sexual drive, dyspareunia, decreased libido 14–36%, etc. [8, 18].

Mental Disorders

IBS patients have also mental symptoms. That includes predominantly depressive symptoms with exhaustion, sleeping problems, loss of appetite, anxiety with nervousness, worrying, rumination, and panic attacks, but these patients are very often in subclinical form [20, 21]. The rate of this mental problem in IBS patients is sometimes more than 90% in some studies [20, 21].

The prevalence studies vary in a large range (all depending on the level of healthcare) from 6% to 70% for depressive, from 5% to 50% for anxiety disorders, and between 0% and 41% for panic disorder who had characteristic episodic vegetative symptoms [8, 20, 21]. Some studies reported an increased prevalence of trauma disorders (e.g., post-traumatic distress) up to 36% [6, 20, 21]. Patients with panic attacks have a risk of IBS up to 47%, with depressive disorders up to 59%, and with generalized anxiety disorder 17–37% [20]. High prevalence is also for patients with eating disorders [20, 21].

A somatoform disorder (SFD) is defined as when a patient has unexplained, persistent, and disabling symptoms accompanied by persistent requests for medical investigations (repeated negative findings and reassurances by doctors that the symptoms have no physical basis). The diagnosis of SFD is also a symptom-based category and tries to avoid etiological assumptions [20–22].

The trait that describes the term somatization is defined as a tendency to experience and communicate psychological distress in the form of somatic symptoms and to seek medical help for them [20–22].

The IBS score is higher on somatization than healthy individuals, and lower in somatoform disorders [23, 24]. Somatization is a significant psychological factor directly associated with IBS severity [24].

In everyday practice, it is important to distinguish the somatic from the psychological part of the disease.

According to the American Psychiatric Association, in 2013, the former category of somatoform disorders was revised and renamed somatic symptom disorder (SSD), and it is defined by three criteria:

1. One or more somatic symptoms that are distressing and/or result in significant disruption of daily life.
2. Excessive thoughts, feelings, or behaviors related to the somatic symptoms or associated health concerns.
3. Disproportionate and persistent thoughts about the seriousness of one's symptoms, persistently high level of anxiety about health or symptoms, or excessive time and energy devoted to these symptoms or health concerns.

We have still no demand for a lack of medical explanation of symptoms. The concept of a somatic symptom disorder describes the common phenomenon that somatic symptoms are combined with psychobehavioral characteristics. The diagnosis can be the primary diagnosis in patients, or it can be the secondary diagnosis in patients who have a defined organic illness [20, 24, 25].

For a while, we have knowledge that the psychological dimension of IBS has clinical relevance. The presence of other somatic (organic and bodily) symptoms beyond the IBS gathers more symptomatology that is associated with higher functional impairment, more psychological distress, and lower quality of life [23].

The presence of psychiatric comorbidity in IBS patients is associated with more severe gastrointestinal symptoms and poorer therapeutic outcomes [20, 26].

There are a lot of publications that describe the evidence that it is rather psychological factors, such as somatization, trait anxiety, maladaptive coping, and catastrophizing, than somatic factors that correlate with the severity of IBS and poorer outcomes [26]. But we also know that the severe IBS symptoms are not related to their other bodily symptoms [26].

Central nervous processes could modulate signals from the periphery as suggested by Rapps et al. The central modulates peripheral input and can underlie the conscious experience of symptoms [25].

So, visceral and other pains are not only seen as pure sensations but also as a homoeostatic emotion. This emotion indicates disturbances in the body and its interaction with the environment.

For that reason, IBS, other FSSs, and somatoform disorders could be conceptualized as disorders of interception (disorders of the sense of the physiological condition of the body) [26, 27].

Etiology and Pathophysiology of IBS and Relations to Comorbidity

The potential mechanisms involved in gut dysfunction, visceral sensation, and at least two symptoms are an epithelial barrier, microbiota in the gut, antigens consumed in food, and bile acids that produce dysregulation or abnormal response to sensorial and motoric functions [28]. In this path, the hypothalamus-pituitary and adrenal (HPA) axis, the immune system (IMS), the brain-gut axis (BGA), and enteric systems (ENS) are involved. Psychosocial factors are also involved in this story. So according to this, we have potential biomarkers, psycho-markers for SIC, comorbidity disorders such as anxiety and depression that have an influence on abdominal symptoms, and psychosocial factors such as stress. All of these factors have repercussions on intestinal motility and visceral sensations [28].

Epithelial Barrier

The epithelial barrier, not only as the surface (first barrier and permeability), has the first role in the etiology and pathophysiology process with bacteria and immune response too. Increased permeability was first described in all postinfectious IBS [28, 29] and the IBS-D form of the disease [29]. The morphological and functional changes in intestinal permeability are explained by the abnormal gene and protein expression of tight junction proteins. The expression of occludin and zonula occludens protein 1 is reduced. We also know that the tight junction proteins claudin and cingulin are changed [27]. This is a result of bacteria-mediated and protein-mediated changes (degradation) by low-grade inflammation [28]. Inflammatory mediators, eicosanoids, proteases, and histamine increase the intestinal epithelial permeability. This can include ENS neurons which may amplify this effect of permeability [28] in the intestine and can increase the development of diarrhea and pain and their severity. The increased intervillous spaces are an indication of increased intestinal permeability and development of IBS and the role of food in this process [28].

Bile Acids

The increase of the bile fecal acids in the intestine caused by the excretion and synthesis of serum C4 accelerates intestine transit and induces diarrhea and visceral sensations in IBS. Genes that are involved in bile acid synthesis are associated with colonic transit in the form of IBS-D [30].

Immune Response

The immune response is also included in the IBS development [28, 31]. About one-third of patients with IBD who are in remission have IBS symptoms [28, 31]. The increase of T-cell and mast cell infiltration in the mucosa of the small and large intestines is found in IBS patients [28, 32]. The immune cell activation is present in half of the IBS patients [27, 31]. The role of mast cells is in not only activating but also in the maintenance of low-grade inflammation in these patients [28, 32, 33]. It is also detected that a higher amount of mast cells are present in biopsy supernatants with both histamine and protease level elevation [28, 31, 32]. In the end, the microbiota can play a role in these processes [28].

Neuroimmune in IBS Interactions (Etiological and Pathophysiological)

The neuroimmune interactions are proven after the isolation of some immune modulators in biopsy specimens in the gut in IBS patients [28]. Mast cells and enteroendocrine cells participate in some role in the neural signaling and activation of human ENS neurons. In this process, the mast cell-derived histamine, enteroendocrine-derived serotonin, and protease-dependent mechanism are included [28, 32]. The mast cell-secreted proteases (serine and cysteine) are present in large amounts in the stool of IBS patients [28] and are accused of intestinal hypersensitivity and dilatation in IBS-D patients [28, 32]. But cysteine proteases are augmented in IBS-C also [27]. The increase of proteases correlates with abdominal impaired epithelial permeability and with pain [28]. The nerve stimuli to the brain are conveyed by protease-activated nociceptors via serine protease activation of the least ones [28].

The importance of agonists of the transient receptor potential cation channels (TRPs) which are important in sensory hyperalgesia. The increase in the level of polyunsaturated fatty acids is detected in colon biopsy samples in IBS individuals [28]. Peripheral blood mononuclear cells (PBMC) supernatants cause mechanical hypersensitivity of visceral afferents via tumor necrosis factor and transient cation channel subfamily transient receptor potential cation channels on human and animals type 1 (TRPA 1) in IBS patients. This all has structural implementation to the gut in mucosal sensory fibers, e.g., more than 56% in mucosal neurons and neuronal outgrowth and has an increase in neurite growth and mRNA expression of growth-associated protein 43 (neuromodulin) [28].

Microbiota

The gastrointestinal microbiota is an important ecosystem that inhibits the entire gastrointestinal tract and has an influence on a lot of mechanisms of peristaltic activity immunology response in visceral hypersensitivity etc. [28]. The microbiota is a very complex organic structure in the intestine tract and has individual variability but has also the rules in and influence on all previous elaborated and other mechanisms.

We know the presence of good bacteria in the intestinal tract that have an influence on normal peristalsis, sensitivity, and immune response of the organism [28]. The Clostridiales are significantly depleted, and Ruminococcus torques are enriched in IBS patients. The dysbiosis was also observed in Rome meetings several times [1–7, 28]. The colonization of animals with microbiota from IBS patients can induce visceral hypersensitivity [34]. The diet can have an effect on microbiota and symptoms in IBS patients [28]. The content of fermentable oligosaccharides, disaccharides, monosaccharides and polyols (called FODMAP), and the sweeteners (fructo-oligosaccharides) or fiber (psyllium) can improve symptoms in IBS patients, but not in all of them [1–7, 28, 32].

The important role of microbiota is the degradation of non-digestible components. Fermentation of carbohydrates has a positive effect on the energy supply to intestinal cells and decreases inflammation via short-chain fatty acids [27]. Sometimes, this mechanism goes to wrong way with hyper- or hypoproduction of metabolites, gas production, etc. and worsening of symptoms in IBS patients [28]. Microbiota stimulates regulatory T-cell differentiation and has a balance between pro-inflammatory and anti-inflammatory mechanisms via short-chain fatty acids [28, 32]. Another way is in protein degradation, and an increased level of proteases probably caused by a significant increase in number in one other carbohydrate-utilizing bacteria, Dorea spp., is observed in IBS patients. This is the case in Western eating habits with insufficient protease degradation. Protein inhibitors such as serine are mostly produced by bifidobacteria [28]. Depletion of bifidobacteria is mentioned in IBS patients [28, 32]. Protein degradation produces a lot of substances that negatively influence cell metabolism [28, 32]. Elevation in the number of gamma proteobacteria has a negative influence on bowel symptoms [28, 32].

About 90% of 5-HT is produced by enteroendocrine cells in the gastrointestinal tract. The intestinal bacteria stimulate the mechanism of 5-HT synthesis [28]. Firmicutes phylum is elevated over Bacteroides in IBS patients [28].

Brain and Intestine

As we explained above, the IBS is strictly correlated and overlaps with various mental disorders [20–25, 35].

The brain, autonomic nervous system, and the HPA axis can influence intestinal motility and fluid secretion, intestinal epithelial permeability, and immune function to gut microbiota [21, 28, 32, 34].

All these peripheral manifestations have an influence on the alteration of the brain in their structure and function [21, 28]. So, we can conclude, that it is bidirectional communication, and much of these inflammations are tuned up or down [28]. On functional MR and other images, we can see structural changes and activity changes in gray matter and white matter in various parts of the human brain [20, 27]. Sex differences are detected on such scanning [21, 28]. We can connect these findings to IBS symptoms, manifestations and the forms of IBS including microbiota, immune reaction and changes, and gene expression [21, 28]. The involvement of neurotrophins (nerve growth factor) and brain-derived neurotrophic agents has an influence on hypersensitivity, neuronal survival, maturation, and migration in the peripheral and central nervous system [21]. The massive release of nerve growth factors in the peripheral circulation with an increase of mRNA in the hypothalamus at the same time can have an influence on neuroendocrine response behavioral response after psychosocial stress [21, 28]. Brain-derived neurotrophic agent is found to be elevated in the gut of IBS patients [21]. Serotonin transporter gene polymorphism is related to a higher risk of depression in IBS patients [21]. Polymorphism can affect the serotonergic, adrenergic, and opioidergic systems and is involved in IBS pathophysiology [21, 28].

Genetic and Epigenetic Changes

The genetic and epigenetic changes and disturbances have an influence on the pathogenesis of IBS and suggest disturbed intestinal barrier function [28].

The silencing of the microRNSA-29 and amplifying mir-199 expression can have important therapeutic implications for some selected IBS patients and their symptoms caused by increased intestinal permeability or hypersensitivity. Genes that have an influence on epithelial barrier function encoding proteins (Cadelhin-CDH1), cell division cycle 42, the immune system (IL6, IL10, and TNF) encoding cytokines, and neuronal signal transduction, neuroexophilin, and sodium voltage-gated channel alpha-subunit were studied. A small study has shown the association of IBS and locus chromosome 10 [27, 28]. Mutations in genes have also been shown to be associated with IBS (solute carrier family 67 member and 5-HT receptor—5HTR3A, HTR3E, and HTR4) [28]. Genes included in bole acid synthesis (Klotho-beta), fibroblast growth factor, and G protein-coupled bile acid receptor 1 are associated with faster colon transport time in IBD-D patients and correlate to the colonic transit response to chenodeoxycholic acid in IBS-C [28]. Epigenetics are important in IBS patients with different expression profiles of mRNA-29a and others in the intestinal mucosa, and regulation of NK factor, claudin, NK correlated to permeability, etc. [28]. Diminished miR-199 correlates with upregulation of TPRV1 and visceral hypersensitivity [28]. The 5-HT receptor genes are associated with IBS-D. The disturbed expression regulation of mRNA leads to IBD. The miR-150 is associated with IBD and pain, with an effect on colonic musculature function [28].

Therapy of IBS

Adequate therapy of IBS alone or in combination with other comorbidity conditions' therapy protocols is needed as the first step in the medication of IBS patients [28]. The routine therapy of IBS depends on the form of the disease, but according to the pathophysiological mechanisms explained above, the therapy includes the use of the lifestyle form (exercise) and eating habits (including fiber diet and excluding the substances that can provoke IBS symptoms such as fat, food that provoke excessive bile acid secretion—all mechanisms are explained in the above section), use of probiotics (all of them have a positive effect to the regulation of peristaltic activity), use of laxatives (various groups such as osmotic laxatives, emollient, volume expanders, etc.), use of antidiarrheals (inhibitors of peristaltic activity), sometimes the use of prokinetics, and in the most refractory form of the disease, the use of magnesium salts (also is the osmotic laxative). In some patients, the eradication of infection is needed for the regulation of peristaltic activity [28]. In view of pathophysiological investigations, the use of 5-HT antagonists such as alosetron, ramosetron, and ondansetron is effective in IBS-D refractory patients [28]. The therapy of IBS can influence the other comorbidity conditions [28].

Therapy of IBS-Related Comorbidity Conditions

Therapy of Gastrointestinal-Related Comorbidity

Recent therapy of *GERB*, without any radical changes, has been well-known for more than the last 30 years after proton pump inhibitors (PPI) were discovered and are on the market [36–43]. This therapy is polished in that last period [36], but it was proven during the last 30 years that therapy in adequate doses and duration is needed for successful and not-too-expensive therapy (Table 23.1) [36–43]. The dosage and duration depend on clinical condition, degree of symptoms (semi-quantified or quantified by different scoring systems, e.g., DeMeester score and Montreal

Table 23.1 Comorbidity conditions in irritable bowel syndrome and therapy

Comorbidity	Therapy
Gastrointestinal	
Dyspepsia	IPP, H2RA, probiotics, fiber or other diet, neuromodulators (antidepressants, anxiolytics, antipsychotics, visceral analgesics), motilitone, iberogast
GERD	IPP, H2RA, antacids, prokinetics
H. Pylori	Eradication therapy (Maastricht V protocol)
FGID	Probiotics, fiber or other diet, prokinetics, antidepressants
IBD	Diet, 5-ASA, corticosteroids, biological therapy
EPI	Diet, supplement therapy (pancreatin), pain relief, IPP
Extraintestinal disorders	
FMS	Supporting therapy, explanations small working groups, chronic pain courses, exercises, use of actometer, mediators of descending inhibition in the nervous system nonpharmacological therapy, paracetamol, tramadol, pramipexole
CPP	NSAID, adhesiolysis, hysterectomy, SNRIs, antiepileptics acupuncture, peripheral neuromodulators, hormonal therapy
SXD	*Men:* Blood flow, nitric oxide, hormonal influences, inflammatory diseases, alcoholism, depression, fatigue, recreational and other serious drugs, hypoactive sexual disorder, relationship problems, humiliation, sexual aversion, testosterone deficiency, diabetes mellitus, age, arterial hypertension, dyslipidaemia, chronic kidney and liver diseases, psychosocial factors, bicycling, ejaculatory disorders, premature ejaculation, delayed ejaculation, anejaculation, male anorgasmia
	Women: Arterial hypertension, coronary artery disease, dermatologic conditions, diabetes mellitus, gynecological conditions (infections, endometriosis, CPP, pelvic organic prolapse, etc.), arthritis, hypothyroidism, malignancies, neuromuscular disorders, spinal cord injuries, Parkinson disease, pituitary tumor, hyperprolactinaemia and renal failure, menopause
SLD	Changing of habits, exercises, medication, psychological th., pain relief
Mental related	
Anxiety	Anxiolytics and antidepressants
Depression	Anxiolytics and antidepressants (TCAs and SSRIs)

FIGD functional gastrointestinal disorder, *IBD* inflammatory bowel disease, *EPI* exocrine pancreatic insufficiency, *LI* lactose intolerance, *FMS* fibromyalgia syndrome, *CFS* chronic fatigue syndrome, *CPP* chronic pelvic pain, *SXD* sexual dysfunction, *SLD* sleep disturbances

classification of reflux disease) in mild forms, endoscopy findings (degree of esophagitis according to Los Angeles or Savary-Miller score), and at least esophageal manometry and 24 h-Ph-metry findings in severe or unclarified forms of GERB, in the past with other methods such as one of the symptom scores and only endoscopy and esophageal scintigraphy, and in recent times according to Lyon consensus or to Dalbir and Fass, both published in Gut, in 2018 [36, 37, 44–49].

The suggested therapy schedule is lifestyle modification, compliance and adherence assessment, splitting the PPI dose, changing to another PPI, and adding non-PPI medication (H2RA, Gaviscon, baclofen, etc.). If symptoms are improved, the suggestion is to taper down to the lowest dose that controls patient symptoms [36]. If this is not the case, the patient has to double the PPI dose and undergo an upper endoscopy with biopsies to treat mucosal abnormality. After that, the patient has to do esophageal Ph-metry and impedance-pH on treatment [37]. Depending on 24 h esophageal Ph-metry, if abnormal reflux is present, the compliance and lifestyle modification medication should be reevaluated and regulated. Esophageal manometry should be suggested in such patients, and if it is abnormal, the motility abnormality has to be treated [25, 37]. If the manometry is normal or suggests motility disorders caused by reflux, the Ph-metry should be done. If the Ph-metry result is normal but the symptom index is positive, the reflux hypersensitivity is detected and H2RS therapy, endoscopic treatment, anti-reflux surgery, neuromodulators, psychosocial intervention, and complementary medicine should be considered. If the normal Ph test is after manometry and the patient does not have symptoms anymore, the functional heartburn should be diagnosed and followed with medication with neuromodulators, psychological intervention, and complementary medicine [36, 37].

In patients with resistance to therapy or with relapses or in patients who do not have improvement on endoscopy, prolonged or continuous therapy is needed [36, 37].

The outcome depends on an accurate diagnostic procedure. The oesophagitis healing is the basis measure for therapeutic trials. Visible oesophagitis is rarely seen in refractory oesophagitis [36, 37]. That is the reason why the symptom description is important to outcome measurement. Also are in use symptom questionnaires, pictograms, pictograms with visual descriptions of symptoms, visual analog scales, adequate vs. inadequate relief, disease-specific questionnaires and quality-of-life questionnaires, which are called patient-report outcome questionnaires [37].

The *selection of PPI in GERD therapy* depends on the need to avoid medical interactions with other medications in particular patients [50–57]. Some PPIs have the same metabolic pathway as the other medication needed (for other diseases) in this group of patients, and some PPI combinations with other medicaments do not have or have it to a negligible degree (see chapter interactions) [50–57]. Sometimes, it is combined with inhibitors of H2-receptors (H2RA) in prolonged or resistant forms of GERD [50–57].

Chronic constipation, functional constipation is diagnosed according to Rome IV criteria and is treated with prokinetics, probiotics, and a fiber diet [2–7].

Dyspepsia can be organic and functional [2–8]. The dyspepsia can be diagnosed according to Rome IV criteria [2–7]. The etiology and pathophysiology of IBS and dyspepsia have a lot of connection points in a lot of segments (changes in gastrointestinal motility, immunology changes, microbiota, visceral hypersensitivity, stress, chronic visceral pain, and brain-gut axis), and that results in similar principles of therapeutic modality [2–7, 58–66]. Some forms of dyspepsia can overlap with IBS [2–7, 58–66]. Dyspepsia therapy is similar to the therapy of IBS [2–7]. The dyspepsia could be diagnosed according to Rome IV criteria [2–7, 58–66].

The first step in dyspepsia treatment is *Helicobacter pylori* (HP) infection detection and eradication. According to the Maastricht V protocol, we have the best available evidence for recommendations to treat HP infection (Table 23.1). The empirical first-line triple therapy using PPI, clarithromycin, amoxicillin, or metronidazole is suggested in the areas with clarithromycin resistance lower than 15% success, and the eradication rate is in the range of acceptance [67]. The triple therapy consisting of a proton pump inhibitor, amoxicillin, and metronidazole for 14 days is recommended as the first-line therapy and is suggested for the areas with HP resistance to clarithromycin higher than 15%, and the metronidazole resistance is still low [67]. In areas where *H. pylori* resistance is greater than 15% for both clarithromycin and metronidazole, suggested first-line treatment is quadruple bismuth therapy using PPI, clarithromycin, amoxicillin, and nitroimidazole with bismuth for 14 days [67]. If there is a failure of these treatments or an allergy to any of these drugs, further recommendations of the Maastricht V consensus should be followed [67].

Another challenge is to treat symptoms with *PPIs alone*, and therapy with standard or low doses is quite effective in these patients [68–70].

Prokinetics are the gastrointestinal tract motor function stimulators and affect functional dyspepsia patients (Table 23.1). They have a function in beta-blocking of dopamine receptors. They inhibit one acetylcholine enzyme and 5-HT-4 receptors [71].

Itopride improves symptoms in patients with functional dyspepsia of postprandial fullness and satiety [72]. Itopride has antagonistic effects on dopamine D2 receptors by inhibiting acetylcholinesterase.

Acotiamide increases the acetylcholine effect in the enteric nervous system and modulates and improves gastric contractions resulting in improvement of delayed gastric emptying [73]. During the second week of treatment, improvement was achieved under the doses of 100 mg (during 4 weeks of therapy) [73].

Neuromodulators are antidepressants, anxiolytics, antipsychotics, and visceral analgesics (Table 23.1).

This medication has proven value in the treatment of disorders of BGA [74, 75].

Their effects on the central nervous system and at the same time their other effect of modulating *peripheral* neurotransmitters is used in therapy. Their value is in reducing symptom severity and quality of life in patients with these disorders.

In patients who have mildly intense, intermittent symptoms, or symptoms associated with bowel movements, peripheral neuromodulators are successful in therapy [74, 75].

Central neuromodulators are suggested to be added to other therapies in patients with chronic and serious symptoms and are successful in patients with abdominal pain, nausea, and vomiting having extra-intestinal symptoms at the same time [74, 75].

Tricyclic antidepressants should be prescribed in low effective doses (adverse events).

The success of amitriptyline 50 mg daily for 10 weeks has been shown to relieve symptoms [76].

Adding to the standard patient's medication the medication with mirtazapine (15 mg daily during the period of 8 weeks) has shown efficacy in ameliorating early satiety, nutrient tolerance, weight loss, and improving quality of life in patients with dyspepsia [77].

Atypical antipsychotic quetiapine was successful in patients with severe BGA disturbance due to its analgesic effect and increasing the effect of antidepressants [78].

Three times a day, 10 mg of *buspirone* (group of azapirones) for 4 weeks, was effective in reducing dyspeptic symptoms and increasing gastric accommodation in patients with FD, compared to placebo.

It significantly ameliorated postprandial fullness, early satiation, and upper abdominal bloating [79].

The botanical drug *motilitone* has excellent prokinetic effects, gastric fundus relaxation with visceral analgesia, and improvement of dyspeptic symptoms and gastrointestinal in patients with FD [80].

The second botanical drug *iberogast* composed of nine plant extracts acts on various mechanisms, normalizes motility and the microbiota, reduces hypersensitivity and gastric acid hypersecretion, suppresses inflammation in the stomach, and is effective in FD and IBS. Iberogast is well-tolerated for use in patients independent of other comorbidities. Therefore, it has a great advantage of being used because dyspepsia is the most common chronic disorder [81].

The *pancreatic insufficiency* is detected by clinical findings (for exocrine insufficiency pain, fatty stool, weight loss, and endocrine diabetes mellitus) and routine laboratory findings using markers (e.g., fecal elastase test, imaging methods ultrasound, CT, MR, EUS, and eventually ERCP) and is medicated with diet, pain relief medicaments, and pancreatic enzyme supplements according to the international protocol (Table 23.1) [82].

When bile acids are accused of diarrhea or worsening of the IBS-D form of the disease, medication with ursodeoxycholic acid supplements is needed for improvement [28, 31–33].

Lactose intolerance is medicated by the exclusion of lactose from the eating habits [28, 31–33].

Therapy of Extraintestinal-Related Comorbidity

The *FMS* therapy is multimodal and multidisciplinary combining pharmacological and nonpharmacological processes suggested by the Australian group [83]. Nonpharmacological approaches tend to overcome medication therapy because they have more success [83]. Multimodal approach has positive results (Table 23.1). Nonpharmacological therapy is based on supporting therapy, explanations small working groups, chronic pain courses, etc. Exercises (biomechanical approach) monitored by a physical therapist are successful, but daily physical activity supported by an actometer is strongly recommended in this group of patients [83].

The pharmacological approach has a supportive role in symptom management [83]. The drugs should be taken in the lowest doses as it is possible. The use of anti-pain relief drugs and antidepressants should be prescribed in low doses that have effects and for the shortest time period as it is possible [83]. Mediators of descending inhibition in the nervous system include serotonin and noradrenaline, and concentrations are reduced in FM patients [83]. Duloxetine at 60 mg daily is successful in pain relief in 50% of cases. Milnacipran inhibits the reuptake of serotonin and noradrenaline at a recommended dose of 100 mg per day [83]. Antiepileptic drugs are effective like pregabalin in 50% of cases with pain relief [83]. Tramadol, pramipexole, and memantine are also therapy options [83]. There is no evidence of paracetamol efficacy when used alone [83].

The therapy of *CPP* (which represents noncyclic pain perceived to be pelvic and persists for 3–6 months or longer and is unrelated to pregnancy) is treated on a few levels (Table 23.1) [84]. Some of them have probable etiology and do not have an identified cause of symptoms [84]. Acute or chronic neuropathic pain should be treated by a specialist in this area. We have topical analgesics, system analgesics (nonsteroidal anti-inflammatory drugs (NSAIDs)), muscle relaxants, and empiric hormonal therapy [84]. Pelvic floor physical therapy is an option. The trigger point injection therapy is used when the trigger points were found [84]. The next step is nerve blocking [84]. The next option is surgical treatment which relieves pain and sometimes resolves the etiological source of pain in this group of patients, e.g., adhesiolysis and hysterectomy [84]. In this group of patients, neuropathic pain relief with neuromodulators, TCAs, anticonvulsants (e.g., pregabalin and gabapentin), SNRIs, and antiepileptics is an option [84]. Sometimes exercise is recommended [84]. We have fewer benefits from acupuncture peripheral neuromodulators and dietary strategies [84]. Endometriosis should be treated [84]. Adjuvant therapy includes antipsychotics, cannabis, etc. [84]. If there is an infection, it should be treated first [84].

SXD therapy is divided into two segments, sexual dysfunction in men and women [84, 85]. In both, the physiology is different but has some similar points; the same points explained in the part of this chapter, etiology and pathophysiology of IBS [28]. The medical conditions that impact sexual function in women probably are some diseases such as arterial hypertension, coronary artery disease, dermatologic conditions, diabetes mellitus, gynaecological conditions (infections, endometriosis, CPP, pelvic organic prolapse, etc.), arthritis, hypothyroidism, malignancies, neuromuscular disorders, spinal cord injuries, Parkinson disease, pituitary tumor, hyperprolactinemia and renal failure, and menopause, and each of them has to be treated for the final result (Table 23.1) [84].

The SXD in men has neural impact, blood flow, nitric oxide, hormonal influences, inflammatory diseases, alcoholism, depression, fatigue, recreational and other serious drugs, hypoactive sexual disorder, relationship problems, humiliation, sexual aversion, testosterone deficiency, diabetes mellitus, age, arterial hypertension, dyslipidaemia, chronic kidney and liver diseases, psychosocial factors, bicycling, ejaculatory disorders, premature ejaculation, delayed ejaculation, anejaculation, male anorgasmia, etc., and each of them should be treated separately by an educated and well-experienced specialist [85–88].

Therapy of Mental Comorbidity

The relations and overlap of mechanisms of IBS and mental disorders are explained above [2–8, 20–27, 32, 34, 35]. For this reason, therapy for both conditions is needed (Table 23.1), but sometimes IBS therapy in severe and refractory forms of IBS, anxiolytics and antidepressants are needed to release IBS symptoms [2–8, 20–27, 32, 34, 35]. The use of tricyclic antidepressants (TCAs) or selective serotonin reuptake inhibitors (SSRIs) is recommended in pain treatment in patients who have refractory symptoms under antispasmodics medication and after dietary modifications [28]. The mechanisms of antidepressants in IBS patients are explained by both peripheral via histaminergic and cholinergic transmission and via the central way by modulation of visceral sensory afferents and central transmission.

We can conclude that the SSRIs are well-tolerated [28]. Dry mouth, constipation, drowsiness, and fatigue are mentioned during TSA medication [28]. TCAs have better outcome success in IBS-D patients than in the IBS-C patients [28].

Therapy of Depression Related to IBS

In the therapy of depression, we have the option to use TCAs and SSRIs (Table 23.1) [28, 36].

SSRIs are the appropriate first-line options for the treatment of depression alone along with psychotherapeutic interventions. Many patients do not respond to different options or are intolerant to the undesired effects of medications [36]. Other therapy has less success in IBS patients who have depression.

In general, we can say that about 60% of patients with depression have residual impairments even after treatment [36]. Patients who have residual symptoms and functional impairment are at higher risk for relapse of depression. The weakening of the health-related, quality of life effects of depression has an adverse impact on individuals, resulting in academic, interpersonal, social, and occupational impairment. After the person is in remission, depression has higher rates of recurrence in up to 80% of all patients with a chance to become chronic in 20% of patients. After the beginning dose, they should be the lowest, which has success in the therapy [28, 36].

So, the therapy of depression is not to be performed by a gastroenterologist. This therapy will be better performed by a psychiatrist with experience in IBS patients in coordination with a gastroenterologist. It is more and more often that serious gastroenterology departments have a psychologist and psychiatrist in their group [28, 36].

Therapy of Anxiety Related to IBS

In therapy of anxiety (Table 23.1), patients have to be treated according to the anxiety disorder diagnosed by the diagnostic and statistical manual of mental disorder (DSM-5) classification [37]. The used medication is SSRIs, selective serotonin-norepinephrine uptake inhibitors (SNRIs), as the first line of therapy. Other medications include TCAs, calcium modulators, azapirone, and selective and reversible inhibitors of monoaminoxidase (RIMA) [37]. Also, other drugs are in medication protocols such as agomelatine, quetiapine, and vortioxetine, but not in the IBDS patients. In around 75% of the patients, the lower doses are sufficient to have success in these patients [37].

This therapy is also very complex and is out of the gastroenterologist's area of knowledge and experience.

This therapy will be better performed by a psychiatrist with experience in IBS patients in coordination with a gastroenterologist. It is more and more often that serious gastroenterology departments have psychologists and psychiatrists in their group.

Novel Therapy Strategies for IBS

With a clear knowledge of overlapping mechanisms in the etiology and pathophysiology, the new experimental therapy was in development [32]. The targets of these novel therapies are master cell maturation and the development of steam cell factor signaling with blocking C-kit signaling. The target is master cell activation and degranulation and secretion of IgE epsilon receptor signaling.

The experiments with mast cell stabilizers with inhibition of master cell degranulation and corticotropin-releasing factor antagonists were successful too [32]. The neurokinin receptors that block NK1/2/3 antagonists were under investigation [32]. The Syk tyrosine kinase that blocks the epsilon receptor of master cell activators, the targeting master cell mediators with protease-activated receptors, histamine which are protease-activated receptors, and the histamine 1 receptor antagonist were all investigated with high hopes at the mast cell potential therapeutic targets for IBS [32].

References

1. Levy RL, Whitehead WE, Von Korff MR, Feld AD. Intergenerational transmission of gastrointestinal illness behavior. Am J Gastroenterol. 2000;95:451–6.
2. Schmulson M, Drossman D. What is new in Rome IV. J Neurogastroenterol Motil. 2017;23(2):151–63. https://doi.org/10.5056/jnm16214.
3. Drossman DA. Functional gastrointestinal disorders: history, pathophysiology, clinical features and Rome IV. Gastroenterology. 2016;150(6):1262–79. https://doi.org/10.1053/j.gastro.2016.02.032.
4. Stanghellini V, Chan FK, Hasler WL, Malagelada JR, Suzuki H, Tack J, et al. Gastroduodenal disorders. Gastroenterology. 2016;150(6):1380–92. https://doi.org/10.1053/j.gastro.2016.02.011.
5. Stanghellini V, Talley NJ, Chan F. Rome IV—gastroduodenal disorders. Gastroenterology. 2016;150(6):1380–92.
6. Smiren M, Palson OS, Whitehead WE. Update on Rome IC criteria for colorectal disorders: implication for clinical practice. Curr Gastroenterol Rep. 2017;18:15. https://doi.org/10.1007/s11894-017.0554-0.
7. Drossman D. Rome IV—functional GI disorders: disorders of gut-brain interaction. Gastroenterology. 2016;150(6):1257–61. https://doi.org/10.1053/j.gastro.2016.03.035.

8. Sperber AD, Dekel R. Irritable bowel syndrome and co-morbid gastrointestinal and extra-gastrointestinal functional syndromes. J Neurogastroenterol Motil. 2010;16(2):113–9.
9. Valderas JM, Starfield BS, Sailsbury C, Roland M. Defining comorbidity: implications for understanding health and health services. Ann Family Med. 2009;7(4):357–63.
10. Whitehead WE, Palson O, Jones KR. Systematic review of the comorbidity of irritable bowel syndrome with other disorders: what are the causes and implications? Gastroenterology. 2002;122:1140–56.
11. Riedl A, Schmidtmann M, Stengel A, et al. Somatic comorbidities of irritable bowel syndrome: a systematic analysis. J Psychosom Res. 2008;64:573–82.
12. Ford AC, Marwaha A, Lim A, Moayyedi P. Systematic review and meta-analysis of the prevalence of irritable bowel syndrome in individuals with dyspepsia. Clin Gastroenterol Hepatol. 2009;8(5):401–9.
13. Wang A, Liao X, Xiong L, et al. The clinical overlap between functional dyspepsia and irritable bowel syndrome based on Rome III criteria. BMC Gastroenterol. 2008;8:43.
14. Talley NJ, Dennis EH, Schettler-Duncan VA, Lacy BE, Olden KW, Crowell MD. Overlapping upper and lower gastrointestinal symptoms in irritable bowel syndrome patients with constipation or diarrhea. Am J Gastroenterol. 2003;98:2454–9.
15. Lee SY, Lee KJ, Kim SJ, Cho SW. Prevalence and risk factors for overlaps between gastroesophageal reflux disease, dyspepsia, and irritable bowel syndrome: a population-based study. Digestion. 2009;79:196–201.
16. Leeds JS, Hopper D, Shidu R, Simmonette A, Azadbakht N, Hpggard N, Morley S, Sanders DS. Some patients with irritable bowel syndrome may have exocrine pancreatic insufficiency. Clin Gastroenterol Hepatol. 2010;8:433–8.
17. Chang L, Berman S, Mayer EA, et al. Brain responses to visceral and somatic stimuli in patients with irritable bowel syndrome with and without fibromyalgia. Am J Gastroenterol. 2003;98:1354–61.
18. Longstreth G, Preskill DB, Youkeles L. Irritable bowel syndrome in women having diagnostic laparoscopy or hysterectomy. Relation to gynecologic features and outcome. Dig Dis Sci. 1990;35:1285–90.
19. Williams RE, Hartmann KE, Sandler RS, Miller WC, Savitz LA, Steege JF. Recognition and treatment of irritable bowel syndrome among women with chronic pelvic pain. Am J Obstet Gynecol. 2005;192:761–7.
20. Hausteiner-Wiehle C, Henningsen P. Irritable bowel syndrome: relations with functional, mental, and somatoform disorders. World J Gastroenterol. 2014;20(20):6024–30.
21. Fadgyas-Stanculete M, Buga AM, Popa-Wagner A, Dumitrascu DL. The relationship between irritable bowel syndrome and psychiatric disorders: from molecular changes to clinical manifestations. J Mol Psychiatry. 2014;2:4.
22. Henningsen P, Herzog W. Irritable bowel syndrome and somatoform disorders. J Psychosom Res. 2008;64:625–9. https://doi.org/10.1016/j.jpsychores.2008.02.015.
23. World Health Organisation. International Classification of Diseases (ICD). Available from: http://apps.who.int/classifications/icd10/browse/2010/en. Last accessed Nov 15th 2013.
24. van Tilburg MA, Palsson OS, Whitehead WE. Which psychological factors exacerbate irritable bowel syndrome? Development of a comprehensive model. J Psychosom Res. 2013;74:486–92. https://doi.org/10.1016/j.jpsychores.2013.03.004.
25. American Psychiatric Association. Diagnostic and statistical manual of mental disorders (Dsm-5). 5th ed. Arlington: American Psychiatric Publishing; 2013.
26. Vandvik PO, Wilhelmsen I, Ihlebaek C, Farup PG. Comorbidity of irritable bowel syndrome in general practice: a striking feature with clinical implications. Aliment Pharmacol Ther. 2004;20:1195–203. https://doi.org/10.1111/j.1365-2036.2004.02250.x.
27. Rapps N, van Oudenhove L, Enck P, Aziz Q. Brain imaging of visceral functions in healthy volunteers and IBS patients. J Psychosom Res. 2008;64:599–604. https://doi.org/10.1016/j.jpsychores.2008.02.018.

28. Enck P, Azis Q, Barbara G, Farmer AD, Fukudo S, Mayer AE, Niesler B, Quigley EMM, Rajilić-Stojanović M, Schemann M, Schwielle-Kiuntke J, Magnus S, Zipfel S, Spiller RC. Irritable bowel syndrome. Nat Rev Dis Primers. 2:16014. https://doi.org/10.1038/nrdp.2016.14.
29. Bischof SC, et al. Intestinal permeability—a new target for disease prevention and therapy. BMC Gastroenterol. 2014;14:189.
30. Slattery SA, Niaz O, Azziz Q, Ford AC, Farmer AD. Systematic review with meta-analysis: the prevalence of bile acid malabsorption in the irritable bowel syndrome with diarrhoea. Aliment Pharmacol Ther. 2015;42:3–11.
31. Rani RA, Raja RA, Lee YY. Irritable bowel syndrome and inflammatory bowel disease overlap syndrome: pieces of the puzzle are falling into place. Intest Res. 2016;14(4):297–304.
32. Zhang L, Song J, Hou X. Mast cells and irritable bowel syndrome: from the bench to the beside. J Naurogastroenterol Motil. 2016;22(4):181.
33. Bajor A, Tornbolm H, Rudling M, Ung KA, Simren M. Increased colonis bile acid exposure: a relevant factor for symptoms and treatment in IBS. Gut. 2015;64:84–92.
34. Crouzet L, et al. The hypersensitivity to colonic distension of IBS patients can be transferred to rats through their fecal microbiota. Neurogastroenterol Motil. 2013;25:272–82.
35. Lipowski ZJ. Somatization: the concept and its clinical application. Am J Psychiatry. 1988;145:1358–68.
36. Sandhu DS, Fass R. Current trends in the management of gastroesophageal reflux disease. Gut and Liver. 2018;12(1):7–16.
37. Gyawali CP, Kahrilas PJ, Savarino E, Zerbib F, Mion F, Smout AJPM, Vaezi M, Sifrim D, Fox MR, Vela MF, Tutuian R, Tack J, Bredenoord AJ, Pandolfino J, Roman S. Modern diagnosis of GERD: the Lyon consensus. Gut. 2018;67:1–12. https://doi.org/10.1136/gutjnl-2017-314722.
38. Fennerty MB. Strategies for diagnosis and short and long-term treatment: respondent overview. Am J Gastroenterol. 2001;96:27–8.
39. Zagari M, Villa KP, Freston JW. Proton pump inhibitors versus H 2 -receptor antagonists for the treatment of erosive gastroesophageal reflux disease: a cost-cooperative study. Am J Managed Care. 1995;1:247–55.
40. Fass R, Ofman JJ, Gralnek IM, et al. Clinical and economic assessment of the omeprazole test in patients with symptoms suggestive of gastroesophageal reflux disease. Arch Intern Med. 1999;159:2161–8.
41. Dent J. Management of reflux disease. Gut. 2002;50(Suppl. 4):67–71.
42. Klinkenberg-Knol EC, Festen H, Jansen J, et al. Long-term treatment with omeprazole for refractory reflux esophagitis: efficacy and safety. Ann Intern Med. 1994;121:161–7.
43. Klinkenberg-Knol EC. Eleven years' experience of continuous maintenance treatment with omeprazole in GERD patients. Gastroenterology. 1998;114:180.
44. Neto RML, Hetrbella FAM, Schlottmann F, Patti MG. Does DeMeester score still define GERD? Dis Esophagus. 2019;32(5) https://doi.org/10.1093/dote/doy118.
45. Savary M, Miller G. Manuel et Atlas d'Endoscopie. Solothurn (Switzerland): Verlag Gassmann; 1977.
46. Lundell LR, Dent J, Bennett JR, et al. Endoscopic assessment of oesophagitis: clinical and functional correlates and further validation of the Los Angeles classification. Gut. 1999;45:172–80.
47. Dent J. Gastrooesophageal reflux disease. Digestion. 1998;59:433–45.
48. Johnson LF, Demeester TR. Twenty-four-hour pH monitoring of the distal esophagus. A quantitative measure of gastroesophageal reflux. Am J Gastroenterol. 1974;62(4):325–32.
49. Babić Ž, Ugarković B, Ivancević D, Babić D. Dynamic scintigraphy of the esophagus in the evaluation of reflux oesophagitis. Nuklearmedizin. 1990;29(5):204–9.
50. Sachs G, Shin JM. The basis for differentiation of PPIs. Drugs Today. 2004;40(Suppl. A):9–14.
51. Gilard M, Armaud B, Cornily JC, Le Gal G, Lacut K, Le calvez G, Mansourati J, Mottier D, Abrigall JF, Boschat J. Influence of omeprazole on the antiplatlet action of clopidogrel associated with aspirin: the randomized, double-blind OCLA (omeprazole, clopidogrel aspirin) study. J Am Coll Cardiol. 2008;23:26–41.
52. Drepper MD, Spahr L, Frossard JL. Clopidogrel and proton pump inhibitors-where do we stand in 2012? WJG. 2012;18:2161–71.

53. Hsu P. New look at antiplatlet agent-related peptic ulcer: an update of orevention and treatment. J Gastroenterol Hepatol. 2012;27:654–61.
54. Dunn SP, Steinbuhl SR, Bauer D, Charmigo RJ, Berger PB, Topol EJ. Impact of proton pump ingibitor therapy on the efficacy of clopidogrel in the CAPRIE and CREDO trials. J Am Heart Assoc. 2013;2:21–11.
55. Lane L, Hennekens C. Proton pump inhibitor and clopidogrel interaction: fact of fiction. Am J Gastroenterol. 2010;105:34–41.
56. Lanza FL, Chan FKL, Quigley EMM. The practice comittee of the American college of gastroenterology. Am J Gastroenterol. 2009;104:728–38.
57. Matula MS, Jilma B, Schror K, Christ G, Hubers K. Effect of proton pump inhibitors on clinical outcome in patients treated with clopidogrel: a systematic review and meta-analysis. J Thromb Haemost. 2010;8:624–264.
58. Goyal R, Guo Y, Mashimo H. Advances in the physiology of gastric emptying. Neurogastroenterol Motil. 201931(4):e13546. https://doi.org/10.1111/nmo.13546.
59. Jacoby DB, Gleich G, Fryer AD. Human eosinophil major basic protein is an endogenous allosteric antagonist at the inhibitory muscarinic M2 receptor. J Clin Invest. 1993;91(4):1314–8. https://doi.org/10.1172/JCI116331.
60. Dent J. Definitions of reflux disease and its separation from dyspepsia. Gut. 2002;50(Suppl. 4):17–20.
61. Shin A, Preidis GA, Shulman R, Kashyap PC. The gut microbiome in adult and pediatric functional gastrointestinal disorders. Clin Gastroenterol Hepatol. 2019;17(2):256–71. https://doi.org/10.1016/j.cgh.2018.08.054.
62. Nakae H, Tsuda A, Matsuoka T, Mine T, Koga Y. Gastric microbiota in the functional dyspepsia patients treated with probiotic yogurt. BMJ Open Gastroenterol. 2016;3(1):e000109. https://doi.org/10.1136/bmjgast-2016-000109.
63. Farmer AD, Aziz Q. Mechanisms of visceral pain in health and functional gastrointestinal disorders. Scand J Pain. 2014;5(2):51–60. https://doi.org/10.1016/j.sjpain.2014.01.002.
64. Greenwood-Van Meerveld B, Johnson AC. Stress-induced chronic visceral pain of gastrointestinal origin. Front Syst Neurosci. 2017;11:86. https://doi.org/10.3389/fnsys.2017.00086.
65. Carabotti M, Scirocco A, Maselli MA, Severi C. The gut-brain axis: interactions between enteric microbiota, central and enteric nervous systems. Ann Gastroenterol. 2015;28(2):203–9.
66. Mayer EA, Gupta A, Kilpatrick LA, Hong JY. Imaging brain mechanisms in chronic visceral pain. Pain. 2015;156(Suppl. 1):S50–63. https://doi.org/10.1097/j.pain.0000000000000106.
67. Malfertheiner P, Mégraud F, O'Morain CA, Gisbert JP, Kuipers EJ, Axon AT, Bazzoli F, Gasbarrini A, Atherton J, Graham DY, Hunt R. Management of Helicobacter pylori infection-the Maastricht V/Florence consensus report. Gut. 2017;66(1):6–30. https://doi.org/10.1136/gutjnl-2016-312288.
68. Suzuki H, Kusunoki H, Kamiya T, Futagami S, Yamaguchi Y, Nishizawa T, et al. Effect of lansoprazole on the epigastric symptoms of functional dyspepsia (ELF study): a multicentre, prospective, randomized, double-blind, placebo-controlled clinical trial. United Eur Gastroenterol J. 2013;1(6):445–52. https://doi.org/10.1177/2050640613510904.
69. Kamiya T, Shikano M, Kubota E. A multicenter randomized trial comparing rabeprazole and itopride in patients with functional dyspepsia in Japan: the NAGOYA study. J Clin Biochem Nutr. 2017;60(2):130–5. https://doi.org/10.3164/jcbn.16-106.
70. Kamada T, Fujimura Y, Gotoh K. A study on the efficacy of proton pump inhibitors in helicobacter pylori-negative primary care patients with dyspepsia in Japan. Gut Liver. 2013;7(1):16–22. https://doi.org/10.5009/gnl.2013.7.1.16.
71. Sheptulin AA, Belousova IB. Modern prokinetics and their role in the treatment of gastroenterological pathology. Klin Med (Mosk). 2016;94(3):178–82.
72. Huang X, Lv B, Zhang S, Fan YH, Meng LN. Itopride therapy for functional dyspepsia: a meta-analysis. World J Gastroenterol. 2012;18(48):7371–7. https://doi.org/10.3748/wjg.v18.i48.7371.

73. Ikeo K, Oshima T, Sei H, Kondo T, Fukui H, Watari J, et al. Acotiamide improves stress-induced impaired gastric accommodation. Neurogastroenterol Motil. 2017;29(4) https://doi.org/10.1111/nmo.12991.
74. Törnblom H, Drossman DA. Psychotropics, antidepressants, and visceral analgesics in functional gastrointestinal disorders. Curr Gastroenterol Rep. 2018;20(12):58. https://doi.org/10.1007/s11894-018-0664-3.
75. Luo QQ, Chen SL. Use of neurotransmitter regulators in functional gastrointestinal disorders based on symptom analysis. J Dig Dis. 2017;18(4):203–6. https://doi.org/10.1111/1751-2980.12472.
76. Talley NJ, Locke GR, Saito YA, Almazar AE, Bouras EP, Howden CW, et al. Effect of amitriptyline and escitalopram on functional dyspepsia: a multicenter, randomized controlled study. Gastroenterology. 2015;149(2):340–9. https://doi.org/10.1053/j.gastro.2015.04.020.
77. Tack J, Ly HG, Carbone F, Vanheel H, Vanuytsel T, Holvoet L, et al. Efficacy of mirtazapine in patients with functional dyspepsia and weight loss. Clin Gastroenterol Hepatol. 2016;14(3):385–92. https://doi.org/10.1016/j.cgh.2015.09.043.
78. Grover M, Dorn SD, Weinland SR, Dalton CB, Gaynes BN, Drossman DA. Atypical antipsychotic quetiapine in the management of severe refractory functional gastrointestinal disorders. Dig Dis Sci. 2009;54(6):1284–91. https://doi.org/10.1007/s10620-009-0723-6.
79. Tack J, Janssen P, Masaoka T, Farré R, Van Oudenhove L. Efficacy of buspirone, a fundus-relaxing drug, in patients with functional dyspepsia. Clin Gastroenterol Hepatol. 2012;10(11):1239–45. https://doi.org/10.1016/j.cgh.2012.06.036.
80. Jin M, Son M. DA-9701 (Motilitone): a multi-targeting botanical drug for the treatment of functional dyspepsia. Int J Mol Sci. 2018;19(12):E4035. https://doi.org/10.3390/ijms19124035.
81. Lapina TL, Trukhmanov AS. Herbal preparation STW 5 for functional gastrointestinal disorders: clinical experience in everyday practice. Dig Dis. 2017;35(Suppl. 1):30–5. https://doi.org/10.1159/000485411.
82. Freedman SD. Options for addressing exocrine pancreatic insufficiency in patients receiving enteral nutrition supplementation. Am J Manag Care Suppl. 2017;23(12):S220–8.
83. Kwiatek R. Treatment of fibromyalgia. Aust Prescr. 2017;40(5):179–83.
84. Tu FF, As-Sanie S. Treatment of chronic pelvic pain in women. Wolters Kluwer; 2019. UpToDate 2020 www:uptodate-com
85. Faubion S, Rullo JE. Sexual dysfunction in women: a practical approach. Am Family Physician. 2015;92(4):281–90.
86. Snyder PJ, Raymond CR. Overview of male sexual dysfunction. Wolters Kluwer. 2019; UpToDate 2020; www:uptodate-com.
87. Faquih AE, Memon RI, Hafeez H, et al. A review of novel antidepressants: a guide for clinicians. Cureus. 2019;11(3):e4185. https://doi.org/10.7759/cureus.4185.
88. Bandelow B, Michaelis S, Wedekind D. Treatment of anxiety disorders. Dialog Clin Neurosci. 2017;19(2):93–107.

Metabolic Disorders 24

Dario Rahelić, Lucija Romić, Marija Martinović, and Sanja Klobučar

Obesity

Obesity presents a major problem in today's society. Its prevalence has risen dramatically all over the world and has led to many devastating consequences. Obesity is a risk factor for many conditions, such as cardiovascular diseases, diabetes, and cancers [1]. It also contributes to many gastrointestinal and hepatic diseases including Barrett's esophagus, nonalcoholic fatty liver disease (NAFLD), gallstones, gastroesophageal reflux disease (GERD), erosive gastritis, acute pancreatitis, inflammatory bowel disease (IBD), polyps, diarrhea, and cancers, such as esophageal adenocarcinoma, hepatocellular carcinoma (HCC), pancreatic cancer, cholangiocarcinoma, and colorectal cancer [2].

Obesity, especially abdominal or visceral obesity, occurs as a part of the metabolic syndrome [3]. Visceral adipose tissue (VAT) secretes cytokines called adipokines. In obese individuals, there is an imbalance between cytokines and increased secretion of interleukin-1, interleukin-6, tumor necrosis alpha (TNF-α), inhibitors

D. Rahelić (✉)
Vuk Vrhovac University Clinic for Diabetes, Endocrinology and Metabolic Diseses, Merkur University Hospital, Zagreb, Croatia

School of Medicine, Catholic University of Croatia, Zagreb, Croatia

Faculty of Medicine, J.J. Strossmayer University of Osijek, Osijek, Croatia

L. Romić · M. Martinović
Vuk Vrhovac University Clinic for Diabetes, Endocrinology and Metabolic Diseses, Merkur University Hospital, Zagreb, Croatia

S. Klobučar
Department of Endocrinology, Diabetes and Metabolic Diseases, University Hospital Centre Rijeka, Rijeka, Croatia
e-mail: sanja.klobucar@uniri.hr

M. Banić, D. Erceg (eds.), *Drug Interactions in Gastroenterology*, Clinical Gastroenterology, https://doi.org/10.1007/978-3-031-69800-2_24

of plasminogen-1 (PAI-1), resistin, and fibrinogen. Leptin and acute phase reactant levels increase and the level of adiponectin decreases. Adipose tissue macrophages (ATMs) produce TNF-α whose levels increase with increasing body fat and obesity [4]. TNF-α induces inactivation of insulin receptors in fat and muscle cells with consequent rise in blood glucose. Increase of lipolysis in adipose tissues induces an elevation of free fatty acids (FFAs) and glycerol concentrations in serum, which disrupts the effect of insulin, leads to increased gluconeogenesis in the liver, and inhibits adiponectin secretion [5].

Gastroesophageal Reflux Disease (GERD) and Barrett's Esophagus

Obesity predisposes to peristaltic dysfunction of the esophagus and increased esophageal acid exposure. Obese individuals have higher estrogen levels which are related to GERD. Gastric acid induces inflammation of the esophageal mucosa and that alternation in function can lead to Barrett's esophagus and esophageal adenocarcinoma [6]. Barrett's esophagus is usually a consequence of chronic GERD which is characterized by the taste of acid in the back of the mouth, heartburn, bad breath, regurgitation, and chest pain [7, 8].

Inflammatory Bowel Disease (IBD)

Inflammatory bowel disease involves two main disorders: ulcerative colitis and Chron's disease. These conditions are chronic inflammatory diseases of the digestive tract. Symptoms may include abdominal pain, cramps, diarrhea, and blood in the stool. About 15–40% of patients with IBD have excess body weight and about 20–40% are obese. Retrospective studies in individuals with ulcerative colitis and Chron's disease have shown different responses to azathioprine. Patients with an initial BMI > 25 kg/m^2 and ulcerative colitis had a higher likelihood of exacerbation. In this study, patients with Chron's disease and BMI > 25 kg/m^2 after discontinuation of azathioprine had a lower rate of subsequent deterioration than individuals with normal BMI [9]. Studies show that obesity is not associated with IBD-related complications. In a cross-sectional study of 846 patients, Pringle and colleagues observed a lower prevalence of complications in obese people compared to patients whose BMI was in the normal range [10]. In longitudinal studies, inferior IBD-related quality of life and high levels of serum C-reactive protein were observed in obese individuals, but there was no difference in the hospitalization, surgery, or emergency department use between obese patients and patients with normal BMI [11]. Despite the increasing rate of obesity in IBD, the impact of obesity on drug absorption, metabolism, and excretion remains poorly understood. Until today there are no such studies that explain the impact of obesity on the efficacy of methotrexate. One retrospective study showed a twofold increase in the loss of response to adalimumab among individuals whose BMI was >30 kg/m^2 compared to normal

BMI [9]. Studies also suggest that infliximab is associated with lower rates of IBD-related hospitalization and abdominal surgery than certolizumab and adalimumab [10].

Acute Pancreatitis

Intra-abdominal adipose tissue is an active secretory organ involved in various metabolic pathways. Pandemic of obesity has increased the incidence of gallstones, diabetes, and hypertriglyceridemia. All these conditions may lead to necrosis and increase the risk of acute pancreatitis [1]. There are several proposed mechanisms through which obesity may initiate acute pancreatitis including cholelithiasis (high cholesterol), hypertriglyceridemia (unmasked primary HTG and secondary HTG), diabetes, drugs, and therapeutic interventions for obesity (weight loss, gastric balloons, and bariatric surgery). Visceral tissue adipocytes are mostly composed of triglycerides. They are hydrolyzed by lipase with consequent release of free fatty acids. Studies that analyzed the composition of pancreatic necrosis showed the presence of oleic acid, linoleic acids, interleukin-1, and interleukin-8. Obesity and a high-fat diet predispose to stones formation in the bile and decrease in circulatory bile acids thus contributing to the development of acute pancreatitis. Hypertriglyceridemia has been shown to induce the formation of microthrombi in the pancreatic vasculature causing ischemia, but therapeutic use of Lactated Ringer's and lipase inhibitors improves outcomes [12].

Type 2 Diabetes

Type 2 diabetes is one of the fastest-growing worldwide chronic diseases affecting more than 366 million people. The number of patients with diabetes are growing due to obesity, urbanization, and sedentary lifestyles. Diabetes affects almost all organ systems in the human body including the gastrointestinal tract. Diabetes-related complications occur throughout the digestive system, from the oral cavity to the anorectal opening. Early recognition is important for appropriate treatment and improvement of life quality [13].

Esophageal Complications

Diabetic neuropathy can affect the lower esophageal sphincter and thoracic esophagus which are formed by the smooth muscle fibers. Neuropathy in type 2 diabetes results in reduced lower sphincter tone and abnormal peristalsis. The prevalence of esophageal dysmotility is high, approximately 63%, and there is no difference between type 1 and type 2 diabetic patients. Gastroesophageal reflux disease also occurs in diabetes and its prevalence is higher in patients with metabolic syndrome. The prevalence could be up to 41% [13].

Gastroparesis

Gastroparesis is one of the most common GI complications of diabetes with delayed gastric emptying [14]. About 27–65% of patients with type 1 diabetes have delayed gastric emptying and about 30% of patients with type 2 diabetes. Risk factors for the development of gastroparesis include the presence of macrovascular and microvascular complications, elevated glycated hemoglobin level, and duration of diabetes more than 10 years. Mechanisms of pathogenesis are multifactorial, uncleared, and poorly understood, but include hyperglycemia, vagal dysfunction, dysmorphic interstitial Cajal cells, oxidative stress, smooth muscle fibrosis, and abnormal macrophage-containing immune infiltrates [14, 15]. Symptoms of gastroparesis are nausea and vomiting, feeling full very quickly when eating, loss of appetite, bloating, weight loss, upper abdominal pain, and heartburn. The vomiting reflex occurs after the main meal, but attacks of vomiting in the acute form of the disease can occur without food. Increased glucovariability as a result of the mismatch of the insulin action and carbohydrate absorption may lead to more time spent in hypoglycemia and hyperglycemia. Treatment of diabetic gastroparesis includes medications to control nausea and vomiting, medications to stimulate the stomach muscles, psychological therapies, dietary modifications, gastric electrical stimulation, and invasive surgical treatment. Metoclopramide is an antiemetic which reduces nausea, postprandial fullness and increases gastroesophageal sphincter tone. Domperidone is similar to metoclopramide with a predominant peripheral mechanism of action. Erythromycin is a motilin receptor agonist which increases the number of gastric contractions. Antiemesis mechanisms of chlorpromazine, promethazine, and prochlorperazine are uncleared [13, 16].

Metabolic Syndrome

Metabolic syndrome (MetS) is a group of metabolic disorders that include centripetal/visceral type of obesity, arterial hypertension, insulin resistance, and atherogenic dyslipidemia. Risks of type 2 diabetes, stroke, cardiovascular diseases, liver steatosis, and carcinoma development increase in parallel with metabolic syndrome. Its prevalence increases due to a large number of obese people and a sedentary lifestyle. Obesity, especially centripetal obesity, is associated with peripheral tissue resistance to the effects of insulin which consequently leads to type 2 diabetes. Different definitions and criteria have been proposed in the last few decades. The World Health Organization created in 1998 the first international definition. They defined metabolic syndrome as the presence of insulin resistance (impaired glucose tolerance, IGT; impaired fasting glucose, IGF; or type 2 diabetes) with two of the following criteria: obesity, arterial hypertension, high triglyceride levels, decreased HDL-cholesterol levels or microalbuminuria. Criteria were also created by IDF (International Diabetes Federation), AHA/NHBLI (American Heart Association/National Heart, Lung, and Blood Institute), and NCEP ATP III (The US National Cholesterol Education Program Adult Treatment Panel III). Pathophysiological mechanisms in MetS are very complex but insulin resistance and centripetal obesity are considered the main causes [3].

Obese people often have metabolic syndrome because obesity is associated with insulin resistance. Visceral adipose tissue produces IL-1, IL-6, TNF-α, and free fatty acids that lead to insulin resistance. Free fatty acids reduce glucose uptake into muscle cells, increase glucose synthesis in the liver, and have a lipotoxic effect on pancreatic beta cells. In patients with insulin resistance, the number of insulin receptors in muscles and adipose tissues are reduced, GLUT-4 expression is altered, and tyrosine kinase and glycogen synthetase activity are reduced. Insulin resistance is also affected by genetic factors so there are people who are obese, but do not have metabolic syndrome. The consequence of insulin resistance in muscles is a decrease in glucose uptake into the cell and an increase in gluconeogenesis in the liver. Furthermore, the condition of long-term hyperinsulinemia leads to beta cell dysfunction which first manifests as IGT and then as type 2 diabetes [17].

Metabolic syndrome is characterized by atherogenic dyslipidemia. Insulin resistance results in increased synthesis of very low-density lipoproteins (VLDL) in the liver which contain mostly triglycerides. VLDL concentration increase in plasma leads to HDL cholesterol decrease due to cholesterol transfer from HDL particle to VLDL. There are two types of LDL particles—large subtype A, and small and dense subtype B. In metabolic syndrome, small and dense LDL particles, which have a higher atherogenic potential, are more common. Patients with arterial hypertension have a higher concentration of plasma insulin than healthy people. Approximately 50% of patients with arterial hypertension have insulin resistance. Insulin affects many processes in the regulation of blood pressure: cation transport, sodium absorption in the kidneys, and sympathetic nervous system activity. Elevated serum insulin levels increase renal sodium absorption and stimulate the sympathetic nervous system [17–19].

Metabolic syndrome is strongly associated with NAFLD whose prevalence increases in line with metabolic syndrome. Pathogenic factor in NAFLD is insulin resistance which can progress to cirrhosis and HCC. Hepatocellular carcinoma is the fifth most common cancer in the world in which its prevalence has increased in the last years [20, 21]. In 2012, the World Health Organization reported that there were approximately 746,000 deaths from liver cancer, making liver cancer the second most common cause of death from cancer [22]. Cirrhosis, metabolic syndrome including obesity and type 2 diabetes, NAFLD, and several inherited disorders (hereditary hemochromatosis, alpha-1 antitrypsin deficiency, and acute intermittent porphyria) lead to primary liver cancer [20, 21]. The risk of HCC is twice as high in patients with T2DM than in those without type 2 diabetes. Studies have shown that HCC mortality is significantly increased in obese individuals. Most patients with NASH who develop HCC are obese men with T2DM and hypertension [23]. HCC is rare among patients without liver disease and more often in populations older than 65 years. Studies have shown that in a large number of patients cirrhosis occurs as a result of NAFLD. Pathophysiological mechanisms of HCC development in patients with NAFLD are not fully clarified. Twenty years ago, Day and James proposed steatohepatitis pathogenesis called the "two-hit" hypothesis. This hypothesis dictated that fatty liver as a result of hepatic lipid accumulation provides a "first hit"-steatosis. "The second hit" is determined by the progression of inflammation, fibrosis, cirrhosis, and HCC [20, 21, 24].

Obesity and insulin resistance stimulate an inflammatory response in which synthesis of adiponectin is reduced and increased release of IL-6, IL-1, TNF-α, and nuclear factor NF-kB.

Decreased adiponectin concentrations and increased leptin concentrations lead to hepatic steatosis, inflammation, and fibrogenesis in obese patients. Also, increased pro-inflammatory cytokines levels lead to histological changes in NASH. Insulin resistance inhibits fatty acid oxidation leading to increased levels of intracellular fatty acids. Microsomal peroxidase leads consequently to DNA damage. Harmful processes, such as oxidative stress and apoptotic pathways contribute to cirrhosis or HCC [25].

Eating Disorders

Eating disorders often occur within the adolescent and young adult population, most often between the ages of 12 and 25, and treatment requires a multidisciplinary approach. A significantly higher occurrence of eating disorders can be found among adolescent women in comparison to men. Eating disorders in more than 90% of the cases appear before the age of 25, which is usually the same age when other chronical gastrointestinal and endocrine diseases are common, and in the end diagnosing the primary cause is more challenging. New studies have shown that gastrointestinal diseases and eating disorders can coexist and might share common molecular pathways. Patients may abuse medications such as insulin or thyroid hormones with the aim of trying to lose weight. Furthermore, the use of corticosteroids leads to weight gain, followed by eating disorders as an end result. Two most common serious conditions are anorexia nervosa (AN) and bulimia nervosa (BN). Previous studies have shown a correlation between eating disorders and diseases such as coeliac disease, inflammatory bowel disease, diabetes, and thyroid disorders, which suggest the possible role of autoimmunity [26]. Patients with eating disorders usually complain about gastrointestinal problems including postprandial fullness and discomfort, abdominal pain and distention, gastric distention, early satiety, nausea, recurrent vomiting, severe constipation, bowel obstruction, and flatulence. In addition, the use of tricyclic antidepressives contributes to constipation in patients experiencing anorexia nervosa [27]. Patients often have an electrolyte imbalance comprising hypokalemia, hypochloremia, and increased bicarbonate levels. Hypokalemia is a serious condition that can lead to cardiac arrhythmias, rhabdomyolysis, muscle weakness or tetany and requires volume repletion and oral or intravenous potassium [28]. Usually, patients with anorexia nervosa have delayed gastric emptying resulting in nausea, vomiting, and gastric fullness. Medications that have effects on delayed gastric emptying are domperidone and cisapride. Because of causing ventricular tachycardia, cisapride is not available in many countries. Several studies have reported complications of rectal prolapse as a consequence of eating disorders, particularly in patients with obstetric trauma, chronic constipation, or elevated intra-abdominal pressure. One study found high levels of amylases that did not require treatment. In many cases, vomiting leads to laxity of the lower esophageal sphincter with consequent GERD and heartburn. Gastric acid acts on the esophagus which can lead to Barrett's esophagus development and can increase the risk of developing adenocarcinoma of the esophagus by 11 times [27].

Celiac disease, or gluten enteropathy, is a chronic disease of the small intestine, which occurs as an immune response of the body to gluten. It results in inflammatory changes in the intestinal mucosa and consequent malabsorption. A large number of patients have silent symptoms of the disease, and by that, the first presentation in adolescents may be failure to thrive. Approximately three million people in the United States have a coeliac disease that is undiagnosed or untreated. Unrecognized coeliac disease can lead to many complications including intestinal lymphoma, progressive bone loss, early osteoporosis, and risk of vertebral and hip fracture. Furthermore, in every patient with an eating disorder, it is important to perform serological screening. Suspected patients are screened with coeliac disease serology which involves a serological test for IgA antibodies to tissue transglutaminase (tTG-IgA) and total IgA. If the serological tests are positive, it is recommended to perform a biopsy of intestinal mucosa. In 2015, studies have shown an association between coeliac disease and eating disorders. Symptoms of anorexia nervosa or bulimia nervosa are constipation or diarrhea, intestinal bloating, and nonspecific gastrointestinal pain [26, 29].

Inflammatory bowel diseases are chronic inflammatory diseases of the digestive tract. Stool calprotectin screening tests should be done on all patients with eating disorders [30]. Calprotectin is a cytosolic protein that is present in the feces during intestinal inflammation [30–34]. The diagnosis of inflammatory bowel disease relies on the identification of history, and physical and laboratory findings. In addition, IBD is diagnosed using an esophagogastroduodenoscopy and ileocolonoscopy with biopsy and imaging studies. From all of the above mentioned, patients with eating disorders can present with different gastrointestinal symptoms and disorders, so a multidisciplinary approach is necessary for diagnosis and treatment [27, 31].

Osteoporosis

Osteoporosis is a metabolic bone disease that leads to bone loss, bone fragility, and damage to the microarchitecture of bone tissue which can lead to fractures with minimal trauma, especially in the thoracic and lumbar spine, wrist, and hip. According to etiology, we distinguish primary and secondary osteoporosis. Primary osteoporosis is divided into idiopathic, postmenopausal, and senile osteoporosis while secondary osteoporosis is the result of other diseases such as endocrine, chronic inflammatory, intestinal diseases, kidney disease, and hematological diseases. The gold standard for estimating bone density is densitometry and the results are interpreted using two scores: *T*-score and *Z*-score. When the *T*-score value is

<−2.5 SD, we can diagnose osteoporosis. For secondary osteoporosis, the *Z*-score is more significant, which represents a deviation of the obtained value from the expected for sex and age, and the value less than −2 SD is suggestive of secondary osteoporosis. FRAX is a fracture risk calculator that estimates fracture risks using a variety of risk factors, among which are also some gastrointestinal diseases that cause secondary osteoporosis [32].

Inflammatory bowel diseases can cause secondary osteoporosis by various mechanisms such as chronic inflammation, decreased absorption of calcium and vitamin D, and the use of glucocorticoids. Chronic inflammatory response can lead to decreased bone density by proinflammatory cytokines which increase the expression of RANKL, which, unlike osteoprotegerin, stimulates bone resorption and osteoclast maturation and activity [33]. Higher concentrations of glucocorticoids stimulate bone resorption and inhibit osteoblast function resulting in decreased new bone synthesis. Also, they reduce intestinal calcium absorption and increase calciuria [32, 34]. Glucocorticoids increase expression of RANKL and decrease osteoprotegerin expression which also leads to osteoclast activation and consequent bone resorption [35]. Since inflammatory bowel disease causes malabsorption of macro and microelements, especially Crohn's disease where inflammation is located in the small intestine, there is also a reduced absorption of calcium in the intestine. Calcium deficiency occurs also because of lactose intolerance in patients with IBD as a result of disruption in the production of lactase [36]. Studies have shown that 15–40% of patients with Crohn's disease have osteoporosis [32, 37]. Patients with inflammatory bowel disease who are on glucocorticoid therapy should take bisphosphonates if the *T*-score is <−1.5 or if they are 65 years or older, regardless of the densitometry finding [38]. In the case that *T*-score is more than −1, it is important to take basic preventive measures (adequate calcium, exercise, smoking cessation, avoid alcohol, minimize corticosteroids, and treat hypogonadism) [39].

Celiac disease is another gastrointestinal condition that can lead to osteoporosis. Due to reduced absorption in the small intestine, calcium and vitamin D deficiencies occur. Also, chronic inflammatory response can cause bone resorption in patients with celiac disease by the increase of pro-inflammatory cytokines [32]. Significant improvement is seen after the administration of food that doesn't contain gluten. In celiac disease, osteoporosis occurs in 15% of patients [40].

Postgastrectomy patients are also at risk for developing osteoporosis. It has been shown that 10–20% of patients develop osteomalacia and 22–42% develop osteoporosis of the lumbar vertebrae L1–L4 and 60% of patients develop osteoporosis of the femoral neck [32]. The pathogenesis of osteoporosis in these patients can be explained by the fact that due to the accelerated passage, food bypasses the duodenum and consequently leads to malabsorption of calcium and vitamin D. It doesn't matter which surgical procedure (Bilroth I or Bilroth II) is used because the risk of osteoporosis is very similar in both of them [41].

In patients with short bowel syndrome, osteoporosis also occurs because of the malabsorption of calcium and vitamin D. When jejunal resection occurs, the ileum compensates for absorptive function by increasing the length but when more than 100 cm of ileum is resected there is no compensatory adaptation of the remaining jejunum. In patients who are diagnosed with short bowel syndrome, osteoporosis occurs in 21–67% of patients [32].

Chronic liver disease can result in osteoporosis by impaired hydroxylation of vitamin D3 which can lead to decreased intestinal absorption of calcium and activation of osteoclasts [42]. In liver cirrhosis, there is a decreased production of IGF-1 which leads to a reduction in the number and activity of osteoblasts. Some proinflammatory cytokines which are seen in cases of chronic liver disease cause the activation of osteoclasts and thereby bone resorption. Also, lower concentrations of serum leptin that are seen in primary biliary cirrhosis can lead to low bone mass because leptin decreases RANKL expression and increases osteoprotegerin expression [43].

Antiresorptive therapy, diet, and physical activity are very important factors in treating osteoporosis in patients who have gastrointestinal diseases. The diet should contain 1200 mg/day of Ca and 800–1000 IU/day of vitamin D. Antiresorptive drugs for the treatment of osteoporosis are bisphosphonates which are effective only if the *T* score is <-2 [32]. Denosumab is a monoclonal antibody that inhibits RANKL and thereby it is also used as a therapy for osteoporosis. Moreover, it is important for the prevention and treatment of osteoporosis that corticosteroids are administered in the lowest dose in patients who have inflammatory bowel disease [44].

Hypothyreosis

Hypothyroidism is a condition of reduced production, secretion, and action of thyroid hormones. Treatment of hypothyroidism is carried out with levothyroxine substitution therapy. Refractory hypothyroidism may occur due to a poor response to levothyroxine treatment, and one of the causes may be gastrointestinal malabsorption. Levels of TSH best demonstrate the response to substitution therapy. T4 absorption was shown to be highest in the upper jejunoileum with 29 ± 14%, slightly lower in the lower jejunoileum, and lowest in the duodenum (15 ± 5%) [45]. Gastric-related malabsorption of levothyroxine may occur due to decreased secretion of gastric acid. Causes of decreased production of gastric acid may be Helicobacter pylori, chronic and atrophic gastritis, and proton pump inhibitors. Studies have shown that the solubility of levothyroxine decreases in an alkaline medium [46]. NH3, which is excreted in H. pylori infection, blocks and neutralizes gastric acid secretion. However, eradication of H. pylori has been shown to partially improve acid secretion and thus improve levothyroxine absorption. Treatment with proton pump inhibitors requires a higher dose of levothyroxine because PPIs increase gastric pH which also leads to poor absorption of T4 [47]. It is known that the consumption of papaya fruit, milk, and calcium carbonate also reduces the absorption of levothyroxine. Gastroparesis is another condition that leads to gastric-related malabsorption of T4 by delayed gastric emptying and adsorption of levothyroxine by residual food in the stomach. Bariatric procedures such as sleeve gastrectomy lead to an increase in gastric pH because of the resection of the gastric fundus and body which contain most of the acid-producing cells [48].

Intestinal-related malabsorption of levothyroxine can happen due to many conditions, and one of them is celiac disease. The damaged mucosa of the small intestine is flattened in celiac disease, and lymphocyte infiltration of lamina propria is also present. All this results in lowering the enzyme of the brush coat (dipeptidase, disaccharase), increased intestinal permeability, motility disorders, bacterial contamination of the intestine, and changes in intestinal pH. Complete clinical remission occurs with the gluten-free diet and thus improved T4 absorption [49].

Another condition that can cause decreased levothyroxine absorption is lactose intolerance. Lactose intolerance occurs due to suboptimal activity of the enzyme lactase in the small intestine. Lactose is unable to degrade into glucose and galactose and therefore accumulates in the intestinal lumen and attracts water [50]. Also, this condition can increase intestinal motility and cause small intestinal bacterial overgrowth. All this can prevent the absorption of levothyroxine. As in celiac disease, lactose-free diet can improve T4 absorption. In some tablet formulations of levothyroxine, a small dose of lactose is seen but studies have shown that only quantities >5 g of ingested lactose are significant for gastrointestinal symptoms [51].

Pancreatic insufficiency can lead to increased fecal losses and elimination of T4 hormone due to decreased secretion of enzyme lipase which results in pancreatic steatorrhea. Liver cirrhosis may cause a poor response to the treatment of hypothyroidism with levothyroxine by reducing the concentration of thyroid-binding globulin and reducing bile secretion. Short bowel syndrome and procedures of bariatric surgery such as Roux-en-Y gastric bypass also prevent the absorption of T4 by reducing intestinal absorptive surface [46, 47].

Other Endocrine Manifestations

Growth Failure

In patients who suffer from inflammatory bowel disease, growth failure occurs at a later stage and is more common in patients who are diagnosed with Crohn's disease (up to 46%) than in patients who have ulcerative colitis (3–10%) [52]. Growth hormone secretion is controlled by two hypothalamic hormones and via two feedback systems. Somatocrinin, which stimulates the release of GH, and somatostatin which inhibits the secretion of growth hormone. The two feedback systems are the short closed loop (between the pituitary gland and hypothalamus) and the long closed loop (hypothalamus-pituitary gland-IGF1). Increased concentration of growth hormone or IGF 1 inhibits GH secretion at the hypothalamus by stimulating the release of somatostatin. In patients with IBD, low IGF 1 values are seen, increased growth hormone resistance, and thereby reduced height velocity. Studies have shown that impaired growth hormone-IGF1 axis is due to a chronic inflammatory response in inflammatory bowel disease mediated by proinflammatory cytokines [39, 53]. Malnutrition is another important cause of growth failure. It occurs due to reduced food intake because patients with IBD have esophagitis and gastritis, so they eat less because of pain and fear of exacerbation of the disease. Malabsorption of fat, proteins, vitamins, and minerals is also a major cause of malnutrition. Glucocorticoids are a part of the treatment in patients who have inflammatory bowel disease and they can significantly affect growth retardation by a number of mechanisms. They increase the levels of somatostatin which inhibits the secretion of growth hormone and interferes with the retention of nitrogen and minerals. Glucocorticoids inhibit the formation of the bones, chondrocyte mitosis, pulsatile GH release, and IGF-I bioactivity. Impairment of collagen synthesis and reduction in the expression of GH receptors are also seen as a result of glucocorticoid treatment. Studies have shown that growth hormone therapy has a reversible effect on glucocorticoid-induced growth retardation [54]. It is very important to conduct screening of children who have inflammatory bowel disease for retardation of growth, i.e., to monitor parameters such as the intake of calories, calcium, and vitamin D, measurement of height, weight, and body mass index, calculation of mid-parental height/centiles, measuring height velocity at the intervals of 4–6-month, and DXA scan to assess bone mineral density [39]. Improvement of growth failure in patients with IBD can be achieved by several mechanisms. First, in patients with malnutrition, supplements of minerals and vitamins are essential as well as an increase in energy intake [55]. Nasogastric tube can be necessary in patients with more severe cases of malnutrition. Infliximab, which belongs to the group of immunomodulators and surgery has also been shown to improve reduced velocity height in patients who have inflammatory bowel disease. As discussed before, growth hormone therapy can be helpful in treating patients who suffer from growth failure if all other measures fail [39].

Hypogonadism

Gonadotropins are follicle-stimulating hormones and luteinizing hormones. They are secreted by gonadotropic cells of the pituitary gland. FSH stimulates follicle growth in the ovary, testicular growth, and spermatogenesis and LH affects ovulation, corpus luteum, Leydig cell stimulation, and steroidogenesis in the ovaries and testes. Their secretion is pulsed and is influenced by GnRH from the hypothalamus, but is also regulated by negative feedback through sex hormones. Hypogonadism in inflammatory bowel disease patients may be the result of various pathogenetic mechanisms. Long-term treatment with glucocorticoids may lead to decreased secretion of gonadotropins and sex hormone-binding globulin and reduced sex hormone secretion by the direct effect of glucocorticoids on gonads [39]. TNF-α and IL-1 are the main proinflammatory cytokines present in inflammatory bowel disease and they inhibit steroidogenesis in the ovaries by inhibiting adenylyl cyclase and post-cAMP sites [56]. As we discussed before, reduced food intake is seen in patients with IBD due to the pain and fear of exacerbation of the disease. There is a hypothesis that restrictive eating will cause decreased leptin secretion from the fat adipocytes and low levels of leptin can inhibit GnRH secretion [57]. It is recommended that IBD patients who suffer from hypogonadism and osteoporosis, especially young men and premenopausal women should take sex hormone replacement therapy [39].

NAFLD

NAFLD is a nonalcoholic fatty liver disease that results in increased synthesis and accumulation of triglycerides in the liver. The disease can progress to nonalcoholic steatohepatitis due to inflammation that may occur as a consequence of cell membrane damage due to lipid peroxidation. The end stages are liver fibrosis, cirrhosis, and hepatocellular carcinoma. Diagnostic indicators of this disease are a reduced AST/ALT ratio, as opposed to alcoholic hepatitis. The gold standard to confirm a diagnosis of nonalcoholic hepatitis is a liver biopsy however an ultrasound method like liver fibroscan has been shown to be much easier to perform and can determine the stages of fibrosis or scarring in the liver.

One of the gastrointestinal diseases that has been shown to be associated with NAFLD is celiac disease. A gluten-free diet and increased intestinal permeability are thought to be major pathogenetic mechanisms leading to nonalcoholic fatty liver disease [58]. The only available treatment for celiac disease is a diet that doesn't contain gluten. Wheat, barley, rye, and oats should be eliminated from the diet. Such a diet contains simple sugars, proteins, saturated fat, and a small amount of complex carbohydrates and fibers which in turn can lead to the development of NAFLD [59]. In celiac disease, changes are most pronounced in the proximal part of the small intestine where subtotal atrophy of the villi and complete flattening of the mucosa occur. A diet with no gluten improves histology of celiac disease, i.e., there is a regression of atrophy and flattening of the intestinal mucosa, which leads to improved intestinal permeability and improved intestinal absorption of a high-calorie diet. Because of the improved intestinal permeability, intestinal bacterial endotoxins such as lipopolysaccharides can cause an enhanced inflammatory response in the liver and also lead to the development of steatosis and nonalcoholic steatohepatitis [58]. On the other side, malnutrition that occurs in celiac disease due to malabsorption can cause abnormal hepatic fat deposition by mitochondrial dysfunction in hepatocytes and decreased fatty acid oxidation in mitochondria [60].

Another condition associated with NAFLD is inflammatory bowel disease. Some pathophysiological mechanisms leading to NAFLD have been mentioned before such as high-calorie intake and reduced fiber intake. This kind of diet can be explained by the fact that patients with IBD have diarrhea and intestinal distension when they eat a lot of fruits, vegetables, and complex carbohydrates [61]. The next mechanism that leads to the development of NAFLD in IBD patients is long-term glucocorticoid therapy. Glucocorticoids have an effect on increased appetite by causing leptin resistance. They stimulate the release of fatty acids from adipose tissue and increase their uptake to the liver. Also, they increase the de novo synthesis of fatty acids from acetyl-CoA and increase gluconeogenesis in the liver [62]. Chronic inflammation in patients with inflammatory bowel disease is a major cause of NAFLD due to proinflammatory cytokines which play a huge role in developing nonalcoholic steatohepatitis.

Nonalcoholic fatty liver disease is associated with a severe form of acute pancreatitis. NAFLD patients are usually obese and have dyslipidemia. Obesity causes a chronic inflammatory response, while dyslipidemia causes the accumulation of free radicals and oxidative stress. These are all mechanisms that can lead to exacerbation of acute pancreatitis in patients who suffer from NAFLD. In addition to obesity and dyslipidemia, nonalcoholic fatty liver disease may directly affect the development of acute pancreatitis as it also causes a systemic inflammatory response which can be confirmed by elevated concentration of C-reactive protein in serum. Systemic inflammatory response in NAFLD occurs due to decreased levels of alfa 1 antitrypsin which has anti-inflammatory effects, increased levels of adipokine, and release of proinflammatory cytokines by the Kupffer cells [63].

Studies also observed that patients with type 2 diabetes have more severe NAFLD than those without diabetes. Patients with obesity, diabetes, and NAFLD have a high risk of HCC development. A large number of patients who have NASH and develop HCC, also have obesity, diabetes, and arterial hypertension. Furthermore, alcohol and smoking have an effect on HCC risk in patients with type 2 diabetes. Therapy used in the treatment of diabetes also has efficacy in NAFLD. Lifestyle change is aimed at weight loss and increased physical activity. Studies have shown that a weight loss of 7% leads to an improvement in liver cell histology. Metformin is the first-line blood-glucose-lowering drug used to treat type 2 diabetes which reduces gluconeogenesis and increases the sensitivity of peripheral tissues to insulin. Thiazolidinediones (pioglitazone) are drugs that bind to PPARγ. They have a positive influence on NAFLD reducing the liver fat content and leading to histological improvement [64]. According to recent studies, glucagon-like peptide 1 (GLP-1) receptor agonists and sodium-glucose cotransporter 2 (SGLT2) inhibitors are expected to ameliorate NASH and NAFLD [65].

References

1. Emerenziani S, Pier Luca Guarino M, Trillo Asensio LM, Altomare A, Ribolsi M, Balestrieri P, et al. Role of overweight and obesity in gastrointestinal disease. Nutrients. 2020;12:111.
2. Su Youn Nam. Obesity-related digestive diseases and their pathophysiology. Gut Liver. 2017;11:323–34.
3. Meigs JB. Metabolic syndrome (insulin resistance syndrome or syndrome X); 2021.
4. Chang M, Yang Z, Sien-Sing Yang SS. Roles of Adipokines in digestive diseases: markers of inflammation, metabolic alteration and disease progression. Int J Mol Sci. 2020;21:8308.
5. Jianping YE. Mechanisms of insulin resistance in obesity. Front Med. 2013;7:14–24.
6. Camilleri M, Malhi H, Acosta A. Gastrointestinal complications of obesity. Gastroenterology. 2017;152(7):1656–70.
7. Corley D, Kubo A. Body mass index and gastroesophageal reflux disease: a systematic review and meta-analysis. Am J Gastroenterol. 2006;101:2619–28.
8. Cook M, Greenwood D, Hardie L, et al. A systematic review and meta-analysis of the risk of increasing adiposity on Barrett's esophagus. Am J Gastroenterol. 2008;103:292–300.

9. Harper JW, Zisman TL. Interaction of obesity and inflammatory bowel disease. World J Gastroenterol. 2016;22(35):7868–81.
10. Singh S, Parambir Dulai S, Zarrinpar A, Ramamoorthy S, Sandborn WJ. Obesity in IBD: epidemiology, pathogenesis, disease course and treatment outcomes. Nat Rev Gastroenterol Hepatol. 2017;14(2):110–21.
11. Seminerio JL, et al. Impact of obesity on the management and clinical course of patients with inflammatory bowel disease. Inflamm Bowel Dis. 2015;21:2857–63.
12. Khatua B, El-Kurdi B, Singh VP. Obesity and pancreatitis. Curr Opin Gastroenterol. 2017;33(5):374–82.
13. Krishnan B, Babu S, Walker J, Walker AB, Pappachan JM. Gastrointestinal complications of diabetes mellitus. World J Diabetes. 2013;4(3):51–63.
14. Hasler WL. Gastroparesis. Curr Opin Gastroenterol. 2012;28:621.
15. Grover M, Farrugia G, Lurken MS, Bernard CE, Faussone Pellegrini MS, Smyrk TC, et al. Cellular changes in diabetic and idiopathic gastroparesis. Gastroenterology. 2011;140:1575–85.
16. Parkman HP, Yates K, Hasler WL, Nguyen L, Pasricha PJ, Snape WJ, et al. Similarities and differences between diabetic and idiopathic gastroparesis. Clin Gastroenterol Hepatol. 2011;9:1056–64.
17. Wisse BE. The inflammatory syndrome: the role of adipose tissue cytokines in metabolic disorders linked to obesity. J Am Soc Nephrol. 2004;15(11):2792–800.
18. Rochlani Y, Venkata Pothineni N, Kovelamudi S, Mehta JL. Metabolic syndrome: pathophysiology, management, and modulation by natural compounds. Ther Adv Cardiovasc Dis. 2017;11(8):215–25.
19. Ruotolo G, Howard BV. Dyslipidemia of the metabolic syndrome. Curr Cardiol Rep. 2000;4(6):494–500.
20. Anstee QM, Reeves HL, Kotsiliti E, Govaere O, Heikenwalder M. From NASH to HCC: current concepts and future challenges. Nat Rev Gastroenterol Hepatol. 2019;16(7):411–28.
21. Schwartz JM, Carithers RL. Epidemiology and risk factors for hepatocellular carcinoma; 2021.
22. Ferlay J, Shin HR, Bray F, Forman D, Mathers C, Parkin DM. Estimates of worldwide burden of cancer in 2008: GLOBOCAN 2008. Int J Cancer. 2010;127(12):2893–917.
23. Stickel F, Hellerbrand C. Non-alcoholic fatty liver disease as a risk factor for hepatocellular carcinoma: mechanisms and implications. Gut. 2010;59(10):1303–7.
24. Golabi P, Rhea L, Henry L, Younossi ZM. Hepatocellular carcinoma and non-alcoholic fatty liver disease. Hepatol Int. 2019;13(6):688–94.
25. Zhang X. NAFLD related-HCC: the relationship with metabolic disorders. Adv Exp Med Biol. 2018;1061:55–62.
26. Avila JT, Park KT, Golden NH. Eating disorders in adolescents with chronic gastrointestinal and endocrine disease. Lancet Child Adolesc Health. 2019;3(3):181–9.
27. Sato Y, Fukudo S. Gastrointestinal symptoms and disorders in patients with eating disorders. Clin J Gastroenterol. 2015;8:255–63.
28. Lasater LM, Mehler PS. Medical complications of bulimia nervosa. Eat Behav. 2001;2(3):279–92.
29. Guandalini S, Assiri A. Celiac disease: a review. JAMA Pediatr. 2014;168:272–8.
30. Yang Z, Clark N, Park KT. Effectiveness and cost-effectiveness of measuring fecal calprotectin in diagnosis of inflammatory bowel disease in adults and children. Clin Gastroenterol Hepatol. 2014;12:253–62.
31. Levine A, Koletzko S, Turner D, et al. ESPGHAN revised Porto criteria for the diagnosis of inflammatory bowel disease in children and adolescents. J Pediatr Gastroenterol Nutr. 2014;58:795–806.
32. Krela-Kaźmierczak I, Szymczak A, Łykowska-Szuber L, Eder P, Linke K. Osteoporosis in gastrointestinal diseases. Adv Clin Exp Med. 2016;25(1):185–90.
33. Hofbauer LC, Schoppet M. Clinical implications of the osteoprotegerin/RANKL/RANK system for bone and vascular diseases. JAMA. 2004;292:490–5.
34. Canalis E. Osteoporosis Int. 2007;18:1319.

35. Swanson C, Lorentzon M, Conaway HH, et al. Glucocorticoid regulation of osteoclast differentiation and expression of receptor activator of nuclear factor-kappaB (NF-kappaB) ligand, osteoprotegerin, and receptor activator of NF-kappaB in mouse calvarial bones. Endocrinology. 2006;147:3613–22.
36. Ratajczak AE, Rychter AM, Zawada A, Dobrowolska A, Krela-Kaźmierczak I. Lactose intolerance in patients with inflammatory bowel diseases and dietary management in prevention of osteoporosis. Nutrition. 2021;82:111043.
37. Ghosh S, Cowen S, Hannan WJ. Low bone mineral density in Crohn's disease, but not in ulcerative colitis, at diagnosis. Gastroenterology. 1994;107:1031–9.
38. Guidelines for osteoporosis in inflammatory bowel disease and celiac disease written and approved by the British Society of Gastroenterology; 2007.
39. Tigas S, et al. Endocrine and metabolic manifestations in inflammatory bowel disease. Ann Gastroenterol. 2012;25:37.
40. Mulder CJ. Celiac disease presenting as severe osteopenia. Hawaii Med J. 2011;70:242–4.
41. Melton, et al. Fracture risk after surgery for peptic ulcer disease: a population-based cohort study. Bone. 1999;25(53):851–60.
42. Van Leeuwen J, van Driel M, van den Bemd G, Pols H. Vitamin D control of osteoblast function and bone extracellular matrix mineralization. Crit Rev Eukaryot Gene Expr. 2001;11:199–226.
43. Handzlik-Orlik G, Holecki M, Wilczyński K, Duława J. Osteoporosis in liver disease: pathogenesis and management. Ther Adv Endocrinol Metab. 2016;7(3):128–35.
44. Elliott R, Kostenuik P, Chen C. Denosumab is a selective inhibitor of human receptor activator of NF-kb ligand (RNKL) that blocks osteoclast formation and function. Osteoporos Int. 2007;18
45. Hays MT. Localization of human thyroxine absorption. Thyroid. 1991;1(3):241–8.
46. Pabla D, Akhlaghi F, Zia H. A comparative pH-dissolution profile study of selected commercial levothyroxine products using inductively coupled plasma mass spectrometry. Eur J Pharm Biopharm. 2009;72(1):105–10.
47. Virili C, Antonelli A, Santaguida MG, Benvenga S, Centanni M. Gastrointestinal malabsorption of thyroxine. Endocr Rev. 2019;40(1):118–36.
48. Padwal R, Brocks D, Sharma AM. A systematic review of drug absorption following bariatric surgery and its theoretical implications. Obes Rev. 2010;11(1):41–50.
49. Tran TH, Smith C, Mangione RA. Drug absorption in celiac disease. Am J Health Syst Pharm. 2013;70(24):2199–206.
50. Bayless TM, Brown E, Paige DM. Lactase nonpersistence and lactose intolerance. Curr Gastroenterol Rep. 2017;19(5):23.
51. Arola H, Tamm A. Metabolism of lactose in the human body. Scand J Gastroenterol Suppl. 1994;202:21–5.
52. Hildebrand H, Karlberg J, Kristiansson B. Longitudinal growth in children and adolescents with inflammatory bowel disease. J Pediatr Gastroenterol Nutr. 1994;18:165–73.
53. Katsanos KH, Tsatsoulis A, Christodoulou D, Challa A, Katsaraki A, Tsianos EV. Reduced serum insulin-like growth factor-1 (IGF-1) and IGF-binding protein-3 levels in adults with inflammatory bowel disease. Growth Hormon IGF Res. 2001;11:364–7.
54. Allen DB, Julius JR, Breen TJ, Attie KM. Treatment of glucocorticoid-induced growth suppression with growth hormone. J Clin Endocrinol Metabol. 1998;83:2824–9.
55. Kleinman RE, Baldassano RN, Caplan A, et al. Nutrition support for pediatric patients with inflammatory bowel disease: a clinical report of the north American Society for Pediatric Gastroenterology, hepatology and nutrition. J Pediatr Gastroenterol Nutr. 2004;39:15–27.
56. Terranova PF, Rice VM. Review: cytokine involvement in ovarian processes. Am J Reprod Immunol. 1997;37:50–63.
57. Warren MP, Voussoughian F, Geer EB, Hyle EP, Adberg CL, et al. Functional hypothalamic amenorrhea: hypoleptinemia and disordered eating. J Clin Endocrinol Metab. 1999;84:873–7.
58. Valvano M, Longo S, Stefanelli G, Frieri G, Viscido A, et al. Celiac disease, gluten-free diet, and metabolic and liver disorders. Nutrients. 2020;12(4):940.

59. Tortora R, Capone P, De Stefano G, Imperatore N, Gerbino N, et al. Metabolic syndrome in patients with coeliac disease on a gluten-free diet. Aliment Pharmacol Ther. 2015;41:352–9.
60. Hoffmanová I, Sánchez D, Tučková L, Tlaskalová-Hogenová H. Celiac disease and liver disorders: from putative pathogenesis to clinical implications. Nutrients. 2018;10(7):892.
61. Magrì S, Paduano D, Chicco F, Cingolani A, Farris C, et al. Nonalcoholic fatty liver disease in patients with inflammatory bowel disease: beyond the natural history. World J Gastroenterol. 2019;25(37):5676–86.
62. Rahimi L, Rajpal A, Ismail-Beigi F. Glucocorticoid-induced fatty liver disease. Diabetes Metab Syndr Obes. 2020;16(13):1133–45.
63. Li X, Guo X, Ji F, Niu J, Gao P. Relationships between metabolic comorbidities and occurrence, severity, and outcomes in patients with acute pancreatitis: a narrative review. Biomed Res Int. 2019;7:146.
64. Tilg H, Moschen AR, Roden M. NAFLD and diabetes mellitus. Nat Rev Hepatol. 2016;14(1):32–42.
65. Sumida Y, Yoneda M, Tokushige K, et al. Antidiabetic therapy in the treatment of nonalcoholic steatohepatitis. Int J Mol Sci. 2020;21(6):1907.

Immune-Mediated Disorders

25

Mirjana Turkalj

Abbreviations

AIE	Autoimmune enteropathy
APC	Antigen-presenting cells
ATD	Autoimmune thyroid disease
CD	Celiac disease
EGID	Eosinophilic gastrointestinal disorders
EoE	Eosinophilic esophagitis
FGID	Functional gastrointestinal disorders
FOXP3	Forkhead box P3
GI	Gastrointestinal
IMIDs	Immune-mediated diseases
IBD	Inflammatory bowel disease
Ig	Immunoglobulin
IL	Interleukin
IPEX	Immune dysfunction, polyendocrinopathy, enteropathy, X-linked
NCGS	Nonceliac gluten sensitivity
NLH	Nodular lymphoid hyperplasia
STAT	Signal transducer and activator of transcription
TH1	T helper lymphocytes type 1.
TH2	T helper lymphocytes type 2
TNF-α	Tumor necrosis factor-alpha

M. Turkalj (✉)
Srebrnjak Children's Hospital, Zagreb, Croatia

Faculty of Medicine, J. J. Strossmayer University of Osijek, Osijek, Croatia

Catholic University of Croatia, Zagreb, Croatia
e-mail: mturkalj@bolnica-srebrnjak.hr

M. Banić, D. Erceg (eds.), *Drug Interactions in Gastroenterology*, Clinical Gastroenterology, https://doi.org/10.1007/978-3-031-69800-2_25

Introduction

Immune responses play a key role in maintaining tissue homeostasis, influencing nearly all systems and organs of the body, such as the gut, skin, lungs, and others. Excessive immune response and chronic inflammation is a key driver in many disorders such as chronic infection, and inflammatory and autoimmune diseases [1].

Immune cells are actively involved in regulating the balance between homeostasis and inflammation and contributing to the maintenance of the health condition. Abnormal innate and adaptive immunities are important factors in the development of immune-mediated disorders (IMDs).For example, dysregulated innate immunity plays a key role in the mechanisms of autoinflammatory disorders, while disturbed adaptive immunity plays a role in celiac disease and autoimmune enteropathy [2]. IMDs which affect the gastrointestinal (GI) tract may compromise GI integrity, interfere with the absorption of nutrients, and cause chronic inflammation [1, 3].

However, IMDs consist of a wide spectrum of gastrointestinal (GI) and extraintestinal disorders. In this chapter, some of the following IMDs with emphasis on the display changes in the immune response will be specifically described:

- Autoimmune enteropathy.
- Celiac disease.
- Food and wheat allergy.
- Eosinophilic gastrointestinal disorders (EGID).
- Eosinophilic esophagitis.
- Inflammatory bowel diseases.
- IMDs in patients with primary immunodeficiency.
- FIGDs.
- Autoinflammatory disorders.

Autoimmune Enteropathy and Autoimmune Gastritis

Autoimmune enteropathy (AIE) is a rare disorder characterized by severe and protracted diarrhea and small intestinal mucosal atrophy resulting from immune-mediated injury. The disease was first described in 1982. The mean features of the disease are chronic diarrhea, malabsorption, small intestinal villous atrophy, lack of response to dietary exclusion, and presence of circulating auto-enteric antibodies [4].

Although AIE is traditionally considered a disease of the small intestine, other sites in the tubular gut may be affected as well. The most common histopathology pattern seen in the small intestine is active enteritis with prominent villous blunting, mononuclear inflammation in the lamina propria, lymphocytic infiltration into deep crypt epithelium (<40 lymphocytes/100 epithelial cells), increased crypt apoptotic bodies, and sometimes with crypt microabscesses. Goblet cells and Paneth cell numbers may be strongly decreased or completely absent. Colon histopathology shows similar abnormalities [5].

Extraintestinal manifestations of AIE can be hypothyroidism, rheumatoid arthritis, nephrotic syndrome, and autoimmune hemolytic anemia. Although it is primarily a pediatric disease, it is now well recognized to occur in adults, as well. AIE appears to result from dysregulation of gut humoral and cellular immunity. Although the pathomechanism of the development of AIE is not fully known, a deficiency or dysfunction in CD4+ and CD25+ regulatory T cells which are involved in the downregulation of immune responses appears to play an important role. Aberrant expression of HLA class II molecules by enterocytes has been described in patients with AIE and circulating autoantibodies to intestinal epithelial cells (goblet cells or enterocytes) are often detected in AIE patients [6].

Genetic mutations in the inherited form of AIE result in T cell overactivity. In patients with the rare X-linked recessive disorder known as IPEX syndrome (immune dysregulation polyendocrinopathy enteropathy X-linked), mutation in the FOXP3 gene (forkhead box p3) in T cells has been found. FOXP3 or a transcriptional regulator is required for normal function and development of regulatory T-cells (Treg). Loss of FOXP3 activity leads to immune overactivity to antigen stimulation and cellular injury via CD4+ T cells. IPEX syndrome manifested early in infancy with insulin-dependent diabetes mellitus, AEI, and skin manifestations such as severe eczema or alopecia. Other genetic mutations that result in T-cell overactivity underlie syndromic forms of AIE such as Autoimmune phenomena, Polyendocrinopathy, Candidiasis, and Ectodermal Dystrophy syndrome (APECED), also known as Autoimmune Polyglandular syndrome (APS-1) [7].

According to recent publications, it was confirmed that autoimmune thyroid disorders, in particular Hashimoto's thyroiditis, are frequently associated with other organ-specific, immune-mediated disorders, such as autoimmune atrophic gastritis or celiac disease. The association of Hashimoto's thyroiditis with autoimmune atrophic gastritis is currently recognized as a part of the polyglandular autoimmune syndromes. It is especially important to emphasize that thyro-entero-gastric autoimmunity may lead to potentially serious consequences like severe anemia, deficiency of micronutrients, and malabsorption, as well as increased risk for malignancies, as well [5, 6, 8].

Celiac Disease

Celiac disease (CD) was the first described gluten-related disorder. It is known that gluten-related disorders also include nonceliac gluten sensitivity (NCGS) and wheat allergy (WA), as well. CD is a multisystem immune-mediated enteropathy which is found in genetically susceptible individuals exposed to dietary gluten present in wheat, barley, and rye. CD has been recognized to be one of the common causes of malabsorption in children as well as in adults. Celiac disease occurs in about 1% of the general population worldwide. Although the prevalence of CD is on the rise, it is still underdiagnosed because CD often manifests with a silent, subtle, or atypical clinical picture. The estimated risk of CD in first-degree relatives is 4–17% and up to 26% in relatives who are homozygous for HLA DQ2or HLA DQ-8 [9].

The primary mechanism involved in CD is related to an inappropriate innate and adaptive immune response to gluten-derived peptides. Gluten is rich in glutamines and prolamines which are incompletely digested into large peptides [10]. These peptides enter into the lamina propria of a small intestine via transcellular and paracellular routes, where the tissue transglutaminase deaminates gliadin increasing its immunogenicity. The deamidated gliadin peptides were processed by the antigen processing cells (APCs) and presented to the T lymphocytes associated with the APCs surface HLA DQ2 or DQ8 molecules. The immunological cascade continues with gliadin-specific CD4-positive T cells which stimulate the production of pro-inflammatory cytokines and the release of metalloproteinases leading to tissue injury. The injury of the small intestinal Villi leads to loss of the absorptive surface area, and the development of symptoms of diarrhea, abdominal pain, and malabsorption of micronutrients, iron, fat-soluble vitamins, vitamin B12, and folic acid [11, 12].

Patients with suspected CD IgG-based testing of IgG anti-TTG or IgG DGP (deamidated gliadin peptide) should be performed. IgA antiendomysial antibodies are highly specific tests (specificity approaches 100%), but are reserved to confirm active celiac disease. Immunoglobulin A (IgA) antitissue transglutaminase (TTG) antibody has a high sensitivity (>95%) and specificity (>95%) and it is recommended as a screening test in patients who do not have concomitant selective IgA deficiency [13].

For the confirmation of the diagnosis of CD, an upper endoscopy with duodenal biopsies should be performed. In patients with CD, characteristic histological feature consists of >25 intraepithelial lymphocytes per 100 enterocytes with elongation of crypts and villous atrophy. Absence of villous atrophy in the presence of IEL is not specific to CD and other causes should be considered [14].

Patients present with a wide spectrum of intestinal and extraintestinal symptoms and are at risk for non-Hodgkin's lymphoma and small intestinal adenocarcinoma, as well. The cornerstone for the treatment of CD is a gluten-free diet. Gluten-free diet improves symptoms, reduces mucosal damage, and eliminates risks for osteoporosis and malignancy. Hidden sources of gluten include contaminated oats, sauces, drug fillers, shared food preparation equipment, and processed meats [13, 14].

Nonceliac Gluten Sensitivity (NCGS)

NCGS is a relatively new recognized clinical entity induced by the ingestion of dietary gluten leading to intestinal and/or extraintestinal symptoms in patients when CD and WA have been excluded and resolved with a gluten-free diet. The symptoms of NCGS may overlap with CD and WA (abdominal pain, bloating, fatigue, headaches, eczema, joint pain, and mood disorders). Patients have a negative IgA TTG and EMA and about 50% may have positive IgG DGP but rarely positive IgA DGP. The endoscopy is almost always normal without Villi atrophy and with mild elevated number of intraepithelial lymphocytes. Up to 50% of patients are homozygous for HLA DQ2 or HLA DQ-8 [11].

The pathogenesis of NCGS is unknown. Sapone A. et al. suggested an important involvement of innate immune response with the activation of toll-like receptors in NCGS pathogenesis. Other studies investigating the pathogenesis of NCGS have suggested elevated number of CD3-positive intraepithelial lymphocytes, increased interferon γ to a gluten challenge suggests gut mucosal activation, as well as increased intestinal permeability [15]. NCGS does not lead to malabsorption and there is no risk of malignancy if left untreated. The goal of treatment is the exclusion of obvious and hidden gluten.

Wheat Allergy

Wheat allergy, especially if manifested by extraintestinal symptoms is not easy to distinguish from other gluten-related disorders, such as celiac disease and NCGS. The wheat allergy can manifest with a very colorful clinical picture such as IgE-mediated anaphylaxis, wheat-dependent exercise-induced anaphylaxis, urticaria, and angioedema or as non-IgE mediated wheat allergy with eosinophilic esophagitis or eosinophilic gastritis. Repeated exposure to wheat flour in pasta factory workers and bakers can induce baker's asthma and baker's rhinitis [16].

Food allergy to wheat as well as other allergic IgE and non-IgE-mediated allergic reactions to food is typically characterized by a T helper type 2 (TH2) lymphocytic inflammation in genetically susceptible individuals. The subsequent cascade of TH2 activation could either lead to an IgE-mediated response with wheat-specific IgE antibodies or a non-IgE-mediated allergy with chronic inflammation of lymphocytes and eosinophils [17].

Currently, the management of WA is based on a wheat diet. Patients should undergo dietary advice and referrals to identify relevant food. Certain therapeutic options in allergic patients including allergen-specific immunotherapy such as oral immunotherapy, sublingual immunotherapy, and epicutaneous immunotherapy are under investigation [16].

Food Allergy

Food allergy is an umbrella term used to describe a variety of adverse, food antigen-driven, immune-mediated diseases which can be manifested in different organs including gastrointestinal tract. The main mechanism includes a breakdown of immunologic tolerance, activation of type 2 immune response, and an impaired mucosal barrier influenced by diverse factors such as diet, infections, changes in gastrointestinal microbiome composition, and genetic and epigenetic factors. Early childhood is recognized as a critical period when these factors have a dominant impact on shaping the immune system and therefore triggering or protecting against the development of food allergy [18].

Gastrointestinal allergic diseases include a spectrum of disorders classified by IgE-mediated, non-IgE-mediated, and mixed IgE-mediated and non-IgE-mediated diseases. Several common pathways in GI allergic diseases have been recognized such as loss of immunologic tolerance including dysregulation of antigen processing and change in function of Treg cells, activation of type 2 immune with domination of Th2 cell responses compared with responses of other T cell subtypes (Treg, TH1, Th17) as well as increased TH2 cytokine production. The Th2 response increases the production of allergen-specific IgE and the production and activation of mast cell, basophil, and eosinophil. The third key event essential for the development of food allergens is an impaired epithelial barrier resulting in increasing encounters of food antigens with immune cells and initiation of epithelial innate immune responses. Finally, collaboration of environmental and genetic factors influences these pathways and promotes or protects against allergic GI disease development [19].

IgE-mediated food allergy may be diagnosed on the basis of a history and physical suggestive of an allergic process and immunological tests including food challenges such as skin prick test, in vitro specific Immunoglobulin E, molecular-based allergy or epitope diagnostics, in vitro flow cytometry-assisted basophile activation test, functional assays or food challenge tests including double-blind placebo-controlled oral food challenge test [20].

Currently, the management of food allergy is based on dietary advice and referrals to identify relevant food allergens, especially for eight of the most common food allergens (milk, egg, peanuts, tree nuts, fish, shellfish, soy, and wheat) [19].

Nonimmunoglobulin E (IgE)-mediated food hypersensitivity includes a spectrum of disorders that predominantly affect the gastrointestinal tract including food protein-induced enterocolitis syndrome allergic proctocolitis, food protein-induced enteropathy, pulmonary hemosiderosis or Heiner syndrome, and cow's milk protein-induced iron deficiency anemia [21].

The symptoms of non-IgE-mediated food hypersensitivity are typically delayed from hours to weeks after ingestion of the culprit food(s). The usual presenting features are profuse emesis and dehydration, blood-streaked protracted diarrhea, and mucous stools with malabsorption. Diagnosis of the non-IgE-mediated food hypersensitivity syndromes can be challenging due to the lack of noninvasive confirmatory tests for most of these disorders and is based on a convincing history and resolution of symptoms with food avoidance [22].

Eosinophilic Gastrointestinal Disorders (EGID)

Eosinophilic gastrointestinal disorders (EGID) are a group of immune-mediated chronic inflammatory disorders triggered by food allergens, characterized by pathologic eosinophilic infiltration of the gastrointestinal tract including esophagus, stomach, small intestine, or colon leading to organ dysfunction and clinical symptoms [23]. These disorders include eosinophilic esophagitis (EoE), eosinophilic gastritis, eosinophilic gastroenteritis, eosinophilic enteritis, and eosinophilic colitis. Symptoms are dependent on the predominant location or organ involved and can be manifested with dysphagia and food impaction, heartburn, abdominal pain, vomiting, nausea, early satiety, diarrhea, and weight loss. Treatment strategies focus on controlling symptoms and bowel inflammation as well as diet of identified food triggers [24].

Eosinophilic Esophagitis (EoE)

Eosinophilic esophagitis (EoE) is an atopic condition of the esophagus resulting from a mixed IgE- and non-IgE-mediated allergic response to food and environmental allergens. Currently seems that non-IgE-mediated mechanisms predominate in EoE. EoE has become increasingly recognized over the last 20 years. The disorder is also referred to as "asthma of the esophagus" given that it shares many clinical and pathophysiologic characteristics with asthma. Risk factors for EoE include atopy and other allergic conditions, e.g., allergic rhinitis, elevated serum immunoglobulin E to common aeroallergens, asthma, and atopic dermatitis. Patients with concomitant EoE and seasonal allergic rhinitis may have more EoE exacerbations during seasons of pollination of aeroallergens. Other risk factors for EoE include alterations in gut barrier function, variation in the nature and timing of aeroallergen exposure, altered microbiome, lack of early exposure to microbes, an *ACE* gene polymorphisms and transforming growth factor-beta polymorphisms, etc. [25, 26].

The pathogenesis of EoE results from an interplay of genetic, immune, and environmental factors which leads to mucosal damage and fibrosis. It is associated with T helper cell-2 (Th2) type immune responses. Elevated levels of the Th2 cytokines interleukin (IL)-4, IL-5, and IL-13, with infiltration of mast cells and eosinophils, have been found in the esophageal biopsies of EoE patients. Eosinophils have a crucial role in the remodeling of esophageal tissues and the development of subepithelial fibrosis. Eosinophils contribute to fibrosis through degranulation and secretion of their granule proteins, such as major basic protein and fibrogenic growth factors (TGF-β) [27, 28].

However, in EoE, eosinophils infiltrate the esophagus, contributing to tissue damage and chronic inflammation. EoE is defined as a disorder characterized by ≥15 eosinophils per high power field and the absence of pathologic gastrointestinal reflux disease with normal pH monitoring study or lack of response to adequate reflux therapy [29]. The majority of patients with EoE have been found to have positive skin prick tests and atopy patch tests for foods and/or aeroallergens. Patients with EoE should be referred to an allergist for optimal management, which may include dietary modifications and pharmacologic agents such as corticosteroids, and for the diagnosis and management of comorbid atopic conditions. Mechanical dilation of the esophagus may also be necessary [30].

Inflammatory Bowel Diseases (IBD)

Inflammatory bowel diseases (IBD) belong to the group of immune-mediated diseases (IMDs) presenting with the primary two forms, Crohn's disease and ulcerative colitis. However, IMDs, consist of a wide spectrum of gastrointestinal and extraintestinal disorders. Dysregulated innate and adaptive immunities are involved in IMDs. There are overlaps in etiopathogenetic pathways, clinical presentations, endoscopic features, and histologic characteristics between classic IBD, autoimmune disorders, and autoinflammatory disorders [31]. Over the second half of the twentieth century, IMDs and IBD markedly increased and since the beginning of the twenty-first century, have been considered in Westernized countries as one of the most prevalent gastrointestinal disorders. In Europe, IBD affects up to 2.2 million patients with an annual incidence ranging between 9 and 15% depending on the geographical area [32].

IBD is chronic and life-threatening inflammatory bowel disease characterized by episodes of inflammation of the intestinal mucosa including Crohn's disease, ulcerative colitis, and IBD-unclassified. IBD is characterized by episodes of abdominal pain, diarrhea, bloody stools, and weight loss. Chronic inflammation of intestinal mucosa is characterized by episodes of exacerbation with the influx of neutrophils and macrophages that produce cytokines, proteolytic enzymes, and free radicals resulting in the reinforcement of inflammation and ulceration. Crohn's disease usually affects the terminal ileum, cecum, perianal area, and colon, but often another region of the intestine in a discontinuous pattern. Ulcerative colitis involves the rectum as well as part of the colon or the entire colon in a continuous pattern. Histological characteristics of Crohn's disease are thickened submucosa, transmural inflammation, fissuring ulceration, and granulomas, while in ulcerative colitis inflammation are limited to the mucosa and submucosa with cryptitis and crypt abscesses [33].

Pathogenesis of IBD is associated with the genetic susceptibility of the host, influence of particular environmental factors such as intestinal microbiota which lead to the development of immunological abnormalities. Associations between genetic and environmental factors (smoking, diet, stress), intestinal microbiota, and proinflammatory and anti-inflammatory immune cells and molecules are continuously investigated and evaluated to understand the pathogenesis of IBD. The immunological dysregulation in IBD is characterized by epithelial damage, enlargement of inflammation driven by intestinal flora, failure of immune regulation to control the inflammatory response with an elevated number of cells infiltrating into the lamina propria including dendritic cells, macrophages, neutrophils, T cells, B lymphocytes. Epithelial integrity of GIT is disturbed with high apoptotic rates, disturbed tight junctions between epithelial cells are disturbed as well, and intestinal epithelial goblet cells are remodeled in IBD patients [34].

In IBD, there is a manifestly increased local production of proinflammatory cytokines such as TNF and TNF-related cytokines and the IL-6 family of cytokines: IL-12, IL-23, IL-17, IL-18, and TGF-β, nonspecific inflammatory mediators, such as leukotrienes, free radicals, and chemokines, which follow the influx of inflammatory cells into the intestinal tissue. The main cells involved in the pathomechanism of IMDs and IBD are CD4+ lymphocytes. However, naïve $CD4^+$ T cells may differentiate into different types of Th cells in the presence of cytokines, including Th1, Th2, Th17, and Th9, and inducible regulatory T (iTreg) cells. The dysfunction of Treg in IBD is usually believed to be due to the defective numbers of Treg or their suppressive function which cannot control the inflammation in intestinal tissue. It has been accepted that Crohn's disease is caused in genetically susceptible individuals by a Th1 immune response and uncontrolled IL-23/Th17 pathway activation to bacterial antigens. On the other side, ulcerative colitis is characterized as a "Th2-like" disease characterized by increased amounts of IL-5 and IL-13. Furthermore, impaired immune responses mediated by Th17 and Treg are implicated in both Crohn's disease and ulcerative colitis, while Th9 cells are predominately included in the pathogenesis of ulcerative colitis [34, 35].

Knowledge of the mechanisms of IBD is crucial to develop novel personalized treatments both for the development of new biomarkers for diagnosis, monitoring, and prediction of disease progress and treatment outcome but also for the development of optimal and new therapeutic options such as TNF alfa inhibitors, NF-κB, and Intercellular adhesion molecule 1 blockers, and other new biologics [36, 37].

Primary Immunodeficiency

Gastrointestinal (GI) disorders present in 5% to 50% of patients with primary immunodeficiencies. This is expected because the gut is the largest lymphoid organ in the body producing large amounts of immunoglobulin and which accommodates numerous lymphocytes. Therefore, it is not surprising that GI disorders are common manifestations in patients with dysfunction in humoral or cellular immunity. The type of immunodeficiency is often suggestive by the nature of infections, e.g., bacterial infections indicate B-cell deficiency, viral or fungal infections indicate T-cell deficiency, and T- and B-cell deficiencies suggest the combined type of immunodeficiency. Many of IMDs patients with PID mimic classic forms of disease such as celiac disease, IBD, or pernicious anemia but differ in pathogenesis and are often unresponsive to conventional therapies [38].

Actually, it is imperative to consider immunodeficiency in any patient with intractable diarrhea, malabsorption, and failure to thrive that is resistant to conventional treatments. Opportunistic or unusual infections in the setting of presumed IMDs should arouse clinical suspicion and immune evaluation and in that case, referring the suspected patient to an immunologist is essential [39].

A clinical history of recurrent infection, atypical histological features that do not fit the usual pattern of disease, and a poor response to conventional therapy should be a signal to search for or exclude primary immunodeficiency. Primary immunodeficiency disorders are relatively common but likely underdiagnosed. Early evaluation and diagnosis of PID in patients with GI symptoms or immune-mediated diseases can prevent potentially irreversible tissue damage. Replacement therapy with immunoglobulins of PID patients in most cases does not prevent or reverse the development of GI disease. It is therefore necessary to administer additional therapies [40].

Functional Gastrointestinal Disorders (FGIDs)

Functional gastrointestinal disorders (FGIDs) are conditions of disordered GI function for which there are no evident structural pathologies. These disorders are diagnosed by patient-reported symptoms, including epigastric pain syndrome, postprandial distress syndrome, irritable bowel syndrome, and functional dyspepsia. It is estimated that over 40% of the general population reports such unexplained abdominal symptoms. Recently, publications in the field suggested an association of activation and an influx of effector cells such as mast cells and eosinophils into the GI tract in the pathogenesis of FGIDs as well as involvement of imbalances in the microbiota and immune responses against dietary components [41].

There are also possible associations between FGIDs and atopy, as well as between FGIDs and nonceliac wheat sensitivity (NCWS). In addition, it seems that T-helper type (Th) 17 cells, in conjunction with Th2 pathways of immune responses are included in the pathogenesis of FGIDs. Reduction in Th1-associated cytokines pathway and increase in Th2-cytokines suggest a disruption to the Th1/Th2 cytokine balance in FGIDs. Homeostatic disruption in the GI tract may drive the loss of Treg cells and ILC3s in favor of a Th17/ILC2-mediated inflammation. Secretion of IL-23 induces naive $CD4^{+}$ T cells to differentiate into Th17 cells, capable of producing IL-17, TNF-α, IL-1β, and IL-6. These cytokines have been reported to be increased in the blood of patients with FGID. Th17 responses have been demonstrated in asthma patients, where Th17 lymphocytes are induced by antigen-presenting cells to release IL-17, which is able to act on the airway epithelium [42, 43].

It is plausible that a subset of patients with FIGDs like asthmatics may have symptoms that result from a Th17-driven immune response. The identification of underlying immune mechanisms in FGIDs represented an important advance in the understanding of these conditions but have not comprehended how these immune pathways are associated with observed changes and clinical pictures [41–43].

Autoinflammatory Disorders

Autoinflammatory diseases or period fever syndromes are a group of rare disorders caused by abnormal activation of the innate immune response and episodes of fever and inflammation. Autoinflammatory diseases such as familial Mediterranean fever, cryopyrin-associated periodic syndromes, deficiency of IL-1-receptor antagonist, and hyper IgD syndrome are caused by changes in genes that regulate the involvement of the innate immune system [44]. The most common symptoms of autoinflammatory disease are fluctuating degrees and recurrent fever. Additional symptoms include abdominal symptoms, joint inflammation, cutaneous signs, and other organ involvement that may lack specificity, making a clinical diagnosis difficult. If disorders are not recognized or not properly controlled, repeated inflammation can lead to the progression and subsidence of potentially fatal deposits of amyloid protein in vital organs [45].

The main mechanism of autoinflammatory disorders includes activation of innate immune cells like monocytes, macrophages, and neutrophils. These cells act as a first line of defense, providing a large array of membrane-bound and intracellular signaling receptors also called pattern-recognition receptors (PRR) which are important for the detection and action against pathogens. These PRRs are vital for danger sensing and recognition of structures expressed by pathogens such as microbial pathogen-associated molecular patterns or PAMPs or damaged cells like non-microbial damage-associated molecular patterns or DAMPs. Recognition of PAMP and DAMP by intracellular sensors leads to remodeling of a multimeric protein called inflammasomes. Inflammasomes are composed of sensor and adapter molecules such as apoptosis-related speck-like proteins containing caspase activation and recruitment domains and effectors molecules such as caspase-1. This pro-Caspase-1 is activated by proteolytic cleavage and further transformed into pro-IL-1β and pro IL-18 to their bioactive form, which is released into the bloodstream. IL-1 receptors sense IL-1β and activate by the NF-κB pathway which is translocated to the nucleus where it promotes the transcription of NF-κB-dependent genes, such as NLRP3, pro-IL-β, pro-IL-18, and IL-6 [46, 47].

References

1. Kurashima Y, Kiyono H. Mucosal ecological network of epithelium and immune cells for gut homeostasis and tissue healing. Annu Rev Immunol. 2017;35:119–47.
2. El Chamy L, Matt N, Ntwasa M, Reichhart JM. The multilayered innate immune defense of the gut. Biom J. 2015;38(4):276–84.
3. Roncarolo MG, Gregori S, Bacchetta R, Battaglia M, Gagliani N. The biology of t regulatory type 1 cells and their therapeutic application in immune-mediated diseases. Immunity. 2018;49:1004–19.
4. Gentile NM, Murray JA, Pardi DS. Autoimmune enteropathy: a review and update of clinical management. Curr Gastroenterol Rep. 2012;14(5):380–5.
5. Montalto M, D'Onofrio F, Santoro L, Gallo A, Gasbarrini A, Gasbarrini G. Autoimmune enteropathy in children and adults. Scand J Gastroenterol. 2009;44:1029–16.
6. Barzaghi F, Passerini L, Bacchetta R. Immune dysregulation, polyendocrinopathy, enteropathy, x-linked syndrome: a paradigm of immunodeficiency with autoimmunity. Front Immunol. 2012;3:211.
7. Bishu S, Arsenescu V, Lee EY, Vargas HD, de Villiers WJ, Arsenescu R. Autoimmune enteropathy with a CD8+ CD7− T-cell small bowel intraepithelial lymphocytosis: case report and literature review. BMC Gastroenterol. 2011;11:131.
8. Singhi AD, Goyal A, Davison JM, Regueiro MD, Roche RL, Ranganathan S. Pediatric autoimmune enteropathy: an entity frequently associated with immunodeficiency disorders. Mod Pathol. 2014;27:543–53.
9. Lionetti E, Castellaneta S, Francavilla R, Pulvirenti A, Tonutti E, Amarri S, et al. Introduction of gluten, HLA status, and the risk of celiac disease in children. N Engl J Med. 2014;371:1295–303.

10. Biesiekierski JR. What is gluten? J Gastroenterol Hepatol. 2017;32(Suppl. 1):78–81.
11. Lebwohl B, Ludvigsson JF, Green PH. Celiac disease and non-celiac gluten sensitivity. BMJ. 2015;351:h4347.
12. Hollon J, Puppa EL, Greenwald B, Goldberg E, Guerrerio A, Fasano A. Effect of gliadin on permeability of intestinal biopsy explants from celiac disease patients and patients with non-celiac gluten sensitivity. Nutrients. 2015;7(3):1565–76.
13. Cianferoni A. Wheat allergy: diagnosis and management. J Asthma Allergy. 2016;9:13–25.
14. Molina-Infante J, Carroccio A. Suspected nonceliac gluten sensitivity confirmed in few patients after gluten challenge in double-blind, placebo-controlled trials. Clin Gastroenterol Hepatol. 2017;15(3):339–48.
15. Leonard MM, Sapone A, Catassi C, Fasano A. Celiac disease and nonceliac gluten sensitivity: a review. JAMA. 2017;318(7):647–56.
16. Elli L, Branchi F, Tomba C, Villalta D, Norsa L, Ferretti F, et al. Diagnosis of gluten related disorders: Celiac disease, wheatallergy and non-celiac gluten sensitivity. World J Gastroenterol. 2015;21(23):7110–9.
17. Pasha I, Saeed F, Sultan MT, Batool R, Aziz M, Ahmed W. Wheat allergy and intolerence; recent updates and perspectives. Crit Rev Food Sci Nutr. 2016;56(1):13–24.
18. Savage J, Johns CB. Food allergy: epidemiology and natural history. Immunol Allergy Clin N Am. 2015;35(1):45–59.
19. Renz H, Allen KJ, Sicherer SH, Sampson HA, Lack G, Beyer K, et al. Food allergy. Nat Rev Dis Prim. 2018;4:17098.
20. Yu W, Freeland DMH, Nadeau KC. Food allergy: immune mechanisms, diagnosis and immunotherapy. Nat Rev Immunol. 2016;16(12):751–65.
21. Nowak-Węgrzyn A, Katz Y, Mehr SS, Koletzko S. Non-IgE-mediated gastrointestinal food allergy. J Allergy Clin Immunol. 2015;135(5):1114–24.
22. Caubet JC, Szajewska H, Shamir R, Nowak-Węgrzyn A. Non-IgE-mediated gastrointestinal food allergies in children. Pediatr Allergy Immunol. 2017;28(1):6–17.
23. Kinoshita Y, Oouchi S, Fujisawa T. Eosinophilicgastrointestinaldiseases—pathogenesis, diagnosis, and treatment. Allergol Int. 2019;68(4):420–9.
24. Zhang M, Li Y. Eosinophilic gastroenteritis: a state-of-the-art review. J Gastroenterol Hepatol. 2017;32(1):64–72.
25. Furuta GT, Katzka DA. Eosinophilic esophagitis. N Engl J Med. 2015;373(17):1640–8.
26. Chen JW, Kao JY. Eosinophilic esophagitis: update on management and controversies. BMJ. 2017;359:j4482.
27. Simon D, Cianferoni A, Spergel JM, Aceves S, Holbreich M, Venter C, et al. Eosinophilic esophagitis is characterized by a non-IgE-mediated food hypersensitivity. Allergy. 2016;71(5):611–20.
28. D'Alessandro A, Esposito D, Pesce M, Cuomo R, De Palma GD, Sarnelli G. Eosinophilic esophagitis: from pathophysiology to treatment. World J Gastrointest Pathophysiol. 2015;6(4):150–8.
29. Schuyler AJ, Wilson JM, Tripathi A, Commins SP, Ogbogu PU, Kruzsewski PG, et al. Specific IgG_4 antibodies to cow's milk proteins in pediatric patients with eosinophilic esophagitis. J Allergy Clin Immunol. 2018;142(1):139–48.
30. Singla MB, Moawad FJ. An overview of the diagnosis and management of eosinophilic esophagitis. Clin Transl Gastroenterol. 2016;7(3):e155.
31. Conway G, Velonias G, Andrews E, Garber JJ, Yajnik V, Ananthakrishnan AN. The impact of co-existing immune-mediated diseases on phenotype and outcomes in inflammatory bowel diseases. Aliment Pharmacol Ther. 2017;45:814–23.
32. Sairenji T, Collins KL, Evans DV. An update on inflammatory bowel disease. Prim Care. 2017;44(4):673–92.
33. de Souza HS, Fiocchi C. Immunopathogenesis of IBD: current state of the art. Nat Rev Gastroenterol Hepatol. 2016;13:13–27.
34. Zhang YZ, Li YY. Inflammatory bowel disease: pathogenesis. World J Gastroenterol. 2014;20(1):91–9.

35. Aggeletopoulou I, Assimakopoulos SF, Konstantakis C, Triantos C. Interleukin 12/interleukin 23 pathway: biological basis and therapeutic effect in patients with Crohn's disease. World J Gastroenterol. 2018;24:4093–103.
36. Frieder J, Kivelevitch D, Haugh I, Watson I, Menter A. Anti-IL-23 and anti-IL-17 biologic agents for the treatment of immune-mediated inflammatory conditions. Clin Pharmacol Ther. 2018;103:88–101.
37. Jeong DY, Kim S, Son MJ, Son CY, Kim JY, Kronbichler A, et al. Induction and maintenance treatment of inflammatory bowel disease: a comprehensive review. Autoimmun Rev. 2019;18(5):439–54.
38. Amaya-Uribe L, Rojas M, Azizi G, Anaya JM, Gershwin ME. Primary immunodeficiency and autoimmunity: a comprehensive review. J Autoimmun. 2019;99:52–72.
39. Schwimmer D, Glover S. Primary immunodeficiency and the gut. Gastroenterol Clin N Am. 2019;48(2):199–220.
40. Agarwal S, Mayer L. Diagnosis and treatment of gastrointestinal disorders in patients with primary immunodeficiency. Clin Gastroenterol Hepatol. 2013;11(9):1050–63.
41. Holtmann G, Shah A, Morrison M. Pathophysiology of functional gastrointestinal disorders: a holistic overview. Dig Dis. 2017;35(Suppl. 1):5–13.
42. Keely S, Walker MM, Marks E, Talley NJ. Immune dysregulation in the functional gastrointestinal disorders. Eur J Clin Investig. 2015;45(12):1350–9.
43. Burns G, Carroll G, Mathe A, Horvat FP, Walker MM, et al. Evidence for local and systemic immune activation in functional dyspepsia and the irritable bowel syndrome: a systematic review. Am J Gastroenterol. 2019;114(3):429–36.
44. Ben-Chetrit E, Gattorno M, Gul A, Kastner DL, Lachmann HJ, Touitou I, et al. Consensus proposal for taxonomy and definition of the autoinflammatory diseases (AIDs): a Delphi study. Ann Rheum Dis. 2018;77:1558–65.
45. Rowczenio D, Shinar Y, Ceccherini I, Sheils K, Gijn MV, Patton SJ, et al. Current practices for the genetic diagnosis of autoinflammatory diseases: results of a European Molecular Genetics Quality Network Survey. Eur J Hum Genet. 2019;27(10):1502–8.
46. Awad F, Assrawi E, Louvrier C, Jumeau C, Georgin-Lavialle S, Grateau G, et al. Inflammasome biology, molecular pathology and therapeutic implications. Pharmacol Ther. 2018;187:133–49.
47. Manthiram Q, Zhou I, Aksentijevich D, KastnerL. The monogenic autoinflammatory diseases define new pathways in human innate immunity and inflammation. Nat Immunol. 2017;18:832–42.

Nervous System Disorders

26

Silvio Bašić, Romana Gjergja Juraški, and Ivana Marković

Introduction

There are several ways how gastrointestinal disorders could provoke neurological dysfunction. Some of the most frequent ones are caused by nutritional deficiency due to malabsorption of different vitamins or other substances like copper. On the other hand, accumulation of toxic metabolites such as ammonia, aromatic amino acids and mercaptans in liver failure frequently results in neurological disturbance. Different gastrointestinal infections such as Tropheryma whipplei, Campylobacter jejunii and hepatitis virus could also be the direct cause or a trigger for a neurological disorder. Moreover, some genetic or immunological/inflammatory gastrointestinal diseases could also present with neurological signs and symptoms.

On the other hand, a distinct number of neurological disorders produce different symptoms of gastrointestinal dysfunction such as obstipation, dysphagia, stomach pain, etc. Hence it is very important for both neurologists and gastroenterologists to be familiar with all conditions which all together could impact neurological and gastrointestinal systems independently of the core pathophysiological process localization.

S. Bašić (✉) · I. Marković
Department of Neurology, Dubrava University Hospital, Zagreb, Croatia

Department of Neurology and Neurosurgery, Faculty of Dental Medicine and Health, J. J. Strossmayer University of Osijek, Osijek, Croatia
e-mail: sbasic@fdmz.hr

R. Gjergja Juraški
Srebrnjak Children's Hospital, Zagreb, Croatia

Faculty of Medicine, J.J. Strossmayer University of Osijek, Osijek, Croatia

M. Banić, D. Erceg (eds.), *Drug Interactions in Gastroenterology*, Clinical Gastroenterology, https://doi.org/10.1007/978-3-031-69800-2_26

The Gut-Brain Axis

During the past few decades, it has been found that there is a complex interaction between the human body and intestinal microbial flora. Besides its physiological function, it has been found that the intestinal microbiome has a bidirectional relationship with various organ systems, particularly the central nervous system (CNS) and hence has a certain impact on brain function and behaviour [1]. A metagenomics analysis of the gut microbiome has shown that each individual harbours at least 160 bacterial species in gastrointestinal system with more than three million microbial genes. The structure of gut microbiota is highly dependent on an individual's genetic predisposition, age, nutrition, physical activity, environmental factors, stress, infection, other diseases and use of antibiotics [1]. The gut-brain axis denotes a bidirectional communication network between the gastrointestinal system, the CNS, the autonomic nervous system (ANS), the enteric nervous system (ENS) and the hypothalamic-pituitary-adrenal axis (HPA). Its role is to monitor and integrate gut functions as well as to link emotional and cognitive centres of the brain with peripheral intestinal functions and mechanisms such as immune activation, intestinal permeability, enteric reflex and enteroendocrine signalling [2]. Both neural and hormonal lines of communication combine to allow the brain to influence the activities of intestinal functional effector cells, such as immune cells, epithelial cells, enteric neurons, smooth muscle cells, interstitial cells of Cajal and enterochromaffin cells [2]. These same cells, on the other hand, are under the influence of the gut microbiota [3]. Gut microbiota could affect CNS through several different mechanisms. Infection caused by gut microbiota causes cytokines to be released into the blood further affecting the innate immune system resulting in alterations of circulatory levels of proinflammatory and anti-inflammatory cytokines, which have a direct impact on brain functions [1]. Activation of the vagus nerve is another way in which microbiota could alternate the function of the nervous system. It could be activated by proinflammatory cytokines or by bacteria themselves [4, 5]. Microbiota metabolites, especially short-chain fatty acids (acetic acid, propionic acid and butyric acid) can directly affect brain physiology. Butyric acid and propionic acid increase the gene expression of tyrosine hydroxylase, an enzyme that limits the rate of synthesis of dopamine and noradrenaline and dopamine-β-hydroxylase, an enzyme that converts dopamine to noradrenaline [6]. They could also affect the function of microglia, induce restoration of microglial malformation and immaturity, affect cytoskeletal integration and stimulate the sympathetic nervous system and mucosal serotonin release [7–12]. Moreover, gut microbiota has the ability to produce diverse neurotransmitters or their precursors. Tryptophan is an amino acid which is an essential precursor for the production of serotonin and kynurenine and gut microbiota appear to play an important role in the metabolism of tryptophan which is known to be associated with clinical depression [1, 13]. It has been observed that gut bacteria can locally produce and release neurotransmitters, including GABA, serotonin, catecholamine and histamine which can deliver signals to the CNS through enterochromaffin cells and enteric nerve receptors [1]. Above mentioned mechanisms have been linked with the development of diverse psychiatric disorders such as anxiety, depression, bipolar disorder and schizophrenia [14, 15]. They have also been linked to certain neurological disorders such as autism spectrum disorder and cognitive decline, but also were linked with the pathogenesis of frequent chronic neurological diseases including multiple sclerosis, Parkinson's disease, Alzheimer's disease glioblastoma and epilepsy [16, 17]. Strong evidence suggests that gut microbiota directly or indirectly affect neuropsychiatric illness and interact with the nervous system by regulating brain chemistry and influencing neuro-endocrine systems. Further studies are required to determine the real impact of this interplay of the gut-brain axis with the pathophysiology of neuropsychiatric disorders and the impact of gut microbiota alterations in the treatment of these chronic conditions. It is worth mentioning that early life perturbations of the developing gut microbiota can impact neurodevelopment and eventually lead to adverse mental health in life [18]. The concept of parallel microbial neural critical windows opens new roads for developing novel microbiota–modulating-based therapeutic interventions in early life to combat neurodevelopmental deficits and brain disorders [18].

Neurological Manifestations in Gastrointestinal Disorders

Coeliac Disease

Over the last 50 years, patients with gluten sensitivity presenting with neurological symptoms have been described more and more [19]. These symptoms predominately include cerebellar ataxia and peripheral neuropathy, but other symptoms of neurological dysfunction such as epileptic seizures or movement disorders have also been observed. The majority of patients with gluten-related disease who present with neurologic complications lack gastrointestinal symptoms. In general, neurological manifestations occur in about 10% of subjects with a confirmed diagnosis of celiac disease (CD) [20]. In the majority of subjects presenting with neurological disease caused by gluten sensitivity, specific antibodies could be detected. Detection of anti-gliadin antibodies (AGA) has been one clue for the diagnosis. But it has been proposed that they have lost much of their diagnostic significance in recent years, due to the introduction of the more sensitive and specific anti-transglutaminase antibodies (TG) [21]. Studies have revealed that distinct subtypes of those antibodies could be found in different conditions linked to gluten sensitivity. In patients with CD, there is a presence of TG 2 antibodies while in patients who predominately present with dermatitis herpetiformis TG 3 antibodies could be found [22]. In patients with neurological manifestations of CD, TG 6 antibodies are predominant but the causative link between neuro-coeliac diseases and circulating TG6 antibodies is still questionable since the same antibodies have been found in patients with multiple sclerosis and amyotrophic lateral sclerosis [19, 23–26]. Regarding neuropathology in gluten sensitivity, degenerative changes of the CNS are prominent, particularly in the cerebellum followed by cerebral cortex, brainstem, spinal cord, deep grey masses and white matter abnormalities [19, 27, 28]. Regarding the observed neuropathology, it is easy to conclude that gluten sensitivity could present with a myriad of neurological signs and symptoms. In more than 50% of patients with neurological disorders of unknown cause gluten sensitivity, assessed by antibody tests, could be detected. The most common of those conditions is progressive cerebellar ataxia, which accounts for up to 40% of idiopathic sporadic ataxia and commonly presents in the absence of gastrointestinal symptoms [29, 30]. Gluten ataxia is associated with high antigliadin antibody titre, hence all patients with sporadic cerebellar ataxia of unknown cause should be considered for this antibody testing [31, 32]. It is estimated that only 10% of all patients with cerebellar ataxia and CD display gastrointestinal symptoms. They usually present with gait and/or limb ataxia, instability, dysarthria, pyramidal signs and altered eye motions [33]. It was supposed that cerebellar ataxia is caused by the cross-reaction of antigliadin antibodies with epitopes on cerebellar Purkinje fibres [34]. Considering that loss of Purkinje cells is irreversible, the timing of diagnosis of gluten ataxia is vital as it is one of the very few treatable causes of sporadic ataxia [29].

Other symptoms of gluten insensitivity/CD include peripheral neuropathy, seizures, impaired cognitive dysfunction, neurological signs and symptoms of vitamin and different movement disorders [33, 35]. A systematic review of the phenomenology of gluten-related movement disorders reported that neurological manifestations, including movement disorders, may precede the diagnosis of gluten sensitivity [36]. It showed that the most frequently observed movement disorders are myoclonus (31%), chorea (11%), tremor (11%), restless leg syndrome (8%), dystonia (6%), Parkinsonism (6%) and tics (6%) and that they may improve or resolve after dietary gluten removal. On the other hand, the same authors reported that ataxia with myoclonus appears to be linked to refractory CD and when observed, there is prompt need for repeat biopsy of the small intestine and often aggressive immunosuppression [36]. Recently, a female patient presenting with paroxysmal non-kinesigenic dyskinesia (PNKD) with silent CD, in whom symptoms completely resolved after the introduction of gluten-free diet, was diagnosed at our Department [37].

Peripheral neuropathy could be detected in up to 50% of patients with CD and it could precede the diagnosis of definite CD [38, 39]. It is predominately a symmetric distal form of sensory neuropathy but could present as pure motor neuropathy, autonomic neuropathy, mononeuritis multiplex and as a Guillain-Barré-like syndrome [39–43]. Hence, gluten insensitivity/CD should be suspected as a potential diagnosis in all patients presenting with peripheral neuropathy of unknown cause. The reported effect of the gluten-free diet in patients with peripheral neuropathy has been controversial with some observations of a positive effect and others with no effect at all [41, 44].

Epilepsy is another neurological disease associated with CD. A specific seizure disorder syndrome has been recorded in CD with bilateral occipital calcification, presenting predominately with focal seizures of temporal and occipital semiology with impaired awareness but also with generalized seizures [45–47]. However, it could also present with a myriad of other seizure types, indistinctive to other epileptic aetiologies and could have no detectable brain pathology on the magnetic resonance imaging. Introduction of gluten-free diet could be useful in seizure control of these patients [48]. Focal, segmental or generalized as well as action or reflex myoclonus had been observed in patients with CD. They are often accompanied by ataxia [49].

Cognitive disturbance, particularly memory impairment could be seen in patients with CD. Other observed symptoms of cognitive dysfunction are amnesia, acalculia, confusion and personality changes [50]. However, patients with CD are not at increased risk for dementia overall [51]. In most patients, a gluten-free diet does not appear to result in an improvement of cognitive function, but in some patients, symptoms appear to ameliorate after removal of dietary gluten [50, 52].

Subclinical CD had been detected in a significant proportion of patients with migraine and it was suggested that in those patients, gluten-free diet could lead to improvement [53]. However, a definite correlation between these two conditions is yet to be established.

Different psychiatric disorders have been associated with CD including anxiety disorders, depressive and mood disorders, attention deficit hyperactivity disorder (ADHD), autism spectrum disorders and schizophrenia [54].

The number of publications on the neurological manifestation of CD in childhood is below those in adults, pointing to the fact that most probably it is an age-dependent phenomenon. About 0–10.7% of CD children exhibited convulsive disorders and 1.1–2.8% of children with epilepsy had CD [55]. The Italian working group on Coeliac Disease and Epilepsy described one of the well-characterized syndromes of epilepsy and CD in children and it includes epilepsy, occipital calcifications and CD, and it rarely improves on gluten-free diet [46].

Despite numerous recommendations in the literature to screen children with neurological problems for CD, or to screen the paediatric population with CD for neurological disorders, there are still contradictive opinions [56–58]. Studies of children with headache and CD reported different prevalence, from 0.35% to 24.8%, and almost all responded well to gluten-free diet [59, 60]. Other rare neurological manifestation in children with CD included ADHD, mental retardation, cerebellar ataxia, ad behaviour disorder [58]. The brain imaging in patients with CD and the longer gluten exposure revealed focal white matter lesions in the brain, but with no correlation with the neurological and electroencephalographic abnormalities [61]. These correlations have been found in children with white matter lesions, neurological dysfunction and CD in up to 20% [59]. Nevertheless, focal white matter lesions in the brain could represent an extraintestinal manifestation of CD because these occur in other chronic, immune-mediated gastrointestinal diseases during childhood. The discrepancy in the frequency of neurological manifestations in adults with CD compared to children with CD could be explained by several mechanisms: shorter duration of CD in children, more symptomatic nature of CD in children and earlier diagnosis, compliance with dietary restrictions in children and the age dependency of autoimmune processes and diseases [55].

In conclusion, CD can present with a myriad of neurological and psychiatric symptoms, even without the evident gastrointestinal disorders. Despite available treatment (gluten-free diet) established neurological dysfunction responds inappropriately and only exceptionally improves with gluten restriction. However, if the condition is early recognized, gluten-free diet could prevent the evolution of serious neurological dysfunction. Hence, there is a necessity for early recognition of CD in patients presenting with neurological symptoms without evident aetiology, but at the same time, there is also the necessity for the early recognition of neurological disturbance in patients with an established diagnosis of CD.

Inflammatory Bowel Disease

Evident neurological manifestations affect approximately one-third of patients with inflammatory bowel disease (IBD), although the number seems to be higher when patients with subclinical or unrecognized neurological impairment are considered [62, 63]. Neurologic involvement has been mainly reported in adults, and information in paediatrics was based primarily on individual case reports. Nevertheless, several studies demonstrate that neurologic and neuropsychiatric morbidity in children and adolescents with IBD is not as rare as previously thought [64, 65]. There are several suggested mechanisms through which neurological damage could occur. Those mechanisms include immunological disturbances that may lead to an autoimmune response against glial-neural components, malabsorption and vitamin deficits, toxicity due to defects in the barrier of the intestinal mucosa, hypercoagulability state due to chronic inflammatory response and opportunistic infections as a consequence of chronic immunosuppression in the treatment. Additionally, neurological symptoms are often adverse events of agents used for the treatment of IBD (steroids, antibiotics, cyclosporine A, methotrexate, thiopurines, anti-TNF agents, vedolizumab and ustekinumab) [66].

Hypercoagulable state due to chronic inflammatory response could result in cerebral thrombotic or thromboembolic complications including cerebral venous thrombosis and ischaemic stroke. Their clinical presentation does not differ from those in patients with other aetiologies. It has been observed that cerebral venous thrombosis including superficial or deep cerebral venous systems is more common in patients with ulcerous colitis than in those with other IBDs. The risk for thrombotic and thromboembolic cerebrovascular disease could be associated with the activity of the disease even though it could be observed also in patients during remission [66–68]. The treatment strategies in acute stages do not differ from general treatment strategies for cerebrovascular disorders. Regarding the fact of increased risk for cerebrovascular events, primary prevention should be performed in all patients during relapses. It includes early mobilization, correct rehydration, vitamin supplementation as well as the use of prophylactic anticoagulants [69]. On the other hand, ischaemic cerebral events could be a consequence of underlying vasculitis since the same could be present in patients with IBD [70]. Hence, in all patients with IBD and ischaemic stroke, cerebral vasculitis must be one of the suspected aetiologies.

Epilepsy in patients with IBD could be a consequence of cerebrovascular disorder, brain toxicity caused by agents used in the treatment of IBD or central nervous system immune disorder due to systemic immune disorder. Thromboembolic events and various vitamin deficiencies such as thiamine and vitamin B12 are mostly responsible for seizures in IBD [70]. Hence, in the case of a new-onset seizure, all patients with IBD should be checked for cerebrovascular pathology as well as for vitamin status. Recently published meta-analysis on the association between systemic autoimmune diseases (including IBD) and epilepsy indicated that patients with systemic autoimmune diseases have 2.5-fold increased risk for epilepsy [71]. There are no specific epilepsy syndromes linked to IBD, all types of seizures including status epilepticus have been reported. Once diagnosed, epilepsy in patients with IBD is treated the same as in all other individuals. When choosing an antiepileptic drug, it is extremely important to avoid antiepileptic drugs with prominent gastrointestinal side effects and those with a potential for pharmacokinetic interactions with agents used for the treatment of IBD.

Peripheral neuropathy (PN) could be commonly seen in patients with IBD [72, 73]. It could be acute or chronic and caused by demyelination or axonal damage, although there is a certain dominance of non-demyelinating versus demyelinating forms [74, 75]. It presents as mononeuropathy, plexopathy, multiple mononeuritis, compressive neuropathy and cranial neuropathy [76]. Underlying causes are different including immunological phenomena, nutritional disturbances, extraintestinal inflammation and also adverse effects of IBD therapeutic agents [75–77].

IBDs have also been associated with demyelinating diseases. There are a number of reports of higher prevalence of multiple sclerosis, with a risk of 50%, in patients with IBD [78–80]. In a small number of patients, demyelinating disease could be a consequence of IBD treatment, especially in those receiving anti-TNFα agents [81]. Besides distinct demyelinating diseases, patients with IBD have a higher prevalence of asymptomatic white matter lesions when compared with healthy subjects [82].

Psychiatric disorders, predominately depression and anxiety, could be frequently observed in adult patients with IBD [83, 84]. In comparison to the general population, there is also a higher prevalence of panic and obsessive-compulsive disorders [85]. Bipolar affective disorder has been also reported to be more frequent in patients with IBD [86]. It has been suggested that gut-brain axis is an important factor in the development of psychiatric disturbances but also that initial psychiatric disturbances throughout the same axis could influence the course of IBD [66].

The neurologic profile of children and adolescents with IBD includes headache, dizziness, hypotonia, ADHD, tics and sensory complaints, while seizures, neuropsychiatric disorders such as obsessive-compulsive disorder, anxiety and learning difficulties are less characteristic [64]. The primary paediatrician, paediatric gastroenterologist and paediatric neurologist should be aware of these neurological features in children with non-recognized IBD, as well as in paediatric patients with diagnosed IBD, because of different pathophysiology and different therapeutic approaches.

Hepatic Encephalopathy

Hepatic encephalopathy (HE) is a syndrome characterized by different aspects of brain dysfunction as a consequence of primary liver disease. It is estimated that it affects 30 to 45% of patients with known cirrhosis; although in a sustained number of patients, it could present with mild symptoms which are easily unrecognized [87, 88]. The exact pathogenesis is still not well understood. Proposed mechanisms include neurotoxicity, inflammatory response and impairment of the brain metabolism or neurotransmission which are a direct consequence of impaired liver function [89]. It could be a consequence of acute liver failure, cirrhosis or due to portosystemic bypass or shunting [90]. Maybe the most known toxic metabolite is ammonia which causes swelling of astrocytes and hence brain oedema [91]. Moreover, ammonia was found to inhibit both excitatory and inhibitory postsynaptic potentials [92]. There is also a presumption that HE leads to impairment of neurotransmission due to changes in the GABAbenzodiazepine-ergic, dopaminergic, serotoninergic and glutamate-ergic neurotransmitter systems; however, the most data regarding dysfunction of neurotransmission have been derived from animal studies, with a lack of data regarding the real impact on human brain [89].

Clinically, HE could present diverse symptoms ranging from mild memory disturbances to cerebral coma. Likewise, neuroradiologically it could present without evident brain pathology or as brain oedema or brain atrophy (predominately cerebellar). In its mildest form, it presents as minimal cognitive impairment affecting orientation, attention, working memory psychomotor speed and visuospatial ability [93]. If not treated, symptoms progress to more prominent psychiatric features such as apathy, irritability, or disinhibition (in advanced stages agitation, confusional state); alterations of consciousness (from somnolence to coma) and focal neurological signs; predominately pyramidal system abnormalities (hypertonia, hyperreflexia and Babinski sign) and asterixis. Signs of extrapyramidal dysfunction (Parkinsonian-like tremor, hypomimia, muscular rigidity, bradykinesia, hypokinesia and dyskinesia) are commonly seen in patients with HE and seizures are very rarely reported [89].

There could be a significant difference in the progression and severity of clinical symptoms in patients with HE. According to the time course of the occurrence of symptoms, HE could be classified as episodic, recurrent and persistent while asterixis had been proposed as the initial sign of overt HE [90]. The West Haven criteria (WHC) are the 'gold standard' for evaluation and gradation of severity of HE. The criteria recognize four grades of HE ranging it from the mildest to the most severe one. Grade I presents patients with a trivial lack of awareness, shortened attention span and euphoria or anxiety. Grade II is characterized by inappropriate behaviour, obvious personality change, disorientation for time, lethargy, or apathy. Grade III is more severe and is characterized by severe disorientation, confusion, bizarre behaviour and somnolence to semi-stupor while grade IV presents the most severe clinical presentation of hepatic encephalopathy—coma [94].

The diagnosis of HE is predominately based on clinical presentation, there are no tests specific for this disorder, especially in the early stages when it could present with only slight cognitive disturbance. In general, the diagnosis of HE could be made only if other possible causes of neurological signs and symptoms have been excluded. However, it should be always suspected in patients with liver disease and new-onset signs or symptoms of neurological dysfunction. It is important to stress that high-blood ammonia levels alone do not add any diagnostic, staging, or prognostic value to HE in patients with chronic liver disease [95]. In all patients with HE, underlying precipitating factors should be detected. There are a proportion of patients with unknown precipitating factors for HE but they are less frequent than those with detectable precipitating factors such as infection, gastrointestinal bleeding, diuretic overdose, electrolyte disorder, constipation, psychoactive medication, dehydration and dietary indiscretion [96]. Precipitating factors could be detected in almost all patients with episodic HE due to cirrhosis. For example, hyponatremia is an independent risk factor for the development of HE in patients with cirrhosis [97]. Correcting precipitating factors is extremely important since in a majority of patients, HE can be treated with just a correction of the precipitating factor.

A scale for grading clinical encephalopathy is useful for assessing encephalopathy in older patients, but is of little value in assessing neonates and infants, particularly in the early stages of encephalopathy [98]. No study has yet been done on the neuropsychiatric function of children with acute hepatic encephalopathy, and also, an age-dependent grading scale is needed. Hepatic encephalopathy in children may progress rapidly in acute liver failure, with coma developing within hours of the earliest detectable signs. Symptoms often resolve if the precipitating factors such as infections, dehydration, variceal bleeding and drug toxicity are treated [98]. Cerebral oedema with brain death is the direct cause of mortality in most children with acute liver failure.

There are no specifically developed drugs for the treatment of HE. Different substances have been used with reported different results regarding their efficacy. Non-absorbable disaccharides (lactulose and lactitol) are recommended as first-line treatment for HE. Recent meta-analysis concluded that there are no observable differences between lactulose and lactitol efficacy in the treatment of HE [99]. It is recommended that the dose of both agents should be titrated in order to maintain two to three stools per day [100, 101]. Lactulose could be continuously used in order to prevent the recurrence of HE. Besides non-absorbable disaccharides, there are other agents which have been used in the treatment of HE. Agents which had shown efficacy are branched-chain amino acids (BCAA), metabolic ammonia scavengers (ornithine phenylacetate and glycerol phenylbutyrate), L-ornithine L-aspartate (LOLA) and polyethylene glycol [102–106]. Antibiotic rifaximin has been showed to be superior to placebo in maintaining remission of HE, especially in patients whose encephalopathy recurred during lactulose treatment [107]. Adequate nutrition with the modulation of nitrogen metabolism is an additional important approach in the management of HE with available guidelines for patients suffering from this condition [108]. Since each episode of overt HE is associated with an increased risk of recurrence and increased one-year mortality, in patients with HE, early diagnosis and adequate treatment are extremely important [90, 94].

Neurological Disorders Due to Nutritional Deficiency in the Setting of Malabsorption

Adequate levels of basic nutrients, vitamins, minerals and trace elements are crucial for the normal functioning of nervous system. Neurological dysfunction in malabsorption syndromes presents with a vast majority of symptoms, which often are subclinical and unrecognized, but if not treated could result in permanent neurological damage. Particularly important for optimal functioning of the nervous system are the B-group vitamins, vitamin E and copper. Disease processes that damage the enteric mucosa and produce malabsorption can trigger neurologic dysfunction both by immune-related processes and by impairing the absorption of essential vitamins and other nutrients [109].

Vitamin B1 (Thiamine) Deficiency

Thiamine deficiency may be a result of poor intake (chronic alcoholism, elderly), poor absorption (malnutrition, gastric bypass surgery and malabsorption syndrome), increased loss (diarrhoea, hyperemesis gravidarum and chronic diuretic use) and increased utilization (pregnancy, lactation and hyperthyroidism) [110]. Relative thiamine deficiency may be seen in high-risk patients during periods of high-carbohydrate intake as is seen with nasogastric feeding, total parenteral nutrition, or intravenous hyperalimentation (glucose administration) [111].

Symptoms of thiamine deficiency include anorexia, irritability, difficulties with short-term memory, vertigo, double vision and confusion. Fatigue and muscle cramps may appear within days to weeks of nutritional deficiency [112]. In the peripheral nervous system, it presents as symmetrical peripheral neuropathy, known as *dry beriberi* [113]. It has characteristics of sensorimotor, distal, axonal neuropathy often associated with calf cramps, muscle tenderness and burning feet. [114, 115]. Symptoms usually begin with distal sensory loss, burning pain, paraesthesia, or muscle weakness in the toes and feet [115]. If left untreated, it can evolve into sensorimotor neuropathy in the hands. Symptoms usually develop gradually over weeks to months, but sometimes they may manifest rapidly over a few days mimicking Guillain-Barré syndrome [116]. Thiamine deficiency may also present as cranial neuropathy (hoarseness, tongue and facial weakness); hence, it is one of the differential diagnoses in patients with cranial mononeuropathies [117].

The most impressive clinical presentation of thiamine deficiency is Wernicke's encephalopathy (WE) which is characterized by a triad of ocular abnormalities (ophthalmoplegia, nystagmus), confusion and gait ataxia [109, 118]. A distinct number of patients who survive WE will develop amnestic confabulatory syndrome characterized by severe anterograde and retrograde amnesia (with preserved other aspects of cognitive functioning) known as Korsakoff syndrome. In such cases, the entity is known as Wernicke-Korsakoff syndrome. In severe cases, WE can lead to coma or death. WE is most frequently seen in chronic alcoholics but also in patients with malabsorption of thiamine or with poor dietary intake (diets primarily high in polished rice/processed grains). It has also been reported in patients with peptic ulcer disease (due to severe gastric mucosal lesions) and following bariatric surgery [109, 119]. Regarding neuroradiological findings, the most common abnormalities seen in patients with WE are symmetric changes in the thalamus, mammillary bodies, periaqueductal area and tectal plate [120]. There is a broad spectrum of conditions which could be included in the differential diagnosis of brain lesions seen in thiamine deficiency (CNS lymphoma, variant Creutzfeldt-Jakob disease, paraneoplastic encephalitis, Miller-Fisher syndrome, multiple sclerosis, Behçet disease, etc.).

Thiamine has a crucial role as an essential nutrient for infant development. Therefore, in children, thiamine deficiency presents with acute symptoms and very rapid onset, and in the vast majority of cases, it affects infants who are breastfed by thiamine-deficient mothers or with thiamine-deficient formulas. Infantile thiamine deficiency (ITD) manifests after 2–3 weeks of thiamine deprivation with initially milder symptoms (refusal to eat, vomiting and irritability), followed by rapid deterioration, with a high fatality rate. Newborns who are severely thiamine-deprived may develop infantile beriberi. This disorder is rare in developed countries, as it can be easily treated with thiamine supplementation. It is a concern in developing countries where the symptoms of deficiency can progress to convulsions, ataxia, paralysis and heart failure and fatality occurs. The children who survive thiamine deficiency-related WE continue to live with developmental disabilities such as severe epilepsy, language impairment, loss of motor function and mental retardation [121].

Recently, thiamine-based treatments have gained attention as a therapy for other neurological disorders linked to mitochondrial dysfunction, such as autistic spectrum disorder (ASD). A subset of children with ASD has been characterized by pyruvate dehydrogenase (PDH) deficiency and mitochondrial dysfunction suggesting that thiamine deficiency may also ensue in PDH deficits or that a borderline thiamine intake would compound the preexistent PDH deficit [122]. One study found a direct correlation between thiamine intake and depressive symptoms in Spanish school children [123].

Treatment: 50–300 mg/d of thiamine in adults (intravenous, intramuscular and oral). Higher doses may be required in patients with WE [99]. In children, less severe cases can be treated with early thiamine supplementation. In general, therapeutic recommended doses for children are 10–25 mg/d IV or IM for 2 weeks, or 10–50 mg/d orally, followed by 5–10 mg/d for 1 month.

It is extremely important to bear in mind that intravenous glucose overload in patients with initial thiamine deficiency may consume the available thiamine in the body and precipitate an acute WE. Hence, intravenous thiamine must be administered prior to intravenous administration of glucose, especially in patients with a high risk of thiamine deficiency.

Vitamin B3 (Niacin) Deficiency

Niacin deficiency has been known under the name *pellagra*. It could be a consequence of niacin malabsorption or it can develop in the setting of deficiency of the essential amino acid tryptophan, which is a precursor of niacin [124]. Although pellagra is primarily seen in young people in areas where diets are based mainly on corn (Africa and India), it also occurs in Western societies in alcoholics, patients with malabsorption syndromes, or as a consequence of eating disorders such as anorexia nervosa [125]. Niacin deficiency has been observed in patients with Crohn's disease, in an immunocompromised patient with colitis due to cytomegalovirus, in a setting of small intestinal bacterial overgrowth with consequent malabsorption and malabsorption secondary to amyloidosis [109]. Classic clinical features of pellagra consist of the triad of dermatitis, diarrhoea and dementia, but all together could be seen in only a small number of patients [126]. Early symptoms are predominantly neuropsychiatric including apathy, inattention, irritability and depression. Without treatment, symptoms can progress to stupor or coma [127]. Other niacin/tryptophan deficit symptoms comprise headache, vertigo, myoclonus, tremor, rigidity, weakness, dysphagia, seizures as well as all other symptoms resembling those observed in neurodegenerative diseases [128, 129]. Dementia in niacin deficiency is similar to Alzheimer's disease and includes psychosis, disorientation, memory loss and confusion, which can regress by niacin supplementation [130].

Parkinson's disease (PD) is a neurodegenerative disorder that may be influenced by diet and nutrition. It is a consequence of the death of dopamine neurons within the substantia nigra leading to symptoms characteristic for extrapyramidal system dysfunction—reduced movement (bradykinesia/akinesia), rigidity and tremor. Only in a minority of patients PD can be attributed to known genetic cause and in majority of patients PD is considered to be sporadic, with a suspected influence of several environmental factors. One of proposed hypotheses in PD development is that the dopamine neurons are compromised through oxidative stress, and more recently, it has been suggested that this oxidative stress may originate in the gastrointestinal tract, leading to neuronal damage [131]. Patients with PD have been shown to have increased intestinal permeability as well as α-synuclein aggregates and higher levels of oxidative stress in the gastrointestinal tract. It has been suggested that diets high in saturated fat from animal sources may have a negative impact on neuronal health, whereas unsaturated fats and foods containing antioxidants may be protective, by reducing inflammation and oxidation [132]. Niacin intake has been suggested to play both protective and detrimental roles in PD and a reduced risk of PD has been associated with higher consumption of foods containing niacin [125, 133, 134]. It has been reported that niacin supplementation in patients with PD could result in easing of the symptoms; however, altering the course of PD through dietary means still remains difficult and further experimentation is needed to determine whether this modulation is impactful [131]. Huntington's disease (HD) is an autosomal dominant neurodegenerative disease characterized by involuntary movements, abnormalities in gait, posture and balance, dementia and other cognitive impairments [135]. Several studies, indeed, have put forward a beneficial effect of niacin in HD by prevention of oxidative stress and inhibition of neuronal death in the striatum. Other studies have reported opposite effects such as worsening of motor performance. Hence, there is still no consensus regarding the role of niacinin, the modification of the natural course of HD [129].

Headache, especially migraine and tension-type headache, is one of the leading causes of disability worldwide. When administrated orally, intramuscularly, or intravenously, niacin has therapeutic effects in headache management but it has still not been implemented in everyday clinical practice [129]. Niacin dysmetabolism may be linked with depression, anxiety, schizophrenia, bipolar disorders and psychological distress, although the exact link and the influence of niacin on psychiatric symptoms has not yet been established.

Unexplained progressive encephalopathy in alcoholics that is not responsive to thiamine should raise the possibility of niacin deficiency [136]. Moreover, alcoholics with encephalopathy may receive thiamine and pyridoxine without niacin which may trigger an encephalopathy caused by niacin deficiency [111]. Moreover, niacin deficiency should be considered in any patient deficient in vitamin B12 or vitamin B1 whose cognition does not improve with supplementation [127].

Pellagra occurs rarely below the age of 15 years and never in infants and young children [137]. Pellagra can be very rarely discovered in malabsorption syndromes of paediatric population (e.g. jejunoileitis, gastroenterostomy, subtotal gastrectomy and Crohn's disease), due to impaired absorption of tryptophan and niacin [138]. In Hartnup disease, malabsorption of amino acids, such as tryptophan, occurs due to the defect in the neutral brush-border system, and such cases were discovered through the findings of aminoaciduria [139].

Treatment: Oral nicotinic acid in a dose of 50 mg three times a day or parenteral doses of 25 mg three times a day is used for treatment of symptomatic patients [111].

Vitamin B6 (Pyridoxine) Deficiency

Pyridoxine deficiency is rare in isolation and is usually found in association with other B vitamin deficiencies such as folic acid and vitamin B12 [140]. Pyridoxine deficiency has been attributed to inadequate gastrointestinal absorption (celiac disease, inflammatory bowel disease and bariatric surgery), hepatic dysfunction (chronic alcohol abuse) and drug interaction or antagonism (isonicotinic acid hydrazide, cycloserine, hydralazine and penicillamine). At risk are also pregnant and lactating women and elderly individuals.

In infants, pyridoxine deficiency rarely may clinically present as Pyridoxine-dependent epilepsy which is a rare genetic disorder characterized by intractable seizures which start within the first weeks to months. Seizures respond abruptly to large daily supplements of pyridoxine. It is a consequence of mutations in ALDH7A1 gene [141]. There are also reports of paediatric patients with infantile spasms being successfully treated with B6 supplementation [142].

In adults, symptoms of pyridoxine deficiency are rare, even with low levels. It may represent with numbness, paraesthesia, or burning pain in the feet which then ascends to the legs and eventually to hands. Neurological examination reveals a length dependent polyneuropathy with decreased distal sensation, reduction of deep tendon reflexes, ataxia and mild distal weakness [125]. It has also been linked with depression and anxiety.

Treatment: 50–100 mg of pyridoxine daily (oral); pyridoxine supplementation in patients on isoniazid [127]. Excess consumption has been associated with a pure sensory peripheral neuropathy or ganglionopathy characterized by sensory ataxia, areflexia, impaired cutaneous and deep sensations and positive Romberg sign [143, 144].

Vitamin B12 (Cobalamin) Deficiency

Methylcobalamin is present in animal and dairy products and is synthesized by specific microorganisms. For methylcobalamin supply, humans depend on nutritional intake. Since methylcobalamin is only found in animal products, strict vegan diets lack methylcobalamin and must be supplemented [127]. Although the cause of methylcobalamin deficiency is often unknown, most patients with clinically expressed methylcobalamin deficiency have malabsorption related to intrinsic factor (IF). It is very common in the elderly, in patients after partial gastrectomy and bariatric surgery and in patients taking H2 blockers (acid reduction therapy) and metformin (especially prolonged use) [109, 143, 144]. Methylcobalamin deficiency has been observed in 5–20% of older adults and up to 40% of older adults have low serum methylcobalamin levels [145].

Neurologic manifestations may be the earliest and often the only manifestation of methylcobalamin deficiency, regardless of a normal haematological picture [109, 146]. The striking feature of methylcobalamin deficiency in neurological system is a myelopathy known as subacute combined degeneration. Histopathological studies have showed breakdown and vacuolization of central nervous system myelin followed by axonal degeneration and gliosis located predominately in cervical and thoracic spinal cord and axonal polyneuropathy in peripheral nervous system [111, 147]. It represents spastic paraparesis, extensor plantar response and impaired proprioception and vibration sense. Additional features include, peripheral neuropathy (acute), optic neuropathy, cognitive impairment, memory disturbance, psychosis and rarely delirium [111]. The neuropathy associated with methylcobalamin deficiency usually begins with sensory symptoms in the feet. Sometimes the sensory symptoms and signs first appear in the upper extremities (numb hand syndrome) [127]. It is worth mentioning that in patients with methylcobalamin deficiency, serum methylcobalamin levels could be normal but additional analysis of serum metabolites methylmalonic acid (MMA) and total homocysteine (Hcy) could reveal the underlying deficiency, especially in patients with low normal range of serum methylcobalamin (300–400 pg/ml) and clinical suspicion on deficiency [111, 127]. When interpreting these results, it is always necessary to exclude other causes that can cause abnormal levels of methylcobalamin, MMA and Hcy (pregnancy, folate deficiency, myeloma, HIV infection, etc.) [111]. Magnetic resonance imaging (MRI) abnormalities include a signal change in the subcortical white matter, posterior and lateral columns, contrast enhancement involving the dorsal or lateral columns, brain and cerebellum T2-hyperintensities, decreased signal on T1-weighted images of the dorsal column and rarely diffuse white matter abnormalities suggestive of a leukoencephalopathy. Lesions may show improvement with vitamin replacement [111].

Since vitamin B12 is essential for development of the central nervous system, nutritional vitamin B12 deficiency in infancy is common in countries with low intake of animal products. Neurological signs may be expected in infants who are exclusively breastfed and who receive inadequate amounts of vitamin B12. Hypotonia and neurodevelopmental delay are the most commonly reported signs in infants and clinical improvement is evident after vitamin supplementation [148]. Vitamin B12 deficiency can lead to dizziness and syncope, because it is important for the production of adrenaline from noradrenaline and it is an essential cofactor involved in myelin degradation and in the synthesis of catecholamine. A cause-and-effect relationship has also been suggested between syncope and postural orthostatic tachycardia syndrome in B12 deficiency [148]. Since nervous symptoms can precede anaemia in months, patients with neurological symptoms should be carefully evaluated in terms of vitamin B12 deficiency with or without associated anaemia.

Treatment: Cyanocobalamin (intramuscular) 1000 μg twice weekly for 2 weeks (or 100 μg twice weekly for 2 weeks), followed by weekly for 2 months and monthly thereafter or cyanocobalamin (intramuscular) 1000 μg daily for the first week, followed by weekly for the first month, then monthly thereafter [111].

Vitamin B9 (Folic Acid) Deficiency

Folic acid deficiency may be seen with bowel disorders associated with malabsorption such as tropical sprue, celiac disease, bacterial overgrowth syndrome, giardiasis, inflammatory bowel disease, after gastric surgery, in patients with atrophic gastritis or those taking acid-suppressive therapy, aminopterin, methotrexate, pyrimethamine, trimethoprim and triamterene [111]. Folic acid deficiency rarely exists in the pure state; it is often associated with a deficiency of other nutrients. Hence, the attribution of neurologic manifestations to folate deficiency requires exclusion of all other potential causes. There is no specific neurologic syndrome associated with folic acid deficiency, although some clinical studies report effects on cognition and mood, particularly depression [149]. In pregnant women, folate deficiency could result in the development of foetal malformation—neural tube defect.

Therapy: Oral folate 1 mg three times a day followed by a maintenance dose of 1 mg a day; for acutely ill patients 1–5 mg/d (parenteral); supplementation with 0.4 mg/d in women in childbearing as for prophylaxis against neural tube defects [111].

Vitamin E Deficiency

Vitamin E deficiency could be acquired or genetic. Acquired vitamin E deficiency could be a result of chronic fat malabsorption or could be seen in association with abetalipoproteinaemia [150]. Fat malabsorption is the most frequent cause of vitamin E deficiency. It could be seen in patients with biliary disease (chronic cholestasis), pancreatic dysfunction, inflammatory bowel disease, cystic fibrosis, biliary atresia, blind loop syndrome, bowel irradiation and extensive small bowel resection as well as after partial or total gastrectomy [109, 111]. Acquired vitamin E deficiency is also most observed in paediatric chronic diseases impending ileal resorption of fat-soluble vitamins, such as cystic fibrosis, Crohn's disease, cholestatic liver disease, or short bowel syndrome [151].

Genetic cause of vitamin E deficiency could be seen in individuals with an autosomal recessive disorder of vitamin E absorption (due to a mutation in an α-tocopherol transfer protein gene) which clinically presents very similarly to Friedriech's ataxia [109]. Those patients present with ataxia, disturbances of coordination, dysarthria, bilateral extensor plantar responses, impaired proprioception, pes cavus and scoliosis [152]. Ataxia with vitamin E deficiency manifests in late childhood or early teens and it is frequently associated with head titubation or dystonia, and less with cardiomyopathy [151]. Since there is a great similarity, in all patients presenting with signs of Friedriech's ataxia, vitamin E levels should be determined during the diagnostic process.

Other symptoms seen in patients with vitamin E deficiency are myopathy and neuropathy and movement disorders such as tremors or myoclonus [109]. It is worth mentioning that symptoms of vitamin E deficiency could present with a significant delay comprising several years after the beginning of the malabsorption syndrome [153]. The most vulnerable patients are patients who undergo total or partial gastrectomy. Ueda et al. observed that the tendency of vitamin E levels to decrease is observed during the postoperative period (up to 50 months) and that serum vitamin E levels normalize upon oral administration of vitamin E, followed by improvement of neurological symptoms [154].

Treatment: Vitamin E ranging from 200 mg/d to 200 mg/kg/d (oral, intramuscular); supplementation of bile salts in some patients [111].

Vitamin A Deficiency

Nutritional deficiency of vitamin A is seen in people using a diet consisting predominantly of grains lacking b-carotene (rice) but it could be a consequence of fat malabsorption in conditions such as celiac disease, pancreatitis, sprue, cystic fibrosis, biliary atresia and cholestatic liver disease [111]. Regarding neurological symptoms, vitamin A deficiency causes night blindness, whilst vitamin A toxicity (in cases of excess vitamin A ingestion) could cause headache, insomnia, irritability, papilloedema and pseudotumour cerebri [111].

Vitamin A deficiency is the leading cause of preventable childhood blindness and increases the risk of death from common childhood illnesses such as diarrhoea. Periodic, high-dose vitamin A supplementation is a proven low-cost intervention which has been shown to reduce all-cause mortality by 12 to 24 per cent, and therefore it is an important program in support of efforts to reduce child mortality [155, 156].

Treatment: Oral vitamin A supplementation is undertaken to normalize plasma levels [111].

Vitamin D Deficiency

Causes of vitamin D deficiency include malabsorption as seen in celiac disease, Crohn's disease, cholestatic liver disease and extensive small bowel resection; advanced liver or kidney disease (can decrease the active form of vitamin D); use of antiepileptic drugs phenobarbital and phenytoin (inhibition of vitamin D hydroxylation in the liver) and inadequate sun exposure. Vitamin D deficiency can cause a proximal myopathy that often exists in association with osteomalacia, pathologic fractures and bone pain, tetany (due to severe hypocalcaemia) and cutaneous hyperalgesia resistant to antidepressants and opiates but responsive to vitamin D repletion [99]. An inverse association between vitamin D (both dietary intake and blood levels) and the risk of developing multiple sclerosis has been reported [157, 158].

The role of vitamin D in brain development, brain function and neuroplasticity has been confirmed by different experimental and clinical studies, and morphological changes in the brain related to vitamin D deficiency were evaluated in a meta-analysis of a few studies [159].

Severe vitamin D deficiency in children can lead to symptomatic hypocalcaemia, which can result in seizures, osteomalacia, or rickets. Rickets involve bone demineralization that occurs in areas adjacent to the growth plate [160]. The exact prevalence of rickets is unknown. However, case reports and case series of documented rickets suggest this problem still exists today [160]. Rickets may be caused by reasons other than nutritional vitamin D deficiency (e.g. calcium and phosphorus deficiency, inherited forms of hypophosphatemic rickets and vitamin D receptor mutations).

Treatment: Vitamin D can be given orally as vitamin D2 or vitamin D3. 400 IU of vitamin D per day is adequate to prevent deficiency in individuals with minimal sun exposure. In patients with clinical deficiency, up to 50,000 IU weekly may be required [111]. In the case administration of high doses of vitamin D, associated secondary hyperparathyroidism and hypercalcaemia should not be overlooked.

Copper Deficiency

Acquired dietary copper deficiency is rare and most frequently it is seen in patients after gastric surgery, but it could also be a complication of total parenteral or enteral nutrition. Copper deficiency can be seen in association with nephrotic syndrome, glomerulonephritis and enteropathies associated with malabsorption. Excessive intakes of zinc have also been suggested as a cause of copper deficiency with neurological manifestations. Both zinc and copper bind to metallothionein in the enterocytes. Excessive zinc intake leads to upregulation of these complexes and copper has a higher affinity for these receptors than zinc leading copper to displace zinc. The zinc is then absorbed into the bloodstream and the copper/metallothionein complex remains in the enterocyte and is excreted in the faeces following normal sloughing of these cells [111]. Copper deficiency has been reported to cause either myelopathy or myeloneuropathy, similar to vitamin B12 deficiency [111, 161]. It presents with sensory ataxia and spastic gait. Peripheral neuropathy without myelopathy, CNS demyelination, myopathy with myelopathy, optic neuropathy with myelopathy, optic neuritis with peripheral neuropathy, sensory ganglionopathy and cognitive impairment have also been described in association with copper deficiency. Since copper and vitamin B12 deficiency may coexist, neurologic deterioration in patients with a history of B12-related myelopathy who have normal B12 levels while on replacement therapy should be suspected for copper deficiency [111]. Besides deficiency, low serum copper could be seen in patients with Wilson disease, in whom it is accompanied by low serum ceruloplasmin levels and other symptoms specific to the condition, including signs of neurological as well as liver dysfunction.

Copper deficiency, like zinc deficiency, is also more likely to develop in premature infants, but it usually does not cause any clinical problems and copper supplementation is unnecessary.

Menkes disease, occipital horn syndrome and X-linked distal hereditary motor neuropathy are genetic disorders of copper metabolism with a broad spectrum of neurological symptoms. Menkes disease is an X-linked neurodegenerative disease of impaired copper transport characterized by severe copper deficiency, but the incidence of this condition is extremely low, and it is rarely encountered in ordinary paediatric practice. Children with the classic form of Menkes disease usually present at 2–3 months of age with the following: loss of developmental milestones, profound truncal hypotonia and epilepsy [162, 163]. Children with milder variants may have minimal neurological symptoms with normal intelligence or only mild intellectual disability and autonomic dysfunction. An ATP7A variant with a missense mutation T994I in the sixth transmembrane domain is associated with distal motor neuropathy [164].

Treatment: Oral elemental copper 8 mg/d for a week, 6 mg/d for the second week, 4 mg/d for the third week and 2 mg/d thereafter [111].

Neurological Symptoms of Specific Gastrointestinal Infectious Diseases

Hepatitis Virus

First link between hepatitis virus and neurological dysfunction was observed during World War I when Hurst reported the first case of acute polyneuropathy complicating hepatitis [165]. Until today, different neurological syndromes have been observed in patients with distinct types of hepatitis virus infection.

Hepatitis E

Hepatitis E virus (HEV) is the most common cause of hepatitis worldwide [166]. The illness usually affects young adults and is usually self-limiting, except in pregnant women where the mortality is 25% [167]. There is a difference in the frequency of genotypes of HEV between developed and developing countries, with a predominance of genotypes 1 and 2 in developing countries and genotypes 3 and 4 in developed countries. In developing countries, HEV is an obligate human pathogen transmitted by ingestion of faecal contaminated water while in developed countries, it is largely a porcine zoonosis [167]. The symptoms of HEV infection are indistinguishable from other forms of hepatitis and most patients with acute hepatitis are asymptomatic. In fact, there are an increasing number of patients with primary neurological illnesses in whom HEV has been diagnosed [167]. Neurological manifestations are the most frequent extrahepatic complications of HEV with a frequency from 5.5 to 8% [168, 169]. The most frequent neurological manifestations of HEV are Guillain-Barré syndrome (GBS), neuralgic amyotrophy, encephalitis, myelitis, myositis, vestibular neuritis, peripheral neuropathy, Bell's palsy and mononeuritis multiplex [167].

GBS or acute inflammatory demyelinating polyradiculoneuropathy (AIDP) is a peripheral nervous system condition which could be seen mostly 2–4 weeks after a benign respiratory or gastrointestinal illness (predominately Campylobacter infection). In recent years, HEV, as well as prior HEV infection, has been observed in patients with GBS, with a reported prevalence of 5–8% [170–173]. Classically, the patient presents with foot paraesthesia/dysesthesia (tingling) which progresses upwards and is followed by ascending and symmetrical low extremity muscle weakness. Patients often report the weakness as having 'rubbery legs'. During this time, symptoms progress cranially and can affect the upper extremities, truncal and respiratory muscles as well as cranial nerves. Time to the clinical dysfunction nadir is around ten days and could last up to 4 weeks, when a plateau phase (characterized by unchanging symptoms) starts. After 2–4 weeks, a gradual recovery starts [174, 175]. The average time for full clinical recovery is around 6 months. Respiratory muscle palsy, which makes this diagnosis life-threatening, could be seen in around one-third of patients. Those patients should be treated in intensive care units (ICU). Sometimes AIDP can present with cranial nerve affection at the very beginning of the disease. In those cases, it is known as Miller-Fisher syndrome [176]. Patients presenting with a GBS have flaccid paraparesis on the neurological exam (low extremities weakness with absent reflexes), and in those presenting with cranial nerve involvement, neurological presentation depends on the affected nerve (facial palsy, dysarthria, dysphagia, ophtalmoplegia, or pupillary disturbance). GBS is diagnosed regarding clinical presentation, history data, CSF findings (albumino-cytologic dissociation, i.e. elevated proteins with normal cell count), electromyography (EMG) and nerve conduction studies (NCS). It is very important to know that needle EMG may be normal in acute nerve lesions, hence normal EMG finding at the very beginning of the disease does not rule out GBS. The syndrome has been successfully treated in most patients by intravenous immunoglobulin (IVIG) or therapeutic plasma exchange (TPE) which are both equally effective. Additional important step in treating patients with GBS is an early and intensive physical therapy. Unfortunately, there is a reported 2–12% mortality rate. With experienced ICU management, it is less than 5% and depends on the severity of several factors including age group, the severity of weakness autonomic dysfunction, pulmonary complications, hypokalaemia, bleeding and the need for mechanical ventilation [177–179].

Neuralgic amyotrophic is a neurological condition characterized by painful mononeuropathy or multiple mononeuropathies in the upper extremity followed by rapid progression of motor weakness and sensory loss [180]. In a study performed on Dutch and UK patients with neuralgic amyotrophy, acute HEV infection was detected in 10% of patients [181]. In patients with HEV, it typically presents as a bilateral disorder in middle-aged men, affecting any part of the brachial plexus in a patchy manner with occasional lumbosacral and phrenic nerve involvement. Prognosis is less favourable than in patients without HEV infection [167].

Other, rarely reported neurological complications of HEV include encephalitis, meningitis or myelitis, demyelinating polyneuropathy, painful neuropathy, mononeuritis multiplex, Bell's palsy vestibular neuritis and myositis [167]. Since there is no proven causal treatment for the HEV, all treatment procedures are based on supportive care and symptomatic therapy.

Sporadic reports of neurological manifestations occurring in association with childhood HEV infection also included transverse myelitis, Guillain-Barré syndrome, meningoencephalitic seizures, oculomotor palsy, Bell's palsy and pseudotumour cerebri [182–187]. However, the pathophysiology of these manifestations and the causal relation with HEV infection remain ambiguous [188]. In conclusion, HEV infection should be considered in all neurological disturbances associated with abnormal liver tests.

Hepatitis C

Chronic hepatitis C has been reported to be associated with neurological and psychiatric disorders in up to 50% of the cases [189]. They often do not correlate with the severity of the primary disease [190]. The most frequent HCV-associated neurological conditions are cerebrovascular events, encephalopathy, myelitis, encephalomyelitis, autoimmune disorders and cognitive impairment whilst frequent psychiatric conditions include depression, anxiety and fatigue [191, 192]. Acute and chronic cerebrovascular disease could be frequently seen in patients with chronic HCV infection and this is supposed to be a consequence of mixed cryoglobulinaemia [192]. A strong association between HCV infection and stroke has been repeatedly reported with an odds ratio from 1.76 to 9.61 and a hazard ratio around 1.2 [193–197]. A meta-analysis published in 2013 indicated a significantly increased risk of stroke (OR = 1.97; 95%CI: 1.64–2.30) in association with HCV infection [198]. In patients with chronic HCV infection, stroke occurs at a younger age, and serum HCV RNA levels have a negative impact on the outcome [199]. It is still unclear how HCV infection predisposes cerebrovascular disease. The proposed mechanisms, which are linked to chronic inflammation, are carotid plaque destabilization with subsequent rupture and thromboembolism, arterial remodelling, development and accelerated progression of atherosclerosis [189]. Occlusive cerebrovascular disease in patients with HCV infection is mainly a consequence of a vasculitis (mixed cryoglobulinaemia, antiphospholipid syndrome and ANCA-associated vasculitis) and it can present as an acute or subacute encephalopathy. Moreover, HCV infection has an influence on other risk factors for cerebrovascular disease such as lipidaemia and glucose-insulin homeostasis [189].

HCV infection has been linked to central nervous system inflammation with different clinical patterns including leukoencephalitis, encephalomyelitis, transverse myelitis and acute disseminated encephalomyelitis [200–203]. It has been suggested that HCV infection triggers demyelination through immune-mediated mechanisms comprising B-cell proliferation and production of monoclonal and polyclonal autoantibodies (including antinuclear antibodies, anti-SSA/anti-SSB, anti-smooth muscle antibodies, antineutrophil cytoplasmic antibodies, anti-ganglioside GM1 and anti-sulphatide antibodies), activation of autoreactive T cells and cross-reactive responses against structural neural and non-neural polypeptides [189]. Hence, in all patients presenting with a demyelinating disease of the central or peripheral nervous system, HCV infection should be excluded.

HCV infection has also been linked with clinical and subclinical demyelinating peripheral neuropathies [204, 205]. Mechanisms underlying neuropathy in HCV are likely due to inflammation and cryoglobulinaemia [206]. Peripheral neuropathies have been observed mostly in patients with HCV-related mixed cryoglobulinaemia, with a prevalence of up to 86%, but it has been also observed in patients without cryoglobulinaemia [207]. The clinical presentation is often as a sub-acute distal, symmetric, sensory or sensorimotor polyneuropathy, although asymmetrical sensory impairment has also been reported [208–210]. Moreover, small fibre sensory polyneuropathy (SFSN), characterized by burning feet and tingling sensation, is the most frequent neuropathy observed in patients with mild cryoglobulinaemia syndrome [211].

Guillain-Barré syndrome is less frequently seen in patients with HCV infection than in patients with HEV infection [212]. Similarly, chronic inflammatory demyelinating polyneuropathy (CIDP) is also rarely observed in patients with HCV.

Cognitive dysfunction has been listed as one of the neurological symptoms in patients with chronic HCV infection. It affects executive function with relatively preserved motor performance and visuospatial function [213]. It could clinically present as difficulties with numbers, sustained attention, psychomotor speed and learning memory [214]. The majority of studies have demonstrated relatively mild impairments of attention, concentration and working memory. While some reports suggested that cognitive test performance was associated with fibrosis stage on liver biopsy, others have revealed that impairments in attention and concentration could affect up to 50% of non-cirrhotic HCV patients [215–217]. However, in studies with strict exclusion criteria, in order to reduce confounding factors, there were no significant cognitive disturbances in patients with HCV when compared to controls [218, 219]. It has been observed that cognitive impairment in HCV-infected patients is highly correlated with IQ and premorbid cognitive ability [220]. The literature clearly demonstrates evidence of neurocognitive impairment in patients with chronic HCV infection, but it is still not clear whether these impairments can be attributed, wholly or in part, to the virus itself [221].

The most frequent psychiatric symptoms in patients with HCV are 'brain fog' (overall feeling of mental fogginess including forgetfulness, concentration problems and confusion), fatigue, weakness, depression and anxiety. Depression and/or anxiety have been reported in about one-third of HCV-infected patients [195, 215].

Clinically apparent acute HCV infection has been very rarely reported in children and adolescents, and fatigue is the main neurologic symptom, along with jaundice. When children and adolescents develop chronic hepatitis C infection, they also very rarely have extrahepatic manifestations [222].

Hepatitis A

Extrahepatic manifestations in hepatitis A are less common than in other types of hepatitis. Hepatitis A virus causes an acute, self-limited infection. Extrahepatic, including neurological manifestations are more frequently seen in patients with a protracted course of the acute infection [223]. Neurological manifestations of hepatitis A comprise optic neuritis, encephalitis, meningoencephalitis, meningitis, Guillain-Barré syndrome, chronic inflammatory demyelinating polyradiculoneuropathy (CIDP), sensory neuropathy, mononeuropathy, mononeuropathy multiplex, myasthenia gravis, myopathy, polymyositis and transverse myelitis (TM), including also longitudinal transverse myelitis (LETM) [224–226]. Treatment of HAV infection is supportive and symptomatic and data regarding treatment of neurological manifestations are limited.

In the absence of fulminant disease, neurological syndrome in children have been observed only rarely in association with hepatitis A. Guillain Barré syndrome has been reported to occur 3 days to 2 weeks after the onset of hepatitis A, as have myeloradiculopathy, vertigo, mononeuritis, meningoencephalitis and exacerbation of multiple sclerosis [227].

Hepatitis B

Chronic active hepatitis B can cause peripheral neuropathies via vascular or immune-mediated mechanisms [228, 229]. Observed neuropathies comprise vascular neuropathies, demyelinating neuropathies such as CIDP and Guillain-Barré syndrome and occasionally chronic immune-mediated, non-vasculitic mononeuropathy multiplex. Acute neuropathy could be also seen during acute HBV infection, but it is extremely rare [230].

Children infected early in life are most likely to develop chronic hepatitis B infection. Neonatal hepatitis B virus infection is usually acquired during delivery. It is usually asymptomatic but can cause chronic subclinical disease in later childhood or adulthood. Symptomatic infection in the early life causes lethargy, failure to thrive, along with jaundice, abdominal distention and clay-coloured stools. Pregnant women should be tested for HBsAg during an early prenatal visit. Neonates whose mothers are HBsAg-positive should be given 1 dose of HBIG 0.5 mL IM within 12 h of birth. Neonates whose mothers have unknown HBsAg status at the time of delivery should also receive their first dose of vaccine within 12 h of birth [231].

Additionally, HBV vaccination may induce hypersensitivity and autoimmune reactions in susceptible individuals and healthy subjects. Autoimmune neurological conditions including myelitis, optic neuritis, GBS and multiple sclerosis have been reported in patients following HBV vaccination [232].

Treatment of Neurological Complications of Hepatitis

Treatment of neurological complications depends on the symptomatology and pathology (i.e. demyelinating neuropathy, cerebrovascular disease, etc.) and it does not differ from the standard of care in the treatment of other patients with the same conditions. The most important step in the treatment is early diagnosis and adequate treatment and control of the primary infection.

Whipple Disease

Whipple disease is an infectious disease caused by T. whipplei, the gram-positive actinobacteria [233]. The pathogen was firstly observed in the small intestine and subsequently also in the CNS, heart, synovium, lymph nodes, lung and liver [234, 235]. The disease itself is rare and is most frequently confined to North America and Europe. Typical clinical manifestations comprise diarrhoea, abdominal pain, weight loss and joint pain [236]. Central nervous system involvement was confirmed by detecting PAS-positive material in ventricular ependymal nodules and in perivascular accumulations [237]. Most frequently reported neurological symptoms include dementia, ophtalmoplegia, myoclonus, insomnia, hyperphagia and polydipsia [238]. Headache, focal seizures, ataxia, disorientation and memory disturbance have also been observed. The combination of convergence nystagmus with palatal, tongue and mandibular movements called oculomasticatory myorhythmia has been considered pathognomonic, but it is not present in all patients [152]. In the absence of pathognomonic signs, obtaining the diagnosis could be challenging. Neuroradiologically, lesions localized in hypothalamus, cingulate gyrus, basal ganglia, insular cortex and cerebellum and CFS analysis are indicative for inflammatory conditions. It has been treated with chloramphenicol and trimethoprim-sulphamethoxazole with gaze palsies and nystagmus as the most therapy-responsive signs of neurological dysfunction [152].

Gastrointestinal Symptoms in Neurological Disorders

There are two distinct groups of neurological disorders which could present with gastrointestinal symptoms—defects of gastrointestinal system innervation and primary disorders of the nervous system in which gastrointestinal symptoms are one part of clinical presentation.

Defects of Gastrointestinal System Innervation

Defects of gastrointestinal system innervation are achalasia and Hirschprung's disease. Achalasia characterized by an absence of peristalsis in the oesophageal body accompanied by a failure of relaxation of the lower oesophageal sphincter is usually a primary disorder but could be a consequence of other diseases such as Chagas' disease. Underlying pathology observed on biopsy consists of loss of ganglion cells with substantial destruction of myenteric nerves accompanied by an inflammatory reaction. The way in which the disease evolves remains unclear [152]. On the other hand, Hirschprung's disease is characterized by the absence of parasympathetic ganglion cells of the intramural plexus in the distal segment of bowel, primarily caused by incomplete migration of neurenteric ganglion cells from the neural crest to the most distal part of the gut [152, 239]. It presents at birth or soon after with obstipation and gaseous abdominal distension.

Dysphagia

The most frequent gastrointestinal symptom seen in patients with neurologic disorders is dysphagia. Due to the complexity of central and peripheral nervous system control of swallowing as well as mandatory coordination of different structures involved in the act of swallowing, there are numerous regions and structures in the nervous system in which dysfunction could lead to dysphagia. Those regions and structures comprise cortical areas and their efferent pathway, the brainstem motor or sensory nuclei, lower cranial nerves in their distal course, neuromuscular junction and striated muscle components involved in swallowing. In most patients with neurogenic dysphagia, other signs and symptoms of neurological dysfunction are evident, but there are rare patients in whom dysphagia could be the leading and the only symptom of underlying neurological disease.

Due to high incidence and prevalence, stroke is the leading neurological cause of dysphagia. It is estimated that up to 64% of all stroke patients suffer from dysphagia [152]. It is more frequently seen in patients with stroke localized within the medulla oblongata but is also present in patients with unilateral or bilateral hemispheric strokes. It was observed that the occurrence of dysphagia in acute stroke does not appear to depend on the size or the site of the lesion. It is usually transient and full recovery of swallowing occurs in almost 90% of patients within 2 weeks [240]. Even though cerebrovascular disease is the most frequent cause of hemispheric and brainstem lesions, other conditions could produce brainstem dysfunction and hence dysphagia. These conditions include multiple sclerosis, brainstem tumours, Arnold Chiari malformation type 1 and syringobulbia. The specific group of neurological disorders in which dysphagia could be one of the prominent symptoms are neuromuscular disorders. Amyotrophic lateral sclerosis (ALS), a neurodegenerative disease involving upper and lower motoneuron could primarily present with bulbar symptoms, i.e. dysphagia, dysarthria, difficulty chewing and dysphonia (a bulbar form of ALS). Affection of lower motoneuron in Guillain-Barré syndrome or other cranial neuropathies could also result in difficulties in swallowing, but these conditions are rarely seen. On the other hand, dysphagia has been estimated to be a prominent symptom in at least one-third of patients with myasthenia gravis [152]. It could be also seen in patients with primarily muscle diseases such as inclusion body myositis, polymyositis, myotonic dystrophy, oculopharyngeal muscular dystrophy as well as in patients with neurodegenerative disorders especially in patients with Parkinson's disease, Huntington's and Wilson's disease, progressive supranuclear palsy and Alzheimer's disease. It is estimated that more than 80% of patients with Parkinson's disease have dysphagia but, as a rule, it is mild and has little or no effect on the patient's nutritional status [240].

Patients with neurogenic dysphagia tend to have difficulty in the early phases of swallowing in contrast to those with mechanical obstruction who tend to sense obstruction beneath the sternum or xiphoid [241].

Management of neurogenic dysphagia is focused primarily on prevention of pulmonary aspiration and maintenance of adequate alimentation. Oral feeding should be encouraged, especially in patients with mild forms of dysphagia. In patients with severe dysphagia, food intake may be via gastrostomy tube feeding. In cases of severe, permanent dysphagia in which the patient is considered for long-term enteral feeding, percutaneous endoscopic gastrostomy (PEG) tube feeding should be considered. In the management and rehabilitation of dysphagia, interdisciplinary approaches (including neurologist, nurse, therapist, gastroenterologist and otorhinolaryngologists when needed) are essential.

Besides conservative management, in certain patients, surgical treatment—cricopharyngeal myotomy has been shown to be effective. Prior to the procedure, two conditions must be fulfilled—failure of relaxation of the pharyngeal sphincter (demonstrated on video fluoroscopy) with preserved the oral phase of swallowing (lip seal, voluntary initiation of swallowing and the propulsive action of the tongue) [240].

Disorders of Gastric and Intestinal Motility

Gastric and intestinal motility could be affected with a primarily neurological disorder or muscular disorder. Disturbances of small and large bowel motility, when seen in neurogenic disorders, are associated with autonomic neuropathy and are particularly common in diabetes mellitus. It can present both with constipation or diarrhoea and may alternate [152]. Primary muscle disorders can lead to dysphagia (for example, with polymyositis or oculopharyngeal dystrophy) or defects of large bowel motility (for example, with Duchenne's muscular dystrophy). In patients with myotonic dystrophy, diarrhoea and abdominal cramps are common, but also megacolon, intestinal pseudoobstruction, abnormal and sustained contraction of the internal and external anal sphincters could be seen [242–244]. Constipation is relatively uncommon [152]. On the other hand, in patients with Duchenne's muscular dystrophy, various gastrointestinal symptoms including diarrhoea and constipation could be seen [152].

Vomiting

Isolated vomiting is an extremely rare presentation of neurological disorder; it is almost invariably associated with other neurological symptoms or signs. Several different structures are involved in the act of vomiting, including area postrema (in the floor of the fourth ventricle), reticular formation, brainstem nuclei, vagal nerve, vestibular system and corticobulbar fibres. Hence, lesions of the mentioned structures could present with vomiting accompanied by other neurological symptoms. Vomiting could be frequently seen in patients with vestibular disorders (Meniere's disease, vestibular neuronitis) and persistent vomiting with or without nausea could be seen in low brainstem lesions. In patients with raised intracranial pressure, vomiting may be sudden and forceful, and is often preceded by severe nausea [245]. Vomiting could be also seen in patients with migraine headaches and abdominal epilepsy.

Migraine

Migraine is a primary headache which is frequently accompanied by nausea and vomiting. According to the classification of headaches (ICHD-3), recurrent gastrointestinal disturbance without headache is an episodic syndrome that may be associated with migraine [246]. Previous terms such as chronic abdominal pain; functional abdominal pain; functional dyspepsia; irritable bowel syndrome and functional abdominal pain syndrome have been interchanged with the term recurrent gastrointestinal disturbance which is characterized by recurrent episodic attacks of abdominal pain and/or discomfort, nausea and/or vomiting, occurring infrequently, chronically or at predictable intervals [246]. Diagnostic criteria that have to be fulfilled are at least five attacks with distinct episodes of abdominal pain and/or discomfort and/or nausea and/or vomiting which could not be attributable to another disorder with normal gastrointestinal examination and evaluation [246]. Recurrent gastrointestinal disturbance can present as cyclical vomiting syndrome or abdominal migraine. Cyclical vomiting syndrome (CVS) is characterized by recurrent episodic attacks of intense nausea and vomiting that may be associated with pallor and lethargy, usually stereotypical in the individual and with predictable timing of episodes. There is complete resolution of symptoms between attacks and history and physical examination do not show signs of gastrointestinal disease. It typically occurs in childhood and is a self-limiting episodic condition [246]. This disorder affects girls more than boys (55:45), typically begins just prior to primary school, can resolve during adolescence although some will persist into adulthood and most are predicted to develop migraines. Most children are also affected by multiple comorbid complaints, especially anxiety, fatigue or limited stamina, postural orthostatic tachycardia syndrome (POTS) and chronic daily nausea. The pathophysiology appears to involve aberrant brain-gut and cellular pathways including migraine pathways, autonomic and hypothalamic-pituitary-adrenal axis hyper-reactivity and mitochondrial dysfunction. CVS in children remains a devastating disorder because of frequent hospitalizations, multiple comorbidities and poor quality of life. Because the response to treatment is heterogeneous, clinicians often trial several different preventative strategies including NK1 antagonists, amitriptyline, anticonvulsants, Ca2 + -channel blockers and other TCA antidepressants [247]. However, CVS is increasingly recognized in adults, beginning either in childhood or in adulthood.

Diagnostic criteria for cyclical vomiting syndrome comprise [246]:

(a) At least five attacks of intense nausea and vomiting, fulfilling criteria B and C.
(b) Stereotypical in the individual patient and recurring with predictable periodicity.
(c) All of the following:
  - Nausea and vomiting occur at least four times per hour.
  - Attacks last for ≥1 h, up to 10 days.
  - Attacks occur ≥1 week apart.
(d) Complete freedom from symptoms between attacks.
(e) Not attributed to another disorder.

Another condition classified as recurrent gastrointestinal disturbance is abdominal migraine. This is an idiopathic disorder seen mainly in children, characterized by recurrent attacks of moderate to severe midline abdominal pain, associated with vasomotor symptoms, nausea and vomiting, lasting 2–72 h. Patients are completely normal between episodes. It is important to note that headache does not occur during these episodes. As in previous condition history, physical exam and investigations do not show signs of gastrointestinal disease or disorder [246].

Diagnostic criteria comprise [246]:

(a) At least five attacks of abdominal pain, fulfilling criteria B–D.
(b) Pain has at least two of the following three characteristics:
  - Midline location, periumbilical or poorly localized.
  - Dull or 'just sore' quality.
  - Moderate or severe intensity.
(c) At least two of the following four associated symptoms or signs:
  - Anorexia.
  - Nausea.
  - Vomiting.
  - Pallor.

(d) Attacks last 2–72 h when untreated or unsuccessfully treated.
(e) Complete freedom from symptoms between attacks.
(f) Not attributed to another disorder.

Abdominal Epilepsy

Abdominal epilepsy is an uncommon epilepsy syndrome which predominately presents with paroxysmal gastrointestinal symptoms. These symptoms are direct presentation of abnormal excessive or synchronous neuronal activity in the brain. Besides gastrointestinal symptoms, abdominal epilepsy comprises also CNS manifestations. Gastrointestinal manifestations include paroxysmal abdominal pain in most cases, followed by nausea and/or vomiting, less frequently bloating and diarrhoea [248, 249]. Reported CNS manifestations include confusion, fatigue, headache, dizziness postictal lethargy, drowsiness, blindness, paraesthesia and convulsion [249, 250]. Headache in patients with abdominal epilepsy is often difficult to differentiate from migraine. In such cases, EEG may be helpful, since patients with abdominal epilepsy usually have specific EEG abnormalities, particularly of a temporal lobe seizure disorder [251]. However, changes in EEG are not mandatory, since up to 40–50% of patients with epileptic disorders may have one or more normal inter-ictal EEG [248, 252]. Therefore, a normal EEG does not exclude epileptic disorder. On the other hand, more than 10% of normal people may have non-specific EEG abnormalities and approximately 1% may have 'epileptiform paroxysmal activity' without seizures [253]. Hence, EEG could be helpful in the diagnostic process but is not a procedure on which we could completely rely on in making decisions while diagnosing abdominal epilepsy. Besides migraine, irritable bowel syndrome is another differential diagnosis which should be ruled out. Abdominal epilepsy may be distinguished from the latter condition by the presence of altered consciousness during some of the episodes, a tendency towards tiredness after an episode and in certain cases EEG abnormalities [249, 254].

Although there are no official criteria for the diagnosis of abdominal epilepsy, proposed criteria often mentioned in the literature comprise (1) paroxysmal gastrointestinal manifestations of undetermined origin after thorough evaluation including laboratory, radiographic and endoscopy testing; (2) symptoms originated from the CNS; (3) an abnormal electroencephalogram (EEG) findings relatively specific for epileptic seizures; (4) a sustained improvement of symptoms by antiepileptic medication [255].

Prior to establishing the diagnosis of abdominal epilepsy, gastrointestinal disease should be ruled out. History details such as paroxysmal episodes of gastrointestinal symptoms are highly indicative of abdominal epilepsy. It is important to distinguish abdominal epilepsy itself from abdominal auras preceding other major seizure manifestations of temporal or parieto-occipital epilepsy [256]. Information of subjective signs such as epigastric rising sensation, déjà vu, jamais vu and olfactory sensation should be inspected. All these features are characteristic of temporal lobe seizure, as well as are gastrointestinal symptoms in abdominal epilepsy.

Treatment of abdominal epilepsy does not differ from the treatment of other types of epilepsy. The mainstay is antiepileptic drug. Moreover, one of the proposed criteria for the diagnosis is a sustained response to anticonvulsants [255]. The choice of medication is based on guidelines regarding the treatment of focal epilepsy as well as patient features (age, comorbidities, co-medication, etc.). The prognosis of abdominal epilepsy is generally good, as it is in other types of epilepsy. In most patients, antiepileptic drug brings relief in gastrointestinal symptoms.

In conclusion, abdominal epilepsy is a rare entity, what can be easily mistaken or misdiagnosed as gastrointestinal, maybe more frequently as a psychiatric disorder often resulting in a number of unnecessary investigations. However, when the proper diagnosis is established, the condition could be easily and successfully treated in the majority of patients.

References

1. Kim YK, Shin C. The microbiota-gut-brain axis in neuropsychiatric disorders: pathophysiological mechanisms and novel treatments. Curr Neuropharmacol. 2018;16(5):559–73. https://doi.org/10.2174/1570159X15666170915141036.
2. Carabotti M, Scirocco A, Maselli MA, Severi C. The gut-brain axis: interactions between enteric microbiota, central and enteric nervous systems. Ann Gastroenterol. 2015;28(2):203–9.
3. Mayer EA, Savidge T, Shulman RJ. Brain-gut microbiome interactions and functional bowel disorders. Gastroenterology. 2014;146(6):1500–12. https://doi.org/10.1053/j.gastro.2014.02.037.
4. Bluthé RM, Walter V, Parnet P, Layé S, Lestage J, Verrier D, et al. Lipopolysaccharide induces sickness behaviour in rats by a vagal mediated mechanism. C R Acad Sci III. 1994;317(6):499–503.
5. Goehler LE, Gaykema RP, Opitz N, Reddaway R, Badr N, Lyte M. Activation in vagal afferents and central autonomic pathways: early responses to intestinal infection with Campylobacter jejuni. Brain Behav Immun. 2005;19(4):334–44. https://doi.org/10.1016/j.bbi.2004.09.002.
6. Nankova BB, Agarwal R, MacFabe DF, La Gamma EF. Enteric bacterial metabolites propionic and butyric acid modulate gene expression, including CREB-dependent catecholaminergic neurotransmission, in PC12 cells—possible relevance to autism spectrum disorders. PLoS One. 2014;9(8):e103740. https://doi.org/10.1371/journal.pone.0103740.
7. Erny D, Hrabě de Angelis AL, Jaitin D, Wieghofer P, Staszewski O, David E, et al. Host microbiota constantly control maturation and function of microglia in the CNS. Nat Neurosci. 2015;18(7):965–77. https://doi.org/10.1038/nn.4030.
8. de Almeida LM, Funchal C, Gottfried C, Wajner M, Pessoa-Pureur R. Propionic acid induces cytoskeletal alterations in cultured astrocytes from rat cerebral cortex. Metab Brain Dis. 2006;21(1):51–62.
9. Huuskonen J, Suuronen T, Nuutinen T, Kyrylenko S, Salminen A. Regulation of microglial inflammatory response by sodium butyrate and short-chain fatty acids. Br J Pharmacol. 2004;141(5):874–80. https://doi.org/10.1038/sj.bjp.0705682.
10. Kimura I, Inoue D, Maeda T, Hara T, Ichimura A, Miyauchi S, et al. Short-chain fatty acids and ketones directly regulate sympathetic nervous system via G protein-coupled receptor 41 (GPR41). Proc Natl Acad Sci U S A. 2011;108(19):8030–5. https://doi.org/10.1073/pnas.1016088108.

11. Grider JR, Piland BE. The peristaltic reflex induced by short-chain fatty acids is mediated by sequential release of 5-HT and neuronal CGRP but not BDNF. Am J Physiol Gastrointest Liver Physiol. 2007;292(1):G429–37. https://doi.org/10.1152/ajpgi.00376.2006.
12. Rothhammer V, Borucki DM, Tjon EC, Takenaka MC, Chao CC, Ardura-Fabregat A, et al. Microglial control of astrocytes in response to microbial metabolites. Nature. 2018;557(7707):724–8. https://doi.org/10.1038/s41586-018-0119-x.
13. Ogawa S, Fujii T, Koga N, Hori H, Teraishi T, Hattori K, et al. Plasma L-tryptophan concentration in major depressive disorder: new data and meta-analysis. J Clin Psychiatry. 2014;75(9):e906–15. https://doi.org/10.4088/JCP.13r08908.
14. Huang TT, Lai JB, Du YL, Xu Y, Ruan LM, Hu SH. Current understanding of gut microbiota in mood disorders: an update of human studies. Front Genet. 2019;10:98. https://doi.org/10.3389/fgene.2019.00098.
15. Bastiaanssen TFS, Cowan CSM, Claesson MJ, Dinan TG, Cryan JF. Making sense of … the microbiome in psychiatry. Int J Neuropsychopharmacol. 2019;22(1):37–52. https://doi.org/10.1093/ijnp/pyy067.
16. Ma Q, Xing C, Long W, Wang HY, Liu Q, Wang RF. Impact of microbiota on central nervous system and neurological diseases: the gut-brain axis. J Neuroinflammation. 2019;16(1):53. https://doi.org/10.1186/s12974-019-1434-3.
17. Dahlin M, Prast-Nielsen S. The gut microbiome and epilepsy. EBioMedicine. 2019;44:741–6. https://doi.org/10.1016/j.ebiom.2019.05.024.
18. Borre YE, O'Keeffe GW, Clarke G, et al. Microbiota and neurodevelopmental windows: implications for brain disorders. Trends Mol Med. 2014;20(9):509–16. https://doi.org/10.1016/j.molmed.2014.05.002.
19. Mulder CJJ, Rouvroye MD, van Dam AM. Transglutaminase 6 antibodies are not yet mainstream in neuro-coeliac disease. Dig Liver Dis. 2018;50(1):96–7. https://doi.org/10.1016/j.dld.2017.10.001.
20. Ghezzi A, Zaffaroni M. Neurological manifestations of gastrointestinal disorders, with particular reference to the differential diagnosis of multiple sclerosis. Neurol Sci. 2001;22(8):S117–22. https://doi.org/10.1007/s100720100048.
21. Bizzaro N, Tonutti E. Anti-gliadin antibodies. In: Shoenfeld Y, Gershwin ME, Meroni PL, editors. Autoantibodies. 2nd ed. Amsterdam: Elsevier; 2007. p. 451–6. https://doi.org/10.1016/B978-0-444-52763-9.X5000-8.
22. Sardy M, Karpati S, Merkl B, Paulsson M, Smyth N. Epidermal transglutaminase (TGase 3) is the autoantigen of dermatitis herpetiformis. J Exp Med. 2002;195:747–57. https://doi.org/10.1084/jem.20011299.
23. Hadjivassiliou M, Mäki M, Sanders DS, Williamson CA, Grünewald RA, Woodroofe NM, et al. Autoantibody targeting of brain and intestinal transglutaminase in gluten ataxia. Neurology. 2006;66:373–7. https://doi.org/10.1212/01.wnl.0000196480.55601.3a.
24. Zis P, Rao DG, Sarrigiannis PG, Aeschlimann P, Aeschlimann DP, Sanders DS, et al. Transglutaminase 6 antibodies in gluten neuropathy. Dig Liver Dis. 2017;49:1196–200. https://doi.org/10.1016/j.dld.2017.08.019.
25. Gadoth A, Nefussy B, Bleiberg M, Klein T, Artman I, Drory VE. Transglutaminase 6 antibodies in the serum of patients with amyotrophic lateral sclerosis. JAMA Neurol. 2015;72:676–81. https://doi.org/10.1001/jamaneurol.2015.48.
26. Cristofanilli M, Gratch D, Pagano B, McDermott K, Huang J, Jian J, Bates D, et al. Transglutaminase-6 is an autoantigen in progressive multiple sclerosis and is upregulated in reactive astrocytes. Mult Scler. 2017;23(13):1707–15. https://doi.org/10.1177/1352458516684022.
27. Kinney HC, Burger PC, Hurwitz BJ, Humans JC, Grant JP. Degeneration of the central nervous system associated with celiac disease. J Neurol Sci. 1982;53:9–22. https://doi.org/10.1016/0022-510X(82)90076-4.
28. Collin P, Pirttilä T, Nurmikko T, Somer H, Erilä T, Keyriläinen O. Celiac disease, brain atrophy, and dementia. Neurology. 1991;41:372–5.

29. Hamidian Y, Togha M, Nafisi S, Dowlatshahi S, Jahromi SR, Moghadam NB, et al. Antigliadin antibody in sporadic adult ataxia. Iran J Neurol. 2012;11(1):16–20.
30. Wong D, Dwinnel M, Schulzer M, Nimmo M, Leavitt BR, Spacey SD. Ataxia and the role of antigliadin antibodies. Can J Neurol Sci. 2007;34(2):193–6. https://doi.org/10.1017/s031716710000603x.
31. Barton SH, Murray JA. Celiac disease and autoimmunity in the gut and elsewhere. Gastroenterol Clin N Am. 2008;37(2):411–28. https://doi.org/10.1016/j.gtc.2008.02.001.
32. Lin CY, Wang MJ, Tse W, Pinotti R, Kuo SH. Serum anti-gliadin antibodies and the risk of cerebellar ataxias: a systematic review and meta-analysis. J Neurol Neurosurg Psychiatry. 2018;89(11):1174–80. https://doi.org/10.1136/jnnp-2018-318215.
33. Casella G, Santilli I, Di Bella C, Crisafulli V, Villanacci V, Baldini V, et al. Cerebellar ataxia, celiac disease and non-celiac gluten sensitivity. Arch Neurosci. 2017;4(2):e44187. https://doi.org/10.5812/archneurosci.44187.
34. Finelli PF, McEntee WJ, Ambler M, Kestenbaum D. Adult celiac disease presenting as cerebellar syndrome. Neurology. 1980;30(3):245–9. https://doi.org/10.1212/wnl.30.3.245.
35. Freeman HJ. Neurological disorders in adult celiac disease. Can J Gastroenterol. 2008;22(11):909–11. https://doi.org/10.1155/2008/824631.
36. Vinagre-Aragón A, Zis P, Grunewald RA, Hadjivassiliou M. Movement disorders related to gluten sensitivity: a systematic review. Nutrients. 2018;10(8):1034. https://doi.org/10.3390/nu10081034.
37. Bago Rožanković P, Rožanković M, Romić ZČ, Bašić S. Paroxismal non-kinesigenic dyskinesia and hemidystonia associated with silent celiac disease. Clin Neurol Neurosurg. 2019;188:105586. https://doi.org/10.1016/j.clineuro.2019.105586. [Epub ahead of print]
38. Cicarelli G, Della Rocca G, Amboni M, Ciacci C, Mazzacca G, Filla A, et al. Clinical and neurological abnormalities in adult celiac disease. Neurol Sci. 2003;24(5):311–7. https://doi.org/10.1007/s10072-003-0181-4.
39. Chin RL, Sander HW, Brannagan TH, Green PH, Hays AP, Alaedini A, et al. Celiac neuropathy. Neurology. 2003;60:1581–5. https://doi.org/10.1212/01.wnl.0000063307.84039.c7.
40. Usai P, Usai Satta P, Lai M, Corda MG, Piras E, Calcara C, et al. Autonomic dysfunction and upper digestive functional disorders in untreated adult celiac disease. Eur J Clin Investig. 1997;27(12):1009–15. https://doi.org/10.1046/j.1365-2362.1997.2340781.x.
41. Kaplan JG, Pack D, Horoupian D, De Souza T, Brin M, Schaumburg H. Distal axonopathy associated with chronic gluten enteropathy: a treatable disorder. Neurology. 1988;38(4):642–5. https://doi.org/10.1212/wnl.38.4.642.
42. Gupta V, Kohli A. Celiac disease associated with recurrent Guillain Barre syndrome. Indian Pediatr. 2010;47(9):797–8. https://doi.org/10.1007/s13312-010-0105-3.
43. Pacitto A, Paglino A, Di Genova L, Leonardi A, Farinelli E, Principi N, et al. Celiac disease presenting with peripheral neuropathy in children: a case report. Int J Environ Res Public Health. 2017;14(7):785. https://doi.org/10.3390/ijerph14070785.
44. Luostarinen L, Himanen SL, Luostarinen M, Collin P, Pirttila T. Neuromuscular and sensory disturbances in patients with well-treated celiac disease. J Neurol Neurosurg Psychiatry. 2003;74:490–4. https://doi.org/10.1136/jnnp.74.4.490.
45. Molteni N, Bardella MT, Baldassarri AR, Bianchi PA. Celiac disease associated with epilepsy and intracranial calcifications: report of two patients. Am J Gastroenterol. 1988;83(9):992–4.
46. Gobbi G, Bouquet F, Greco L, Lambertini A, Tassinari CA, Ventura A, et al. Celiac disease, epilepsy, and cerebral calcifications. The Italian Working Group on Celiac Disease and Epilepsy. Lancet. 1992;340(8817):439–43. https://doi.org/10.1016/0140-6736(92)91766-2.
47. Arroyo HA, De Rosa S, Ruggieri V, de Davila MT, Fejerman N. Epilepsy, occipital calcifications, and oligosymptomatic celiac disease in childhood. J Child Neurol. 2002;17(11):800–6. https://doi.org/10.1177/08830738020170110801.
48. Bashiri H, Afshari D, Babaei N, Ghadami MR. Celiac disease and epilepsy: the effect of gluten-free diet on seizure control. Adv Clin Exp Med. 2016;25(4):751–4. https://doi.org/10.17219/acem/43585.

49. Nikpour S. Neurological manifestations, diagnosis, and treatment of celiac disease: a comprehensive review. Iran J Neurol. 2012;11(2):59–64.
50. Hu WT, Murray JA, Greenaway MC, Parisi JE, Josephs KA. Cognitive impairment and celiac disease. Arch Neurol. 2006;63(10):1440–6. https://doi.org/10.1001/archneur.63.10.1440.
51. Lebwohl B, Luchsinger JA, Freedberg DE, Green PH, Ludvigsson JF. Risk of dementia in patients with celiac disease: a population-based cohort study. J Alzheimers Dis. 2016;49(1):179–85. https://doi.org/10.3233/JAD-150388.
52. Lurie Y, Landau DA, Pfeffer J, Oren R. Celiac disease diagnosed in the elderly. J Clin Gastroenterol. 2008;42(1):59–61. https://doi.org/10.1097/01.mcg.0000247995.12087.7b.
53. Gabrielli M, Cremonini F, Fiore G, Addolorato G, Padalino C, Candelli M, et al. Association between migraine and celiac disease: results from a preliminary case-control and therapeutic study. Am J Gastroenterol. 2003;98(3):625–9. https://doi.org/10.1111/j.1572-0241.2003.07300.x.
54. Jackson JR, Eaton WW, Cascella NG, Fasano A, Kelly DL. Neurologic and psychiatric manifestations of celiac disease and gluten sensitivity. Psychiatry Q. 2012;83(1):91–102. https://doi.org/10.1007/s11126-011-9186-y.
55. Lerner A. New therapeutic strategies for celiac disease. Autoimmun Rev. 2010;9(3):144–7. https://doi.org/10.1016/j.autrev.2009.05.002.
56. Zelnik N, Pacht A, Obeid R, Lerner A. Range of neurologic disorders in patients with celiac disease. Pediatrics. 2004;113(6):1672–6. https://doi.org/10.1542/peds.113.6.1672.
57. Mavroudi A, KaratzaE PT, Panteliadis C, Spiroglou K. Succesful treatment of epilepsy and celical disease with gluten free diet. Pediatr Neurol. 2005;33(4):292–5. https://doi.org/10.1016/j.pediatrneurol.2005.05.010.
58. Diaconu G, Burlea M, Grigore I, Anton DT, Trandafir LM. Celiac disease with neurologic manifestations in children. Rev Med Chir Soc Med Nat Iasi. 2013;117(1):88–94.
59. Ruggieri M, Incorpora G, Polizzi A, Parano E, Spina M, Pavone P. Low prevalence of neurologic and psychiatric manifestations in children with gluten sensitivity. J Pediatr. 2008;152(2):244–9. https://doi.org/10.1016/j.jpeds.2007.06.042.
60. Cakir D, Tosun A, Polat M, Celebisoy N, Gokben S, Aydogdu S, Yagci RV, Tekgul H. Subclinical neurological abnormalities in children with celiac disease receiving a gluten-free diet. J Pediatr Gastroenterol Nutr. 2007;45(3):366–9. https://doi.org/10.1097/MPG.0b013e31806907e8.
61. Kieslich M, Errazuriz G, Posselt HG, Moeller-Hartmann W, Zanella F, Boegles H. Brain white matter lesions in coeliac disease: a prospective studyof 75 diet-treated patients. Pediatrics. 2001;108(2):E21. https://doi.org/10.1542/peds.108.2.e21.
62. Geissler A, Andus T, Roth M, Kullmann F, Caesar I, Held P, et al. Focal white-matter lesions in brain of patients with inflammatory bowel disease. Lancet. 1995;345(8954):897–8. https://doi.org/10.1016/s0140-6736(95)90013-6.
63. Lindgren S, Lilja B, Rosén I, Sundkvist G. Disturbed autonomic nerve function in patients with Crohn's disease. Scand J Gastroenterol. 1991;26(4):361–6. https://doi.org/10.3109/00365529108996495.
64. Ben-Or O, Zelnik N, Shaoul R, Pacht A, Lerner A. The neurologic profile of children and adolescents with inflammatory bowel disease. J Child Neurol. 2015;30(5):551–7. https://doi.org/10.1177/0883073814521296.
65. Chams S, Badran R, El Sayegh S, Chams N, Shams A, Hussein IH. Inflammatory bowel disease: looking beyond the tract. Int J Immunopathol Pharmacol. 2019;33:2058738419866567. Published online 2019. https://doi.org/10.1177/2058738419866567.
66. Plata-Bello J, Acosta-López S. Neurological manifestations of inflammatory bowel disease, new concepts in inflammatory bowel disease. Batool Mutar Mahdi: IntechOpen; 2018. https://doi.org/10.5772/intechopen.73017. Available from: https://www.intechopen.com/books/new-concepts-in-inflammatory-bowel-disease/neurological-manifestations-of-inflammatory-bowel-disease. Acessed on Nov 2, 2019
67. Zezos P, Kouklakis G, Saibil F. Inflammatory bowel disease and thromboembolism. World J Gastroenterol. 2014;20(38):13863–78. https://doi.org/10.3748/wjg.v20.i38.13863.

68. Grainge MJ, West J, Card TR. Venous thromboembolism during active disease and remission in inflammatory bowel disease: a cohort study. Lancet. 2010;375(9715):657–63. https://doi.org/10.1016/S0140-6736(09)61963-2.
69. Dentali F, Douketis JD, Gianni M, Lim W, Crowther MA. Meta-analysis: anticoagulant prophylaxis to prevent symptomatic venous thromboembolism in hospitalized medical patients. Ann Intern Med. 2007;146(4):278–88. https://doi.org/10.7326/0003-4819-146-4-200702200-00007.
70. Casella G, Tontini GE, Bassotti G, Pastorelli L, Villanacci V, Spina L, et al. Neurological disorders and inflammatory bowel diseases. World J Gastroenterol. 2014;20(27):8764–82. https://doi.org/10.3748/wjg.v20.i27.8764.
71. Lin Z, Si Q, Xiaoyi Z. Association between epilepsy and systemic autoimmune diseases: a meta-analysis. Seizure. 2016;41:160–6. https://doi.org/10.1016/j.seizure.2016.08.003.
72. Benavente L, Morís G. Neurologic disorders associated with inflammatory bowel disease. Eur J Neurol. 2011;18(1):138–43. https://doi.org/10.1111/j.1468-1331.2010.03095.x.
73. Lossos A, River Y, Eliakim A, Steiner I. Neurologic aspects of inflammatory bowel disease. Neurology. 1995;45(3 Pt 1):416–21. https://doi.org/10.1212/wnl.45.3.416.
74. Morís G. Inflammatory bowel disease: an increased risk factor for neurologic complications. World J Gastroenterol. 2014;20(5):1228–37. https://doi.org/10.3748/wjg.v20.i5.1228.
75. Gondim FAA, Grannagan TH, Sander HW, Chin RL, Latov N. Peripheral neuropathy in patients with inflammatory bowel disease. Brain. 2005;128(4):867–79. https://doi.org/10.1093/brain/awh429.
76. Pfeiffer RF. Gastroenterology and neurology. Continuum (Minneap Minn): Lifelong Learn Neurol. 2017;23(3):744–61. https://doi.org/10.1212/CON.0000000000000484.
77. Deepak P, Stobaugh DJ, Sherid M, Sifuentes H, Ehrenpreis ED. Neurological events with tumour necrosis factor alpha inhibitors reported to the Food and Drug Administration adverse event reporting system. Aliment Pharm Ther. 2013;38(4):388–96. https://doi.org/10.1111/apt.12385.
78. Rang EH, Brooke BN, Hermon-Taylor J. Association of ulcerative colitis with multiple sclerosis. Lancet. 1982;2(8297):555. https://doi.org/10.1016/s0140-6736(82)90629-8.
79. Kosmidou M, Katsanos AH, Katsanos KH, Kyritsis AP, Tsivgoulis G, Christodoulou D, et al. Multiple sclerosis and inflammatory bowel diseases: a systematic review and meta-analysis. J Neurol. 2017;264(2):254–9. https://doi.org/10.1007/s00415-016-8340-8.
80. Gupta G, Gelfand JM, Lewis JD. Increased risk for demyelinating diseases in patients with inflammatory bowel disease. Gastroenterology. 2005;129(3):819–26. https://doi.org/10.1053/j.gastro.2005.06.022.
81. Ramos-Casals M, Perez-Alvarez R, Diaz-Lagares C, Cuadrado MJ, Khamashta MA, BIOGEAS Study Group. Autoimmune diseases induced by biological agents: a double-edged sword? Autoimmun Rev. 2010;9(3):188–93. https://doi.org/10.1016/j.autrev.2009.10.003.
82. Dolapcioglu C, Guleryuzlu Y, Uygur-Bayramicli O, Ahishali E, Dabak R. Asymptomatic brain lesions on cranial magnetic resonance imaging in inflammatory bowel disease. Gut Liver. 2013;7(2):169–74. https://doi.org/10.5009/gnl.2013.7.2.169.
83. Graff LA, Walker JR, Bernstein CN. Depression and anxiety in inflammatory bowel disease: a review of comorbidity and management. Inflamm Bowel Dis. 2009;15(7):1105–18. https://doi.org/10.1002/ibd.20873.
84. Nowakowski J, Chrobak AA, Dudek D. Psychiatric illnesses in inflammatory bowel diseases—psychiatric comorbidity and biological underpinnings. Psychiatr Pol. 2016;50(6):1157–66. https://doi.org/10.12740/PP/62382.
85. Walker JR, Ediger JP, Graff LA, Greenfeld JM, Clara I, Lix L, et al. The Manitoba IBD cohort study: a population-based study of the prevalence of lifetime and 12-month anxiety and mood disorders. Am J Gastroenterol. 2008;103(8):1989–97. https://doi.org/10.1111/j.1572-0241.2008.01980.x.
86. Eaton WW, Pedersen MG, Nielsen PR, Mortensen PB. Autoimmune diseases, bipolar disorder, and non-affective psychosis. Bipolar Disord. 2010;12(6):638–46. https://doi.org/10.1111/j.1399-5618.2010.00853.x.

87. Butterworth RF. Editorial: rifaximin and minimal hepatic encephalopathy. Am J Gastroenterol. 2011;106(2):317–8. https://doi.org/10.1038/ajg.2010.460.
88. Bismuth M, Funakoshi N, Cadranel JF, Blanc P. Hepatic encephalopathy: from pathophysiology to therapeutic management. Eur J Gastroenterol Hepatol. 2011;23(1):8–22. https://doi.org/10.1097/MEG.0b013e3283417567.
89. Ferenci P. Hepatic encephalopathy. Gastroenterol Rep. 2017;5(2):138–47. https://doi.org/10.1093/gastro/gox013.
90. Bajaj JS, Cordoba J, Mullen KD, Amodio P, Shawcross DL, Butterworth RF, et al. Review article: the design of clinical trials in hepatic encephalopathy—an International Society for Hepatic Encephalopathy and Nitrogen Metabolism (ISHEN) consensus statement. Aliment Pharmacol Ther. 2011;33:739–47. https://doi.org/10.1111/j.1365-2036.2011.04590.x.
91. Görg B, Schliess F, Häussinger D. Osmotic and oxidative/nitrosative stress in ammonia toxicity and hepatic encephalopathy. Arch Biochem Biophys. 2013;536(2):158–63. https://doi.org/10.1016/j.abb.2013.03.010.
92. Raabe W. Effects of hyperammonemia on neuronal function: NH_4^+, IPSP and Cl^--extrusion. Adv Exp Med Biol. 1993;341:71–82. https://doi.org/10.1007/978-1-4615-2484-7_7.
93. Amodio P, Montagnese S, Gatta A, Morgan MY. Characteristics of minimal hepatic encephalopathy. Metab Brain Dis. 2004;19(3–4):253–67. https://doi.org/10.1023/b:mebr.0000043975.01841.de.
94. Vilstrup H, Amodio P, Bajaj J, Cordoba J, Ferenci P, Mullen KD, et al. Hepatic encephalopathy in chronic liver disease: 2014 Practice Guideline by the American Association for the Study of Liver Diseases and the European Association for the Study of the Liver. Hepatology. 2014;60(2):715–35. https://doi.org/10.1002/hep.27210.
95. Lockwood AH. Blood ammonia levels and hepatic encephalopathy. Metab Brain Dis. 2004;19(3–4):345–9. https://doi.org/10.1023/b:mebr.0000043980.74574.eb.
96. Weissenborn K. Hepatic encephalopathy: definition, clinical grading and diagnostic principles. Drugs. 2019;79(Suppl. 1):5–9. https://doi.org/10.1007/s40265-018-1018-z.
97. Guevara M, Baccaro ME, Torre A, Gómez-Ansón B, Ríos J, Torres F, et al. Hyponatremia is a risk factor of hepatic encephalopathy in patients with cirrhosis: a prospective study with time-dependent analysis. Am J Gastroenterol. 2009;104(6):1382–9. https://doi.org/10.1038/ajg.2009.293.
98. Toney NA, Bell MJ, Belle SH, Hardison RM, Rodriguez-Baez N, Loomes KM, Vodovotz Y, Zamora R, Squires RH, Pediatric Acute Liver Failure Study Group. Hepatic encephalopathy in children with acute liver failure: utility of serum neuromarkers. J Pediatr Gastroenterol Nutr. 2019;69(1):108–15. https://doi.org/10.1097/MPG.0000000000002351.
99. Gluud LL, Vilstrup H, Morgan MY. Non-absorbable disaccharides versus placebo/no intervention and lactulose versus lactitol for the prevention and treatment of hepatic encephalopathy in people with cirrhosis. Cochrane Database Syst Rev. 2016;4:CD003044. https://doi.org/10.1002/14651858.CD003044.pub3.
100. Conn HO. The hepatic encephalopathies. In: Conn HO, editor. Hepatic encephalopathy: syndromes and therapies. Bloomington. IL: Medi Ed Press; 1994. p. 1–12.
101. Morgan MY, Alonso M, Stanger LC. Lactitol and lactulose for the treatment of subclinical hepatic encephalopathy in cirrhotic patients. A randomised, cross-over study. J Hepatol. 1989;8(2):208–17. https://doi.org/10.1016/0168-8278(89)90009-3.
102. Park JG, Tak WY, Park SY, Kweon YO, Jang SY, Lee YR, et al. Effects of branched-chain amino acids (BCAAs) on the progression of advanced liver disease: a Korean nationwide, multicenter, retrospective, observational, cohort study. Medicine (Baltimore). 2017;96(24):e6580. https://doi.org/10.1097/MD.0000000000006580.
103. Jover-Cobos M, Noiret L, Sharifi Y, Jalan R. Ornithine phenylacetate revisited. Metab Brain Dis. 2013;28(2):327–31. https://doi.org/10.1007/s11011-013-9391-5.
104. Rockey DC, Vierling JM, Mantry P, Ghabril M, Brown RS Jr, Alexeeva O, et al. Randomized, double-blind, controlled study of glycerol phenylbutyrate in hepatic encephalopathy. Hepatology. 2014;59(3):1073–83. https://doi.org/10.1002/hep.26611.

105. Butterworth RF, McPhail MJW. L-Ornithine L-Aspartate (LOLA) for hepatic encephalopathy in cirrhosis: results of randomized controlled trials and meta-analyses. Drugs. 2019;79(Suppl. 1):31–7. https://doi.org/10.1007/s40265-018-1024-1.
106. Shehata HH, Elfert AA, Abdin AA, Soliman SM, Elkhouly RA, Hawash NI, Soliman HH. Randomized controlled trial of polyethylene glycol versus lactulose for the treatment of overt hepatic encephalopathy. Eur J Gastroenterol Hepatol. 2018;30(12):1476–81. https://doi.org/10.1097/MEG.0000000000001267.
107. Bass NM, Mullen KD, Sanyal A, Poordad F, Neff G, Leevy CB, et al. Rifaximin treatment in hepatic encephalopathy. N Engl J Med. 2010;362(12):1071–81. https://doi.org/10.1056/NEJMoa0907893.
108. Amodio P, Bemeur C, Butterworth R, Cordoba J, Kato A, Montagnese S, et al. The nutritional management of hepatic encephalopathy in patients with cirrhosis: ISHEN practice guidelines. Hepatology. 2013;58(1):325–36. https://doi.org/10.1002/hep.26370.
109. Pfeiffer RF. Neurologic manifestations of malabsorption syndromes. Handb Clin Neurol. 2014;120:621–32. https://doi.org/10.1016/B978-0-7020-4087-0.00042-5.
110. Attaluri P, Castillo A, Edriss H, Nugent K. Thiamine deficiency: an important consideration in critically ill patients. Am J Med Sci. 2018;356(4):382–90. https://doi.org/10.1016/j.amjms.2018.06.015.
111. Kumar N. Neurologic presentations of nutritional deficiencies. Neurol Clin. 2010;28(1):107–70. https://doi.org/10.1016/j.ncl.2009.09.006.
112. Blass J. Vitamin and nutritional deficiencies. In: Siegel GJ, Agranoff BW, Albers RW, Molinoff PB, editors. Basic neurochemistry. 5th ed. New York: Raven Press; 1994. p. 749–60. https://doi.org/10.1002/jnr.490390418.
113. Wiley KD, Gupta M. Vitamin B1 thiamine deficiency (Beriberi). StatPearls; 2019. [Cited 2019 Nov 23]. Available from: https://www.ncbi.nlm.nih.gov/books/NBK537204/
114. Ohnishi A, Tsuji S, Igisu H, Murai Y, Goto I, Kuroiwa Y, et al. Beriberi neuropathy. Morphometric study of sural nerve. J Neurol Sci. 1980;45(2–3):177–90.
115. Koike H, Misu K, Hattori N, Ito S, Ichimura M, Ito H, et al. Postgastrectomy polyneuropathy with thiamine deficiency. J Neurol Neurosurg Psychiatry. 2001;71(3):357–62. https://doi.org/10.1136/jnnp.71.3.357.
116. Murphy C, Bangash IH, Varma A. Dry beriberi mimicking the Guillain-Barre syndrome. Pract Neurol. 2009;9(4):221–4. https://doi.org/10.1136/jnnp.2009.182097.
117. Saperstein DB, Barohn RJ. Polyneuropathy caused by nutritional and vitamin deficiency. In: Dyck P, editor. Peripheral neuropathy. Philadelphia: Elsevier; 2005. p. 2051–62.
118. Sechi GP, Serra A. Wernicke's encephalopathy: new clinical settings and recent advances in diagnosis and management. Lancet Neurol. 2007;6(5):442–55. https://doi.org/10.1016/S1474-4422(07)70104-7.
119. Uruha A, Shimizu T, Katoh T, Yamasaki Y, Matsubara S. Wernicke's encephalopathy in a patient with peptic ulcer disease. Case Rep Med. 2011;2011:156104. https://doi.org/10.1155/2011/156104. Epub 2011 Jun 28
120. Zuccoli G, Pipitone N. Neuroimaging findings in acute Wernicke's encephalopathy: review of the literature. AJR Am J Roentgenol. 2009;192(2):501–8. https://doi.org/10.2214/AJR.07.3959.
121. Dhir S, Tarasenko M, Napoli E, Gulivi C. Neurological, psychiatric and biochemical aspects of thiamine deficiency in children and adults. Front Psych. 2019;10:207. https://doi.org/10.3389/fpsyt.2019.00207.
122. Gu F, Chauhan V, Kaur K, Brown WT, LaFucci G, Weigel J, et al. Alterations in mitochondrial DNA copy number and the activities of electron tramnsport chain complexes and pyruvate dechydrogenase in the frontal cortex from subjects with autism. Transl Psychiatry. 2013;3(9):e299. https://doi.org/10.1038/tp.2013.68.
123. Rubio-Lopez N, Morales-Suarez-Varela M, Pico Y, Livianos-aldana L, Llopis-Gonzales A. Nutrient intake and depression symptoms in Spanish children: the ANIVA study. Int J Environ Res Public Health. 2016;13(3):352. https://doi.org/10.3390/ijerph13030352.

124. Lanska DJ. Chapter 30: Historical aspects of the major neurological vitamin deficiency disorders: the watersoluble B vitamins. Handb Clin Neurol. 2010;95:445–76. https://doi.org/10.1016/S0072-9752(08)02130-1.
125. Williams A, Ramsden D. Nicotinamide: a double edged sword. Parkinsonism Relat Disord. 2005;11(7):413–20. https://doi.org/10.1016/j.parkreldis.2005.05.011.
126. Spivak JL, Jackson DL. Pellagra: an analysis of 18 patients and a review of the literature. Johns Hopkins Med J. 1977;140(6):295–309.
127. Hammond N, Wang Y, Dimachkie MM, Barohn RJ. Nutritional neuropathies. Neurol Clin. 2013;31(2):477–89.
128. Weathers AL, Lewis SL. Rare and unusual ... or are they? Less commonly diagnosed encephalopathies associated with systemic disease. Semin Neurol. 2009;29(2):136–53. https://doi.org/10.1055/s-0029-1213734.
129. Gasperi V, Sibilano M, Savini I, Catani MV. Niacin in the central nervous system: an update of biological aspects and clinical applications. Int J Mol Sci. 2019;20(4):974. https://doi.org/10.3390/ijms20040974.
130. Morris MC, Schneider JA, Tangney CC. Thoughts on B-vitamins and dementia. J Alzheimers Dis. 2006;9(4):429–33. Available from: https://www.ncbi.nlm.nih.gov/pmc/articles/PMC3428233/
131. Fricker RA, Green EL, Jenkins SI, Griffin SM. The Influence of nicotinamide on health and disease in the central nervous system. Int J Tryptophan Res. 2018;11:1178646918776658. https://doi.org/10.1177/1178646918776658.
132. Rasmussen HE, Piazza BR, Forsyth CB, Keshavarzian A. Nutrition and gastrointestinal health as modulators of Parkinson's disease. In: Folkerts G, Garssen J, editors. Pharma-nutrition: an overview. New York: Springer International Publishing; 2014. p. 213–43.
133. Hellenbrand W, Boeing H, Robra BP, Seidler A, Vieregge P, Nischan P, et al. Diet and Parkinson's disease II: A possible role for the past intake of specific nutrients results from a self-administered food-frequency questionnaire in a case-control study. Neurology. 1996;47(3):644–50. https://doi.org/10.1212/wnl.47.3.644.
134. Fall PA, Fredrikson M, Axelson O, Granérus AK. Nutritional and occupational factors influencing the risk of Parkinson's disease: a case-control study in southeastern Sweden. Mov Disord. 1999;14(1):28–37. https://doi.org/10.1002/1531-8257(199901)14:1<28::aid-mds1007>3.0.co;2-o.
135. Testa CM, Jankovic J. Huntington disease: a quarter century of progress since the gene discovery. J Neurol Sci. 2019;396:52–68. https://doi.org/10.1016/j.jns.2018.09.022.
136. Serdaru M, Hausser-Hauw C, Laplane D, Buge A, Castaigne P, Goulon M, et al. The clinical spectrum of alcoholic pellagra encephalopathy. A retrospective analysis of 22 cases studied pathologically. Brain. 1988;111(Pt 4):829–42. https://doi.org/10.1093/brain/111.4.829.
137. Patnaik R, Chowdary TN, Sesikeran B, Satyanath RV, Udaykumar P. Nutrition and the skin. In: Valia RG, Valia AR, editors. IADVL textbook of dermatology. 3rd ed. Mumbai: Bhalani Publishing House; 2008. p. 1275–7.
138. Thappa DM, Karthikeyan K. Pellagra in an alcoholic. Indian J Dermatol. 2002;47(3):173–5.
139. Patel AB, Prabhu AS. Hartnup disease. Indian J Dermatol. 2008;53:31–2.
140. Brown MJ, Beier K. Vitamin B6 deficiency (pyridoxine). StatPearls; 2019. [Cited 2019 Dec 1]. Available from: https://www.ncbi.nlm.nih.gov/books/NBK470579/
141. Mills PB, Footitt EJ, Mills KA, Tuschl K, Aylett S, Varadkar S, et al. Genotypic and phenotypic spectrum of pyridoxine-dependent epilepsy (ALDH7A1 deficiency). Brain. 2010;133(Pt 7):2148–59. https://doi.org/10.1093/brain/awq143.
142. Pietz J, Benninger C, Schafer H, et al. Treatment of infantile spasms with high-dosage vitamin B6. Epilepsia. 1993;34(4):757–63. https://doi.org/10.1111/j.1528-1157.1993.tb00458.x.
143. Schaumburg H, Kaplan J, Windebank A, Vick N, Rasmus S, Pleasure D, et al. Sensory neuropathy from pyridoxine abuse. A new megavitamin syndrome. N Engl J Med. 1983;309(8):445–8. https://doi.org/10.1056/NEJM198308253090801.
144. Parry GJ, Bredesen DE. Sensory neuropathy with low-dose pyridoxine. Neurology. 1985;35(10):1466–8. https://doi.org/10.1212/wnl.35.10.1466.

145. Leishear K, Boudreau RM, Studenski SA, Ferrucci L, Rosano C, de Rekeneire N, et al. Relationship between vitamin B12 and sensory and motor peripheral nerve function in older adults. J Am Geriatr Soc. 2012;60(6):1057–63. https://doi.org/10.1111/j.1532-5415.2012.03998.x.
146. Voukelatou P, Vrettos I, Kalliakmanis A. Neurologic symptoms as the only manifestation of B12 deficiency in a young patient with normal hematocrit, MCV, peripheral blood smear and homocysteine levels. Oxf Med Case Rep. 2016;2016(12):omw091. https://doi.org/10.1093/omcr/omw091.
147. Weir DG, Baillieres SJM. The biochemical basis of the neuropathy in cobalamin deficiency. Baillieres Clin Haematol. 1995;8(3):479–97. https://doi.org/10.1016/s0950-3536(05)80217-3.
148. Serin HM, Arslan EA. Neurological symptoms of vitamin B12 deficiency: analysis of pediatric patients. Acta Clin Croat. 2019;58(2):295–302. https://doi.org/10.20471/acc.2019.58.02.13.
149. Reynolds EH. Folic acid, ageing, depression, and dementia. BMJ. 2002;324(7352):1512–5. https://doi.org/10.1136/bmj.324.7352.1512.
150. Kayden HJ. The neurologic syndrome of vitamin E deficiency: a significant cause of ataxia. Neurology. 1993;43(11):2167–9. https://doi.org/10.1212/wnl.43.11.2167.
151. Jayadev S, Bird TD. Hereditary ataxias: overview. Genet Med. 2013;15(9):673–83. https://doi.org/10.1038/gim.2013.28.
152. Perkin GD, Murray-Lyon I. Neurology and the gastrointestinal system. J Neurol Neurosurg Psychiatry. 1998;65:291–300. Available from: https://pdfs.semanticscholar.org/9928/9dbc6242ed3228aa91efebde83d87dab956e.pdf
153. Weder B, Meienberg O, Wildi E, Meier C. Neurologic disorder of vitamin E deficiency in acquired intestinal malabsorption. Neurology. 1984;34(12):1561–5. https://doi.org/10.1212/wnl.34.12.1561.
154. Ueda N, Suzuki Y, Rino Y, Takahashi T, Imada T, Takanashi Y, et al. Correlation between neurological dysfunction with vitamin E deficiency and gastrectomy. J Neurol Sci. 2009;287(1–2):216–20. https://doi.org/10.1016/j.jns.2009.07.020.
155. Stevens GA, Bennett JE, Hennocq Q, Lu Y, De-Regil LM, Rogers L, et al. Trends and mortality effects of vitamin A deficiency in children in 138 low-income and middle-income countries between 1991 and 2013: a pooled analysis of population-based surveys. Lancet Glob Health. 2015;3(9):e528–36. https://doi.org/10.1016/S2214-109X(15)00039-X.
156. Imdad A, Mayo-Wilson E, Herzer K, Bhutta ZA. Vitamin A supplementation for preventing morbidity and mortality in children from 6 months to 5 years of age. Cochrane Database Syst Rev. 2017;2017(3):CD008524. https://doi.org/10.1002/14651858.CD008524.pub3.
157. Munger KL, Zhang SM, O'Reilly E, Hernán MA, Olek MJ, Willett WC, et al. Vitamin D intake and incidence of multiple sclerosis. Neurology. 2004;62(1):60–5. https://doi.org/10.1212/01.wnl.0000101723.79681.38.
158. Munger KL, Levin LI, Hollis BW, Howard NS, Ascherio A. Serum 25-hydroxyvitamin D levels and risk of multiple sclerosis. JAMA. 2006;296(23):2832–8. https://doi.org/10.1001/jama.296.23.2832.
159. Annweiler T, Montero-Odasso M, Bartha R, Beauchet O. Vitamin D and brain volumetric changes: systematic review and meta-analysis. Maturitas. 2014;78(1):30–9. https://doi.org/10.1016/j.maturitas.2014.02.013.
160. Misra M, Pacaud D, Petryk A, Collett-Solberg PF, Kappy M, and on behalf of the Drug and Therapeutics Committee of the Lawson Wilkins Pediatric Endocrine Society. Vitamin D deficiency in children and its management: review of current knowledge and recommendations. Pediatrics. 2008;122(2):398–417. https://doi.org/10.1542/peds.2007-1894.
161. Kumar N. Copper deficiency myelopathy (human swayback). Mayo Clin Proc. 2006;81(10):1371–84. https://doi.org/10.4065/81.10.1371.
162. Bahi-Buisson N, Kaminska A, Nabbout R, Barnerias C, Desguerre I, De Lonlay P, et al. Epilepsy in Menkes disease: analysis of clinical stages. Epilepsia. 2006;47(2):380–6. https://doi.org/10.1111/j.1528-1167.2006.00432.x.

163. Prasad AN, Levin S, Rupar CA, Prasad C. Menkes disease and infantile epilepsy. Brain Dev. 2011;33(10):866–76. https://doi.org/10.1016/j.braindev.2011.08.002.
164. Yi L, Kaler SG. Interaction between the AAA ATPase p97/VCP and a concealed UBX domain in the copper transporter ATP7A is associated with motor neuron degeneration. J Biol Chem. 2018;293(20):7606–17. https://doi.org/10.1074/jbc.RA117.000686.
165. Hurst A. Medical diseases of the war. 3rd ed. Baltimore: Williams & Wilkins Co.; 1943. p. 328.
166. Kamar N, Dalton HR, Abravanel F, Izopet J. Hepatitis E virus infection. Clin Microbiol Rev. 2014;27(1):116–38. https://doi.org/10.1128/CMR.00057-13.
167. Mclean BN, Gulliver J, Dalton HR. Hepatitis E virus and neurological disorders. Pract Neurol. 2017;17(4):282–8. https://doi.org/10.1136/practneurol-2016-001588.
168. Woolson KL, Forbes A, Vine L, Beynon L, McElhinney L, Panayi V. Extra-hepatic manifestations of autochthonous hepatitis E infection. Aliment Pharmacol Ther. 2014;40(11–12):1282–91. https://doi.org/10.1111/apt.12986.
169. Kamar N, Bendall RP, Peron JM, Cintas P, Prudhomme L, Masuy JM, et al. Hepatitis E virus and neurologic disorders. Emerg Infect Dis. 2011;17(2):173–9. https://doi.org/10.3201/eid1702.100856.
170. van den Berg B, van der Eijk AA, Pas SD, Hunter JG, Madden RG, Tio-Gillen AP, et al. Guillain-Barré syndrome associated with preceding hepatitis E virus infection. Neurology. 2014;82(6):491–7. https://doi.org/10.1212/WNL.0000000000000111.
171. Fukae J, Tsugawa J, Ouma S, Umezu T, Kusunoki S, Tsuboi Y. Guillain-Barré and Miller Fisher syndromes in patients with anti-hepatitis E virus antibody: a hospital-based survey in Japan. Neurol Sci. 2016;37(11):1849–51. https://doi.org/10.1007/s10072-016-2644-4.
172. GeurtsvanKessel CH, Islam Z, Mohammad QD, Jacobs BC, Endtz HP, et al. Hepatitis E and Guillain-Barré syndrome. Clin Infect Dis. 2013;57(9):1369–70. https://doi.org/10.1093/cid/cit512.
173. Stevens O, Claeys KG, Poesen K, Saegeman V, Van Damme P. Diagnostic challenges and clinical characteristics of hepatitis E virus associated Guillain-Barré syndrome. JAMA Neurol. 2017;74(1):26–33. https://doi.org/10.1001/jamaneurol.2016.3541.
174. Hughes RA, Rees JH. Clinical and epidemiologic features of Guillain-Barré syndrome. J Infect Dis. 1997;176(Suppl. 2):S92–8. https://doi.org/10.1086/513793.
175. El Mhandi L, Calmels P, Camdessanché JP, Gautheron V, Féasson L. Muscle strength recovery in treated Guillain-Barré syndrome: a prospective study for the first 18 months after onset. Am J Phys Med Rehabil. 2007;86(9):716–24. https://doi.org/10.1097/PHM.0b013e31813e0b67.
176. Lo YL. Clinical and immunological spectrum of the Miller Fisher syndrome. Muscle Nerve. 2007;36(5):615–27. https://doi.org/10.1002/mus.20835.
177. Alshekhlee A, Hussain Z, Sultan B, Katirji B. Guillain-Barré syndrome: incidence and mortality rates in US hospitals. Neurology. 2008;70(18):1608–13. https://doi.org/10.1212/01.wnl.0000310983.38724.d4.
178. van den Berg B, Bunschoten C, van Doorn PA, Jacobs BC. Mortality in Guillain-Barré syndrome. Neurology. 2013;80(18):1650–4. https://doi.org/10.1212/WNL.0b013e3182904fcc.
179. Netto AB, Taly AB, Kulkarni GB, Rao UG, Rao S. Mortality in mechanically ventilated patients of Guillain Barré syndrome. Ann Indian Acad Neurol. 2011;14(4):262–6. https://doi.org/10.4103/0972-2327.91942.
180. Seror P. Neuralgic amyotrophy. An update. Joint Bone Spine. 2017;84(2):153–8. https://doi.org/10.1016/j.jbspin.2016.03.005.
181. van Eijk JJ, Madden RG, van der Eijk AA, Hunter JG, Reimerink JH, Bendall RP, et al. Neuralgic amyotrophy and hepatitis E virus infection. Neurology. 2014;82(6):498–503. https://doi.org/10.1212/WNL.0000000000000112.
182. Mandal K, Chopra N. Acute transverse myelitis following hepatitis E virus infection. Indian Pediatr. 2006;43(4):365–6.
183. Kamani P, Baijal R, Amarapurkar D, Gupte P, Patel N, Kumar P, Agal S. Guillain-Barre syndrome associated with acute hepatitis E. Indian J Gastroenterol. 2005;24(5):216.

184. Kejariwal D, Roy S, Sarkar N. Seizure associated with acute hepatitis E. Neurology. 2001;57(10):1935. https://doi.org/10.1212/WNL.57.10.1935.
185. Yadav KK, Rohatgi A, Sharma SK, Kulshrestha M, Sachdeva S, Pardasani V. Oculomotor palsy associated with hepatitis E infection. J Assoc Physicians India. 2002;50(5):737.
186. Dixit VK, Abhilash VB, Kate MP, Jain AK. Hepatitis E infection with Bell's palsy. J Assoc Physicians India. 2006;54:418.
187. Thapa R, Mallick D, Biswas B. Pseudotumor cerebri in childhood hepatitis E virus infection. Headache: J Head Face Pain. 2009;49:610–1. https://doi.org/10.1111/j.1526-4610.2009.01367.x.
188. Fousekis FS, Mitselos IV, Dimitrios K. Christodoulou extrahepatic manifestations of hepatitis E virus: an overview. Clin Mol Hepatol. 2020;26(1):16–23. https://doi.org/10.3350/cmh.2019.0082.
189. Adinolfi LE, Nevola R, Lus G, Restivo L, Guerrera B, Romano C, et al. Chronic hepatitis C virus infection and neurological and psychiatric disorders: an overview. World J Gastroenterol. 2015;21(8):2269–80. https://doi.org/10.3748/wjg.v21.i8.2269.
190. Fletcher NF, McKeating JA. Hepatitis C virus and the brain. J Viral Hepat. 2012;19(5):301–6. https://doi.org/10.1111/j.1365-2893.2012.01591.x.
191. Monaco S, Ferrari S, Gajofatto A, Zanusso G, Mariotto S. HCV-related nervous system disorders. Clin Dev Immunol. 2012;2012:236148. https://doi.org/10.1155/2012/236148.
192. Origgi L, Vanoli M, Carbone A, Grasso M, Scorza R. Central nervous system involvement in patients with HCV-related cryoglobulinemia. Am J Med Sci. 1998;315(3):208–10. https://doi.org/10.1097/00000441-199803000-00012.
193. Enger C, Forssen UM, Bennett D, Theodore D, Shantakumar S, McAfee A. Thromboembolic events among patients with hepatitis C virus infection and cirrhosis: a matched-cohort study. Adv Ther. 2014;31(8):891–903. https://doi.org/10.1007/s12325-014-0138-4.
194. Gutierrez J, Elkind MSV. Chronic inflammatory diseases and stroke: evidence for heterogeneous mechanisms. Ann Neurol. 2012;72:S6–7. https://doi.org/10.1002/ana.23669.
195. Liao CC, Su TC, Sung FC, Chou WH, Chen TL. Does hepatitis C virus infection increase risk for stroke? A population-based cohort study. PLoS One. 2012;7(2):e31527. https://doi.org/10.1371/journal.pone.0031527.
196. Hsu CS, Kao JH, Chao YC, Lin HH, Fan YC, Huang CJ, Tsai PS. Interferon-based therapy reduces risk of stroke in chronic hepatitis C patients: a population-based cohort study in Taiwan. Aliment Pharmacol Ther. 2013;38(4):415–23. https://doi.org/10.1111/apt.12391.
197. Adinolfi LE, Restivo L, Guerrera B, Sellitto A, Ciervo A, Iuliano N, Rinaldi L, Santoro A, Li Vigni G, Marrone A. Chronic HCV infection is a risk factor of ischemic stroke. Atherosclerosis. 2013;231(1):22–6. https://doi.org/10.1016/j.atherosclerosis.2013.08.003.
198. Huang H, Kang R, Zhao Z. Hepatitis C virus infection and risk of stroke: a systematic review and meta-analysis. PLoS One. 2013;8(11):e81305. https://doi.org/10.1371/journal.pone.0081305.
199. Lee MH, Yang HI, Wang CH, Jen CL, Yeh SH, Liu CJ, et al. Hepatitis C virus infection and increased risk of cerebrovascular disease. Stroke. 2010;41(12):2894–900. https://doi.org/10.1161/STROKEAHA.110.598136.
200. Zandman-Goddard G, Levy Y, Weiss P, Shoenfeld Y, Langevitz P. Transverse myelitis associated with chronic hepatitis C. Clin Exp Rheumatol. 2003;21(1):111–3.
201. Mariotto S, Ferrari S, Monaco S. HCV-related central and peripheral nervous system demyelinating disorders. Inflamm Allergy Drug Targets. 2014;13(5):299–304. https://doi.org/10.2174/1871528113666140908113841.
202. Sacconi S, Salviati L, Merelli E. Acute disseminated encephalomyelitis associated with hepatitis C virus infection. Arch Neurol. 2001;58(10):1679–81. https://doi.org/10.1001/archneur.58.10.1679.
203. Sim JE, Lee JB, Cho YN, Suh SH, Kim JK, Lee KY. A case of acute disseminated encephalomyelitis associated with hepatitis C virus infection. Yonsei Med J. 2012;53(4):856–8. https://doi.org/10.3349/ymj.2012.53.4.856.

204. Mapoure NY, Budzi MN, Eloumou SAFB, Malongue A, Okalla C, et al. Neurological manifestations in chronic hepatitis C patients receiving care in a reference hospital in sub-Saharan Africa: a cross-sectional study. PLoS One. 2018;13(3):e0192406. https://doi.org/10.1371/journal.pone.0192406.
205. Santoro L, Manganelli F, Briani C, Giannini F, Benedetti L, Vitelli E, et al. Prevalence and characteristics of peripheral neuropathy in hepatitis C virus population. J Neurol Neurosurg Psychiatry. 2006;77(5):626–9. https://doi.org/10.1136/jnnp.2005.081570.
206. Nemni R, Sanvito L, Quattrini A, Santuccio G, Camerlingo M, Canal N. Peripheral neuropathy in hepatitis C virus infection with and without cryoglobulinaemia. J Neurol Neurosurg Psychiatry. 2003;74(9):1267–71. https://doi.org/10.1136/jnnp.74.9.1267.
207. Bonetti B, Scardoni M, Monaco S, Rizzuto N, Scarpa A. Hepatitis C virus infection of peripheral nerves in type II cryoglobulinaemia. Virchows Arch. 1999;434(6):533–5. https://doi.org/10.1007/s004280050380.
208. Gemignani F, Melli G, Inglese C, Marbini A. Cryoglobulinemia is a frequent cause of peripheral neuropathy in undiagnosed referral patients. J Peripher Nerv Syst. 2002;7(1):59–64. https://doi.org/10.1046/j.1529-8027.2002.02007.x.
209. Gemignani F, Brindani F, Alfieri S, Giuberti T, Allegri I, Ferrari C, Marbini A. Clinical spectrum of cryoglobulinaemic neuropathy. J Neurol Neurosurg Psychiatry. 2005;76(10):1410–4. https://doi.org/10.1136/jnnp.2004.057620.
210. Paoletti V, Donnarumma L, De Matteis A, Mammarella A, Labbadia G, Musca A, et al. Peripheral neuropathy without cryoglobulinemia in patients with hepatitis C virus infection. Panminerva Med. 2000;42(3):175–8.
211. Herrmann DN, Ferguson ML, Pannoni V, Barbano RL, Stanton M, Logigian EL. Plantar nerve AP and skin biopsy in sensory neuropathies with normal routine conduction studies. Neurology. 2004;63(5):879–85. https://doi.org/10.1212/01.wnl.0000137036.26601.84.
212. Bezerra ME, Harumi JA, Shinosaki JM, Pedroso JL, Henriques de Aquino CC, et al. Hepatitis C virus: a rare manifestation—remitting relapsing central and peripheral demyelination. Neurol India. 2011;59:114–6. Available from: http://www.neurologyindia.com/text.asp?2011/59/1/114/76889
213. Weissenborn K, Krause J, Bokemeyer M, Hecker H, Schuler A, Ennen JC. Hepatitis C virus infection affects the brain-evidence from psychometric studies and magnetic resonance spectroscopy. J Hepatol. 2004;41(5):845–51. https://doi.org/10.1016/j.jhep.2004.07.022.
214. Iriana S, Curry MP, Afdhal NH. Neurologic manifestations of hepatitis C virus infection. Clin Liver Dis. 2017;21(3):535–42. https://doi.org/10.1016/j.cld.2017.03.008.
215. Yarlott L, Heald E, Forton D. Hepatitis C virus infection, and neurological and psychiatric disorders—a review. J Adv Res. 2017;8(2):139–48. https://doi.org/10.1016/j.jare.2016.09.005.
216. Hilsabeck RC, Perry W, Hassanein TI. Neuropsychological impairment in patients with chronic hepatitis C. Hepatology. 2002;35(2):440–6. https://doi.org/10.1053/jhep.2002.31257.
217. Hilsabeck RC, Hassanein TI, Carlson MD, Ziegler EA, Perry W. Cognitive functioning and psychiatric symptomatology in patients with chronic hepatitis C. J Int Neuropsychol Soc. 2003;9(6):847–54. https://doi.org/10.1017/S1355617703960048.
218. McAndrews MP, Farcnik K, Carlen P, Damyanovich A, Mrkonjic M, Jones S. Prevalence and significance of neurocognitive dysfunction in hepatitis C in the absence of correlated risk factors. Hepatology. 2005;41(4):801–8. https://doi.org/10.1002/hep.20635.
219. Cordoba J, Flavia M, Jacas C, Sauleda S, Esteban JI, Vargas V. Quality of life and cognitive function in hepatitis C at different stages of liver disease. J Hepatol. 2003;39(2):231–8. https://doi.org/10.1016/s0168-8278(03)00189-2.
220. Abrantes J, Torres DS, de Mello CE. Patients with hepatitis C infection and normal liver function: an evaluation of cognitive function. Postgrad Med J. 2013;89(1054):433–9. https://doi.org/10.1136/postgradmedj-2012-131185.
221. Fontana RJ, Bieliauskas LA, Back-Madruga C, Lindsay KL, Kronfol Z, Lok AS. Cognitive function in hepatitis C patients with advanced fibrosis enrolled in the HALT-C trial. J Hepatol. 2005;43(4):614–22. https://doi.org/10.1016/j.jhep.2005.04.006.

222. Squires JE, Balistreri WF. Hepatitis C virus infection in children and adolescents. Hepatol Commun. 2017;1(2):87–98. https://doi.org/10.1002/hep4.1028.
223. Maria HS, John TB. Hepatitis A. In Mark F, Lawrence SF, Lawrence JB. Sleisenger and Fordtran's gastrointestinal and liver disease. vol. 78. Philadelphia: Elsevier, 2016. p. 1302–1308.
224. Geetika B, Varrinder SS, Charlene KM. A rare presentation of hepatitis A infection with extrahepatic manifestations. Case Rep Gastrointest Med. 2014;2014:286914. https://doi.org/10.1155/2014/286914.
225. Jo S, Baek JH, Jeon J, Lee SA. Encephalomyelitis by hepatitis A virus infection. Neurology. 2017;88(Suppl. 16):P3.305.
226. Chonmaitree P, Methawasin K. Transverse myelitis in acute hepatitis A infection: the rare co-occurrence of hepatology and neurology. Case Rep Gastroenterol. 2016;10:44–53. https://doi.org/10.1159/000444013.
227. Hazarika D. Clinical spectrum of hepatitis A infection in children: an overview. Pediatr Infect Dis. 2011;3(1):7–12. https://doi.org/10.1016/S2212-8328(11)80003-2.
228. Guillevin L, Lhote F, Cohen P, Sauvaget F, Jarrousse B, Lortholary O, et al. Polyarteritis nodosa related to hepatitis B virus. A prospective study with long-term observation of 41 patients. Medicine (Baltimore). 1995;74(5):238–53. https://doi.org/10.1097/00005792-199509000-00002.
229. Tsukada N, Koh CS, Inoue A, Yanagisawa N. Demyelinating neuropathy associated with hepatitis B virus infection. Detection of immune complexes composed of hepatitis B virus surface antigen. J Neurol Sci. 1987;77(2–3):203–16. https://doi.org/10.1016/0022-510x(87)90123-7.
230. Kappus MR, Sterling RK. Extrahepatic manifestations of acute hepatitis B virus infection. Gastroenterol Hepatol. 2013;9(2):123–6.
231. Terrault NA, Lok ASF, McMahon BJ, Chang KM, Hwang JP, Jonas JP, et al. Update on prevention, diagnosis, and treatment of chronic hepatitis B: AASLD 2018 hepatitis B guidance. Hepatology. 2018;67(4):1560–99. https://doi.org/10.1002/hep.29800.
232. Geier MR, Geier DA. A case-series of adverse events, positive re-challenge of symptoms, and events in identical twins following hepatitis B vaccination: analysis of the Vaccine Adverse Event Reporting System (VAERS) database and literature review. Clin Exp Rheumatol. 2004;22:749–55.
233. Relman DA, Schmidt TM, MacDermott RP, Falkow S. Identification of the uncultured bacillus of Whipple's disease. N Engl J Med. 1992;327(5):293–301. https://doi.org/10.1056/NEJM199207303270501.
234. Fredricks DN, Relman DA. Cultivation of Whipple bacillus: the irony and the ecstasy. Lancet. 1997;350:1262–3.
235. Keren DF, Weisburger WR, Yardley JH, Salyer WR, Arthur RR, Charache P. Whipple's disease: demonstration by immunofluorescence of similar bacterial antigens in macrophages from three cases. Johns Hopkins Med J. 1976;139(2):51–9.
236. Keren DF. Whipple's disease: the causative agent defined. Its pathogenesis remains obscure. Medicine (Baltimore). 1993;72(5):355–8.
237. Sieracki JC. Whipple's disease: observations on systemic involvement. AMA Arch Pathol. 1958;66(4):464–7.
238. Misbah SA, Mapstone NP. Whipple's disease revisited. J Clin Pathol. 2000;53(10):750–5. https://doi.org/10.1136/jcp.53.10.750.
239. Bodian M, Stephens FD, Ward BCH. Hirschsprung's disease and idiopathic megacolon. Lancet. 1949;1(6540):6–11. https://doi.org/10.1016/s0140-6736(49)90340-2.
240. Bakheit AMO. Management of neurogenic dysphagia. Postgrad Med J. 2001;77(913):694–9. https://doi.org/10.1136/pmj.77.913.694.
241. Keane JR. Neurologic symptoms mistaken for gastrointestinal disease. Neurology. 1998;50(4):1189–90. https://doi.org/10.1212/wnl.50.4.1189.
242. Goldberg HI, Sheft DJ. Esophageal and colon changes in myotonia dystrophica. Gastroenterology. 1972;63(1):134–9.

243. Brunner HG, Hamel BCJ, Rieu P, Höweler CJ, Peter FTM. Intestinal pseudo-obstruction in myotonic dystrophy. J Med Genet. 1992;29:791–3. Available from: https://www.ncbi.nlm.nih.gov/pmc/articles/PMC1016174/pdf/jmedgene00025-0033.pdf
244. Schuster MM, Tow DE, Sherbourne DH. Anal sphincter abnormalities characteristic of myotonic dystrophy. Gastroenterology. 1965;49(6):641–8.
245. Parkes JD. A neurologist's view of nausea and vomiting. In: Davis CJ, Lake-Bakaar GV, Grahame-Smith DG, editors. Nausea and vomiting: mechanisms and treatment. Berlin, Heidelberg: Springer; 1986. p. 160–6. https://doi.org/10.1007/978-3-642-70479-6.
246. Headache Classification Committee of the International Headache Society (IHS). The international classification of headache disorders, 3rd edition (beta version). Cephalalgia. 2013;33(9):629–808. https://doi.org/10.1177/0333102413485658.
247. Li BU. Managing cyclic vomiting syndrome in children: beyond the guidelines. Eur J Pediatr. 2018;177(10):1435–42. https://doi.org/10.1007/s00431-018-3218-7.
248. Murai T, Kinoshita M. Acute diarrhea as a manifestation of abdominal epilepsy. IntechOpen; 2019. https://doi.org/10.5772/intechopen.86719. Available from: https://www.intechopen.com/online-first/acute-diarrhea-as-a-manifestation-of-abdominal-epilepsy. [Cited 2019 Dec 5]
249. Dutta SR, Hazarika I, Chakravarty BP. Abdominal epilepsy, an uncommon cause of recurrent abdominal pain: a brief report. Gut. 2007;56(3):439–41. https://doi.org/10.1136/gut.2006.094250.
250. Tiamkao S, Pratipanawatr T, Jitpimolmard S. Abdominal epilepsy: an uncommon of non-convulsive status epilepticus. J Med Assoc Thail. 2011;94(8):998–1001.
251. Peppercorn MA, Herzog AG. The spectrum of abdominal epilepsy in adults. Am J Gastroenterol. 1989;84(10):1294–6.
252. Binnie CD, Prior PF. Electroencephalography. J Neurol Neurosurg Psychiatr. 1994;57(11):1308–19. https://doi.org/10.1136/jnnp.57.11.1308.
253. Niedermeyer E, Lpes da Silva F. Electroencephalography: basic principles, clinical applications, and related fields. Philadelphia, London: Lippincott Williams & Wilkins; 2005. p. 1309.
254. Zarling EJ. Abdominal epilepsy: an unusual cause of recurrent abdominal pain. Am J Gastroenterol. 1984;79(9):687–8.
255. Zinkin NT, Peppercorn MA. Abdominal epilepsy. Best Pract Res Clin Gastroenterol. 2005;19(2):263–74. https://doi.org/10.1016/j.bpg.2004.10.001.
256. Foldvary-Schaefer N, Unnwongse K. Localizing and lateralizing features of auras and seizures. Epilepsy Behav. 2011;20(2):160–6. https://doi.org/10.1016/j.yebeh.2010.08.034.

Further Reading

Yang YX, Metz DC. Safety of proton pump inhibitor exposure. Gastroenterology. 2010;139(4):1115–27. https://doi.org/10.1053/j.gastro.2010.08.023.

Reinstatler L, Qi YP, Williamson RS, Garn JV, Oakley GP. Association of biochemical B12 deficiency with metformin therapy and vitamin B12 supplements: the National Health and Nutrition Examination Survey, 1999–2006. Diabetes Care. 2012;35(2):327–33. https://doi.org/10.2337/dc11-1582.

Part V

Comedication and Drug Interactions in Gastroenterology

Acid-Related Disorders

27

Marinko Marušić, Mia Knobloch, and Matej Paić

Introduction

Diseases of the upper gastrointestinal tract are very common and have a vast impact on healthcare systems worldwide. Acid-related disorders include gastroesophageal reflux disease (GERD), peptic ulcer disease (PUD), Zollinger-Ellison syndrome, gastritis (and dyspepsia), but acid suppressants are also used in treating H. pylori infection and prophylaxis of stress and nonsteroidal anti-inflammatory drugs (NSAIDs)-induced ulcer disease. Those conditions are highly prevalent in general population studies, ranging from 10% to 20% for GERD [1] and from 0.1% to 0.19% for PUD based on hospitalization data [2]. Total prevalence of acid-reducing drug usage could be even higher considering many of those patients opt for self-treatment and do not seek medical advice [3]. Instead, they reach for many of the drugs available over the counter. Total prevalence of these conditions increases with advanced age [4] as does comorbidity, and many of those disorders require long-term or prolonged treatment which also increases interaction potential. There are many possible mechanisms for increasing prevalence pertaining to age-related physiologic changes affecting the oropharynx, the esophagus, the stomach, and the small intestine [4]. With increasing age also rises the prevalence of H. pylori

M. Marušić (✉)
Department of Gastroenterology and Hepatology, Sveti Duh University Hospital, Zagreb, Croatia

Faculty of Medicine, J. J. Strossmayer University of Osijek, Osijek, Croatia

Faculty of Health Studies, University of Rijeka, Rijeka, Croatia
e-mail: marinko.marusic1@zg.t-com.hr

M. Knobloch · M. Paić
Department of Gastroenterology and Hepatology, Sveti Duh University Hospital, Zagreb, Croatia

M. Banić, D. Erceg (eds.), *Drug Interactions in Gastroenterology*, Clinical Gastroenterology, https://doi.org/10.1007/978-3-031-69800-2_27

infection, the use of NSAIDs, and general use of other medications. That is why it is important to know all the possible mechanisms of drug-drug interactions between acid-reducing agents and other groups of drugs our patient may use concomitantly. In this chapter, we will use a systematic approach to review all of the possible interactions we could encounter while using acid suppressants.

Polypharmacy

Something we always have to consider when prescribing medications is to do no harm and that every drug can be a double-edged sword. There are a plethora of prescription medications at our disposal as well as over-the-counter agents and other herbal and food supplements. It is as necessary as it is challenging to keep in mind all of the possible drug-drug interactions we can encounter. They vary from mild, clinically insignificant to severe and even life-threatening interactions. Elderly patients are at special risk for adverse reactions as they often take many different medications on everyday basis. With age also rises the number of chronic diseases such as cardiovascular conditions, diabetes, hypertension, renal failure, and many others. It is also evident that age-related changes in pharmacodynamics and pharmacokinetics contribute to adverse interactions, as well as factors such as differences in genetics, and other environmental changes, interpersonal differences, nutritional status, comorbid conditions, etc. Some studies report around 30% of adverse reactions affect the population over 65 years, with an average of 4–8, 5 taken drugs per patient [5, 6]. The numbers are perhaps even higher considering many interactions remain unrecognized. It is worth mentioning the appropriate usage of acid-reducing drugs, especially proton pump inhibitors as they are often prescribed inappropriately which relates to concomitant usage of other drugs [7]. Caution is also advised with H2 receptor antagonists as we recently witnessed FDAs (Food and Drug Administration) request for withdrawal of all prescription and over-the-counter (OTC) ranitidine preparations because of N-nitrosodimethylamine (NDMA) contamination. NDMA is a probable human carcinogen which can be found in ranitidine at low levels (as in some food and water) but increases with storage time, even under normal storage conditions [8]. There are thousands of possible drug interactions and memorizing all of them would be unrealistic. In this chapter, we will give a short summary of the most important drug interactions pertaining to acid-reducing drugs. We will emphasize the specific interactions for each group of acid-reducing agents with possible drugs used for treating cardiovascular, cerebrovascular, psychiatric, infective, inflammatory, and many other conditions we can encounter.

Mechanisms of Drug-Drug Interactions

Acid-reducing agents can interact with other drugs by affecting their absorption, metabolism, or elimination (see also Chap. 5).

Absorption

After oral administration, drugs are systemically absorbed through the gastrointestinal tract into bloodstream and distributed to the site of action. The extent of absorption is determined by the gastrointestinal characteristics of the patient. The intrinsic physicochemical properties of the medication are important factors for oral absorption, including stability, permeability, lipophilicity, particle size, shape, and physical form of the active pharmaceutical ingredient and formulation [9, 10].

It is important to know the physiologic gastrointestinal pH to understand the action of acid-reducing agents. In the fasting state, gastric pH is 1.0–3.5 and in the fed state 3.0–7.0. The pH in the small intestine is 6.0–8.0 and in the colon 5.5–8.0 [11–13].

When gastric pH is raised by acid-reducing agents, the solubility of weak acids generally increases and the solubility of weak bases decreases [14]. Most clinically meaningful drug-drug interactions caused by acid-reducing agents through this mechanism are with weak bases.

There are many oral dosage forms which include immediate-release and modified-release dosage forms. Immediate-release dosage forms dissolve rapidly after oral administration and for this formulation, the acid-base characteristics of the substrate medication are important in determining its solubility or chemical stability in gastric fluid [15]. Modified-release dosage forms include extended-release and delayed-release forms. Extended-release forms usually do not interact with acid-reducing agents because of the lack of involvement of pH components in drug release. Whereas delayed-release forms have an enteric-coated surface which passes through gastric fluid untouched and is dissolved in a higher pH environment of the intestine. Acid-reducing agents can raise gastric pH above 6.0 which can lead to premature release of drugs formulated in a delayed-release dosage form [16].

Polyvalent cations (aluminum, magnesium, and calcium cations) in antacid formulations can form insoluble chelate complexes with other medications reducing their bioavailability. Sodium bicarbonate is the only metal ion-containing antacid that is not subject to chelation-based drug-drug interaction [15].

Antacids containing magnesium are known to cause rapid gastrointestinal transit which accelerates the rate of absorption of some medications and often have diarrhea as a side effect. That is why they are no longer used alone but in combination with other antacids, e.g., aluminum [15].

Metabolism

Approximately 80% of medications are metabolized by cytochrome (CYP), a heme-containing protein [17]. CYPs are primarily membrane-associated proteins located either in the inner membrane of mitochondria or in the endoplasmic reticulum of cells. When talking about acid-reducing agents, CYP1A2, CYP2C9, CYP2C19, CYP2D6, and CYP3A4 are the most important from drug-drug interaction standpoint [17]. H2RAs and PPI can act either as inhibitors or inducers of CYP enzymes

[18], with CYP inhibition, based on competitive inhibition, as more common cause of drug-drug interaction. Induction of CYP enzymes results in either increased activity of prodrug or heightened elimination of the drug itself but is less commonly seen in drug-drug interaction.

Elimination

Organic cation transporters (OCTs) are expressed throughout the body, but OCT2 is primarily localized in the proximal tubule of the kidney. OCT2 can be inhibited by H2RAs, which may lead to decreased renal excretion of the substrate and increased systemic exposure and potential toxicity [19].

Urinary pH is a major factor in the renal excretion of medications. Urine alkalization was observed after 7 days of ingestion of antacids—aluminum and magnesium hydroxide. In alkaline urine, the renal clearance of weakly acidic drug is increased which may lead to reduced efficacy of those medications, whereas the excretion of weakly basic drugs is decreased causing possible toxic concentrations in organism [20, 21].

Most recommendations regarding drug-drug interaction are based on studies on the pharmacokinetic behavior of various drugs in healthy young volunteers. It must be kept in mind that drug behavior in study subjects varies considerably from clinical situations where patient age, diet, gastrointestinal motility, and other drugs play significant roles.

Antacids

Antacids consist of basic substances coupled with a cation. They directly neutralize gastric acid, providing a quick onset of action and a short duration of acid suppression of approximately 2 h. The possible mechanisms underlying DDIs (drug-drug interactions) for antacids are gastric pH elevation, chelation, gastrointestinal motility, and urine alkalization. Sodium bicarbonate is the only antacid containing a metal ion that is not known to chelate with substrate medications [22]. Magnesium-containing antacids may promote gastric emptying and accelerate the rate of absorption [15].

H2RA

Cimetidine was the first available H2 antagonist and thus one of the most studied. It undergoes liver metabolism and can be involved in significant drug interactions if not used cautiously. It shows to inhibit the activity of CYP1A2, CYP2C, CYP2D6, and CYP3A [23]. Ranitidine has less pronounced binding and therefore inhibits the P-450 enzyme superfamily than cimetidine [24, 25]. Famotidine is the newest of H2 receptor antagonists, so far with a good drug-drug interaction profile, perhaps due to being less studied than the two aforementioned, but more importantly, it does not significantly bind to cytochrome P450 isoenzymes.

PPIs

PPI may interfere with drug absorption through increasing gastric pH, as well as through induction or inhibition of the enzymes of the cytochrome P450 superfamily. Variation in their metabolism through different forms of CYP P450 yields unique interaction profiles for each specific PPI. Omeprazole is the prototypical PPI and one of the most investigated on the market with the most studied interactions. Almost completely goes through phase I drug metabolizing enzymes, CYP 450 superfamily, particularly CYP2C19, and to a much lesser extent CYP3A4. It is known to reversibly inhibit CYP2C19 and CYP2C9 as well as induce CYP1A2. Esomeprazole is a mixture of (S) and (R) isomers of omeprazole, so it is expected to have a similar drug interaction profile. Esomeprazole, as well as omeprazole, undergoes CYP2C19- and CYP3A4-mediated metabolisms, but has ten times greater affinity for CYP2C19; however, the rate of esomeprazole metabolism is three times slower than for omeprazole. That is why it has more pronounced acid suppression. On the other hand, pantoprazole shows relatively lower affinity for CYP2C19 and CYP3A4 and undergoes phase II metabolism via sulfotransferase conjugation so it has less potential interactions compared to other proton pump inhibitors [26, 27]. Lansoprazole and rabeprazole undergo primarily CYP2C19 and CYP3A4 isoenzymes metabolism, but rabeprazole has a low affinity for CYP isoenzymes, so those metabolic pathways are of much lesser importance than for other proton pump inhibitors [28], especially as it is mainly nonenzymatically metabolized to its thioether form [28]. CYP2C19 inhibition of rabeprazole is half the inhibition strength of omeprazole [29]. According to that rabeprazole has a good adverse reaction profile, although new studies are needed to investigate rabeprazole thioether metabolite impact on CYP isoenzymes family [30].

1. Cardiovascular Drugs
   (a) Beta-Blockers
      - Antacids

        Several studies have been conducted studying the effects of antacids on propranolol, metoprolol, and atenolol. Two similar studies showed different results on aluminum hydroxide influence on propranolol. One study demonstrated a decreased bioavailability of propranolol [31], while in the other study significant changes in plasma concentrations could not be demonstrated [32]. Aluminum-induced change in gastric emptying may be responsible for decreased absorption, rather than a physical drug-antacid interaction [33]. Metoprolol demonstrated an increased bioavailability of 11%, while atenolol demonstrated a decreased bioavailability of 33% in co-administration with aluminum hydroxide [34]. So far, no published human studies demonstrated a significant interaction between beta blockers and magnesium-containing antacids.

        Potential interactions between beta-blockers and antacids could exist but no firm clinical evidence has so far been demonstrated.

- H2RA

  There are numerous studies on beta-blockers and their use with cimetidine. Propranolol was shown to have lowered clearance [35] resulting in higher serum concentration and lower resting heartbeat [36–38] and the same effect was observed with metoprolol [39] and labetalol [40]. Increase in serum concentration of atenolol was observed but without the impact on beta-adrenoreceptor blocking effect [41]. Sedman [42] postulated that those effects were, not only induced metabolically, but also with decreased first-pass hepatic extraction by cimetidine but some later studies showed cimetidine has no significant effect on hepatic blood flow [43, 44]. Propranolol has no interactions with ranitidine [45–47], as well as atenolol [48]. Regarding ranitidine and metoprolol interaction, it was shown that although it can raise plasma concentration of metoprolol [48, 49], exercise-induced heart rate was not affected by concomitant ranitidine [39, 50], indicating no pharmacodynamic albeit pharmacokinetics interference.

- PPIs

  Metoprolol [51] and propranolol [52] have no significant interactions and can be safely used with omeprazole. Same is observed with lansoprazole and propranolol [53]. No interactions are observed with pantoprazole and metoprolol [54]. Proton pump inhibitors are generally considered safe to use with beta-blocker drugs.

(b) Antihypertensive Drugs

- Antacids

  Although ACEi (angiotensin-converting-enzyme inhibitors) are commonly used drugs to treat hypertension, so far only one study that dealt with antacid and ACEi interaction has been published. The study reported that administration of an aluminum/magnesium-containing antacid reduced the bioavailability of unchanged captopril. The antacid usually retards gastric emptying and elevates the gastric pH which may reduce the bioavailability of ACE inhibitors [55].

  One study investigated the interaction between aluminum/magnesium-containing antacid and olmesartan, an angiotensin receptor blocker. The small reduction in bioavailability has been noted but without clinical significance [56].

- H2RA

  So far it was shown that cimetidine may raise the concentration of calcium channel blockers. As studies showed, more potent blood pressure lowering when combining nifedipine and cimetidine, this combination is best avoided or used cautiously and is a partial consequence of gastric pH lowering, but dominantly due to inhibition of oxidative liver metabolism, decreased hepatic clearance of nifedipine by cimetidine cytochrome P-450 inhibition. Caution is warranted as well with cimetidine and diltiazem [57], carvedilol [58], and felodipine [59] as it can increase their serum concentrations. On the other hand, concomitant use of ranitidine and nifedipine has no pharmacodynamic nor pharmacokinetic consequences [60]. No unanimous results of cimetidine and verapamil interactions are published, as there are studies which showed the considerate effect of cimetidine on verapamil pharmacokinetics and pharmacodynamics in studies from Mikus and Stuber [61] . However, others found no alterations in verapamil pharmacokinetics or harmacodynamics parameters [62]. Given the lack of interactions, ranitidine is the drug of choice when concurrent cardiovascular drugs are used [60].

- PPIs
  No effect of nifedipine was observed with concomitant use of omeprazole [63] or pantoprazole [64]. Omeprazole can affect amlodipine metabolism which potentiates its blood pressure impact [65]. While searching the literature, we found no published interactions between ACEi and proton pump inhibitors.

(c) Antiarrhythmic Drugs

- Antacids
  The investigations suggest that interaction between digoxin and magnesium trisalicylate may not be significant in most clinical situations [66].
- H2RA
  Studies have shown no effect of cimetidine on digoxin absorption [67] and even though there are limited changes in digoxin concentrations when used concomitantly, they are of no clinical significance. Amiodarone, however, should not be used with cimetidine because of higher serum concentrations of this antiarrhythmic [68]. The effect of cimetidine competition for tubular secretion with other basic substances was observed with procainamide and N-acetylprocainamide when used with cimetidine [69, 70] and was dose-dependent, so caution is advised when using it concomitantly. Even more significant are cimetidine metabolism effects in the elderly, for example, toxicity of quinidine [60]. Similarly, as cimetidine but to a lesser extent, procainamide showed dose-dependent increase in AUC (*area under the curve*—represents the total drug exposure across time) and lower renal excretion when used with ranitidine, and caution or dosage modification is warranted when using these agents together. Unlike cimetidine and ranitidine, studies showed that famotidine does not affect procainamide renal excretion [71]. Lidocaine clearance was significantly decreased by using cimetidine so it should be given in reduced doses if used with cimetidine [72–74], contrary to ranitidine which did not show interference with lidocaine [75, 76].
- PPIs
  Digoxin showed an increase in AUC when used with omeprazole, but without clinical significance [77, 78]. As is the case with all proton pump inhibitors, pantoprazole and rabeprazole can increase digoxin absorption, but this interaction is clinically insignificant [79]. There were no interactions observed with omeprazole and lansoprazole when used with ivabradine [80].

Table 27.1 Cardiovascular drugs and acid-reducing agents

Drug	Antacid		H2RA		PPI
	Aluminum hydroxide	Magnesium hydroxide	Cimetidine	Ranitidine	
Propranolol	+	–	+	–	–
Metoprolol	+	–	+	–	–
Atenolol	+	–	–	–	–
Captopril	+		/		–
Olmesartan	–		/		/
Nifedipine	/		+	–	–
Amlodipine	/		/	/	+ Omeprazole
Diltiazem	/		+	–	/
Carvedilol	/		+	–	/
Felodipine	/		+	–	/
Digoxin	– Magnesium trisalicylate		–	/	–
Amiodarone	/		+	/	/
Lidocaine	/		+	–	/
Procainamide/N-acetylprocainamide	/		+	+	/
Ivabradine	/		/		– Omeprazole – Lansoprazole

+ there is significant interaction, – no significant interaction, / no relevant studies
H2RA histamine 2 receptor antagonist, *PPI* proton pump inhibitors

All aforementioned interactions between cardiovascular drugs and acid-reducing agents are systematically shown in Table 27.1.

2. Hematologic Drugs
   (a) Antiplatelet Drugs
      - Antacids
        Clopidogrel can be safely used with antacids [81]. Other significant studies with other antiplatelet drugs have not been conducted.
      - H2RA
        Famotidine does not influence platelet function on clopidogrel and same is observed with ranitidine which can be safely used with either prasugrel or clopidogrel [82] as it showed no clinically significant impact on the area under the plasma concentration-time curve (AUC). It appears that all H2RA but cimetidine [83], which is a potent CYP2C19 inhibitor, are safe to use with clopidogrel.
      - PPIs
        Antiaggregation therapy with clopidogrel has significant interactions with omeprazole because clopidogrel has to be activated through CYPC219, an enzyme inhibited by omeprazole. This interaction is observed even if splitting doses by 12 h, so this combination must be avoided [84]. It is also advised to avoid esomeprazole usage with clopidogrel as it affects its active compound metabolism, the same way it was

observed with omeprazole (inhibition of CYP2C19 needed to convert clopidogrel to active component). Unlike omeprazole, pantoprazole can be safely used with clopidogrel [85]. Although lansoprazole slightly decreases prasugrel AUC, so far it has not shown diminished platelet aggregation inhibition [86]. On the other hand, clopidogrel concentration when used concomitantly with lansoprazole has not been changed, but the clinically insignificant reduction of platelet inhibition was observed [87]. Nevertheless, both clopidogrel and prasugrel can be cautiously used with lansoprazole. There have been various information regarding clopidogrel when used concomitantly with rabeprazole, but so far it seems that unlike omeprazole and esomeprazole, rabeprazole does not affect clopidogrel's antiplatelet effects [88, 89].

(b) Anticoagulation Drugs

- Antacids

  Coadministration of magnesium or aluminum hydroxide did not alter the plasma concentrations or pharmacologic action of warfarin [90, 91] nor rivaroxaban [92].

- H2RA

  Warfarin must be avoided with cimetidine therapy as it causes hypersaturation with warfarin that could cause hemorrhages [93–95]. Excessive anticoagulation is the result of competitive inhibition of warfarin metabolism by cimetidine confirmed by number of studies [96–99]. This interaction is pronounced only with the less potent stereoisomer of warfarin. Similarly as cimetidine, ranitidine shows warfarin interference by increasing AUC significantly and in that way prothrombin time as well [100]. Coadministration of ranitidine has no appreciable effects on rivaroxaban [92].

- PPIs

  As far as warfarin therapy is concerned, although omeprazole decreases warfarin clearance, it mostly affects its lesser potent R-isomer [101]. That explains why this interaction is not of clinical significance [102, 103], nevertheless caution is advised and therapy must be monitored. Esomeprazole has the same effect observed with omeprazole in altering the (R)-warfarin (less potent isomer) metabolism. Because it does not affect the more potent (S)-warfarin, no clinically significant interactions were observed with esomeprazole. There are no interactions between warfarin and lansoprazole [104], rabeprazole [105], and pantoprazole [106]. Generally, proton pump inhibitors can be used with warfarin therapy, even though a slight increase in coagulation parameters can be noted but is mostly safe and clinically insignificant. There is limited information about novel anticoagulant drugs and their use with proton pump inhibitors, but they seem to be generally safe when used concomitantly at least for rivaroxaban, apixaban, dabigatran, and pantoprazole [107, 108]. All aforementioned interactions between hematologic drugs and acid-reducing agents are systematically shown in Table 27.2.

Table 27.2 Hematologic drugs and acid-reducing agents

Drug	Antacid	H2RA			PPI				
		Cimetidine	Ranitidine	Famotidine	Ome	Esom	Panto	Lanso	Rabe
Clopidogrel	–	+	–	–	+	+	–	–	–
Prasugrel	/	/	–	/	/	/	/	–	/
Warfarin	–	+	+		–	–	–	–	–
Rivaroxaban	–	/	–	/	/	/	–	/	/
Apixaban	/	/			/	/	–	/	/
Dabigatran	/	/			/	/	–	/	/

+ there is significant interaction, – no significant interaction, / no relevant studies
H2RA histamine 2 receptor antagonist, *PPI* proton pump inhibitors, *ome* omeprazole, *esom* esomeprazole, *panto* pantoprazole, *lanso* lansoprazole, *rabe* rabeprazole

3. Anti-Inflammatory Drugs
   - Antacids

     NSAIDs are the most commonly used analgesics for acute or short-term pain as well as anti-inflammatory agents for chronic inflammatory diseases. These medications cause dyspepsia and upper gastrointestinal mucosal damage so there is a common coadministration of antacids with NSAIDs. Antacids containing only aluminum hydroxide or a mixture of aluminum and magnesium hydroxides cause no change or clinically insignificant reduction in the AUC of most NSAIDs. As an exception, antacids reduce the AUCs of indomethacin [109]. Magnesium hydroxide and sodium bicarbonate may enhance the rate and in some cases the extent of intestinal absorption of some NSAIDs. Some reports showed that the coadministration of these two antacids increases the early plasma concentrations and sometimes AUC of naproxen [110] and ibuprofen [111]. Magnesium hydroxide neutralizes gastric pH and accelerates gastric emptying, it may increase the solubility of weakly acidic drugs and promote more rapid transit to the jejunum where most of the drug absorption takes place. In contrast, aluminum hydroxide prolongs gastric emptying. Taken together, the clinical relevance of drug-drug interaction between NSAIDs and some described antacids is not clear.

     In several studies, it has been reported that concomitant administration of antacids and prednisone reduces both C_{max} and AUC by 40% [112–115] but since these studies measured only serum concentrations of prednisolone, which is a metabolite of prednisone, the clinical relevance of DDI remains unclear.
   - H2RA

     Several interactions were found with cimetidine and NSAIDs. It was shown to increase the area under the plasma concentration time for piroxicam, indomethacin, flurbiprofen, sulindac, oxaprozin, and aspirin [116]. Results for aspirin were inconsistent and the same is noted for cimetidine studies on interactions with ibuprofen and ketoprofen [117] but nevertheless, those interactions seem to be clinically insignificant [118, 119]. Nizatidine can also be used safely with ibuprofen [120]. Ranitidine showed a better interaction profile with NSAIDs, although it was also prone to increasing oxaprozine concentrations [121]. So far it shows that cyclosporine used concomitantly with cimetidine could lead to an increase in serum creatinine but not cyclosporine concentrations [122]. As inulin clearance was not affected by cimetidine, this could be the result of tubular secretion inhibition on cationic substances as cimetidine may show competition for renal tubular secretion with other basic substances. No interactions are observed between cimetidine and prednisolone [123].

- PPIs

  Proton pump inhibitors are generally thought to be safe to use with NSAIDs. Studies showed pantoprazole can be used with diclofenac [124], naproxen [125], and piroxicam [125]. Cyclosporin should be cautiously used with omeprazole as there are studies showing that it can increase cyclosporine concentration in heart transplant patients [126] but that effect was not seen in controlled trials in patients with renal transplant [127]. Phenazone can be used safely with lansoprazole [128] as is the case with prednisolone [129].

  All aforementioned interactions between anti-inflammatory drugs and acid-reducing agents are systematically shown in Table 27.3.

4. Oral Antidiabetic Drugs
   - Antacids

     Coadministration of magnesium hydroxide as milk of magnesia, but not aluminum hydroxide, may accelerate the rate of absorption of the nonmicronized form of glibenclamide [130, 131] and tolbutamide [132]. Similar situation is with glipizide, only the fractional AUC increases significantly [133, 134] but the total AUCs are not altered significantly, so the antacids may increase the rate, but not the extent, of absorption of these drugs.
   - H2RA

     Metformin is not metabolized but undergoes urine excretion which can be affected by cimetidine and thus can elevate the risk for lactic acidosis due to increased serum concentration of metformin [135]. Renal clearance of metformin was also decreased with ranitidine [136]. Famotidine was shown to increase metformin bioavailability albeit with an increase in renal clearance, but no effect was observed in area under the curve concentration time and is preferred H2RA in those on metformin therapy [137]. Sulfonylureas preparations (i.e., glibenclamide, gliclazide, and tolbutamide) should not be used

Table 27.3 Anti-inflammatory drugs and acid-reducing agents

Drug	Antacid	H2RA		PPI
		Cimetidine	Ranitidine	
NSAID	–	–	/	–
Prednisolone	Unclear interaction	–	/	–
Cyclosporine	/	/	–	Unclear interaction

+ there is significant interaction, – no significant interaction, / no relevant studies

H2RA histamine 2 receptor antagonist, *PPI* proton pump inhibitors

with cimetidine as it will result in increased plasma levels and could lead to hypoglycemia [138].

- PPIs

  Studies showed that pantoprazole and rabeprazole can significantly increase the metformin plasma exposure but without effect on glucose levels [139]. There are no considerate interactions between pantoprazole and glibenclamide [140] as well as between esomeprazole with glibenclamide or tolbutamide [141] at therapeutic doses (confirmed by animal models). There are a few studies suggesting that supratherapeutic doses of omeprazole [142], lansoprazole [143], and pantoprazole [144] can prolong hypoglycemia induced by sulfonylureas in animal studies, but are considered safe when used at their therapeutic rate. However, caution is needed when prescribing sulfonylureas with PPIs.

  All aforementioned interactions between oral antidiabetic drugs and acid-reducing agents are systematically shown in Table 27.4.

5. CNS Agents
   - Antacid

     Many CNS agents (including levodopa, ondansetron, phenytoin, sulpiride, benzodiazepines, lithium carbonate, sertindole, and ziprasidone) were studied in numerous studies for possible DDIs with antacids but no clinically relevant DDIs have been reported so far [145–156].
   - H2RA

     Cimetidine should be used cautiously with concurrent psychiatric drugs as many possible interactions are noted. It should not be used with diazepam as it significantly increases its serum concentration [157–159] and can cause marked and prolonged sedation. On the other hand, lorazepam and oxazepam can be used safely with cimetidine as they undergo glucuronidation, a process independent of cytochrome P-450 [160]. Ranitidine can also be used safely when combined with lorazepam and diazepam [161, 162]. Phenytoin concentration rises when coadministered with cimetidine [163–165] or ranitidine [166], and this combination should not be used, or if needed, with monitoring of the drug concentration. Other anticonvulsant agent which shows interference with cimetidine is carbamazepine [167], as this combination can be toxic and lead to changes in consciences, dizziness, vomiting, and nystagmus.

Table 27.4 Oral antidiabetic drugs and acid-reducing agents

Drug	Antacid		H2RA	IPP	
	Aluminum hydroxide	Magnesium hydroxide	Cimetidine	Pantoprazole	Esomeprazole
Glibenclamide	–	+	+	–	–
Tolbutamide	–	+	+	/	–
Gliclazide	/	/	+	/	/
Metformin	/		+	/	/

+ there is significant interaction, – no significant interaction, / no relevant studies
H2RA histamine 2 receptor antagonist, *PPI* proton pump inhibitors

Significant increase in area under the curve concentration was observed when combining triazolam and alprazolam with cimetidine [168], so monitoring or reducing the dosage of those drugs is warranted. There is one report of clozapine toxicity when used with cimetidine [169] but further investigations are needed. Tricyclic antidepressant imipramine and its biologically active metabolite desipramine show increased bioavailability when used with cimetidine [170], so practice caution with these agents. Although cimetidine can lead to a slight increase in systemic exposure of escitalopram, this is clinically irrelevant as is the case with cimetidine and mirtazapine [171]. Midazolam concentrations are raised when administered with cimetidine and ranitidine [172, 173] which can lead to a more pronounced hypnotic effect of this benzodiazepine. Later H2 antagonist famotidine does not show interaction with diazepam nor with phenytoin [174].

- PPIs

  One of the more important interactions with omeprazole is the considerate reduction of diazepam clearance [175, 176], pronounced in extensive (normal) S-mephenytoin 49-hydroxylase (CYP2C19) metabolizer phenotype. No such interaction was seen in slow metabolizers as both drugs then undergo different paths of transformation [177]. No interactions are observed with other benzodiazepines that undergo glucuronidation such as lorazepam, oxazepam, and temazepam [178]. Selective serotonin reuptake inhibitors such as citalopram and escitalopram showed significantly higher serum concentrations when used with omeprazole, esomeprazole, and lansoprazole [179], but more so with the two aforementioned as they are more potent inhibitors of CYP2C19. There are studies suggesting omeprazole increases phenytoin plasma concentration and half-life [180], but others found no alterations in plasma levels while using omeprazole in therapeutic doses (20 mg daily) [181]. Esomeprazole was shown to increase the AUC of diazepam, and although this renders of clinical insignificance, concomitant use could lead to accumulation of diazepam and cause motor discoordination and vigilance disruption [182, 183]. The same is noted for phenytoin metabolism, as a 10 to 15% increase of plasma concentration with concomitant administering with esomeprazole was seen, but this interaction is disregarded of clinical significance. Pantoprazole can be safely used with carbamazepine [184], and both pantoprazole and lansoprazole can be used with diazepam [185, 186] and phenytoin [187, 188] as well as rabeprazole and phenytoin [189].

  All aforementioned interactions between CNS agents and acid-reducing agents are systematically shown in Table 27.5.

6. Antimicrobial Agents
   (a) Antibiotics
   - Antacids

     Coadministration of aluminum hydroxide interferes with the absorption of chlortetracycline [190] and antacid-containing aluminum and magnesium hydroxides interfere with the absorption of tetracycline, doxycycline, and demeclocycline by approximately 90% compared with

Table 27.5 CNS agents and acid-reducing agents

Drug	Antacid	H2RA			PPI				
		Cimetidine	Ranitidine	Famotidine	Ome	Esom	Panto	Lanso	Rabe
Diazepam	–	+	–	–	+	±	–	–	/
Lorazepam	/	–	–	/	–	/	/	/	/
Triazolam	/	+	/	/	/	/	/	/	/
Alprazolam	/	+	/	/	/	/	/	/	/
Oxazepam	–	–	/	/	–	/	/	/	/
Phenytoin	–	+	+	–	±	–	–	–	–
Carbamazepine	/	+	/	/	/	/	–	/	/
Alprazolam	/	+	/	/	/	/	/	/	/
Midazolam	/	+	+	/	/	/	/	/	/
Escitalopram	/	–	/	/	+	+	+	+	/
Mirtazapine	/	–	/	/	/	/	/	/	/
Imipramine/ desipramine	/	+	/	/	/	/	/	/	/

+ there is significant interaction, – no significant interaction, / no relevant studies
H2RA histamine 2 receptor antagonist, *PPI* proton pump inhibitors, *ome* omeprazole, *esom* esomeprazole, *panto* pantoprazole, *lanso* lansoprazole, *rabe* rabeprazole

respective control values [191] . Therefore, tetracycline analogues are susceptible to DDIs with antacids so concomitant administration should be avoided although reasonable explanation for this phenomenon is difficult to find.

Coadministration of aluminum and magnesium hydroxides with ciprofloxacin reduced C_{max} and AUC of this antibacterial drug by 90% [192]. Magnitudes of reduction in AUC and C_{max} are >50% for some of the fluoroquinolones so the concomitant administration is not advised.

In general, coadministration of antacids and first- or second-generation cephalosporins (e.g., cephalexin and cefixime) shows no significant changes in the AUC. However, some third-generation cephalosporins (e.g., cefpodoxime proxetil) have significantly reduced AUC in coadministration with aluminum and magnesium hydroxides [193] whereas antacids have no significant effects on the AUC of cefteram pivoxil [194] or cefetamet pivoxil [195]. Coadministration of antacids has no significant effect on the AUCs of amoxicillin and clavulanic acid [196, 197].

The coadministration of antacids and clindamycin reduces the C_{max} by 67% and AUC by 23%, which indicates that the rate but not the extent of absorption may be clinically significantly reduced [198]. There are no clinically significant DDIs between antacids and azithromycin [199], erythromycin [200], linezolid [201], sulfamethoxazole, and trimethoprim [202].

- H2RA

  Orally administered penicillin can be safely used with H2RA [203], contrary to oral cephalosporins such as cefpodoxime and cefuroxime which should not be used with H2RA as they will significantly decrease their absorption [193]. These should be separated by at least 2 h if used concomitantly. Even though cimetidine does not affect quinolone absorption, it can lead to decreased renal clearance as cimetidine inhibits renal tubular secretion of quinolones [204]. Cimetidine was also shown to decrease the bioavailability of pefloxacin [205] and enoxacin [206]. There are inconclusive results of the cimetidine effect on tetracycline ranging from no impact on plasma concentration to decreased plasma concentration of tetracycline [207–210]. There is no effect of cimetidine on cotrimoxazole and ampicillin absorption [211, 212] and those can be used concomitantly. No unanimous results are yet published regarding metronidazole and cimetidine interactions [213–215].

- PPIs

  Orally administered penicillin can be safely used with PPIs [203]. Clarithromycin and omeprazole used together increase the plasma concentration of each other thus perhaps helping in H. pylori eradication [216]. Combination of omeprazole and cefuroxime or cefpodoxime must be avoided. Omeprazole can be safely used with ciprofloxacin [217] and metronidazole [218]. Pantoprazole can be used with clarithromycin [219] and coadministration of omeprazole and amoxicillin and bacampicillin is also considered safe [77].

  All aforementioned interactions between antibiotics and acid-reducing agents are systematically shown in Table 27.6.

(b) Antiviral drugs

- Antacids

  Available data show no clinically significant interaction between antacids and antiviral drugs such as fosamprenavir [220], atazanavir [221], raltegravir, lersivirine [222, 223], oseltamivir, and valaciclovir [224, 225].

Table 27.6 Antibiotics and acid-reducing agents

Drug	Antacid	H2RA	PPI
Tetracycline	+	±	/
Ciprofloxacin	+	/	–
Cephalexin	–	/	/
Cefixime	–	/	/
Cefpodoxime proxetil	+	+	+
Cefterampivoxil	–	/	/
Amoxicillin	–	–	–
Clindamycin	–	/	/
Azithromycin	–	/	/
Linezolid	–	/	/
Metronidazole	/	±	–
Clarithromycin	/	/	–

+ there is significant interaction, – no significant interaction, / no relevant studies

H2RA histamine 2 receptor antagonist, *PPI* proton pump inhibitors

- H2RA
  Atazanavir should be administered separately of H2 antagonists (cimetidine, famotidine, ranitidine, or nizatinide) as it will otherwise interfere with its absorption [226, 227]. H2-receptor antagonists and their concurrent use with didanosin [228], etravirine [229], tenofovir, abacavir, lamivudine, emtricitabine, or maraviroc is considered safe [230]. Regarding acyclovir, it was observed that cimetidine can increase AUC significantly in those receiving high-dose acyclovir therapy [231]. Famciclovir on the other hand can be safely used with cimetidine [232].
- PPIs

Significant interactions are noted between PPIs and protease inhibitors atazanavir [233], nelfinavir [234], indinavir [235], lopinavir and ritonavir [236], and simeprevir [237]. Caution is especially advised with omeprazole. Using omeprazole with protease inhibitors, atazanavir and nelfinavir, significantly decreases their availability and is best avoided [238]. There are some studies suggesting that boosted atazanavir (with ritonavir) can overcome this interaction, but PPIs in general and atazanavir combination are best avoided [238]. On the other hand, raltegravir shows increased solubility at higher pH, so combination with PPIs must be monitored [239] although this was well tolerated and without adverse effects. Protease inhibitors and concomitant use of omeprazole are even more complex when we add ritonavir into consideration which has better solubility at lower pH and is used to boost other protease inhibitors via CYP3A4 inhibition. It was shown that omeprazole potentiates CYP3A4 inhibition of ritonavir by inhibiting P-glycoprotein and thus increases its effect on saquinavir and indinavir [240]. Indinavir alone, on the other hand in concomitant usage with omeprazole shows decreased exposure [238]. Etravirine can be safely used with all proton pump inhibitors [241], unlike rilpivirine which should not be used with PPIs (esomeprazole, lansoprazole, omeprazole, pantoprazole, rabeprazole) [242]. As with H2RA, proton pump inhibitors are considered safe to use with tenofovir, abacavir, lamivudine, emtricitabine, or maraviroc [230].

All aforementioned interactions between antiviral drugs and acid-reducing agents are systematically shown in Table 27.7.

(c) Antifungal drugs
- Antacids
  When antifungal drugs itraconazole and ketoconazole are prescribed for systemic fungal infection, it may be advisable to avoid using antacids or space out the dosing intervals since ketoconazole was associated with 40% reduction of AUC [243] and itraconazole with 66% [244].
  In contrast, other antifungal drugs (fluconazole [245], posaconazole [246], and genaconazole [247]) were not associated with clinically relevant changes in the AUC when administered together with antacids.
- H2RA
  Ketoconazole, itraconazole, and fluconazole should not be used with cimetidine as it will decrease their absorption [248–250] and the same is applied to ranitidine coadministered with ketoconazole [251]. These interactions can

Table 27.7 Antiviral drugs and acid-reducing agents

Drug	Antacid	H2RA				PPI
		Cimetidine	Famotidine	Ranitidine	Nizatinide	
Abacavir	/	–				–
Atazanavir	–	+				+
Emtricitabine	/	–				–
Nelfinavir	/	/				+
Indinavir	/	/				+
Simeprevir	/	/				+
Etravirine	/	–				–
Rilpivirine	/	/				+
Oseltamivir	–	/				/
Lamivudine	/	–				–
Ritonavir	/	/				+
Tenofovir	/	–				–
Maraviroc	/	–				–
Acyclovir	/	+	/	/	/	/

+ there is significant interaction, – no significant interaction, / no relevant studies
H2RA histamine 2 receptor antagonist, *PPI* proton pump inhibitors

Table 27.8 Antifungal drugs and acid-reducing agents

Drug	Antacid	H2RA		IPP
		Cimetidine	Ranitidine	
Ketoconazole	+	+	+	+
Itraconazole	+	/		+
Fluconazole	–	/		+
Terbinafine	/	+	/	/

+ there is significant interaction, – no significant interaction, / no relevant studies
H2RA histamine 2 receptor antagonist, *PPI* proton pump inhibitors

be avoided by splitting doses by one to 2 h. Cimetidine can also interact with another antifungal agent, terbinafine, but it is shown to decrease its clearance by inhibition of the CYP1A2 isoenzyme, which leads to a rise in concentration of terbinafine [252].

- PPIs
  Itraconazole and ketoconazole as weak bases are better absorbed in an acidic medium so PPIs are generally not advised to use concomitantly [253–255]. This can be partially avoided if using these agents together with an acidic beverage (i.e., Coca-Cola) [256] or if using itraconazole in the form of a solution [257]. By contrast, fluconazole absorption is less susceptible to changes in gastric pH, but fluconazole was shown to significantly increase serum concentration of omeprazole [258].
  All aforementioned interactions between antifungal drugs and acid-reducing agents are systematically shown in Table 27.8.

Sucralfate

Sucralfate is a sulfated polysaccharide, sucrose octasulfate, complexed with aluminum hydroxide. It prevents acute, chemically induced mucosal damage and heals chronic ulcers without altering gastric acid or pepsin secretion or significantly buffering acid [259, 260]. Similar to aluminum-containing antacids, sucralfate stimulates angiogenesis and the formation of granulation tissue, possibly due to growth factor binding [259]. Aluminum hydroxide mediates some of the actions of sucralfate, but the sucrose octasulfate moiety may also have a role by contributing sulfhydryl groups to reduce oxidant damage to epithelial cells. Sucralfate has few adverse effects [260], it can bind to other drugs if taken simultaneously. Similar to antacids, significant aluminum retention only occurs in patients with renal failure [261]. Sucralfate can also bind to phosphate and lead to hypophosphatemia [262]. Combining sucralfate and antacids can potentially amplify these effects.

Sucralfate may decrease the serum concentration of bisphosphonate derivates, furosemide, digoxin, dolutegravir, elvitegravir, raltegravir, ketoconazole, penicillamine, quinidine, quinolones, tetracyclines, sulpiride, so they should be administered separately in order to minimize the impact of this interaction [263].

Bismuth

Bismuth does not inhibit or neutralize gastric acid. The role of bismuth preparations (e.g., bismuth subcitrate and bismuth subsalicylate (BSS)) is limited to part of a quadruple antibiotic therapy regimen in H. pylori-positive ulcers. In the colon, bismuth salts react with hydrogen sulfide to form bismuth sulfide, which blackens the stools. Bismuth toxicity is rare with colloidal bismuth subcitrate (CBS) or BSS [264, 265]. Bismuth absorption varies with the specific form of bismuth; absorption is much greater with CBS than with BSS or bismuth subnitrate [266, 267].

Coadministration of histamine-2 receptor antagonists increases bismuth absorption from CBS, but not from BSS or bismuth subnitrate [268]. Bismuth should be avoided or serum bismuth concentrations monitored in patients with renal failure [261]. The subsalicylate moiety in BSS is converted to salicylic acid and absorbed; however, salicylate in the absence of the acetyl group does not inhibit platelet function or appear to share the same high risk of aspirin for gastrointestinal bleeding [269–272]. However, the salicylate from BSS will raise serum salicylate levels and can cause salicylate toxicity, and combination with other salicylate products should therefore be avoided.

Possible major drug-drug interactions are noted between oral carbonic anhydrase inhibitors (acetazolamide [273], brinzolamide [274], dichlorphenamide [275], dorzolamide [276], and methazolamide [277]) and the large doses of salicylates, including bismuth subsalicylate, which may rarely result in severe metabolic acidosis and/or salicylate toxicity.

Bismuth salicylate may increase the risk of bleeding when taken with antiplatelet and anticoagulant drugs, so the coadministration with clopidogrel, prasugrel, warfarin, apixaban, dabigatran, enoxaparin, and rivaroxaban should be careful [278].

Ciprofloxacin bioavailability will not be significantly decreased by single doses of bismuth subsalicylate when the two medications are administered simultaneously [279]. On the other hand, the bioavailability of doxycycline was significantly reduced by 37% and 51%, respectively, when subsalicylate bismuth was given simultaneously and as a multiple-dose regimen before doxycycline [280].

Prostaglandin Analogue

Misoprostol is a 15-deoxy-15-hydroxy-16-methyl analogue of prostaglandin E1. Prostaglandins, particularly of the E and I group, inhibit acid secretion by selectively reducing the ability of the parietal cell to generate cyclic adenosine monophosphate in response to histamine [281]. Prostaglandins also enhance mucosal defense mechanisms [282].

Concomitant administration of antacids can reduce the bioavailability of misoprostol acid, the active metabolite of misoprostol. The mechanism of interaction is unknown. In 12 study subjects, coadministration of misoprostol with antacid reduced the bioavailability of misoprostol acid by 16% relative to fasting. Clinical trials of misoprostol conducted with concomitant antacid use suggest that this effect is not clinically important [283, 284]. Magnesium-containing antacids can exacerbate misoprostol-induced diarrhea, so if an antacid is needed, one that contains aluminum or calcium should be prescribed.

The use of misoprostol with other oxytocic agents like dinoprostone is contraindicated because it may stimulate uterine hypertonus, which can lead to uterine rupture or cervical laceration, particularly in the presence of an undilated or poorly dilated cervix [285].

Not many studies have been conducted on misoprostol drug-drug interaction, so it is an open field for further investigation.

References

1. Dent J, El-Serag HB, Wallander MA, Johansson S. Epidemiology of gastro-oesophageal reflux disease: a systematic review. Gut. 2005;54:710.
2. Sung JJ, Kuipers EJ, El-Serag HB. Systematic review: the global incidence and prevalence of peptic ulcer disease. Aliment Pharmacol Ther. 2009;29:938.
3. Shaw MJ, Fendrick AM, Kane RL, et al. Self-reported effectiveness and physician consultation rate in users of over-the counter histamine-2 receptor antagonists. Am J Gastroenterol. 2001;96:673–6.
4. Greenwald DA. Aging, the gastrointestinal tract, and risk of acid-related disease. Am J Med. 2004;117(5):8–13.
5. Marengoni A, et al. Understanding adverse drug reactions in older adults through drug–drug interactions. Eur J Intern Med. 2014;25(9):843–6.

6. Hohl CM, et al. Polypharmacy, adverse drug-related events, and potential adverse drug interactions in elderly patients presenting to an emergency department. Ann Emerg Med. 2001;38(6):666–71.
7. Pasina L, et al. Prevalence and appropriateness of drug prescriptions for peptic ulcer and gastro-esophageal reflux disease in a cohort of hospitalized elderly. Eur J Intern Med. 2011;22(2):205–10.
8. FDA Advises Consumers, patients and health care professionals after new FDA studies show risk to public health. FDA Requests Removal of All Ranitidine Products (Zantac) from the Market. https://www.fda.gov/news-events/press-announcements/fda-requests-removal-all-ranitidine-products-zantac-market. Accessed 11 June 2020.
9. Bergström CAS, Holm R, Jørgensen SA, Andersson SBE, Artursson P, Beato S, et al. Early pharmaceutical profling to predictoral drug absorption: current status and unmet needs. Eur J Pharm Sci. 2014;57:173–99.
10. Lahner E, Annibale B, DelleFave G. Systematic review: impaired drug absorption related to the co-administration of antisecretory therapy. Aliment Pharmacol Ther. 2009;29(12):1219–29.
11. Sjögren E, Abrahamsson B, Augustijns P, Becker D, Bolger MB, Brewster M, et al. In vivo methods for drug absorption—comparative physiologies, model selection, correlations with in vitro methods (IVIVC), and applications for formulation/API/excipient characterization including food efects. Eur J Pharm Sci. 2014;57:99–151.
12. Fallingborg J. Intraluminal pH of the human gastrointestinal tract. Dan Med Bull. 1999;46(3):183–96.
13. Evans DF, Pye G, Bramley R, Clark AG, Dyson TJ, Hardcastle JD. Measurement of gastrointestinal pH profiles in normal ambulant human subjects. Gut. 1988;29(8):1035–41.
14. Zhang L, Wu F, Lee SC, Zhao H. pH-dependent drug–drug interactions for weak base drugs: potential implications for new drug development. Clin Pharmacol Ther. 2014;96(2):266–77.
15. Ogawa R, Echizen H. Clinically significant drug interactions with antacids: an update. Drugs. 2011;71(14):1839–64.
16. Allen LV Jr, Popovich NG, Ansel HC. Ansel's pharmaceutical dosage forms and drug delivery systems, ninth edition. J Pharm Technol. 2010;26(3):167–8.
17. Zanger UM, Schwab M. Cytochrome P450 enzymes in drug metabolism: regulation of gene expression, enzyme activities, and impact of genetic variation. Pharmacol Ther. 2013;138(1):103–41.
18. Humphries TJ, Merritt GJ. Review article: drug interactions with agents used to treat acid-related diseases. Aliment Pharmacol Ther. 1999;13(S3):18–26.
19. Giacomini KM, Huang SM, Tweedie DJ, Benet LZ, Brouwer KL, Chu X, et al. Membrane transporters in drug development. Nat Rev Drug Discov. 2010;9(3):215–36.
20. Gibaldi M, Grundhofer B, Levy G. Effect of antacids on pH of urine. Clin Pharmacol Ther. 1974;16(3):520–5.
21. Prescott LF. Mechanisms of renal excretion of drugs (with special reference to drugs used by anaesthetists). Br J Anaesth. 1972;44(3):246–51.
22. Maton PN, Burton ME. Antacids revisited: a review of their clinical pharmacology and recommended therapeutic use. Drugs. 1999;57(6):855–70.
23. Welage LS, Rosemary RB. Drug interactions with antiulcer agents: considerations in the treatment of acid-peptic disease. J Pharm Pract. 1994;7(4):177–95.
24. Henry BA, MacDonald LA, Kitelington G, Bill GD, Longman MJS. Cimetidine and ranitidine comparison of effects on hepatic drug metabolism. Br Med J. 1980;281:775.
25. Breen KJ, Bury R, Desmond PV, Mostfond ML, Morphelt B, Westwood B, Shaw RG. Effects of cimetidine and ranitidine on hepatic drug metabolism. Clin Pharmacol Ther. 1982;31:297.
26. Meyer UA. Metabolic interactions of the proton-pump inhibitors lansoprazole, omeprazole and pantoprazole with other drugs. Eur J Gastroenterol Hepatol. 1996;8(1):21S–5S.
27. Radhofer-Welte S. Pharmacokinetics and metabolism of the proton pump inhibitor pantoprazole in man. Drugs Today. 1999;35(10):765–72.
28. Gerson LB, Triadafilopoulos G. Proton pump inhibitors and their drug interactions: an evidence-based approach. Eur J Gastroenterol Hepatol. 2001;13(5):611–6.

29. Ishizaki T, Chiba K, Manabe K, Koyama E, Hayashi M, Yasuda S, et al. Comparison of the interaction potential of a new proton pump inhibitor, E3810, versus omeprazole with diazepam in extensive and poor metabolizers of S-mephenytoin 49-hydroxylation. Clin Pharmacol Ther. 1995;58:155–64.
30. Li XQ, et al. Comparison of inhibitory effects of the proton pump-inhibiting drugs omeprazole, esomeprazole, lansoprazole, pantoprazole, and rabeprazole on human cytochrome P450 activities. Drug Metab Dispos. 2004;32(8):821–7.
31. Dobbs IH, Skoutakis VA, Acchardo SR. Effects of aluminium hydroxide on the absorption of propranolol. CUIT Ther Res. 1976;21:887–92.
32. Hong CY, Hu SC, Lin SJ, et al. Lack of influence of aluminium hydroxide on the bioavailability and beta-adrenoceptor blocking activity of propranolol. Int J Clin Pharmacol Ther Toxicol. 1985;23:244–6.
33. McElnay JC, Temple DJ. The use of buccal partitioning as a model to examine the effects of aluminium hydroxide gel on the absorption of propranolol. Br J Clin Pharmacol. 1982;13:399–403.
34. Regardh CG, Lundborg P, Persson BA. The effect of antacid, metoclopramide, and propantheline on the bioavailability of metoprolol and atenolol. Biopharm Drug Dispos. 1981;2:79–87.
35. Freely J, Wilkinson GR, Wood AJJ. Reduction of liver blood flow and propranolol metabolism by cimetidine. N Engl J Med. 1981;304:692–5.
36. Heagerty AM, Donovan MA, Castleden CM, Pohl JF, Pate L, Hedges A. Influence of cimetidine on the pharmacokinetics of propranolol. Br Med J. 1981;282:1917–9.
37. Donovan MA, Heagerty AM, Pate L, Castleden M, Pohl JEF. Cimetidine and bioavailability of propranolol (letter). Lancet. 1981;I:164.
38. Reimann IW, Klotz U, Siems B, Frolich JC. Cimetidine increases steady state plasma levels of propranolol. Br J Clin Pharmacol. 1981;12:785–90.
39. Kirch W, Kohler H, Spahn H, Mutschler E. Interaction of cimetidine with metoprolol, propranolol, or atenolol. Lancet. 1981;II:531–2.
40. Daneshmend TK, Roberts CJC. Cimetidine and the bioavailability of labetalol (letter). Lancet. 1981;I:565.
41. Houtzagers JJ, Streurman O, Regardh CG. The effect of pretreatment with cimetidine on the bioavailability and disposition of atenolol and metoprolol. Br J Clin Pharmacol. 1982;14:67–72.
42. Sedman AJ. Cimetidine-drug interactions. Am J Med. 1984;76(1):109–14.
43. Bauer LA, McDonnell N, Horn JR, et al. Single and multiple doses of oral cimetidine do not change liver blood flow in humans. Clin Pharmacol Ther. 1990;48:195–200.
44. Lewis JH. Hepatic effects of drugs used in the treatment of peptic ulcer disease. Am J Gastroenterol. 1987;82(10):987–1003.
45. Heagerty AM, Castleden CM, Patel L. Failure of ranitidine to interact with propranolol. Br Med J. 1982;284:1304.
46. Palel L, Weerasuriya K. Effect of cimetidine and ranitidine 509 on propranolol clearance. Br J Clin Pharmacol. 1983;15:152.
47. Reimann W, Klotz U, Frohlich JE. Effects of cimetidine on steady state propranolol kinetics. Clin Pharmacol Ther. 1982;32:749.
48. Spahn H, Mutschler E, Kirch W, Ohnhaus EE, Janisch HD. Influence of ranitidine on plasma metoprolol and atenolol concentrations. Br Med J. 1983;286(6377):1546–7.
49. Kelly JG, Shanks RG, McDevitt DG. Influence of ranitidine on plasma metoprolol concentrations. Br Med J. 1983;287(6400):1218–9.
50. Desmond PV, Marshford ML, Harman PJ, Morphett BJ, Breen KJ, Wang YM. Decreased oral warfarin clearance after ranitidine and cimetidine. Clin Pharmacol Ther. 1984;35(3):338–41.
51. Andersson T, Lundborg P, Reg CG. Lack of effect of omeprazole treatment on steady-state plasma levels of metoprolol. Eur J Clin Pharmacol. 1991;40(1):61–5.
52. Henry D, et al. Propranolol steady-state pharmacokinetics are unaltered by omeprazole. Eur J Clin Pharmacol. 1987;33(4):369–73.

53. Karol MD, Locke CS, Cavanaugh JH. Lack of interaction between lansoprazole and propranolol, a pharmacokinetic and safety assessment. J Clin Pharmacol. 2000;40(3):301–8.
54. Koch HJ, Hartmann M, Bliesath H, Huber R, Steinijans VW, Mascher H, et al. Pantoprazole has no influence on steady state pharmacokinetics and pharmacodynamics of metoprolol in healthy volunteers. Int J Clin Pharmacol Ther. 1996;34:420–3.
55. Mantyla R, Mannisto PT, Vuorela A, et al. Impairment of captopril bioavailability by concomitant food and antacid intake. Int J Clin Pharmacol Ther Toxicol. 1984;22:626–9.
56. Laeis P, Puchler K, Kirch W. The pharmacokinetic and metabolic profile of olmesartan medoxomil limits the risk of clinically relevant drug interaction. J Hypertens. 2001;19(1):21–32.
57. Winship LC, McKenney JM, Wright JT Jr, Wood JH, Goodman RP. The effect of ranitidine and cimetidine on single-dose diltiazem pharmacokinetics. Pharmacotherapy. 1985;5(1):16–9. https://doi.org/10.1002/j.1875-9114.1985.tb04451.x.
58. Vanderhoff BT, Ruppel HM, Amsterdam PB. Carvedilol: the new role of beta-blockers in congestive heart failure. Am Fam Physician. 1998;58(7):1627.
59. Todd PA, Faulds D. Felodipine. Drugs. 1992;44(2):251–77.
60. Baciewicz AM, Baciewicz FA Jr. Effect of cimetidine and ranitidine on cardiovascular drugs. Am Heart J. 1989;118(1):144–54.
61. Mikus G, Eichelbaum M, Fischer C, Gumulka S, Klotz U, Kroemer HK. Interaction of verapamil and cimetidine: stereochemical aspects of drug metabolism, drug disposition and drug action. J Pharmacol Exp Therapeut. 1990;253(3):1042–8.
62. Abernethy DR, Schwartz JB, Todd EL. Lack of interaction between verapamil and cimetidine. Clin Pharmacol Ther. 1985;38(3):342–9.
63. Soons PA, van den Berg G, Danhof M, van Brummelen P, Jansen JB, Lamers CB, et al. Influence of single- and multiple-dose omeprazole treatment on nifedipine pharmacokinetics and effects in healthy subjects. Eur J Clin Pharmacol. 1992;42:319–24.
64. Bliesath H, Huber R, Steinijans VW, Koch HJ, Kunz K, Wurst W. Pantoprazole does not interact with nifedipine in man under steady-state conditions. Int J Clin Pharmacol Ther. 1996;34:51–5.
65. Dorofeeva MN, Shikh EV, Sizova ZM, Shindryaeva NN, Lapidus NI. Effect of omeprazole on antihypertensive efficacy of amlodipine in patients with comorbid pathology—arterial hypertension and acid-dependent disease. Electron J Gen Med. 2018;15(4):23–5.
66. Cooke J, Smith JA. Absence of interaction of digoxin with antacids under clinical conditions. Br Med J. 1978;2:1166–967.
67. Jordaens L, Hoegaerts J, Belpaire F. Non-interaction of cimetidine with digoxin absorption. Acta Clin Belg. 1981;36:109–10.
68. Hogan C, Landau S, Tepper D, Somberg J. Cimetidine-amiodarone interaction. J Clin Pharmacol. 1988;28:909.
69. Kosoglou T, Vlasses PH. Drug interactions involving renal transport mechanisms: an overview. DICP Ann Pharmacother. 1989;23:116–23.
70. Somogyi A, Bochner F. Dose and concentration dependent effect of ranitidine on procainamide disposition and renal clearance in man. Br J Clin Pharm. 1984;18:175–81.
71. Klotz U, Arwela P, Rosenkranz B. Famotidine, a new HI receptor antagonist, does not affect hepatic elimination of diazepam or tubular secretion of procainamide. Eur J Clin Pharmaco1. 1985;28:671–5.
72. Freely J, Wilkinson GR, McAllister CB, Wood AJJ. Increased toxicity and reduced clearance of lidocaine by cimetidine. Ann Intern Med. 1982;96:592–4.
73. Knapp AB, Maguire W, Keren G, et al. The effect of cimetidine administration on serum lidocaine levels in man (abstr). Am J Cardiol. 1982;49:1026.
74. Knapp AB, Maguire W, Keren G, et al. The cimetidine-lidocaine interaction. Ann Intern Med. 1983;98:174–7.
75. Jackson EJ, et al. Effects of histamine-2 receptor blockade on lidocaine kinetics. Clin Pharmacol Therapeut. 1985;37(5):544–8.

76. Feely J, Guy E. Lack of effect of ranitidine on the disposition of lidocaine. Br J Clin Pharmacol. 1983;15:378–9.
77. Andersson T. Omeprazole drug interaction studies. Clin Pharmacokinet. 1991;21(3):195–212. https://doi.org/10.2165/00003088-199121030-00004.
78. Oosterhuis B, Jonkman JHG. Omeprazole: pharmacology, pharmacokinetics and interactions. Digestion. 1989;44:9–17.
79. Hartmann M, Huber R, Bliesath H, Steinijans VW, Koch HJ, Wurst W, et al. Lack of interaction between pantoprazole and digoxin at therapeutic doses in man. Int J Clin Pharmacol Ther. 1996;34:67–S71.
80. Portoles A, Calvo A, Terleira A, et al. Lack of pharmacokinetic interaction between omeprazole or lansoprazole and ivabradine in healthy volunteers: an open-label, randomized, crossover, pharmacokinetic interaction clinical trial. J Clin Pharmacol. 2006;46(10):1195–203.
81. Plavix (clopidogrel bisulfate) FDA Drug Safety Communication, FDA Date: 11/17/2009, https://www.pdr.net/fda-drug-safety-communication/plavix?druglabelid=525&id=5223. Accessed 14 June 2020.
82. Small DS, Farid NA, Li YG, Ernest CS II, Payne CD, Salazar DE, Winters KJ. Effect of ranitidine on the pharmacokinetics and pharmacodynamics of prasugrel and clopidogrel. Curr Med Res Opin. 2008;24(8):2251–7.
83. Lin SL, Chang HM, Liu CP, Chou LP, Chan JW. Clinical evidence of interaction between clopidogrel and proton pump inhibitors. World J Cardiol. 2011;3(5):153–64. https://doi.org/10.4330/wjc.v3.i5.153.
84. Bates ER, Lau WC, Angiolillo DJ. Clopidogrel–drug interactions. J Am Coll Cardiol. 2011;57(11):1251–63.
85. Angiolillo DJ, Gibson CM, Cheng S, et al. Differential effects of omeprazole and pantoprazole on the pharmacodynamics and pharmacokinetics of clopidogrel in healthy subjects: randomized, placebo-controlled, crossover comparison studies. Clin Pharmacol Ther. 2011;89(1):65–74.
86. Small DS, et al. Effects of the proton pump inhibitor lansoprazole on the pharmacokinetics and pharmacodynamics of prasugrel and clopidogrel. J Clin Pharmacol. 2008;48(4):475–84.
87. Frelinger AL, Lee RD, Mulford DJ, et al. A randomized, 2-period, crossover design study to assess the effects of dexlansoprazole, lansoprazole, esomeprazole, and omeprazole on the steady-state pharmacokinetics and pharmacodynamics of clopidogrel in healthy volunteers. J Am Coll Cardiol. 2012;59:1304–11.
88. Wu J, Jia LT, Shao LM, et al. Drug–drug interaction of rabeprazole and clopidogrel in healthy Chinese volunteers. Eur J Clin Pharmacol. 2013;69:179–87.
89. Funck-Brentano C, Szymezak J, Steichen O, et al. Effects of rabeprazole on the antiplatelet effects and pharmacokinetics of clopidogrel in healthy volunteers. Arch Cardiovasc Dis. 2013;106:661–71.
90. Ambre JJ, Fischer LJ. Effect of coadministration of aluminum and magnesium hydroxides on absorption of anticoagulants in man. Clin Pharmacol Ther. 1973;14(2):231–7.
91. Robinson DS, Benjamin DM, McCormack JJ. Interaction of warfarin and nonsystemic gastrointestinal drugs. Clin Pharmacol Ther. 1971;12(3):491–5.
92. Kubitza D, Becka M, Zuehlsdorf M, et al. Effect of food, an antacid, and the H2 antagonist ranitidine on the absorption of BAY 59-7939 (rivaroxaban), an oral, direct factor Xa inhibitor, in healthy subjects. J Clin Pharmacol. 2006;46(5):549–58.
93. Kerley B, Ali M. Cimetidine potentiation of warfarin action (letter). Can Med Assoc J. 1982;126:116.
94. Silver BA, Bell WR. Cimetidine potentiation of the hypoprothrombinemic effect of warfarin. Ann Intern Med. 1979;90:348–9.
95. Wallin BA, Jacknowitz A, Raich PC. Cimetidine and effect of warfarin (letter). Ann Intern Med. 1979;90:993.
96. Serlin MJ, Challinger M, Park BK, Turcan PA, Breckenridge AM. Cimetidine potentiates the anticoagulant effect of warfarin by inhibition of drug metabolism. Biochem Pharmacol. 1980;29:1971–2.

97. Puurunen J, Sotaniemi E, Pelkonen O. Effect of cimetidine on microsomal drug metabolism in man. Eur J Clin Pharmacol. 1980;18:185–7.
98. Puurunen J, Sotaniemi E, Pelkonen O. Cimetidine inhibits microsomal drug metabolism in man (abstr). Naunyn Schmiedeberg's Arch Pharmacol. 1979;308:R24.
99. Rendic S, Sunjic V, Toso R, Kajfez F, Ruf HH. Interaction of cimetidine with liver microsomes. Xenobiotica. 1979;9:555–64.
100. Desmond PV, Marshford ML, Harman PJ, Morphett BJ, Breen KJ, Wang YM. Decreased oral warfarin clearance after ranitidine and cimetidine. Clin Pharmacol Ther. 1984;35:338–41.
101. Sutfin T, et al. Stereoselective interaction of omeprazole with warfarin in healthy men. Ther Drug Monit. 1989;11(2):176–84.
102. Unge P, Svedberg LE, Nordgren A, et al. A study of the interaction of omeprazole and warfarin in anticoagulated patients. Br J Clin Pharmacol. 1992;34(6):509–12. https://doi.org/10.1111/j.1365-2125.1992.tb05656.x.
103. Uno T, et al. The role of cytochrome P2C19 in R-warfarin pharmacokinetics and its interaction with omeprazole. Ther Drug Monit. 2008;30(3):276–81.
104. Gremse DA. Lansoprazole: pharmacokinetics, pharmacodynamics and clinical uses. Expert Opin Pharmacother. 2001;2(10):1663–70.
105. Humphries TJ, Nardi RV, Spera AC, et al. Coadministration of rabeprazole sodium (E3810) does not affect the pharmacokinetics of anhydrous theophylline or warfarin. Gastroenterology. 1996;110:A138.
106. Duursema L, Muller FO, Schall R, et al. Lack of effect of pantoprazole on thepharmacodynamics and pharmacokinetics of warfarin. Br J Clin Pharmacol. 1995;39(6):700–3.
107. Bolek T, Samoš M, Škorňová I, et al. Does proton pump inhibition change the on-treatment anti-Xa activity in xabans-treated patients with atrial fibrillation? A pilot study. J Thromb Thrombolysis. 2019;47(1):140–5. https://doi.org/10.1007/s11239-018-1748-5.
108. Stangier J, Stähle H, Rathgen K, et al. Pharmacokinetics and pharmacodynamics of the direct oral thrombin inhibitor dabigatranin healthy elderly subjects. Clin Pharmacokinet. 2008;47:47–59.
109. Galeazzi RL. The effect of an antacid on the bioavailability of indomethacin. Eur J Clin Pharmacol. 1977;12(1):65–8.
110. Segre EJ, Sevelium H, Varady J. Letter: Effects of antacids on naproxen absorption. N Engl J Med. 1974;291(11):582–3.
111. Neuvonen PJ. The effect of magnesium hydroxide on the oral absorption of ibuprofen, ketoprofen and diclofenac. Br J ClinPharmacol. 1991;31(3):263–6.
112. Albin H, Vincon G, Demotes-Mainard F, et al. Effect of aluminium phosphate on the bioavailability of cimetidine and prednisolone. Eur J Clin Pharmacol. 1984;26(2):271–3.
113. Bergrem H, Djoseland O, Jervell J, et al. Immunosuppressive treatment policies. (A) Glucocorticoids: absorption of prednisolone, I: the effect of fasting, food, and food combined with antacids. Scand J Urol Nephrol Suppl. 1981;64:167–73.
114. Tanner AR, Caffin JA, Halliday JW, et al. Concurrent administration of antacids and prednisone: effect on serum levels of prednisolone. Br J Clin Pharmacol. 1979;7(4):397–400.
115. Uribe M, Casian C, Rojas S, et al. Decreased bioavailability of prednisone due to antacids in patients with chronic active liver disease and in healthy volunteers. Gastroenterology. 1981;80(4):661–5.
116. Dixon JS, Page MC. Interactions between non-steroidal anti-inflammatory drugs and H2-receptor antagonists or prostaglandin analogues. Rheumatol Int. 1991;11:13–8.
117. Verbeeck RK, Corman CL, Wallace SM, et al. Single and multiple dose pharmacokinetics of enteric coated ketoprofen: effect of cimetidine. Eur J Clin Pharmacol. 1988;35:521–7.
118. Li G, Treiber G, Klotz U. The Ibuprofen-Cimetidine Interaction. Drug Invest. 1989;1:11–7. https://doi.org/10.1007/BF03259161.
119. Evans AM, Nation RL, Sansom LN. Lack of effect of cimetidine on the pharmacokinetics of R (−)- and S (+)- ibuprofen. Br J Clin Pharmacol. 1989;28(2):143–9.
120. Forsyth DR, Jayasinghe KSA, Roberts CJC. Do nizatidine and cimetidine interact with ibuprofen? Eur J Clin Pharmacol. 1988;35:85–8.

121. Scavone JM, Greenblatt DJ, Matlis R, Harmatz JS. Interaction of oxaprozin with acetaminophen, cimetidine, and ranitidine. Eur J Clin Pharmacol. 1986;31(3):371–4.
122. Pachon J, Lorber MI, Bia MJ. Effects of H2-receptor antagonists on renal function in cyclosporine treated renal transplant patients. Transplantation. 1989;47:254–9.
123. Morrison PJ, Rogers HJ, Bradbrook ID, Parsons C. Concurrent administration of cimetidine and enteric-coated prednisolone: effect on plasma levels of prednisolone. Br J Clin Pharmacol. 1980;10:87–9.
124. Bliesath H, Huber R, Steinijans VW, Koch HJ, Wurst W, Mascher H. Lack of pharmacokinetic interaction between pantoprazole and diclofenac. Int J Clin Pharmacol Ther Toxicol. 1996;34:152–6.
125. Andersson T, Bredberg E, Naesdal I, Wilson I. Lack of drug–drug interaction between three different non-steroidal antiinflammatory drugs and omeprazol. Eur J Clin Pharmacol. 1998;54:399–404.
126. Reichenspurner H, Meiser BM, Muschiol F, et al. The influence of gastrointestinal agents on resorption and metabolism of cyclosporine after heart transplantation: experimental and clinical results. J Heart Lung Transpl. 1993;12(6 Pt 1):987–92.
127. Blohme I, Idstrom JP, Andersson T. A study of the interaction between omeprazole and cyclosporine in renal transplant patients. Br J Clin Pharmacol. 1993;35(2):156–60.
128. St Peter JV, Awni WM, Granneman GR, et al. The effects of lansoprazole on the disposition of antipyrine and indocyanine green in normal human subjects. Am J Ther. 1995;2(8):561–8.
129. Cavanaugh JH, Karol MD. Lack of pharmacokinetic interaction after administration of lansoprazole or omeprazole with prednisone. J Clin Pharmacol. 1996;36(11):1064–71.
130. Neuvonen PJ, Kivisto KT. The effects of magnesium hydroxide on the absorption and efficacy of two glibenclamide preparations. Br J Clin Pharmacol. 1991;32(2):215–20.
131. Zuccaro P, Pacifici R, Pichini S, et al. Influence of antacids on the bioavailability of glibenclamide. Drugs Exp Clin Res. 1989;15(4):165–9.
132. Kivisto KT, Neuvonen PJ. Effect of magnesium hydroxide on the absorption and efficacy of tolbutamide and chlorpropamide. Eur J Clin Pharmacol. 1992;42(6):675–9.
133. Kivisto KT, Neuvonen PJ. Differential effects of sodium bicarbonate and aluminium hydroxide on the absorption and activity of glipizide. Eur J Clin Pharmacol. 1991;40(4):383–6.
134. Kivisto KT, Neuvonen PJ. Enhancement of absorption and effect of glipizide by magnesium hydroxide. Clin Pharmacol Ther. 1991;49(1):39–43.
135. Seo JH, Da YL, Hong CW, et al. Severe lactic acidosis and acute pancreatitis associated with cimetidine in a patient with type 2 diabetes mellitus taking metformin. Intern Med. 2013;52(19):2245–8.
136. Cho SK, Chung JY. The MATE1 rs2289669 polymorphism affects the renal clearance of metformin following ranitidine treatment. Int J Clin Pharmacol Ther. 2016;54(4):253–62.
137. Pakkir Maideen NM, Jumale A, Balasubramaniam R. Drug Interactions of Metformin Involving Drug Transporter Proteins. Adv Pharm Bull. 2017;7(4):501–5. https://doi.org/10.15171/apb.2017.062.
138. Holstein A, Beil W, Kovacs P. CYP2C metabolism of oral antidiabetic drugs-impact on pharmacokinetics, drug interactions and pharmacogenetic aspects. Expert Opin Drug Metab Toxicol. 2012;8(12):1549–63. https://doi.org/10.1517/17425255.2012.722619.
139. Kim A, Chung I, Yoon SH, et al. Effects of proton pump inhibitors on metformin pharmacokinetics and pharmacodynamics. Drug Metab Dispos. 2014;42(7):1174–9. https://doi.org/10.1124/dmd.113.055616.
140. Walter-Sack IE, Bliesath H, Stötzer F, et al. Lack of pharmacokinetic and pharmacodynamic interaction between pantoprazole and glibenclamide in humans. Clin Drug Investig. 1998;15(3):253–60.
141. Swamy VK, Shankaraiah MM, Jyothi TM, et al. A study on drug-drug interaction of esomeprazole and anti-diabetic drugs. J Young Pharm. 2010;2(4):424–7.
142. Kumar V, Rao NV, Setty SR. Influence of omeprazole on hypoglycaemic activity of glibenclamide and tolbutamide in normal albino rabbits. Acta Pharm Sci. 2000;42(4)

143. Rajendra SV, Raghaveergupta PS, Joshi VG, et al. Influence of lansoprazole on hypoglycaemic activity of oral antidiabetic agents in healthy albino rats. Acta Pharm Turcica. 2004;46:95–9.
144. Babitha S, Swamy S, Karegouda GL. A study on the drug-drug interaction of pantaprazole with glipizide. Hyderabad: 57th Ind Pharm Congress; 2005. p. 252.
145. Shader RI, Ciraulo DA, Greenblatt DJ, et al. Steady-state plasma desmethyldiazepam during long-term clorazepate use: effects of antacids. Clin Pharmacol Ther. 1982;31(2):180–3.
146. Greenblatt DJ, Allen MD, MacLaughlin DS, et al. Diazepam absorption: effect of antacids and food. Clin Pharmacol Ther. 1978;24(5):600–9.
147. Leon AS, Spiegel HE. The effect of antacid administration on the absorption and metabolism of levodopa. J Clin Pharmacol N Drugs. 1972;12(7):263–7.
148. Goode DL, Newton DW, Ueda CT, et al. Effect of antacid on the bioavailabiity of lithium carbonate. Clin Pharm. 1984;3(3):284–7.
149. Payne K, Mattheyse FJ, Liebenberg D, et al. The pharmacokinetics of midazolam in paediatric patients. Eur J Clin Pharmacol. 1989;37(3):267–72.
150. Bozigian HP, Pritchard JF, Gooding AE, et al. Ondansetron absorption in adults: effect of dosage form, food, and antacids. J Pharm Sci. 1994;83(7):1011–3.
151. Carter BL, Garnett WR, Pellock JM, et al. Effect of antacids on phenytoin bioavailability. Ther Drug Monit. 1981;3(4):333–40.
152. Chapron DJ, Kramer PA, Mariano SL, et al. Effect of calcium and antacids on phenytoin bioavailability. Arch Neurol. 1979;36(7):436–8.
153. Wong SL, Linnen P, Mack R, et al. Effects of food, antacid, and dosage form on the pharmacokinetics and relative bioavailability of sertindole in healthy volunteers. Biopharm Drug Dispos. 1997;18(6):533–41.
154. Shinkuma D, Hamaguchi T, Kobayashi M, et al. The bioavailability of sulpiride taken as a film-coated tablet with sodium bicarbonate, cimetidine, natural orange juice or hydrochloric acid. Int J Clin Pharmacol Ther Toxicol. 1989;27(10):499–502.
155. Kroboth PD, Smith RB, Rault R, et al. Effects of end-stage renal disease and aluminum hydroxide on temazepam kinetics. Clin Pharmacol Ther. 1985;37(4):453–9.
156. Wilner KD, Hansen RA, Folger CJ, et al. The pharmacokinetics of ziprasidone in healthy volunteers treated with cimetidine or antacid. Br J Clin Pharmacol. 2000;49(Suppl. 1):57S–60S.
157. Klotz U, Reimann I. Delayed clearance of diazepam due to cimetidine. N Engl J Med. 1980;302:1012–4.
158. Klotz U, Antilla VJ, Reimann I. Cimetidine/diazepam interaction (letter). Lancet. 1979;II:699.
159. Ruffalo RL, Thompson JF. Effect of cimetidine on the clearance of benzodiazepines. N Engl J Med. 1980;303:753–4.
160. Patwardhan RV, Yarborough GW, Desmond PV, et al. Cimetidine spares the glucuronidation of lorazepam and oxazepam. Gastroenterology. 1980;79:912–6.
161. Abernethy DR, Greenblatt DJ, Eshelman FN, Shader RI. Ranitidine does not impair oxidative or conjugative metabolism: noninteraction with antipyrine, diazepam, and lorazepam. Clin Pharmacol Ther. 1984;35(2):188–92.
162. Klotz U, Reimann IW, Ohnhaus EE. Effect of ranitidine on the steady state pharmacokinetics of diazepam. Eur J Clin Pharmacol. 1983;24(3):357–60.
163. Neuvonen PJ, Tokola RA, Kaste M. Cimetidine-phenytoin interaction: effect on serum phenytoin concentration and antipyrine test. Eur J Clin Pharmacol. 1981;21(3):215–20.
164. Hetzel DJ, Bochner F, Hallpike JF, et al. Cimetidine interaction with phenytoin. Br Med J. 1981;282:1512.
165. Neuvonen PJ, Tokola R, Kaste M. Cimetidine interaction with phenytoin (letter). Br Med J. 1981;283:501.
166. Tse CT, Akinwande KI, Biallowons K. Phenytoin concentration elevation subsequent to ranitidine administration. Ann Pharmacother. 1993;27(12):1448–51.
167. Telerman-Toppet N, Duret ME, Cöers C. Cimetidine interaction with carbamazepine. Ann Intern Med. 1981;94(4 pt 1):544. https://doi.org/10.7326/0003-4819-94-4-544_2.

168. Abernethy DR, Greenblatt DJ, Divoll D, et al. Interaction of cimetidine with the triazolobenzodiazepines alprazolam and triazolam. Psychopharmacology. 1983;80(3):275–8.
169. Szymanski S, Lieberman JA, Picou D, et al. A case report of cimetidine-induced clozapine toxicity. J Clin Psychiatry. 1991;52(1):21–2.
170. Abernethy DR, Greenblatt DJ, Shader RI. Imipramine-cimetidine interaction: impairment of clearance and enhanced absolute bioavailability. J Pharmacol Exp Ther. 1984;229(3):702–5.
171. Sitsen JM, Maris FA, Timmer CJ. Concomitant use of mirtazapine and cimetidine: a drug-drug interaction study in healthy male subjects. Eur J Clin Pharmacol. 2000;56(5):389–94. https://doi.org/10.1007/s002280000174.
172. Fee JP, Collier PS, Howard PJ, Dundee JW. Cimetidine and ranitidine increase midazolam bioavailability. Clin Pharmacol Ther. 1987;41(1):80–4. https://doi.org/10.1038/clpt.1987.13.
173. Kirch W, Hoensch H, Janisch HD. Interactions and non-interactions with ranitidine. Clin Pharmacokinet. 1984;9(6):493–510. https://doi.org/10.2165/00003088-198409060-00002.
174. Humphries TJ. Famotidine: a notable lack of drug interactions. Scand J Gastroenterol Suppl. 1987;134:55–60. https://doi.org/10.3109/00365528709090142.
175. Caraco Y, Tateishi T, Wood AJ. Interethnic difference in omeprazole's inhibition of diazepam metabolism. Clin Pharmacol Ther. 1995;58:62–72.
176. Andersson T, Andren K, Cederberg C, et al. Effect of omeprazole and cimetidine on plasma diazepam levels. Eur J Clin Pharmacol. 1990;39:51–4.
177. Zomorodi K, Houston JB. Diazepam–omeprazole inhibition interaction: an in vitro investigation using human liver microsomes. Br J Clin Pharmacol. 1996;42(2):157–62.
178. Worth LJ, Blyth CC, Booth DL, et al. Optimizing antifungal drug dosing and monitoring to avoid toxicity and improve outcomes in patients with haematological disorders. Intern Med J. 2008;38(6b):521–37. https://doi.org/10.1111/j.1445-5994.2008.01726.x.
179. Gjestad C, Westin AA, Skogvoll E, Spigset O. Effect of proton pump inhibitors on the serum concentrations of the selective serotonin reuptake inhibitors citalopram, escitalopram, and sertraline. Ther Drug Monit. 2015;37(1):90–7. https://doi.org/10.1097/FTD.0000000000000101.
180. Gugler R, Jensen JC. Omeprazole inhibits oxidative drug metabolism. Studies with diazepam and phenytoin in vivo and 7-ethoxycoumarin in vitro. Gastroenterology. 1985;89(6):1235–41.
181. Andersson T, Lagerström PO, Unge P. A study of the interaction between omeprazole and phenytoin in epileptic patients. Ther Drug Monit. 1990;12(4):329–33. https://doi.org/10.1097/00007691-199007000-00005.
182. Drewelow B, Schaffler K, Reitmeir P. Superior interaction profile of pantoprazole vs esomeprazole after single dose diazepam regarding pharmacodynamic (PD) and kinetic (PK) parameters. Can J Gastroenterol. 2006;20(Suppl. A):144.
183. Drewelow B, Schaffler K, Reitmeir P, et al. Effects of multiple-dose esomeprazole and pantoprazole on diazepam pharmacokinetic profile and pharmacodynamic effects on cognitive and psychomotor function in healthy volunteers. Arzneimittelforschung. 2010;60(8):483–91.
184. Huber R, Bliesath H, Hartmann M, et al. Pantoprazole does not interact with the pharmacokinetics of carbamazepine. Int J Clin Pharmacol Ther. 1998;36:521–4.
185. Gugler R, Hartmann M, Rudi J, et al. Lack of pharmacokinetic interaction of pantoprazole with diazepam in man. Br J Clin Pharmacol. 1996;42:249–52.
186. Lefebvre RA, Flouvat B, Karolac-Tamisier S, Moerman E, Van Ganse E. Influence of lansoprazole treatment on diazepam plasma concentrations. Clin Pharmacol Ther. 1992;52(5):458–63.
187. Middle MV, MuÈller FO, Schall R, Groenewoud G, Hundt HK, Huber R, et al. No influence of pantoprazole on the pharmacokinetics of phenytoin. Int J Clin Pharmacol Ther. 1996;34(Suppl. 1):S72–5.
188. Karol MD, Locke CS, Cavanaugh JH. Lack of pharmacokinetic interaction between lansoprazole and intravenously administered phenytoin. J Clin Pharmacol. 1999;39(12):1283–9.
189. Humphries TJ. A review of the drug–drug interaction potential of rabeprazole sodium based on CYP-450 interference or absorption effects. Digestion. 1998;59(Suppl. 3):76.
190. Waisbren BA, Hueckel JS. Reduced absorption of aureomycin caused by aluminum hydroxide gel. Proc Soc Exp Biol Med. 1950;73(1):73–4.

191. Rosenblatt JE, Barrett JE, Brodie JL, et al. Comparison of in vitro activity and clinical pharmacology of doxycycline with other tetracyclines. Antimicrob Agents Chemother (Bethesda). 1966;6:134–41.
192. Höffken G, Borner K, Glatzel PD, et al. Reduced enteral absorption of ciprofloxacin in the presence of antacids [letter]. Eur J Clin Microbiol. 1985;4(3):345.
193. Saathoff N, Lode H, Neider K, et al. Pharmacokinetics of cefpodoximeproxetil and interactions with an antacid and an H2 receptor antagonist. Antimicrob Agents Chemother. 1992;36(4):796–800.
194. Shimada J, Saito A, Shiba K, et al. Effects of antacids on absorption, excretion and metabolism of cefterampivoxil [in Japanese]. Jpn J Antibiot. 1990 Aug;43(8):1353–70.
195. Blouin RA, Kneer J, Ambros RJ, et al. Influence of antacid and ranitidine on the pharmacokinetics of oral cefetametpivoxil. Antimicrob Agents Chemother. 1990;34(9):1744–8.
196. Deppermann KM, Lode H, Hoffken G, et al. Influence of ranitidine, pirenzepine, and aluminum magnesium hydroxide on the bioavailability of various antibiotics, including amoxicillin, cephalexin, doxycycline, and amoxicillin-clavulanic acid. Antimicrob Agents Chemother. 1989;33(11):1901–7.
197. Staniforth DH, Clarke HL, Horton R, et al. Augmentin bioavailability following cimetidine, aluminum hydroxide and milk. Int J Clin Pharmacol Ther Toxicol. 1985;23(3):154–7.
198. Albert KS, DeSante KA, Welch RD, et al. Pharmacokinetic evaluation of a drug interaction between kaolinpectin and clindamycin. J Pharm Sci. 1978;67(11):1579–82.
199. Chandra R, Liu P, Breen JD, et al. Clinical pharmacokinetics and gastrointestinal tolerability of a novel extended-release microsphere formulation of azithromycin. Clin Pharmacokinet. 2007;46(3):247–59.
200. Yamreudeewong W, Scavone JM, Paone RP, et al. Effect of antacid coadministration on the bioavailability of erythromycin stearate. Clin Pharm. 1989;8(5):352–4.
201. Grunder G, Zysset-Aschmann Y, Vollenweider F, et al. Lack of pharmacokinetic interaction between linezolid and antacid in healthy volunteers. Antimicrob Agents Chemother. 2006;50(1):68–72.
202. Gupta KC, Desai NK, Satoskar RS, et al. Effect of pectin and kaolin on bioavailability of co-trimoxazole suspension. Int J Clin Pharmacol Ther Toxicol. 1987;25(6):320–1.
203. Pai MP, Momary KM, Rodvold KA. Antibiotic drug interactions. Med Clin. 2006;90(6):1223–55.
204. Sorgel F, Granneman GR, Stephan U, et al. Effect of cimetidine on the pharmacokinetic of temafloxacin. Clin Pharmacokinet. 1992;22(Suppl. 1):75–82.
205. Janknegt R. Drug interactions with quinolones. J Antimicrob Chemother. 1990;26(Suppl. D):7–29.
206. Gugler R, Allgayer H. Effects of antacids on the clinical pharmacokinetics of drugs: an update. Clin Pharmacokinet. 1990;18:210–9.
207. Powell JR, Donn KH. The pharmacokinetic basis for H2-antagonist drug interactions: concepts and implications. J Clin Gastroenterol. 1983;5(Suppl. 1):95–113. https://doi.org/10.1097/00004836-198312001-00010.
208. Cole JJ, Charles BG, Ravenscroft PJ. Interaction of cimetidine with tetracycline absorption. Lancet. 1980;2(8193):536. https://doi.org/10.1016/s0140-6736(80)91860-7.
209. Garty M, Hurwitz A. Effect of cimetidine and antacids on gastrointestinal absorption of tetracycline. Clin Pharmacol Ther. 1980;28:203–7.
210. Fisher P, House F, Inns P, Morrison PJ, Rogers HJ, Bradbrook ID. Effect of cimetidine on the absorption of orally administered tetracycline. Br J Clin Pharmacol. 1980;9:153–8.
211. Rogers HJ, James CA, Morrison PJ, Bradbrook ID. Effect of cimetidine on oral absorption of ampicillin and cotrimoxazole. J Antimicrob Chemother. 1980;6:297–300.
212. Richards DA. Comparative pharmacodynamics and pharmacokinetics of cimetidine and ranitidine. J Clin Gastroenterol. 1983;5(Suppl. 1):81–90. https://doi.org/10.1097/00004836-198312001-00008.
213. Gugler R, Jensen JC. Interaction between cimetidine and metronidazole. N Engl J Med. 1983;309(24):1518–9. https://doi.org/10.1056/NEJM198312153092412.

214. Eradiri O, Jamali F, Thomson AB. Interaction of metronidazole with phenobarbital, cimetidine, prednisone, and sulfasalazine in Crohn's disease. Biopharm Drug Dispos. 1988;9(2):219–27. https://doi.org/10.1002/bod.2510090210.
215. Loft S, Døssing M, Sonne J, Dalhof K, Bjerrum K, Poulsen HE. Lack of effect of cimetidine on the pharmacokinetics and metabolism of a single oral dose of metronidazole. Eur J Clin Pharmacol. 1988;35(1):65–8. https://doi.org/10.1007/BF00555509.
216. Furuta T, Ohashi K, Kobayashi K, Iida I, Yoshida H, Shirai N, et al. Effects of clarithromycin on the metabolism of omeprazole in relation to CYP2C19 genotype status in humans. Clin Pharmacol Ther. 1999;66:265–74.
217. Washington C, Hou E, Hughes N, Berner B. Effect of omeprazole on bioavailability of an oral extended-release formulation of ciprofloxacin. Am J Health Syst Pharm. 2006;63(7):653–6. https://doi.org/10.2146/ajhp050355.
218. David FL, Da Silva CM, Mendes FD, et al. Acid suppression by omeprazole does not affect orally administered metronidazole bioavailability and metabolism in healthy male volunteers. Aliment Pharmacol Ther. 1998;12(4):349–54. https://doi.org/10.1046/j.1365-2036.1998.00298.x.
219. Calabresi L, Pazzucconi F, Ferrara S, Di Paolo A, Tacca MD, Sirtori C. Pharmacokinetic interactions between omeprazole/pantoprazole and clarithromycin in health volunteers. Pharmacol Res. 2004;49(5):493–9. https://doi.org/10.1016/j.phrs.2003.10.010.
220. Ford SL, Wire MB, Lou Y, et al. Effect of antacids and ranitidine on the single-dose pharmacokinetics of fosamprenavir. Antimicrob Agents Chemother. 2005;49(1):467–9.
221. Kaul S, Olszyk C, Ji P, et al. Pharmacokinetics of didanosine enteric coated capsules co-administered with atazanavir or atazanavir/ritonavir [abstract no. 648]. In: 12th Conference on retroviruses and opportunistic infections; 2005 Feb 22–25; Boston, MA, 2005.
222. Vourvahis M, Banerjee S, LaBadie R, et al. Lack of a clinically relevant effect of an antacid on the pharmacokinetics of lersivirine. Antimicrob Agents Chemother. 2010;54(5):2209–11.
223. Kiser JJ, Bumpass JB, Meditz AL, et al. Effect of antacids on the pharmacokinetics of raltegravir in human immunodeficiency virus-seronegative volunteers. Antimicrob Agents Chemother. 2010;54(12):4999–5003.
224. Snell P, Oo C, Dorr A, et al. Lack of pharmacokinetic interaction between the oral anti-influenza neuraminidase inhibitor prodrug oseltamivir and antacids. Br J Clin Pharmacol. 2002;54(4):372–7.
225. de Bony F, Bidault R, Peck R, Posner J. Lack of interaction between valaciclovir, the L-valyl ester of acyclovir, and Maalox antacid. J Antimicrob Chemother. 1996;37(2):383–7. https://doi.org/10.1093/jac/37.2.383.
226. Agarwala S, Thal G, Nettles R, Bertz R. Further information on the administration of h2-receptor antagonists with atazanavir. J Acquir Immune Defic Syndr. 2006;42(4):516. https://doi.org/10.1097/01.qai.0000221687.75434.b4.
227. Dahri K, Lum E. Atazanavir and acid-lowering therapy. Can J Hosp Pharm. 2008;61(1)
228. Knupp CA, Graziiano FM, Dixon RM, et al. Pharmacokinetic interaction study of didanosine and ranitidine in patients seropositive for human immunodeficiency virus. Antimicrob Agents Chemother. 1992;36:2075–9.
229. Schöller-Gyüre M, Kakuda TN, De Smedt G, et al. A pharmacokinetic study of etravirine (TMC125) co-administered with ranitidine and omeprazole in HIV-negative volunteers. Br J Clin Pharmacol. 2008;66(4):508–16. https://doi.org/10.1111/j.1365-2125.2008.03214.x.
230. Lewis JM, Stott KE, Monnery D, Seden K, Beeching NJ, Chaponda M, Khoo S, Beadsworth MB. Managing potential drug-drug interactions between gastric acid-reducing agents and antiretroviral therapy: experience from a large HIV-positive cohort. Int J STD AIDS. 2016;27(2):105–9.
231. De Bony F, Tod M, Bidault R, On NT, Posner J, Rolan P. Multiple interactions of cimetidine and probenecid with valaciclovir and its metabolite acyclovir. Antimicrob Agents Chemother. 2002;46(2):458–63. https://doi.org/10.1128/aac.46.2.458-463.2002.

232. Perry CM, Wagstaff AJ. Famciclovir: a review of its pharmacological properties and therapeutic efficacy in herpesvirus infections. Drugs. 1995;50(2):396–415. https://doi.org/10.2165/00003495-199550020-00011.
233. Kis O, Walmsley SL, Bendayan R. In Vitro and In Situ evaluation of pH-dependence of atazanavir intestinal permeability and interactions with acid-reducing agents. Pharm Res. 2014;31:2404–19.
234. Fang AF, Damle BD, LaBadie RR, et al. Significant decrease in nelfinavir systemic exposure after omeprazole coadministration in healthy subjects. Pharmacotherapy. 2008;28:42–50.
235. Burger DM, Hugen PW, Kroon FP, et al. Pharmacokinetic interaction between the proton pump inhibitor omeprazole and the HIV protease inhibitor indinavir. AIDS. 1998;12:2080–2.
236. Overton ET, Tschampa JM, Klebert M, et al. The effect of acid reduction with a proton pump inhibitor on the pharmacokinetics of lopinavir or ritonavir in HIV-infected patients on lopinavir/ritonavir-based therapy. J Clin Pharmacol. 2010;50:1050–5.
237. Ouwerkerk-Mahadevan S, Snoeys J, Peeters M, et al. Drug-drug Interactions with the NS3/4A Protease Inhibitor Simeprevir. Clin Pharmacokinet. 2015;55(2):197–208.
238. McCabe SM, Smith PF, Ma Q, Morse GD. Drug interactions between proton pump inhibitors and antiretroviral drugs. Expert Opin Drug Metab Toxicol. 2007;3(2):197–207. https://doi.org/10.1517/17425255.3.2.197.
239. Iwamoto M, Wenning LA, Nguyen B-Y, et al. Effects of omeprazole on plasma levels of raltegravir. Clin Infect Dis. 2009;48:489–92.
240. Tappouni HL, Rublein JC, Donovan BJ, et al. Effect of omeprazole on the plasma concentrations of indinavir when administered alone and in combination with ritonavir. Am J Health Syst Pharm. 2008;65(5):422–8. https://doi.org/10.2146/ajhp070226.
241. Scholler-Gyure M, Kakuda TN, De Smedt G, et al. A pharmacokinetic study of etravirine (TMC125) co-administered with ranitidine and omeprazole in HIV–volunteers. Br J Clin Pharmacol. 2008;66:508–16.
242. Hughes CA, Robinson L, Tseng A, MacArthur RD. New antiretroviral drugs: a review of the efficacy, safety, pharmacokinetics, and resistance profile of tipranavir, darunavir, etravirine, rilpivirine, maraviroc, and raltegravir. Expert Opin Pharmacother. 2009;10(15):2445–66. https://doi.org/10.1517/14656560903176446.
243. Brass C, Galgiani JN, Blaschke TF, et al. Disposition of ketoconazole, an oral antifungal, in humans. Antimicrob Agents Chemother. 1982;21(1):151–8.
244. Lohitnavy M, Lohitnavy O, Thangkeattiyanon O, et al. Reduced oral itraconazole bioavailability by antacid suspension. J Clin Pharm Ther. 2005;30(3):201–6.
245. Thorpe JE, Baker N, Bromet-Petit M. Effect of oral antacid administration on the pharmacokinetics of oral fluconazole. Antimicrob Agents Chemother. 1990;34(10):2032–3.
246. Courtney R, Radwanski E, Lim J, et al. Pharmacokinetics of posaconazolecoadministered with antacid in fasting or nonfasting healthy men. Antimicrob Agents Chemother. 2004;48(3):804–8.
247. Kosoglou T, Perentesis GP, Affrime MB, et al. The effect of antacid and cimetidine on the oral absorption of the antifungal agent SCH 39304. J Clin Pharmacol. 1990;30(7):638–42.
248. Van der Meer JWM, Keuning JJ, Scheijgrond HW, Heykants J, Van Cutsem J, Brugmans J. The influence of gastric acidity on the bioavailability of ketoconazole. J Antimicrob Chemother. 1980;6:552–4.
249. Katz HI. Possible drug interactions in oral treatment of onychomycosis. J Am Podiatr Med Assoc. 1997;87(12):571–4. https://doi.org/10.7547/87507315-87-12-571.
250. Katz HI. Drug interactions of the newer oral antifungal agents. Br J Dermatol. 1999;141(Suppl. 56):26–32. https://doi.org/10.1046/j.1365-2133.1999.00011.x.
251. Piscitelli SC, Goss TF, Wilton JH, et al. Effects of ranitidine and sucralfate on ketaconazole bioavailability. Antimicrob Agents Chemother. 1991;35:1765–71.
252. Shear N, Drake L, Gupta AK, Lambert J, Yaniv R. The implications and management of drug interactions with itraconazole, fluconazole and terbinafine. Dermatology. 2000;201(3):196–203. https://doi.org/10.1159/000018488.

253. Heaton A. High frequency of itraconazole prescriptions with potentially interacting medications in a large health care plan. J Manag Care Spec Pharm. 2002;8:199–203.
254. Jaruratanasirikul S, Sriwiriyajan S. Effect of omeprazole on the pharmacokinetics of itraconazole. Eur J Clin Pharmacol. 1998;54(2):159–61.
255. Humphries TJ, Nardi RV, Spera AC, Lazer JD, Laurent AL, Spanyers SA. Coadministration of rabeprazolesodium (E3810) and ketoconazole results in a predictable interaction with ketoconazole. [Abstract]. Gastroenterology. 1996;110(4):138.
256. Chin TW, Loeb M, Fong IW. Effects of an acidic beverage (Coca-Cola) on absorption of ketoconazole. Antimicrob Agents Chemother. 1995;39(8):1671–5. https://doi.org/10.1128/aac.39.8.1671.
257. Itraconazole oral solution package insert. Titusville (NJ): Janssen Pharmaceutica Inc; February 1997.
258. Kang BC, Yang CQ, Cho HK, Suh OK, Shin WG. Influence of fluconazole on the pharmacokinetics of omeprazole in healthy volunteers. Biopharm Drug Dispos. 2002;23(2):77–81. https://doi.org/10.1002/bdd.291.
259. Tarnawski A, Tanoue K, Santos AM, Sarfeh IJ. Cellular and molecular mechanisms of gastric ulcer healing. Is the quality of mucosal scar affected by treatment? Scand J Gastroenterol Suppl. 1995;210:9.
260. Soll AH, Weinstein WM, Kurata J, McCarthy D. Nonsteroidal anti-inflammatory drugs and peptic ulcer disease. Ann Intern Med. 1991;114(4):307.
261. Gladziwa U, Koltz U. Pharmacokinetic optimisation of the treatment of peptic ulcer in patients with renal failure. Clin Pharmacokinet. 1994;27(5):393.
262. Chines A, Pacifici R. Antacid and sucralfate-induced hypophosphatemic osteomalacia: a case report and review of the literature. Calcif Tissue Int. 1990;47(5):291.
263. Sucralfate:Drug information—UpToDate. Accsessed: 10 June 2020.
264. Gorbach SL. Bismuth therapy in gastrointestinal diseases. Gastroenterology. 1990;99(3):863.
265. Wagstaff AJ, Benfield P, Monk JP. Colloidal bismuth subcitrate. A review of its pharmacodynamic and pharmacokinetic properties, and its therapeutic use in peptic ulcer disease. Drugs. 1988;36(2):132.
266. Nwokolo CU, Gavey CJ, Smith JT, Pounder RE. The absorption of bismuth from oral doses of tripotassium dicitrato bismuthate. Aliment Pharmacol Ther. 1989;3(1):29.
267. Nwokolo CU, Prewett EJ, Sawyer AM, et al. Lack of bismuth absorption from bismuth subnitrate (Roter) tablets. Eur J Gastroenterol Hepatol. 1990;2:433.
268. Nwokolo CU, Prewett EJ, Sawyerr AM, Hudson M, Pounder RE. The effect of histamine H2-receptor blockade on bismuth absorption from three ulcer-healing compounds. Gastroenterology. 1991;101(4):889.
269. Sweeney JD, Hoernig LA. Hemostatic effects of salsalate in normal subjects and patients with hemophilia A. Thromb Res. 1991;61(1):23.
270. Danesh BJ, McLaren M, Russell RI, Lowe GD, Forbes CD. Comparison of the effect of aspirin and choline magnesium trisalicylate on thromboxane biosynthesis in human platelets: role of the acetyl moiety. Haemostasis. 1989;19(3):169.
271. Cohen A. Fecal blood loss and plasma salicylate study of salicylsalicylic acid and aspirin. J Clin Pharmacol. 1979;19(4):242.
272. Torgyán S, Ady E, Wagner L, Neumann T, Béres G, Csányi M. Reduction of indomethacin-induced gastrointestinal blood loss by sodium salicylate in man. Int J Clin Pharmacol Biopharm. 1978;16(12):610.
273. Drug Interactions between acetazolamide and bismuth subsalicylate. https://www.drugs.com/drug-interactions/acetazolamide-with-bismuth-subsalicylate-86-0-391-0.html?professional=1. Accessed 14 June 2020.
274. Drug Interactions between bismuth subsalicylate and brinzolamide ophthalmic. https://www.drugs.com/drug-interactions/bismuth-subsalicylate-with-brinzolamide-ophthalmic-391-0-411-0.html?professional=1. Accesed 14 June 2020.

275. Drug Interactions between bismuth subsalicylate and dichlorphenamide. https://www.drugs.com/drug-interactions/bismuth-subsalicylate-with-dichlorphenamide-391-0-868-0.html?professional=1. Accesed: 14 June 2020.
276. Drug Interactions between bismuth subsalicylate and dorzolamide ophthalmic. https://www.drugs.com/drug-interactions/bismuth-subsalicylate-with-dorzolamide-ophthalmic-391-0-930-0.html?professional=1. Accesed 14 June 2020.
277. Drug Interactions between bismuth subsalicylate and methazolamide. https://www.drugs.com/drug-interactions/bismuth-subsalicylate-with-methazolamide-391-0-1580-0.html?professional=1. Accesed 14 June 2020.
278. Bismuth subsalicylate Drug Interactions. https://www.drugs.com/drug-interactions/bismuth-subsalicylate-index.html. Accessed 20 June 2020.
279. Rambout L, Sahai J, Gallicano K, Oliveras L, Garber G. Effect of bismuth subsalicylate on ciprofloxacin bioavailability. Antimicrob Agents Chemother. 1994;38(9):2187–90. https://doi.org/10.1128/aac.38.9.2187.
280. Ericsson CD, Feldman S, Pickering LK, Cleary TG. Influence of subsalicylate bismuth on absorption of doxycycline. JAMA. 1982;247(16):2266–7.
281. Chen MC, Amirian DA, Toomey M, Sanders MJ, Soll AH. Prostanoid inhibition of canine parietal cells: mediation by the inhibitory guanosine triphosphate-binding protein of adenylate cyclase. Gastroenterology. 1988;94(5 Pt 1):1121.
282. Feldman M. Prostaglandins and gastric ulcers: from seminal vesicle to misoprostol (Cytotec). Am J Med Sci. 1990;300(2):116.
283. Karim A, Rozek LF, Smith ME, Kowalski KG. Effects of food and antacid on oral absorption of misoprostol, a synthetic prostaglandin E1 analog. J Clin Pharmacol. 1989;29:439–43.
284. Product Information. Arthrotec (diclofenac-misoprostol). Searle, Skokie, IL.
285. Drug Interactions between dinoprostone topical and misoprostol. https://www.drugs.com/drug-interactions/dinoprostone-topical-with-misoprostol-895-0-1641-0.html?professional=1. Accessed 14 June 2020.

28 Intestinal Inflammation: Conventional Anti-Inflammatory Drugs

Alen Biščanin, Petra Ćaćić, and Marko Banić

Introduction

Inflammatory bowel diseases [IBD], including the syndrome of colitis represent the paradigm of intestinal inflammation, and the prevalence of IBD in some western, highly industrialized countries has reached almost 0.5% in these populations.

Before the mid of twentieth century, the incidence of ulcerative colitis was significantly higher than the incidence of Crohn's disease, and recent data suggests that the incidence of Crohn's disease is growing rapidly, approaching that of ulcerative colitis. Time-trend analysis also showed a significant increase in the overall IBD incidence, over time [1].

Taking into account the relatively stable genetic background of the human population, the increase in IBD incidence reflects the influence of environmental exposure or exposome. Very important notion is the difference in IBD phenotype across the age spectrum, with the environment playing the greater role in cohort of elderly onset IBD that represents 15% of patients with IBD. According to the results of clinical and translational studies, the genetic background plays a major role in the onset of the disease during infancy and childhood, especially in the cases of monogenic/oligogenic disease [2].

A. Biščanin (✉) · P. Ćaćić
Department of Gastroenterology and Hepatology, Sestre Milosrdnice University Hospital Center, Zagreb, Croatia

M. Banić
Division for IBD and Clinical Nutrition, Department of Gastroenterology, Hepatology and Clinical Nutrition, Dubrava University Hospital, Zagreb, Croatia

School of Medicine, University of Zagreb, Zagreb, Croatia

School of Medicine, University of Rijeka, Rijeka, Croatia
e-mail: mbanic@kbd.hr

M. Banić, D. Erceg (eds.), *Drug Interactions in Gastroenterology*, Clinical Gastroenterology, https://doi.org/10.1007/978-3-031-69800-2_28

Inflammatory bowel diseases represent complex and life-long inflammatory disorders and therapeutic approaches may vary between clinicians and between practices in different countries. In order to overcome this problem and aiming to unify the balanced therapeutic approaches and modalities for IBD, the guidelines have been developed on the local, national, and international levels. The several guidelines and topical reviews (European Crohn's and Colitis Organization—ECCO, American College of Gastroenterology—ACG, American Gastroenterology Association—AGA, British Society of Gastroenterology—BSG) have strived to cover the field of diagnosis, management (medical and surgical), treatment of special situations (penetrating/fistulizing disease, complicated disease with strictures and loss of intestinal function, extraintestinal complications), approach to opportunistic infections, and surveillance of the patients during the course of the disease. Noteworthy, modern civilization, medicine, and healthcare are challenged by an increasing number of elderly, a fact that implies polypharmacy, due to growing comorbidity and co-medication in the elderly population. All these lead to an increased risk of clinically significant drug interactions in the elderly. The results of a Swedish study, published a quarter of a century ago observed that the average number of prescriptions in elderly outpatients was more than five [3]. Since that time, the growth of the therapeutic armamentarium has exceeded beyond the expectations of health professionals. In light of this, the risks of clinically significant drug interactions strongly influence the patient's outcomes and related healthcare costs. Thus, the special clinical challenge represents the avoidance of significant drug interactions in children and elderly, immunocompromised, and cancer patients. Drug interactions in pediatric gastroenterology and oncology patients are beyond the scope of this book.

The current therapeutic armamentarium for treating intestinal inflammation in IBD in clinical practice encompasses conventional agents (5-ASA derivatives, corticosteroids, immunomodulators—thiopurines and methothrexate, calcineurin inhibitors, and antibiotics) and newly designed biologics and small molecules. In treating the symptoms, the antisecretory agents (histamine H2 antagonists and proton pump inhibitors), antidiarrheals, antispasmodic agents, bile acid sequestrants, and analgesics (NSAIDs) can be also used, episodically. In general, the therapeutic approach in adult patients should also consider the biological age of the individual patients.

In regard to the use of conventional drugs during the course of IBD, the therapeutic regimens are combined and sequential, and the specific combinations are not effective in all patients. On the other hand, the specific combination of conventional drugs does not represent the adequate therapeutic regimen in variable disease extent and in all phases of disease activity, during the biological course of the disease in an individual patient. However, conventional drugs and their combinations represent the mainstay of therapy for IBD patients with mild to moderate disease. Basic mechanisms of drug interactions in regard to the use of conventional anti-inflammatory therapy with other drugs include the effects on absorption, distribution, metabolism, and elimination, so-called pharmacokinetic interactions (see also Chaps. 9 and 13). Pharmacodynamic interactions include synergistic or antagonistic effects, and clinically significant idiosyncratic reactions are quite rare [4].

5-ASA Compounds

Mesalamine

Therapeutic Indication and Dose Range

Mesalamine, also known as mesalazine or 5-aminosalicylic acid (5-ASA), is a medication used to treat mild to moderate ulcerative colitis (UC). Novel meta-analyses and ECCO guidelines positioned it as obsolete in the treatment of Crohn's disease (CD) [5]. Nowadays various formulations of oral and topical drugs are available. In treatment of the active form of UC, recommended doses are as follows: 1 g of mesalamine suppository once daily (with or without oral mesalamine) for proctitis; combination of mesalamine enema >1 g and oral mesalamine ≥2.4 g per day in case of left-sided or extensive colitis. Daily oral doses shouldn't exceed 4 g. Remission maintenance doses are 2 g/day of oral mesalamine and 3 g/week in divided doses for rectal treatment.

Pathophysiologic Mechanisms

Although the exact mechanism of action remains poorly elucidated, it is supposed that mesalamine acts directly/locally to the inflamed intestinal mucosa, while systemic drug products are meant to be connected with side effects. Studies suggest mesalamine inhibits the production of cytokines and leukotrienes by interfering with cyclooxygenase and lipoxygenase pathways. It also may play an important role in the activation and proliferation of T cells and may have a strong antioxidant effect [6]. Mesalamine and other noncompound salicylic acid derivatives (e.g., acetylsalicyilc acid) tend to absorb in the upper part of gastrointestinal [GI] tract. In order to deliver mesalamine molecules to the distal part of GI tract, a few different pharmacoengineering solutions have been adopted (Table 28.1) [7]. Time-dependent formulations are encapsulated with ethylcellulose semi-permeable membrane making active substances being slowly released from duodenum to the rectum. Coat of pH-dependent formulations dissolves at pH higher than 6 or 7, depending on the product, thus delivering a higher concentration of mesalamine to the distal ileum and colon. Multimatrix system (MMX) is a technology based on a double-layer capsule. Outer lipophilic layer dissolves at the terminal ileum after which the inner hydrophilic matrix reacts with intestinal fluid and swells to form a viscous gel mass, maintaining a controlled release of active substance throughout the entire colon.

Table 28.1 Pharmacoengineering solutions in order to deliver mesalamine molecules to the distal part of gastrointestinal tract

Time-dependent formulations	pH-dependent formulations	Multimatrix system	Azo-bonded prodrugs
Pentasa®	Asacol®	Mezavant®	Sulfasalazine
	Mesren®	Lialda®	Olsalazine
	Salofalk®	Mezavant XL®	Balsalazide
	Mesasal®		
	Claversal®		

Topical formulations, suppositories, enemas, and rectal foams are appropriate for distal colitis and proctitis.

After contact with the intestinal mucosa mesalamine is partially absorbed and metabolized into N-acetyl mesalamine. Acetylated mesalamine is mostly eliminated by kidney and nonacetylated by feces.

Clinical Aspects and Drug Interactions

According to guidelines, complete blood count, liver enzymes, and renal function [including urinalysis] should be assessed prior to initiation of 5-ASA products and 14 days after the introduction of therapy. In the following 2–3 months, regular monthly examinations should be done. If there are no side effects, periodic controls should be arranged every 3 months.

Gastric Acid Suppression Medications: Mesalamine

Antacids, histamine H2 receptor antagonists, and proton pump inhibitors (PPI) can interfere with all oral Ph-dependent formulations and MMX. According to studies, H2 antagonists and PPIs can elevate intragastric pH over 6 for 17–23% of a 24-h period [8, 9]. That can cause significant coat dissolving in the upper part of the GI tract so very few mesalamine would reach the colon. On the other side, agents that lower colonic pH [e.g., lactulose], can disturb absorption in the opposite direction—pH will remain low throughout the whole GI tract, so pH-dependent mesalamine formulations will be excreted intact.

In case of indication for concomitant use, try to avoid mesalamine administration during period of peak PPI acid-suppressing effects.

Varicella Virus-Containing Vaccines: 5-ASA Derivatives

Although a rare finding, Rey's syndrome is greater among children given salicylate during varicella virus infection. Albeit, there is no strong evidence showing 5-ASA derivatives can interfere with varicella vaccines, manufacturers recommend avoiding salicylates for at least 6 weeks after vaccination [10, 11].

Anticoagulants: 5-ASA Derivatives

Concomitant administration of 5-ASA and high- or low-molecular weight heparins may increase the risk of bleeding. Studies have shown contradictory information on the antiplatelet effect of nonacetylated salicylates. Interestingly, IBD patients seem to have higher baseline platelet activation and 5-ASA derivatives may decrease it [12]. It remains unknown whether it is due to direct antiplatelet or therapeutic effects.

If there is a need for concomitant administration of 5-ASA derivatives and heparins, increased bleeding monitoring is recommended.

Although 5-ASA derivatives may increase the adverse/toxic effects of vitamin K antagonists, no action is required except with sulfasalazine. Namely, some case reports described decreased [13] while others reported an increase [14] in INR after introducing sulfasalazine in patients on chronic warfarin therapy. Thereby, consider performing INR testing more frequently in those patients.

Nonsteroidal Anti-Inflammatory Agents [NSAIDs]: 5-ASA Derivatives

Though real incidence remains unknown, studies suggest 5-ASA products may cause interstitial nephritis [15]. Combination with well-known nephrotoxic agents such as NSAIDs may enhance this effect. It is recommended to frequently monitor all patients on concomitant NSAIDs and 5-ASA derivatives therapy for the development of nephrotoxicity, especially those with renal impairment.

Thiopurine Analogs: 5-ASA Derivatives

Studies showed that 5-ASA agents, sulfasalazine and olsalazine, may decrease the metabolism of thiopurine analogs and enhance their toxicity [16, 17]. It seems both agents inhibit thiopurine methyltransferase (TPMT), so special vigilance is warranted among patients with low or absent TMPT activity.

Cardiac Glycosides: 5-ASA Derivatives

Cardiac glycosides are a group of agents with a narrow therapeutic range and 5-ASA derivatives can decrease their serum concentration [18]. It is recommended to monitor serum concentrations of cardiac glycosides in case of initiation, discontinuation, or dose changing of 5-ASA derivatives.

Myelosuppressive Agents: Mesalamine

Mesalamine prescribing information caution on enhanced myelosuppressive effect in case of concomitant use with myelosuppressive agents. Close monitoring of bone marrow toxicity and associated complications is necessary.

Sulfasalazine

Therapeutic Indication, Dose Range, and Pathophysiologic Mechanisms

Sulfasalazine is azo-bonded prodrug compound of mesalamine and sulfapyridine. The drug is activated in the colon where azoreductase containing colonic bacteria cleaves azo-bond and releases mesalamine. Albeit, sulfapyridine moiety tends to have some anti-inflammatory effects, it is mostly connected with side effects in the therapy of UC. In contrast to mesalamine, this derivative showed a small effect of borderline statistical significance in the therapy of CD [5]. In case of acute attacks, the recommended therapy is 4–8 g divided into four equal doses per day. The maintenance dosage is 500 mg four times per day [19].

Clinical Aspects and Drug Interactions

Sulfasalazine is contraindicated in patients allergic to salicylates or sulfonamides, and in patients with porphyria. Special cautiousness is necessary in patients with known glucose 6 phosphate dehydrogenase deficiency [19]. Sulfasalazine can cause reversible oligospermia. Sperm count is usually normalized 2–3 months after drug withdrawal. For precaution measures and drug interactions connected with mesalamine, see previous section. Chemical interactions connected with a sulfapyridine moiety of sulfasalazine are:

Sulfonylurea Derivatives: Sulfasalazine

Biochemical similarity between insulin secretagogues and sulfasalazine is a probable cause of interactions among those groups. Namely, sulfasalazine can induce hypoglycemia in patients taking derivatives of sulfonylurea, so blood glucose should be regularly monitored [19].

Folate: Sulfasalazine

Absorption and metabolism of folate, its activated form 5-methyltetrahydrofolate (5-MTHF) as well as synthetic folic acid, are highly influenced by sulfasalazine [20]. IBD patients are at a greater risk of folate deficiency due to inflammation, so additional decrement caused by sulfasalazine may seriously endanger those patients. It is necessary to closely monitor the response to folic acid supplementation, especially in pregnant women.

Immunosuppressants: Sulfasalazine

Sulfasalazine is a potentially hepatotoxic agent [19] and its toxicity can be enhanced when administered with other liver-toxic drugs such as methotrexate [21]. When used together, there is also a higher incidence of GI side effects, especially nausea. If there is an indication of concomitant use of these two molecules, intensify monitoring for hepatotoxicity.

Sulfasalazine can significantly decrease the serum concentration of cyclosporine [22], so frequent monitoring of cyclosporine serum concentration is recommended.

Voxilaprevir: Sulfasalazine

Sulfasalazine should be discontinued in a patient who starts voxilaprevir therapy. Pharmacokinetic studies revealed voxilaprevir can increase serum concentrations of BCRP/ABCG2 substrates [23], and sulfasalazine is one of them.

Local Anesthetics: Sulfasalazine

Both, sulfasalazine and local anesthetics, are potentially methemoglobinemia precipitating agents. Patients suffering glucose 6 phosphate deficiencies or idiopathic methemoglobinemia are under a greater risk [24]. Careful monitoring for methemoglobinemia (e.g., hypoxia, cyanosis) is endorsed.

Other Clinically Significant Drug Interactions of Sulfasalazine Are Described with

Lasmiditan, methenamine, riluzole, tolvaptan, eltrombopag, nitric oxide, osimertinib, regorafenib, rolapitant, sodium nitrite, tafamidis, teriflunomide, etanerecept, dapsone, tedizolid (additional information: https://www.webmd.com/interaction-checker/default.htm).

Olsalazine

Therapeutic Indication, Dose Range, and Pathophysiologic Mechanisms

Olsalazine is also a prodrug, a compound of two molecules of mesalamine connected with azo-bond [7]. It is used for the treatment of mild active ulcerative colitis and maintenance of remission, particularly in patients intolerant of a sulfa moiety of sulfasalazine. A single dose should not exceed 1 g, and the daily dose should be titrated up to 3 g daily over 1 week. Due to molecular splitting in colon hyperosmolar, diarrhea is a profound side effect which can be minimized by taking drugs with food [25].

Special warning, precautions, and drug interactions are described in the section Mesalamine.

Balsalazide

Therapeutic Indication, Dose Range, and Pathophysiologic Mechanisms

Balsalazide consists of mesalamine and 4-aminobenzoyl-β-alanine molecule linked with azo-bond. Indication, special warning, precautions, and drug interactions are same as with other 5-ASA compounds (see previous section).

Topical Corticosteroids

Budesonide

Therapeutic Indication and Dose Range

Budesonide is a potent topical steroid used for induction of remission in patients with mild to moderate CD and UC [5] as well as microscopic colitis [26]. Location and extension of disease determine preferable drug formulation. In the case of UC, prescribing budesonide as add-on therapy to 5-ASA agents may prove beneficial in achieving remission [27]. Budesonide is absolutely indicated in 5-ASA nonresponders or drug intolerance.

Therapeutic dose for oral formulation is 9 mg once daily [or divided into 3 equal doses], and for rectal foams, enemas and suppositories 2 mg per day. Maximum duration of treatment shouldn't exceed 8 weeks. As with all steroids, budesonide needs to be tapered before complete discontinuation of the medication. Recommended scheme is: induction dose, 9 mg, during 4 weeks, followed by 3 mg reduction every 4 weeks (9, 6, 3 mg).

Pathophysiologic Mechanisms

Oral budesonide is available in the market in the form of pH and time-dependent formulation as well as MMX (for detailed information, see 5-ASA section).

Although the exact mechanism of action remains unknown, it is thought budesonide acts directly on the gut mucosa. After absorption, it undergoes extensive first-pass elimination via CYP3A4 making its hydroxylated metabolites negligible corticosteroid active [28]. Nonmetabolized molecules have significantly less impact on suppression of hypothalamic pituitary adrenal axis and immune cells, even in systemic corticosteroid equivalent doses.

Clinical Aspects and Drug Interactions

Special cautiousness is necessary for patients with hepatic cirrhosis, peptic ulcers, arterial hypertension, diabetes, osteoporosis, and tuberculosis. In the case of long-term administration, systemic side effects such as adrenal suppression, Cushing syndrome, decrease in bone density, and psychiatric disorders may occur.

Saluretics: Budesonide

Nonpotassium-sparing diuretics and budesonide have a synergistic effect on potassium excretion in the kidney. It is important to have that in mind when introducing potassium replacement therapy [26].

Antacids: Budesonide

As budesonide oral formulations are pH-dependent, any change in hydrogen ion concentration may interrupt drug pharmacodynamics. Consider separating the dose by 2 or more hours to minimize the interaction.

Vaccines: Corticosteroids

Vaccines containing live or attenuated microorganisms should be avoided during corticosteroid therapy because of the high risk of infection. On the other side, vaccination with inactivated vaccines can be diminished by the immunosuppressive effect of corticosteroids. If the patient is vaccinated with inactive vaccine during or 2 weeks prior to initiation of immunosuppressive therapy, revaccination should be done at least 3 months after drug discontinuation [29]. Similar recommendations are stated in intravesical BCG prescribing information.

Bile Acid Sequestrants: Oral Corticosteroids

Studies have shown that bile acid sequestrants can decrease the absorption of oral corticosteroids [30]. The suggested mechanism of interaction is the intraluminal binding of corticosteroids to sequestrants. Separating the administration of those agents by 2 or more hours can reduce the risk of interaction. According to colesevalm prescribing information, this time should be prolonged to 1 h prior or 4 h after sequestrants intake.

CYP3A4: Budesonide

As a CYP3A4 substrate, metabolism of budesonide is highly influenced by CYP3A4 inducers, inhibitors, and other competitive substrates.

Concomitant administration of budesonide and CYP3A4 inhibitors (see Table 28.2) should be avoided. Data showed ketoconazole, a strong CYP3A4

Table 28.2 CYP3A4 inhibitors

CYP3A4 inhibitors	CYP3A4 inducers	CYP3A4 substrates
Atazanavir, ceritinib, clarithromycin, cobicistat, darunavir, idelalisib, indinavir, itraconazole, ketoconazole [systemic], lopinavir, mifepristone, nefazodone, nelfinavir, ombitasvir, paritaprevir, simeprevir, ritonavir, ombitasvir, paritaprevir, and dasabuvir, posaconazole, saquinavir, telithromycin, tucatinib, voriconazole, aprepitant, conivaptan, crizotinib, diltiazem, dronedarone, duvelisib, erythromycin [systemic], fedratinib, fluconazole, fosamprenavir, fosnetupitant, grapefruit juice, imatinib, isavuconazonium sulfate, lefamulin, letermovir, netupitant, nilotinib, ribociclib, schisandra, verapamil	Aminoglutethimide, bexarotene, bosentan, carbamazepine, dexamethasone,efavirenz, fosphenytoin, griseofulvin, modafinil, nafcillin, nevirapine, oxcarbazepine, phenobarbital, phenytoin, primidone, rifabutin, rifampin, rifapentine, St. John's wort	Alfentanil, almotriptan, alprazolam, amiodarone, amlodipine, atazanavir, atorvastatin, bromocriptine, buprenorphine, bupropion, carbamazepine, clarithromycin, clonazepam, clopidogrel, colchicine, cyclophosphamide, ciclosporin, dihydroergotamine, diltiazem, donepezil, doxorubicin, dutasteride, eplerenone, ergotamine, erythromycin, fentanyl, finasteride, fosamprenavir, imatinib, levomethadyl, loperamide, lopinavir, loratadine, midazolam, mifepristone, nifedipine, oxycodone, paclitaxel, pioglitazone, quetiapine, ranolazine, repaglinide, ritonavir, sildenafil, simvastatin, sirolimus, tacrolimus, tadalafil, tamoxifen, tamsulosin, testosterone, verapamil, zolpidem

inhibitor, can cause sixfold increase in systemic budesonide exposure [26]. Cushing syndrome has been observed in patients taking budesonide and CYP3A4 inhibitors [31, 32]. If those combinations are inevitable, close monitoring for signs and symptoms of corticosteroid excess is mandatory.

Although most of CYP3A4 activity is presented in hepatocytes, this enzyme is also expressed in enterocytes. Thus, CYP3A4 inducers (see Table 28.2) may decrease both, systemic and local exposure to budesonide which may require higher corticosteroid doses.

Impact of other CYP3A4 (see Table 28.2) substrates on the metabolism of budesonide depends on the affinity of both agents. Before introducing any of these, please check individual interaction for each medication (https://www.webmd.com/interaction-checker/default.htm).

Other Clinically Significant Drug Interactions of Budesonide Are Described with

Aldesleukin, cladribine, conivaptan, fusidic acid, idelalisib, pimecrolimus, tacrolimus, upadacitinib, natalizumab, baricitinib, fingolimod, hyaluronidase, leflunomide, mifepristone, nivolumab, roflumilast, sipuleucel-T, stiripentol, aprepitant, clofazimine, coccidioides immitis skin test, corticorelin, deferasirox, denosumab, duvelisib, erdafitinib, fosaprepitant, fosnetupitant, larotrecitinib, netupitant, ocrelizumab, ozanimod, palbociclib, pidotimod, ritodrine, siponimod, tertomotide, trastuzumab, idebenone, luliconazole, piperaquine, pranlukast, echinacea (additional information: https://www.webmd.com/interaction-checker/default.htm).

Beclomethasone

Therapeutic Indication and Dose Range

Beclomethasone is a topical steroid, indicated for the treatment of active UC as add-on therapy to 5-ASA compounds or as a single therapy in 5-ASA nonresponders [33, 34]. Although, some data suggest beclomethasone may be beneficial in remission maintenance in mild to moderate CD [35], head-to-head studies with budesonide revealed its inferiority [36]. Therapeutic dose of beclomethasone is 5 mg per day for 4 weeks.

Pathophysiologic mechanisms, precaution measures, side effects, and drug interactions declared in Budesonide section are completely applicable to beclomethasone.

Systemic Corticosteroids

Therapeutic Indication and Dose Range

Prednisone, prednisolone, and methylprednisolone are systemic corticosteroids with a wide range of indications. They differ according to glucocorticoid and

Table 28.3 Glucocorticoid and mineralocorticoid potency ratio of corticosteroid drugs

	Relative glucocorticoid potency	Relative mineralocorticoid potency
Hydrocortisone	1	1
Prednisone	4	0.8
Prednisolone	4	0.8
Methylprednisolone	5	0.5

mineralocorticoid potency (see Table 28.3). Systemic corticosteroids are a mainstay therapy for induction of remission in moderate to severe CD and UC, as well as mild UC unresponsive to 5-ASA derivatives [5]. The appropriate regime in the case of CD is 0.5–0.75 mg/kg of oral prednisone and prednisolone with a maximum daily dose of 60 mg [37], and up to 48 mg per day of methylprednisolone [38]. Recommended daily dosage for active UC is 0.5–0.75 mg/kg of prednisone and prednisolone, and up to 60 mg of methylprednisolone [38]. Different tapering schemes are used worldwide, and there is neither evidence nor consensus about the superiority of any of them. After 7–10 days of the initial dose of prednisone/prednisolone, it is usually tapered by 5 mg per week, followed by a 2.5 mg decrease every week in doses below 20 mg [39]. Methylprednisolone can be tapered by 4 mg every week, or, in case of faster corticosteroid discontinuation necessity, by 8 mg every week till the dose of 24 mg. Doses below 24 mg should be tapered by 4 mg every week.

Pathophysiologic Mechanisms

After ingestion, corticosteroids are rapidly absorbed and widely distributed in the tissues. Before acting peripherally, prednisone has to be converted into prednisolone in the liver.

Corticosteroids have the potential to completely inhibit the immune system, primarily by activating intracellular receptors and various transcription factors, thus modifying gene expression. They also influence the metabolism of fat, proteins, and carbohydrates as well as the endocrine system. Although minor, prednisone, prednisolone, and methylprednisolone have mineralocorticoid effects, so they can interfere with fluid and electrolyte balance. Systemic corticosteroids are metabolized via the CYP3A4 enzyme and mostly excreted in the urine [39].

Clinical Aspects and Drug Interactions

All corticosteroids have a fast onset of action and a wide range of side effects. Special caution is necessary in patients with arterial hypertension, diabetes, osteoporosis, peptic ulcers, and glaucoma. Corticosteroids may cause Cushing syndrome and adrenal suppression if doses over 6 mg are administered for 3 or more weeks. Psychiatric disturbances have been observed for several weeks after drug introduction. Patients taking corticosteroids are at higher risk of thromboembolic incidents and are more prone to acquire opportunistic infection. In the case of latent tuberculosis, chemoprophylaxis should precede corticosteroid therapy. Passive immunization is mandatory in following 10 days after contact with varicella zoster in nonimmune patients who take, or were exposed to steroids 3 months ago. Exposure to measles should be avoided, otherwise immunoglobulin prophylaxis may be needed. For drug interaction with all types of vaccines and bile acid sequestrants, see section Budesonide.

Antacids: Corticosteroids

Although the antacids' impact on prednisone, prednisolone, and methylprednisolone isn't as profound as on budesonide, studies suggest they may decrease steroid absorption. However, these interactions have been confirmed only between systemic corticosteroids and aluminum/magnesium hydroxide [40] or magnesium trisilicate [41]. Interaction between systemic corticosteroids and PPI or H2 blockers wasn't found.

NSAIDs: Corticosteroids

Both NSAIDs and corticosteroids are well-known gastro erosive agents. Multiple studies have shown corticosteroids have been independently associated with gastrointestinal ulcerations [42, 43]. The incidence is even higher when coadministered with NSAIDs [44]. Probable mechanism of action in both agents is inhibition of prostaglandin synthesis and reduction in protective mucosal secretion. In case of concomitant administration, monitoring for signs and symptoms of upper GI upset is recommended. Although, COX-2 selective NSAIDs have fewer influences on prostaglandin synthesis, the same precaution measures are recommended.

Salicylates: Corticosteroids

There are two types of interaction between salicylates and corticosteroids. Similar to NSAIDs, salicylates can increase the risk of GI ulceration and bleeding when combined with corticosteroids. Albeit, the real mechanism of interaction remains poorly elucidated, corticosteroids may decrease the serum concentration of salicylates [45, 46]. Opposite, salicylate toxicity has been observed after corticosteroid withdrawal [47]. Besides monitoring for upper GI adverse events, salicylate concentration should be assessed after every alternation in corticosteroid therapy.

Cyclosporine: Corticosteroids

Various studies showed discrepant information about the interaction between cyclosporine and systemic corticosteroids. Several studies found a decreased clearance of prednisolone in patients receiving cyclosporine [48, 49] and vice versa, a decrease clearance of cyclosporine in patients taking systemic corticosteroids [50, 51]. There are also few studies that didn't find any change in drug contraction when those agents are given parallel [52–54]. Multiple interaction mechanisms have been proposed, but the exact one still remains unknown. However, monitoring in changes of cyclosporine concentration and the toxic effects of systemic corticosteroids is highly recommended.

CYP3A4: Corticosteroids

Although the interaction of systemic corticosteroids with CYP3A4 inhibitors and inducers (see Table 28.2) is not as prominent as with budesonide and beclomethasone, attention is warranted. Strong CYP3A4 inhibitors may increase plasma levels of corticosteroids, while the concomitant administration with inducers may demand higher doses of corticosteroids due to increased clearance. Before introducing any of these, please check individual interaction for each medication (https://www.webmd.com/interaction-checker/default.htm).

Antimicrobial Agents: Corticosteroids

The amphotericin B hypokalemic effect can be enhanced by concomitant corticosteroid therapy [55]. Cardiac function and serum electrolyte level should be monitored during therapy.

Lower serum isoniazid concentrations have been observed 8.5 h after administration of prednisolone [56]. Thus, reduced effects of isoniazid can be expected in those patients.

Postmarketing surveillance revealed a higher rate of tendonitis and tendon rupture in patients receiving quinolone antibiotics and systemic corticosteroid [57]. Any new-onset tendon or joint pain in those patients should raise suspicion about this pathology. Populations under special risk for this side effect are older patients [58] and recipients of heart, lung, and kidney transplants [59].

Saluretics: Corticosteroids

Thiazide, thiazide-like diuretics, and loop diuretics in combination with corticosteroids may lead to severe potassium depletion [60]. Addition of potassium supplementation or potassium-sparing diuretics may be needed.

Vitamin K Antagonists: Corticosteroids

Multiple studies have shown systemic corticosteroids may enhance the anticoagulation effect of vitamin K antagonists [61–63]. Close INR monitoring is mandatory when those agents are combined.

Calcitriol: Corticosteroids

Impaired intestinal calcium absorption has been observed as a corticosteroid dose-dependent side effect [64–66]. If there is a need for concomitant calcitriol administration, regular monitor for calcium serum concentration is recommended.

Neuromuscular Junction Acting Agents: Corticosteroids

Nondepolarizing neuromuscular blocking agents in combination with corticosteroids increase the risk of myopathy or neuropathy development [67, 68]. Although, this combination should be avoided, in the case of therapeutic necessity, close monitoring for new onset of muscle weakness, loss of deep tendon reflexes, and peripheral sensory deficits should be done.

Interestingly, systemic corticosteroids may also enhance the toxic effect of acetylcholine inhibitors in patients with myasthenia gravis causing exacerbation of muscular weakness [69].

Diltiazem: Corticosteroids

Two small studies on healthy volunteers have shown diltiazem increases methylprednisolone AUC by 1.5 to 2.6 times [70, 71]. Although the real mechanism is unknown, theory suggests diltiazem may inhibit corticosteroid metabolism and transport by CYP3A4 and/or P-glycoprotein inhibition. Regular monitoring for corticosteroids excess is needed.

Other Clinically Significant Drug Interactions of Systemic Corticosteroids Are Described with

Natalimumab, pimecrolimus, tacrolimus, upadacitinib, baricitinib, tofacitinib, aldesleukin, cladribine, dezmopressin, fexinidazole, indium 111 capromab pendetide, macimorelin, mifamurtide, mifepristone, desirudin, aprepitant, axicabtagene ciloleucel, fingolimod, fosaprepitant, hyaluronidase, leflunomide, nivolumab, ritonavir, roflumilast, sipuleucel-T, tisagenlecleucel, androgens, carbimazole, methimazole, coccidioides immitis skin test, corticorelin, cosyntropin, deferasirox, denosumab, estrogen derivatives, indacaterol, mitotane, nicorandil, ocrelizumab, ozanimod, pidotimod, ritodrine, sargramostin, siponimod, somatropin, tertomotide, trastuzumab, urea cycle disorder agents, bupropion, methacoline, progestins, protirelin (additional information: https://www.webmd.com/interaction-checker/default.htm).

Immunosuppressive Drugs

Thiopurines

Therapeutic Indication and Dose Range

Thiopurines, azathioprine (AZA), and 6-mercaptopurine (6-MP, off-label use in IBD) are immunosuppressive antimetabolites, and may be used in Crohn's disease and ulcerative colitis as adjunctive therapy or steroid-sparing agent for maintaining remission [72]. However, their slow onset of action (3 months of therapy, but may take up to 6 months in some patients) precludes the use of thiopurines monotherapy for active disease in the induction phase. Recommended daily dosage for AZA is 1.5–2.5 mg/kg/day and for 6-MP 0.75–1.5 mg/kg/day, both orally in undivided dose once per day. There is no evidence supporting the use of thiopurine monotherapy for the medical treatment of perianal fistulae.

Pathophysiologic Mechanisms

Purine antimetabolites, AZA and 6-MP, are well absorbed following oral administration, moderately bound to serum proteins [30%] and partially dialyzable [73]. After entering the cell, prodrug AZA is quickly metabolized to 6-MP via a nonenzymatic nucleophilic attack by sulfhydryl-containing compounds (Fig. 28.1). 6-MP is subsequently metabolized in the gut and liver through one of three enzymes: thiopurine-S-methyltransferase (TPMT) catalyzes the methylation of 6-MP to an inactive 6-methyl-mercaptopurine; xanthine oxidase catalyzes 6-MP to inactive 6-thiouric acid; hypoxanthine-guanine-phosphoribosyltransferase converts 6-MP to active metabolite 6-thioguanine nucleotides [74, 75]. The immunosuppressive effects of thiopurines are mediated by ribonucleotide synthesis inhibition. Incorporation of 6-thioguanine nucleotides into cellular nucleic acids results with inhibition of lymphocyte proliferation [73]. Second important mechanism of immunomodulation is the induction of T-cell apoptosis by modulating the cell [Rac1] signaling pathway [75]. Genetic polymorphism of TPMT enzyme results in a higher concentration of active metabolite and an increased risk of myelotoxicity [76]. It is estimated that 11% of the population are heterozygous and 0.3% recessive homozygous for TPMT. While heterozygotes have decreased enzyme activity and demand

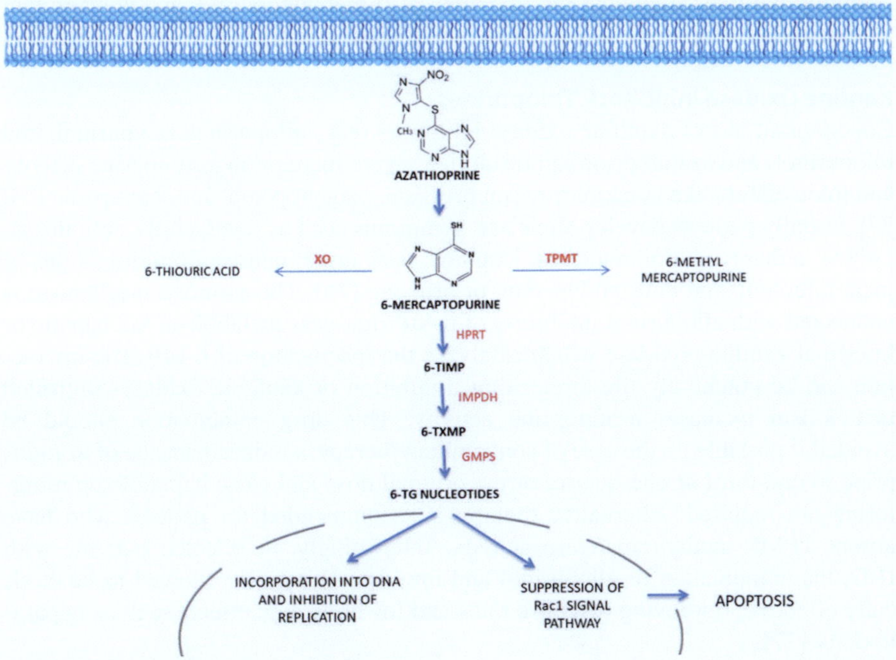

Fig. 28.1 Azathioprine—mechanism of action
XO xanthine oxidase, *TPMT* thiopurine S-methyltransferase, *HPRT* hypoxanthine phosphoribosyl transferase, *TIMP* thioinosine monophosphate, *IMPDH* inosine monophosphate dehydrogenase, *TXMP* thioxanthosine monophosphate, *GMPS* guanosine monophosphate synthetase, *TG NUCLEOTIDES* thioguanine nucleotides

lower doses of medications, recessive homozygotes' TPMT activity is reduced to the extent where further therapy is contraindicated.

Clinical Aspects and Drug Interactions

Side effects of AZA and 6-MP include dose-dependent side effects, like bone marrow suppression and hepatotoxicity, and dose-independent side effects, like pancreatitis, infection, and malignancy [75]. Special cautiousness is necessary in patients on chronic immunosuppression therapy with thiopurines. Pretreatment assessment includes full blood count, liver function tests, renal function tests, TPMT genotypization and optionally, chest X-ray. Full blood count should be done once weekly during the first eight weeks of treatment, and then should be checked every 3 months together with liver function tests [75, 76]. In patients with reduced renal function, a lowered dosage of thiopurines, due to reduced elimination of the active metabolites, may be necessary. Metabolism of azathioprine is also altered in patients with hepatic impairment as a result of reduced conversion into the active form and diminished breakdown to eliminable metabolites [76]. In those patients, dose reduction must be considered.

6-MP: Azathioprine

Azathioprine may potentiate the toxicities of 6-mercaptopurine, and concomitant administration may result in additive adverse effects [76].

Xantine Oxidase Inhibitors: Thiopurines

Concomitant use of xanthine oxidase inhibitors (e.g., allopurinol, oxypurinol, and thiopurinol) and azathioprine can result in a severe increase in azathioprine activity and toxic effects like bone marrow suppression, pancytopenia, and leukopenia [74, 77]. Usually patients develop signs and symptoms such as fever, chills, sore throat, fatigue, lethargy, pallor, anorexia, jaundice, dark urine, nausea, vomiting, signs of local infection, and unusual bleeding or bruising [76]. The assumed mechanism is connected with allopurinol inhibition of 6-MP first-pass metabolism via hepatic or intestinal xanthine oxidase which catalyzes the inactivation of 6-MP. The interaction can be potentially life-threatening. Inhibition of xanthine oxidase-controlled metabolism increases azathioprine activity. This drug combination should be avoided if possible. In the case of concomitant therapy, a reduced dosage of azathioprine to one-third or one-quarter of the original dose and close hematologic monitoring are required. Alternative therapy is recommended for patients who have absent TPMP methyltransferase activity. Interestingly, in selected patients with IBD, the combination of allopurinol and low-dose thiopurine showed to be clinically effective, improving response rates and lowering side effects such as hepatotoxicity [77].

Tofacitinib: Thiopurines

Coadministration of tofacitinib and thiopurines may potentiate the risk of severe infections, lymphoma, and other malignancies [78]; therefore, concurrent use of tofacitinib and potent immunosuppressants should be avoided.

5-ASA Derivatives: Thiopurines

Derivatives of 5-aminosalicylate (e.g., mesalamine, sulfasalazine, balsalazide, olsalazine) may potentiate the pharmacological effects of thiopurines [77]. 5-ASA derivatives inhibit the TPMT enzyme, leading to the myelosuppressive effects of purine antagonist antimetabolites with causal bone marrow suppression after treatment initiation. Patients in whom coadministration of 5-ASA derivatives and thiopurines is planned should be closely monitored for hematologic toxicity [77, 79].

Anti-TNF: Azathioprine

Coadministration of tumor necrosis factor-alpha (TNF-α) blockers with thiopurines increases the risk of infections, serious infections, and sepsis [80]. Concomitant use of TNF-α blockers and immunosuppressants like AZA/6-MP may increase the risk of white blood cell cancer known as hepatosplenic T-Cell lymphoma (HSTCL) [81]. HSTCL was primarily reported in young males receiving combination immunosuppressive treatment for IBD [82]. Further analysis showed HSTCL was connected with AZA monotherapy, while TNF-α inhibitor monotherapy wasn't connected with a higher risk of developing the disease [82]. Because individuals with Crohn's disease may develop lymphoma more likely than the general population, it is challenging to assess the additional risk of combination therapy with TNF-α blockers and azathioprine or mercaptopurine. However, concomitant immunosuppressive therapy with infliximab significantly reduces the incidence of developing infliximab antibodies. Patients on combination therapy should be monitored closely.

Vaccines [Live]: Thiopurines

According to General Recommendations on Immunization of Center for Disease Control and Prevention, vaccination with live vaccines should be avoided during, and at least 3 months after withdrawal of the immunosuppressive drug.

Vaccines [Inactivated]: Thiopurines

Vaccination with inactivated or noninfectious vaccines for immunosuppressed patients is generally safe, but the immunologic response may be diminished or suboptimal due to inhibition of antibody synthesis [83]. Inactivated vaccines can be administered to immunosuppressed patients [except HIV-positive patients] according to the [local] guidelines for healthy patients [83]. Special situations may require higher dosages or more frequent boosters and, possibly, serological testing.

Smallpox Vaccine: Thiopurines

Administration of live smallpox virus, vaccine during immunosuppressant therapy is contraindicated and may be associated with a risk of serious infection [84]. In an immunocompromised patient, replication of vaccine virus may be enhanced. In those patients, immune response is decreased or suboptimal, and adverse reactions are more often. Vaccination should not be administered during immunosuppressive therapy and for at least 3 months after therapy discontinuation [84]. If vaccination occurred prior to immunosuppressive therapy, initiation of immunosuppressive drug should be delayed for at least 2 weeks. Moreover, vaccination should not be administered to household members of immunosuppressed patients. An exception can be made in case of immunosuppressed patients with a high-risk exposure, when the risk of serious complications of the vaccination must be weighed against the risk of potentially serious/fatal smallpox infection [85].

ACE Inhibitors: Thiopurines

Angiotensin-converting enzyme inhibitors and azathioprine may have additive hematologic effects present as anemia, neutropenia or leukopenia, but data are very limited [86, 87]. Patients on concomitant therapy with thiopurines and ACE inhibitors [especially captopril and enalapril] should be regularly monitored for hematologic disorders.

Neuromuscular Acting Agents: Thiopurines

Special care is necessary when azathioprine is given concomitantly with neuromuscular-acting agents. Azathioprine may enhance, reduce or reverse the effects of non-depolarizing muscle relaxants (e.g., Tubocurarine) by an unknown mechanism. Reduction of effects may be related to the inhibition of phosphodiesterase in motor nerve axon terminals [88]. Azathioprine may potentiate the neuromuscular blockade produced by succinylcholine, but data are scarce [76]. Clinical significance is unknown and routine monitoring of the patient is recommended.

Anticoagulants: Thiopurines

Thiopurines may reduce the hypoprothrombinemic response to warfarin and other oral anticoagulants [89]. Pathophysiological mechanisms may be related to enhanced activation or synthesis of prothrombin. Given the interaction potential and the consequence of the therapeutic index of oral anticoagulants, patients should be closely monitored during concomitant therapy with thiopurines, especially following initiation or discontinuation of thiopurine therapy [90].

Antibiotics: Thiopurines

Close therapy monitoring is recommended in case of concomitant administration of thiopurines with trimethoprim and sulfamethoxazole. Higher incidences of neutropenia and thrombocytopenia have been observed among patients receiving thiopurines and sulfamethoxazole–trimethoprim compared to those receiving thiopurines alone [91, 92]. Studies suggest sulfamethoxazole–trimethoprim have bone marrow suppression effect by its antifolate activity [93–96]. Thus, the probable mechanism of this interaction is the synergistic bone marrow suppressive effect of 6-mercaptopurine and sulfamethoxazole–trimethoprim [92].

Other Clinically Significant Drug Interactions of Systemic Corticosteroids Are Described with

BCG (intravesical), cladribine, febuxostat, natalizumab, pimecrolimus, tacrolimus, upadacitinib, baricitinib, echinacea, fingolimod, leflunomide, nivolumab, ribavirin, roflumilast, sipuleucel, coccidioides immitis skin test, cyclophosphamide, denosumab, inebilizumab, ocrelizumab, ozanimod, pidotimod, siponimod, trastuzumab (additional information: https://www.webmd.com/interaction-checker/default.htm).

Methotrexate

Therapeutic Indication and Dose Range

Methotrexate (MTX) is an immunosuppressive drug registered for the treatment of rheumatic arthritis, severe forms of psoriasis vulgaris, and several oncologic conditions. According to ECCO guidelines, its off-label use is recommended as second-line therapy in maintaining remission in steroid-dependent CD [5]. Albeit, one study has tried to position MTX even as induction therapy in steroid-dependent CD, it is strongly limited by concomitant use of steroids [97]. Regarding the long time to respond after drug introduction (for MTX, it is 10 weeks) and only a few imprecision studies available, no agreement was achieved about MTX as CD induction therapy in ECCO Consensus. The same conclusion was reached for UC, due to the heterogeneity and insufficient evidence, there is no recommendation for MTX usage at UC [98].

Recommended induction dose is 25 mg intramuscular once per week during 16 week, followed by a dose reduction to 15 mg once per week. Both parenteral and oral routes of administration can be used during the maintenance dose [5]. In order to reduce MTX toxicity, folic acid is coprescribed between 42 and 48 h after MTX administration.

Pathophysiologic Mechanisms

After oral intake or intramuscular administration, MTX is actively transported across cell membranes and widely distributed into body tissues. In plasma, a considerable amount of MTX is bound to serum proteins. MTX doesn't seem to be highly metabolized before it is excreted by the kidneys. This antimetabolite is a competitive inhibitor of dihydrofolate reductase, the enzyme that converts folate and folic acid into their activated form 5-methyltetrahydrofolate (5-MTHF)—metabolite pivotal for cell replications (Fig. 28.2). Cells mostly affected by this inhibition are those in actively proliferating tissues, such as malignant and immune cells. Inhibition of lymphocyte multiplication seems to be the main mechanism of immunosuppressive and anti-inflammatory effects [99].

Clinical Aspects and Drug Interactions

As agents highly accumulate in the liver and kidney, it shows significant hepatotoxic and nephrotoxic effects. If possible, MTX should be avoided in patients with the previous or current liver disease despite etiology. In case of renal impairment, MTX dose has to be adjusted. If clearance of creatinine is below 30 ml/min, MTX must not be administered. Prolongation of serum half-life is observed in patients with pathological fluid accumulation. Therefore, before MTX therapy is instituted, pleural effusions and ascites should be drained. Although rare, bone marrow

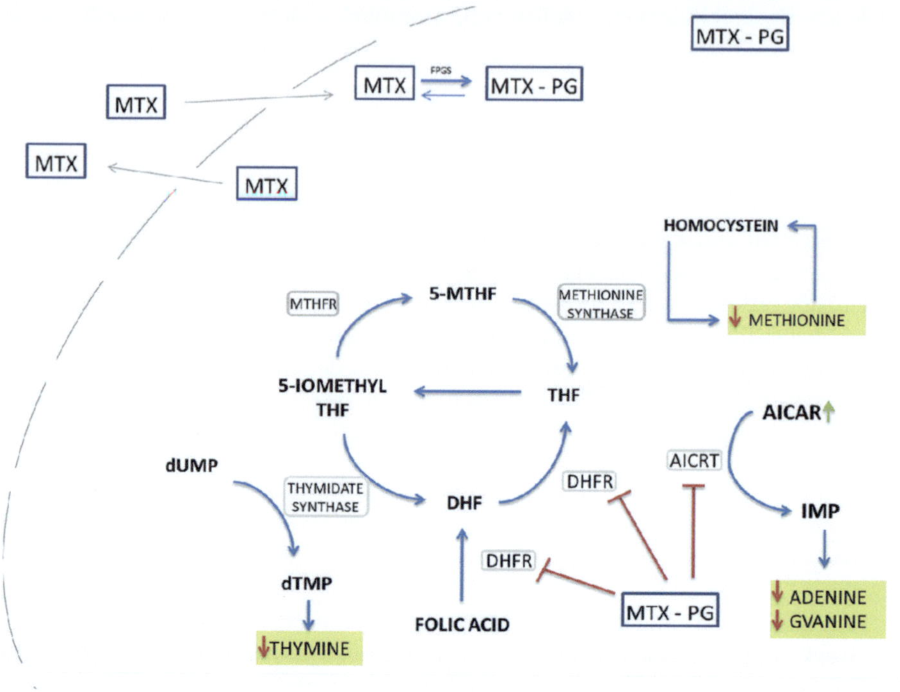

Fig. 28.2 Methotrexate—mechanism of action
After entering the cell, MTX molecule converts to MTX-PG [methotrexate polyglutamate] in order to be selectively retained inside the cell. MTX-PG inhibits DHFR (dihydrofolate reductase) and AICRT (aminoimidazole carboxamide ribonucleotide transformylase) which lead to decreased synthesis of thymine, adenine, guanine as well as methionine. Inhibiting AICRT, it also increases AICAR (aminoimidazole-4-carboxamide ribonucleotide) concentration—molecule with widespread anti-inflammatory effects. (FPGS, folypolyglutamate synthase; DHF, dihydrofolate; THF, tetrahydrofolate; IOMETHYL THF, iomethyl tetrahydrofolate; MTHFR, methyltetrahydrofolate reductase; MTHF, methyltetrahydrofolate; dUMP, deoxyuridine monophosphate; dTMP, deoxythymidine monophosphate; IMP, inosine monophosphate)

depression, leukopenia, and thrombocytopenia may occur during MTX therapy. As an immunosuppressant, MTX is contraindicated in patients with active infectious and immunodeficiency syndrome of any cause. MTX is a well-known teratogenic and abortifacient agent. Contraception for both genders is mandatory during, and at least 6 months after drug withdrawal. MTX is also excreted into breast milk so the drug should be excluded during the lactation period. Having in mind all prior mentioned, pretreatment assessment must include full blood count, electrolytes, liver function tests, renal function tests and urinalysis, chest X-ray, Varicella Zoster, HIV, and hepatitis serology. Two weeks after drug introduction, control full blood count, liver and renal function tests should be done, monthly thereafter. If there is no side effect during a longer period of use, monitoring can be reduced to every 2–3 months [99]. Severe drug interaction of MTX substantially can be seen in combination with other hepatotoxic, nephrotoxic, and myelotoxic drugs.

Vaccination: Methotrexate

According to General Recommendations on Immunization of Center for Disease Control and Prevention, vaccination, either with live or inactivated vaccines, should be avoided during and at least 3 months after withdrawal of the immunosuppressive drug. However, the immunosuppressive effect of MTX seems to be dose-dependent, so the American College of Rheumatology doesn't recommend avoiding any vaccine in patients being treated with low-dose MTX (0.4 mg/kg/week or less) [100].

NSAIDs: Methotrexate

Studies have shown NSAIDs can significantly change MTX pharmacokinetics. Although this effect differs among the different NSAIDs, most of them increase serum concentration of MTX predisposing patients to develop side effects [101]. NSAIDs per se are also hematotoxic and nephrotoxic agents, so combination with MTX can multiply this toxicity. On the other side, some NSAIDs seem to inhibit MTX excretion, whether by inhibiting renal transport or decreasing renal perfusion [102–104]. Labels for dexketoprofen, dexibuprofen, and dipyrone strongly disapprove concomitant use with MTX doses higher than 15 mg/week. In case this coadministration can't be avoided, intensive monitoring for signs of hematologic toxicity, nephrotoxicity, and hepatotoxicity is mandatory.

Salicylates: Methotrexate

It is thought that the same mechanisms, tubular inhibition of MTX excretion and decreased renal perfusion, stand behind salicylate–MTX interaction. Moreover, MTX is a molecule highly bounded to serum albumins, so free serum proportion of the drug may be severely influenced by other competitive albumin-bounding substrates, such as salicylate. Concomitant use of high doses of MTX and salicylates has resulted in lethal pancytopenia [105]. Interestingly, serum MTX concentration doesn't seem to be influenced by prophylaxis doses of salicylates used for the prevention of cardiovascular events. Close monitoring for MTX toxicity is needed when higher doses are used, especially in the case of neoplastic disorders treatment.

5-ASA Derivatives: Methotrexate

Combining sulfasalazine and MTX may lead to severe hepatic impairment [106, 107]. On the other side, mesalamine may enhance the myelosuppressive effect of MTX [108]. Close monitoring for signs and symptoms of hepatic and hematologic toxicity is needed in case of parallel administration.

Proton Pump Inhibitors: Methotrexate

A retrospective study of 79 patients revealed delayed MTX elimination when used with PPIs [109]. Numerous case reports describe the same effect on MTX pharmacokinetics [110–114]. Although the real mechanism of interaction is unknown, some in vitro and animal studies suggest that PPI-mediated inhibition of the BCRP, ABCG2, and/or MRP2 transporters may have an important role [115, 116]. Another proposed mechanism includes PPI-mediated inhibition of hydrogen renal excretion. Namely, MTX is actively secreted with hydrogen ions. Monitor patients for increased MTX toxicity if PPI is used concomitantly, especially when antineoplastic doses are prescribed.

Bile Acid Sequestrants: Methotrexate

Not only cholestyramine can decrease oral MTX absorption, but it has also been used to treat MTX toxicity (after enteral as well as parenteral administration). It seems cholestyramine binds molecules of MTX inside GI tract, therefore inhibiting absorption and enterohepatic circulation [117]. Separating the administration of agents by at least 2 h may minimize the risk of interaction.

Loop Diuretics: Methotrexate

Loop diuretics and MTX are secreted in renal tubules, therefore assumed mechanism of interaction is competitive inhibition in kidneys. Parallel use of drugs leads to an increase in serum concentrations and toxicity of both agents. Loop diuretics achieve therapeutic effects only after they are secreted in the renal tubule, thus decreased therapeutic effect of furosemide has been observed. In case concomitant use can't be avoided, close monitoring is recommended [118].

Theophylline Derivatives: Methotrexate

According to researches, MTX can increase serum theophylline concentration by 20% [21, 119]. Theophylline concentration and dose adjustment should be done after MTX introduction as well as after discontinuation.

Warfarin: Methotrexate

Although there is no strong evidence, few case reports detected higher INR values in patients taking warfarin and MTX as part of combination chemotherapy regimens [120]. The mechanism of any interaction is unclear. However, more often INR controls in patients on concomitant warfarin and MTX therapy could be useful.

Antibiotics: Methotrexate

Many antibiotics may increase MTX serum concentration and toxicity. Therapy modification should be considered with sulfonamide antibiotics. Studies have shown sulfamethoxazole/trimethoprim increase MTX serum concentration and lead predominantly to hematologic toxicity [121]. MTX, sulfamethoxazole, and trimethoprim all possess antifolate activity which may cause a synergistic effect on blood cell formation. Moreover, trimethoprim and sulfamethoxazole, as well as other sulfonamides, seem to displace MTX and its toxic metabolite from serum albumins, thus increasing their concentrations and half-lives [122, 123].

Tetracyclines can also increase MTX serum concentration by reducing MTX clearance [124]. The exact mechanism isn't clear. Albeit this interaction doesn't seem to be clinically significant with antirheumatic doses of MTX, monitoring for MTX toxic effects is recommended in case of tetracycline initiation or dose escalation when higher MTX doses are prescribed.

The authors reported two cases of MTX-ceftriaxone-induced severe neutropenia [125]. Possible mechanisms of interactions are competing for OAT3 transporters in kidneys and MTX competitive displacement from serum albumins. Screening for neutropenia is recommended with concurrent use of MTX and ceftriaxone.

Penicillin antibiotics also seem to increase MTX serum concentration [126–129]. Interaction is more likely if higher doses of both agents are used. Monitoring for MTX toxic effects is recommended when MTX and penicillin antibiotics are used concomitantly. The same effect is observed with concomitant use of ciprofloxacin and MTX [130, 131], thus the same precaution measures are recommended.

Nitrofurantoin, as well as other hepatotoxic drugs, may have a synergistic effect on the liver when combined with MTX. Regular liver function tests should be done in this case.

Natalizumab: Methotrexate

Patients receiving natalizumab must not take immunosuppressants like MTX, azathioprine, 6-mercaptopurine, cyclosporine, and TNF-alpha inhibitors due to increased risk of progressive multifocal leukoencephalopathy and other severe or opportunistic infections [132]. Natalizumab prescribing information also emphasizes the importance of corticosteroid tapering prior to drug introduction.

Tofacitinib: Immunosuppressants

Although concurrent use of tofacitinib and potent immunosuppressants should be avoided, parallel administration of tofacitinib and antirheumatic doses of MTX is permitted [78]. Before introducing this combination of drugs, provide your patient with all necessary information about the potential risk of severe infections.

Other Clinically Significant Drug Interactions of Sulfasalazine Are Described with

Acitretin, cladribine, dipyrone, lasmiditan, foscarnet, nitrous oxide, pimecrolimus, tacrolimus, baricitinib, deferiprone, dichlorphenamide, Echinacea, fingolimod, leflunomide, lenograstim, lipegfilgrastim, nivolumab, palifermin, probenecid, roflumilast, sipuleucel-T, tolvaptan, alitretionin, chloral hydrate, clozapine, phenytoin,alchocol, amiodarone, gemfibrozil, coccidioides immitis skin test, denosumab, eltrombopag, erdafitinib, amphotericin B, ibrutinib, leflunomide, levetiracetam, Licorice, lumacaftor, ivacaftor, mipomersan, nitisinone, ocrelizumab, ozanimod, pidotimod, pretomanid, pyrimethamine, ranolazine, sapropterin, siponimod, tegafur, teriflunomide, tertomotide, promazine, trastuzumab, digoxin, aminoquinolines, upadacitinib, triamteren (additional information: https://www.webmd.com/interaction-checker/default.htm).

Mycophenolate Mofetil

Mycophenolate mofetil (MMF) is an immunosuppressive agent used in combination with ciclosporin and corticosteroids for prophylaxis of acute transplant rejections [133]. It inhibits inosine monophosphate dehydrogenase, an enzyme crucial for de novo guanosine synthesis and DNA replication. In contrast to other human cells, which can use various pathways of purine synthesis, T and B lymphocytes are mostly dependent on de novo synthesis making MMF highly selective for immune cells. Although, animal models [134] and few clinical reports [135, 136] suggest MMF may be useful in patients with CD, ECCO guidelines do not recommend its use in standard practice [137, 138].

Immunomodulatory Agents

Ciclosporin

Therapeutic Indication and Dose Range

Ciclosporin (also known as ciclosporin A, cyclosporin, or cyclosporine) is an immunosuppressant registered for the prevention of graft rejection following solid organ or bone marrow transplantation. ECCO guidelines positioned ciclosporin (CsA), alongside tacrolimus and infliximab, as an off-label medication for management of acute, moderate-to-severe UC refractory to corticosteroids [139, 140]. Standard dose recommended in clinical praxis for above mentioned indication is 2 mg/kg/day [141]. After initial parenteral administration of CsA, switch to oral therapy, as soon as clinical response has been achieved, should be encouraged. Due to numerous side effects, CsA should be discontinued within 6 months during which another, slower-acting immunomodulator, achieves full potential. Available data suggest thiopurines reduce the risk of colectomy when introduced after CsA [142–144]. Only three small, uncontrolled case series have reported the efficacy of intravenous CsA (administered in much higher doses compared to UC, 4–5 mg/kg/day) for the treatment of CD [145–147], while placebo-controlled trials observed no effect [148–150]. Thus, ECCO doesn't recommend its use in patients with CD [137].

Pathophysiologic Mechanism

CsA is a lipophilic peptide consisting of 11 amino acids, highly selective for lymphocytes [151]. After entering lymphocytes cytoplasm, CsA binds to cyclophilin, making complex, which inhibits calcineurin activity—factor crucial for transcription and synthesis of interleukins (IL), particularly IL2, IL3, and IL4, as well as tumor necrosis factor-alpha, granulocyte-macrophage colony-stimulating factor, and interferon-gamma [152] (Fig. 28.3). Lack of those signal molecules inhibits T-cell proliferation making CsA a potent immunosuppressant. All available data suggest that this CsA effect on lymphocytes is completely reversible. In contrast to other cytostatic agents, hemopoiesis and phagocytic cell function are not impaired by CsA [151]. As a lipophilic cyclic molecule, CsA absorption depends upon bile salts and it is mostly absorbed in the small intestine. CsA is extensively metabolized via CYP3A4 enzymes presented both, in gut mucosa and liver, resulting in metabolites with less than 20% of CsA immunosuppressive activity. Poor absorption and extensive biotransformation lead to limited oral bioavailability of CsA. A considerable proportion of drug molecules in serum are bound to albumins and lipoproteins. Drug is mostly excreted via the biliary tract [151, 152].

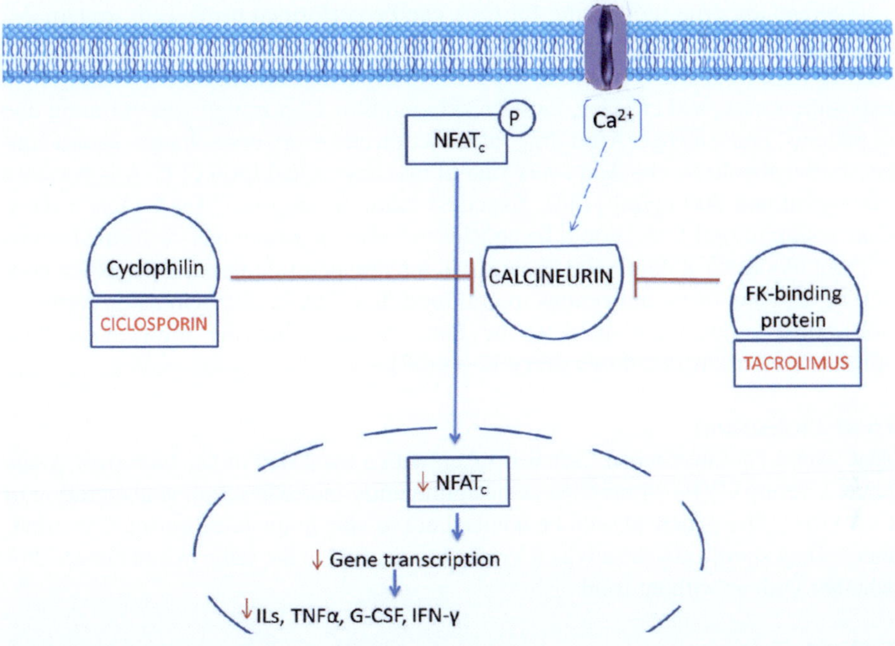

Fig. 28.3 Calcineurin inhibitors—mechanism of action
Calcium ions activate calcineurin which then starts to dephosphorylate the nuclear factor of activated T lymphocyte complex (NFAT$_c$). Dephosphorylated NFAT$_c$ translocate into the cell nucleus and promote transcription of genes encoded for interleukins (ILs), tumor necrosis factor-alpha (TNFα), granulocyte colony-stimulating factor (G-CSF), and interferon gamma (IFN-γ). Ciclosporin inhibits this process, making inert cyclophilin-ciclosporin-calcineurin complex. On the other side, tacrolimus forms FK-binding protein-tacrolimus-calcineurin complex with the same outcome

Clinical Aspects and Drug Interaction

Oral and parenteral drug preparations are available on the market. Regarding the oral formulation, two types of molecule can be used; nonmodified and modified CsA. Advantage of modified CsA, registered as microemulsion formulation, is increased bioavailability due to its absorption independent of bile salt [152].

Common side effects noticed by CsA administration are nephrotoxicity, hypertension, neurotoxicity, metabolic abnormalities (diabetes, dyslipidemia, hyperkalemia, hyperuricemia, hypomagnesemia), infections, and malignancies (squamous cell skin cancer, as well as, benign and malignant lymphoproliferative disorders). If patients already have some of these disorders, other medication should be considered [152]. CsA is also contraindicated if the patient has a history of intolerance or failure of immunomodulator therapy [e.g., azathioprine] and/or biologic agents [153]. After the institution of CsA, the patient must be carefully monitored for all abovementioned disorders: nephrotoxicity, hypertension, neurotoxicity, electrolyte abnormalities, and infections [151]. Every patient should receive prophylaxis against *Pneumocystis* during CsA therapy [153].

Therapeutic drug monitoring for CsA can be performed using 12-h trough, 2-h postdose, or abbreviated area under the time concentration curve [154]. Although studies have shown 2-h postdose drug concentrations correlate more closely with exposure, safety, and efficacy, most centers monitor 12-h trough concentration due to patients' convenience. After drug introduction and every dose change, serum concentration should be checked every one to two days. Goal level of CsA is between 200 ng/ml and 300 ng/ml [144]. Expected "time to response" for CsA is 3 days. Conversion to oral CsA should be considered when a patient has <6 formed stools without blood, no abdominal pain, and can tolerate peroral intake [153]. When converting patients from intravenous to oral modified CsA (a microemulsion formulation), dose adjustments have to be done by doubling the intravenous dose administered in divided doses every 12 h [153].

Food: Ciclosporin

AUC was 13% lower when CsA was taken with a meal rich in fat. Moreover, grape juice, a strong CYP3A4 inhibitor, can significantly increase serum concentration of CsA [151]. The patient should be advised not to take grape juice during CsA treatment. They should also be advised to take medication in the same manner every day, whether with or without food.

CYP3A4: Ciclosporin

As a CYP3A4 substrate, CsA's pharmacokinetics can be strongly influenced by all CYP3A4 inducers, inhibitors, and other substrates [151]. Most clinically significant agents with impact on CYP3A4 are listed in Table 28.2. If the combination of drugs can't be avoided, intensive monitoring of CsA serum concentration and dose adjustment is mandatory.

P-Glycoprotein: Ciclosporin

CsA is a substrate and inhibitor of P-glycoprotein (permeability glycoprotein) also known as multidrug resistance protein 1 (MDR1) or ATP-binding cassette subfamily B member 1 (ABCB1) or cluster of differentiation 243 (CD243). P-glycoprotein is highly distributed along the intestinal epithelium where it pumps xenobiotics back into the lumen. It is also present in liver cells, proximal tubules, and capillary endothelial cells with the main function of excretion of foreign substances. P-glycoprotein inducers may decrease the serum concentration of CsA and inhibitors may cause the opposite effect. The exact effects of different P-glycoprotein substrates depend on their affinity to the transporter. Before CsA introduction, individual drug interaction and the clinical significance of a particular relation should be checked. P-glycoprotein inhibitors, inducers, and substrates are listed in Table 28.4.

Anticoagulants: Ciclosporin

All factor Xa inhibitors are P-glycoprotein substrates, thus, concomitant use with CsA may increase the risk of bleeding among those patients. Interactions between CsA and betrixaban, as well as CsA and edoxaban, are rated as a major, so

Table 28.4 P-glycoprotein inhibitors, inducers, and substrates

P-glycoprotein inducers	P-glycoprotein inhibitors	P-glycoprotein substrates
Apalutamide, carbamazepine, fosphenytoin, lorlatinib, phenytoin, rifampin, St John's wort	Amiodarone, azithromycin (systemic), capmatinib, carvedilol, clarithromycin, cyclosporine (systemic), daclatasvir, dronedarone, elagolix, elagolix, estradiol, norethindrone, elexacaftor, tezacaftor, ivacaftor, eliglustat, erythromycin (systemic), flibanserin, fostamatinib, glecaprevir, pibrentasvir, itraconazole, ivacaftor, ketoconazole (systemic), lapatinib, ledipasvir, neratinib, ombitasvir, paritaprevir, ritonavir, osimertinib, propafenone, quinidine, quinine, ranolazine, ritonavir, rolapitant, simeprevir, tezacaftor, ivacaftor, tucatinib, velpatasvir, vemurafenib, verapamil	Afatinib, aliskiren, amiodarone, bilastine, brentuximab vedotin, carfilzomib, carvedilol, celiprolol, ceritinib, cetirizine (systemic), cimetidine, colchicine, crizotinib, cyclosporine (systemic), dabigatran etexilate, daunorubicin (conventional), daunorubicin (liposomal), desloratadine, dexamethasone (systemic), digitoxin, digoxin, diltiazem, docetaxel, doxorubicin (conventional), erythromycin (systemic), estradiol (systemic), estradiol (topical), etoposide, etoposide phosphate, everolimus, fexofenadine, fosamprenavir, gilteritinib, hydrocortisone (systemic), idarubicin, imatinib, indinavir, irinotecan (conventional), irinotecan (liposomal), ivermectin (systemic), lapatinib, larotrectinib, ledipasvir, lefamulin, letermovir, linagliptin, loperamide, loperamide oxide, loratadine, lovastatin, methotrexate, mitomycin (systemic), morphine (systemic), nadolol, naldemedine, naloxegol, nelfinavir, nicardipine, nintedanib, paclitaxel (conventional), paclitaxel (protein bound), paliperidone, pazopanib, quinidine, quinine, ranitidine (withdrawn from us market), ranolazine, rifampin, rimegepant, riociguat, risperidone, ritonavir, romidepsin, saquinavir, saxagliptin, silodosin, sirolimus, sitagliptin, sofosbuvir, tacrolimus (systemic), temsirolimus, teniposide, tolvaptan, trabectedin, ubrogepant, vemurafenib, venetoclax, verapamil, vinblastine, vincristine, vincristine (liposomal)

anticoagulant dose reduction is recommended (for betrixaban initial single dose of 80 mg should be followed by 40 mg once daily; for edoxaban 30 mg once daily) [155]. On the other side, interactions between CsA and apixaban and CsA and rivaroxaban are rated as moderate, so close monitoring is a suitable precaution measure.

Dabigatran, another P-glycoprotein substrate, should also be avoided during CsA treatment, especially in patients with renal impairment [156].

Statins and Other Hypolipidemic Drugs: Ciclosporin

Although both statins and CsA are CYP3A4 substrates, CsA seems to have a higher affinity to the enzyme. Consequently, concomitant use leads to higher, sometimes even toxic, concentrations of statins. Drug labeling for atorvastatin, simvastatin, fluvastatin, rosuvastatin, lovastatin, pitavastatin, and pravastatin states that concurrent use with CsA should be avoided due to increased risk for statin-related toxicities such as myopathy and rhabdomyolysis [157–160].

CsA can also significantly increase the serum concentration of ezetimibe, an oral inhibitor of cholesterol absorption [also available in combination with statins] [161]. The mechanism of interaction remains unknown.

Drugs Affecting GI Motility: Ciclosporin

Most prokinetic agents decrease CsA absorption. On the other hand, antidiarrheal agents and opioid agonists increase CsA bioavailability. Interestingly, metoclopramide seems to be an exception. Available data suggest the AUC of cyclosporine was increased by an average of 29% when administered with metoclopramide [162]. Although the clinical impact of interaction remains unknown, monitoring of CsA serum concentration is recommended.

Vaccines: Ciclosporin

All recommendations stated in sections "Corticosteroids" and "MTX" about vaccination are completely applicable to CsA.

Hepatitis C Antiviral Agents: Ciclosporin

Concomitant use of CsA and grazoprevir, glecaprevir, pibrentasvir, simeprevir, and voxilaprevir should be strictly avoided.

In a study conducted on a 14 subjects, the average grazoprevir AUC was 15.2 times higher when co-administered with CsA [163]. Similar studies and results are described with glecaprevir, pibrentasvir [164], simeprevir, and voxilaprevir. However, CsA doses lower than 100 mg per day were not associated with a significant increase in serum concentration of glecaprevir and pibrentasvir [164], so this combination can be used with great caution. One case report also described an increment in serum concentration of CsA when coadministered with simeprivir [165].

Pharmacokinetic studies showed ombitasvir/paritaprevir/ritonavir can increase CsA concentration significantly. Probable mechanism of interaction is the dual inhibition of CYP3A4 and P-glycoprotein caused by these antiviral combinations of drugs. If concomitant administration is unavoidable, a reduction of the maintenance dose of CsA by 80% must be undertaken. Close monitoring of renal function and CsA-related side effects should be done.

Although simeprevir can increase serum CsA concentration, this interaction seems significant only for orally administered CsA. Probably, it is due to selective simeprevir inhibition of intestinal CYP3A4 without impact on the hepatic isoform of the enzyme.

Gastric Acid Suppression Medication: Ciclosporine

Data on histamine H_2 receptor antagonist impact on CsA are inconsistent [166, 167]. However, the serum CsA concentration should be measured after H_2-antagonist initiation, withdrawal, or dose change.

Omeprazole may also increase serum CsA concentration [168], although the real mechanism of this interaction remains unknown. Interestingly, this effect wasn't observed with pantoprazole [169].

Antiarrhythmic Drugs: Ciclosporine

According to dronedarone prescribing information, concomitant use with CsA is contraindicated due to severe increases in dronedarone concentration and side effects when combined with CsA. On the other side, studies revealed amiodarone inhibition of CYP3A4 and P-glycoprotein can cause increases in serum CsA concentration despite CsA dose reduction [170, 171]. However, concomitant use of amiodarone and CsA is allowed, but CsA serum level measurement should be done after amiodarone introduction, withdrawal, and/or each dose change in both medications.

Digoxin, P-glycoprotein substrate, is highly influenced by CsA, especially when both agents are taken orally [172]. Case reports describe digoxin toxicity following initiation of CsA [173, 174]. In case of concomitant use, monitoring for digoxin toxicity is mandatory.

Diuretics: Ciclosporin

Hyperkalemia has been associated with CsA even without interaction with other agents. Thus, eplerenone and other potassium-sparing diuretics are contraindicated in combination with CsA.

Loop diuretics (furosemide) were associated with hyperuricemia and gout attacks [175]. The suggested mechanism of interaction is impaired tubular urate clearance caused by CsA. Close monitoring for signs and symptoms of hyperuricemia is recommended.

Natalizumab: Ciclosporin

Please see section "Methotrexate"—"Natalizumab—methotrexate interaction".

Tacrolimus: Ciclosporin

Concomitant use of tacrolimus and CsA should be strictly avoided due to synergistic nephrotoxic effect. Moreover, both agents share common metabolic pathways so unpredicted serum levels of either agent can occur [176, 177].

Mycophenolate Mofetil: Ciclosporin

Therapy modification should be considered in case of concomitant use of MMF and CsA. CsA may decrease the serum concentration of MMF, particularly its active metabolite mycophenolic acid (MPA). The proposed mechanism of interaction is CsA-mediated inhibition of MPA biliary excretion and subsequently decreased MPA enterohepatic recirculation [178, 179].

Tofacitinib: Ciclosporin

Please see section "Methotrexate"—"Tofacitinib—immunosuppressants".

Adalimumab: Ciclosporin

Adalimumab can decrease the serum concentration of CsA, so close monitoring is recommended in case of parallel use [180]. It is thought that decreased cytokine activity caused by adalimumab may increase CYP3A4 synthesis and consequently decrease CsA bioactivity.

Methotrexate: Ciclosporin

Different MTX and CsA toxic effects have been observed when administered concomitantly [181–183]. However, concomitant therapy with reduced doses of CsA seems to be safe and effective [184]. Increased monitoring is recommended.

Sulfasalazine: Ciclosporin

Monitor for decreased CsA concentration during concomitant therapy with sulfasalazine. Observed data suggests a 75% increment in CsA serum concentration after sulfasalazine discontinuations [22].

Other Clinically Significant Drug Interactions of Ciclosporin Are Described with

Aliskiren, bosentan, cladribine, conivaptan, disulfiram, elagolix, enzalutamide, foscarnet, fusidic acid, idelasilib,lercanidipine, lasmiditan, lumacaftor, ivacaftor, methotrimeprazine, mifamurtide, ozanimod, pazopanib, pimozide, revefenacin, rimegepant, topotecan, sirolimus, pimecrolimus, everolimus, upadacitinib, vincristine, afatinib, alpelisib, androgen, azole derivatives, ambrisentan, baricitinib, bilastine, cladribine, dabrafenib, caspofungin, carvedilol, cholic acid, colchicine, chloramphenicol, colesevelam, eluxadoline, doxorubicin, Echinacea, efavirenz, enzalutamide, etoposide, etoposide phosphate, fingolimod, lomitapide, lefamulin, leflunomide, lemborexant, letermovir, mifepristone, mitotane, mitoxantrone, nivolumab, NSAID-s, obeticholic acid, orlistat, ritonavir, roflumilast, repaglinid, rifamycin derivatives, sipuleucel-T, stiripentol, St. John's Wort, triazolam, ubrogepant, venetoclax, allopurinol, acetazolamide, aminoquinolines, aminoglycosides, amphotericin B, angiotensin II receptor blockers, ascorbic acid, aprepitant, armodafinil, azithromycin, barbiturates, bosentan, brentuximab vedotin, calcium channel blockers, celiprolol, clofazimine, clarithromycin, coccidioides immitis skin test, cyclophosphamide, glyburide, dexamethasone, dabigatran, deferasirox, denosumab, dofetilide, dronabinol, duvelisib, eltrombopag, erythromycin, estrogen derivatives, erdafitinib, filmasartan, flibanserin, fosaprepitant, fosnetupitant, fosphenytoin, fluconazole, ganciclovir/valganciclovir, griseofulvin, imatinib, isavuconazonium sulfate, ivacaftor, ivosidenib, imipenem, larotrecitinib, lumateprone, melphalan, metreleptin, minoxidil, modafinil, methylprednisolone, naldemedine, nimodipine, naloxegol, nafcilin, netupitant, norfloxacin, neuromuscular-blocking agent, ocrelizumab, ozanimod, palbociclib, pidotimod, pyrazinamide, prucalopride, quinupristin, ranolazine, rifaximin, phenytoin, prednisolone, prednisone, progestins, sarilumab, sevelamar, sibutramine, silodosin, siltuximab, siponimod, sulfinpyrazone, ticagrelor, ticlopidine, talazoparib, telithromycin, terbinafine, tertomotide, tigecycline, tocilizumab, trastuzumab, somatostatin analogs, sulfonylureas, sulfonamide, vitamin E, angiotensin-converting enzyme inhibitors, ciprofloxacin, levofloxacin, metronidazole,nystatin, tegaserod, temsirolimus, anagliptin, aripiprazole, avatrombopag, bromocriptine, citalopram, eliglustat, fidaxomicin, idebenone, lefamulin, loperamide, luliconazole, micafungin,neratinib, omadacycline, piperaquine, pitolisant, pranlukast, roxithromycin, telotristat ethyl (additional information: https://www.webmd.com/interaction-checker/default.htm).

Tacrolimus

Tacrolimus is macrolide antibiotic with the mechanism of action very similar to CsA (Fig. 28.3). While CsA binds to cyclophilin, tacrolimus binds to FK-binding protein which inhibits further cascade in the same manner as CsA [185]. It also shares the same absorption pathway with CsA. Therefore, tacrolimus has the same therapeutic indication in the treatment of UC as CsA.

Oral, intravenous, and topical preparations of tacrolimus are available on the market. Regarding oral preparations, three different types can be used: immediate-release capsules, extended-release capsules, and extended-release tablets. Special caution is needed when prescribing extended-release formulations because capsules and tablets are not interchangeable. Pharmacokinetics and bioavailability differ vastly, so formulation change may demand dose change as well (different dose adjustment formulas in case of formulation change are available) [152]. Recommended initial dose is 0.01–0.02 mg/kg for intravenous use and 0.1–0.2 mg/kg for oral formulation. Most studies have been conducted based on level of high serum trough concentration of 10–15 ng/ml [186].

All precaution measures, contraindications, and drug interactions previously stated for CsA are completely applicable for tacrolimus.

Sirolimus

Sirolimus, also known as rapamycin, inhibits T cell activation by reducing their sensitivity to interleukin-2 (IL-2) through mTOR inhibition. Although, theoretically sirolimus may be beneficial in modulating immune response in inflammatory bowel disease, qualitative studies are lacking [187, 188]. Thus, sirolimus is not recommended therapy in the management of inflammatory bowel disease.

Thalidomide

Therapeutic Indication and Dose Range

Thalidomide, a drug with a long controversial history, is nowadays registered for the treatment of multiple myeloma [189]. It is also used for treatment of several cutaneous inflammatory disorders. Although there is limited evidence of thalidomide efficacy in the management of IBD, it has also been prescribed to a highly selected cohort of pediatric patients with refractory CD [190–197]. It has been used for induction of remission as well as maintenance therapy, even in patients who do not tolerate or lose their response to biological anti-TNF agents. Regarding its numerous side effects and teratogenicity, close monitoring and appropriate contraception for both genders are mandatory. The recommended starting dose for adolescents is equal to adult dose—50 mg once daily followed by dose adjustment according to response and tolerance. For young children, the suggested dose is 2 mg/kg.

Pathophysiologic Mechanism

According to ATC classification, thalidomide is an immunosuppressant. Its spectrum of activity is yet not fully characterized. It is thought that immunomodulatory, anti-inflammatory, and antineoplastic effects may be due to suppression of TNF-α production, decreased expression of surface adhesion molecule involved in leukocyte migration and antiangiogenic activity. Thalidomide also shows a hypnotic effect, acting as a nonbarbiturate centrally active sedative agent [189].

Thalidomide is available in oral formulation. After absorption, only a minimal proportion of the drug is metabolized by hepatic cytochrome P450, while the vast majority is hydrolyzed by nonenzymatic processes. It is mostly excreted by the urinary system. Thalidomide bioavailability is not significantly influenced by age, gender, renal function, and blood chemistry variables [189].

Clinical Aspects and Drug Interaction

Prior to thalidomide institution, a negative pregnancy test is necessary in all fertile female patients. Also, adequate contraception methods have to be introduced to patients despite their gender. Thalidomide's common side effect is somnolence, thus recommended dosage regime is once daily before bedtime. Most psychiatric adverse effects (vertigo, somnolence, agitation, and anxiety) are dose-dependent [189]. Among other common adverse events significant for pediatric population, is peripheral neuropathy. According to studies by Lazzerini [195, 196] and Felipez [197], prevalence of peripheral neuropathy was 25% and 42%, respectively. If not recognized in time, it may cause irreversible damages [190]. Careful monitoring for paresthesia, dysesthesia, discomfort, abnormal coordination, or weakness is mandatory.

CNS Depressant: Thalidomide

Concomitant use of thalidomide and other CNS depressants is contraindicated as it may have a potential synergistic sedative effect [189]. Aforementioned potentially harmful CNS depressants belong to a different group of medication: anxiolytics, hypnotics, antipsychotics, H_1 antihistamines, opiate derivatives, barbiturates, and alcohol.

Cannabis: Thalidomide

Tetrahydrocannabinol (THC),a major known psychoactive component of cannabis, is a well-known CNS depressant. Its combination with other similarly acting agents, such as thalidomide, may enhance this effect [198, 199]. Recreational drug abuse is more common among younger patients, thus ensure they have all the relevant information about this potentially harmful interaction.

Vaccines: Thalidomide

All recommendations stated in sections "Corticosteroids" and "MTX" about vaccination are completely applicable to thalidomide.

Estrogen Derivatives [Contraceptive]: Thalidomide

Albeit there is a strong theoretical concept about the increased risk of thromboembolism in patients receiving thalidomide and oral contraceptives, real-world data are lacking. Nevertheless, close monitoring for signs and symptoms of thromboembolism is recommended.

Vedolizumab: Thalidomide

According to a vedolizumab summary of product characteristic, any coadministration with anti-TNF agents, including thalidomide, is strictly contraindicated as it may enhance the toxic effects of this monoclonal antibody [200].

Natalizumab: Thalidomide

Natalizumab labeling emphasizes the importance of avoiding the concomitants use with all immunosuppressants due to the increased risk of concurrent infection and adverse effect [132].

Other Clinically Significant Drug Interactions of Sulfasalazine Are Described with

Abatacept, anakinra, azelastine, BCG, bromperidol, canakinumab, cetrolizumab pegol, cladribine, dipyrone, orphenadrine, oxomemazine, paraldehyde, pembrolizumab, pimecrolimus, rilonacept, tocilizumab, upadacitinib, amifostine, baricitinib, blonanserin, chlormethiazole, deferiprone, dexamethasone, droperidol, *Echinacea*, fingolimod, flunitrazepam, leflunomide, lemborexant, methotrimeprazine, nivolumab, obinutuzumab, opioid agonists, oxycodone, perampanel, roflumilast, sipuleucel-T, sodium oxybate, suvorexant, zolpidem, alfuzosin, alizapride, amilsulpiride, benperidol, bisphosphonate derivatives, blood pressure lowering agents, brexanolone, brimonidine, bromopride, cholaramphenicol, clozapine, coccidioides immitis skin test, denosumab, diazoxide, dimethindene, doxylamine, dronabinol, duloxetine, erythropoiesis-stimulating agents, esketamine, hydroxyzine, hypotension-associated agents, inebilizumab, kava kava, levodopa-containing products, lisuride, lofexidine, lormetazepam, magnesium sulfate, metoclopramide, metyrosine, minocycline, molsidomine, nabilone, naftopidil, nicergoline, nicorandil, nitroprusside, ocrelizumab, ozanimod, pamidronate, pentoxifylline, pholcodine, phosphodiesterase 5 inhibitors, pribedil, pramipexole, progestins, promazine, prostacyclin analogues, quinagolide, ropinirole, rotigotine, rufinamide, siponimod, tertomotide, trastuzumab, trimeprazine, zoledronic acid, levodropropizine, mianserin (additional information: https://www.webmd.com/interaction-checker/default.htm).

References

1. Torres J, Bonovas S, Doherty G, Kucharzik T, Gisbert JP, Raine T, et al. ECCO guidelines on therapeutics in Crohn's disease: medical treatment. J Crohns Colitis. 2019;2020:4–22.
2. Harbord M, Eliakim R, Bettenworth D, Karmiris K, Katsanos K, Kopylov U, et al. Third European evidence-based consensus on diagnosis and management of ulcerative colitis. Part 2: Current management. J Crohn's Colitis. 2017:769–84.
3. Ligumsky M, Karmeli F, Sharon P, Zor U, Cohen F, Rachmilewitz D. Enhanced thromboxane A2 and prostacyclin production by cultured rectal mucosa in ulcerative colitis and its inhibition by steroids and sulfasalazine. Gastroenterology. 1981;81(3):444–9.
4. Hawkey CJ, Boughton-Smith NK, Whittle BJR. Modulation of human colonic arachidonic acid metabolism by sulfasalazine. Dig Dis Sci. 1985;30(12):1161–5.
5. Santucci L, Wallace J, Mencarelli A, Farneti S, Morelli A, Fiorucci S. Different sensitivity of lamina propria T-cell subsets to nitric oxide-induced apoptosis explains immunomodulatory activity of a nitric oxide-releasing derivative of mesalamine in rodent colitis. Gastroenterology. 2005;128(5):1243–57.
6. Ahnfelt-Rønne I, Nielsen OH, Christensen A, Langholz E, Binder V, Riis P. Clinical evidence supporting the radical scavenger mechanism of 5-aminosalicylic acid. Gastroenterology. 1990;98(5 Part 1):1162–9.
7. Ye B. Mesalazine preparations for the treatment of ulcerative colitis: are all created equal? World J Gastrointest Pharmacol Ther. 2015;6(4):137.
8. Bell NJV, Burget D, Howden CW, Wilkinson J, Hunt RH. Appropriate acid suppression for the management of gastro-oesophageal reflux disease. Digestion. 1992;51(1):59–67.
9. Blum RA, Shi H, Karol MD, Greski-Rose PA, Hunt RH. The comparative effects of lansoprazole, omeprazole, and ranitidine in suppressing gastric acid secretion. Clin Ther. 1997;19(5):1013–23.
10. MMRVAXPRO (Measles, Mumps and Rubella Vaccine (Live)). Summary of product characteristics (SmPC)—(EMC). Lyon, France: Merck Sharp & Dohme Limited; 2019.
11. Varilrix (varicella-zoster virus). Summary of product characteristics (SmPC)—(EMC). Middlesex, UK: GlaxoSmithKline UK; 2020.
12. Carty M, Rampton. Inhibition of platelet activation by 5-aminosalicylic acid in inflammatory bowel disease. Aliment Pharmacol Ther. 2000;14(9):1169–79.
13. Teefy AM, Martin JE, Kovacs MJ. Warfarin resistance due to sulfasalazine. Ann Pharmacother. 2000;34(11):1265–8.
14. Hall S, Rindone JP. A case of sulphasalazine potentiating the hypoprothombinemic effect of warfarin resulting in bleeding. J Clin Pharm Ther. 2011;36(2):246–8.
15. Gisbert JP, González-Lama Y, Maté J. 5-Aminosalicylates and renal function in inflammatory bowel disease: a systematic review. Inflamm Bowel Dis. 2007;13(5):629–38.
16. Szumlanski C, Weinshilboum R. Sulphasalazine inhibition of thiopurine methyltransferase: possible mechanism for interaction with 6-mercaptopurine and azathioprine. Br J Clin Pharmacol. 1995;39(4):456–9.
17. Lewis LD, Benin A, Szumlanski CL, Otterness DM, Lennard L, Weinshilboum RM, et al. Olsalazine and 6-mercaptopurine-related bone marrow suppression: a possible drug-drug interaction. Clin Pharmacol Ther. 1997;62(4):464–75.
18. Juhl RP, Summers RW, Guillory JK, Blaug SM, Cheng FH, Brown DD. Effect of sulfasalazine on digoxin bioavailability. Clin Pharmacol Ther. 1976;20(4):387–94.
19. Salazopyrin Tablets (sulfasalazine). Summary of product characteristics (SmPC)—(EMC). Kent, UK: Pfizer Limited; 2019.
20. Krogh Jensen M, Ekelund S, Svendsen L. Folate and homocysteine status and haemolysis in patients treated with sulphasalazine for arthritis. Scand J Clin Lab Invest. 1996;56(5):421–9.
21. Methotrexate (methotrexate). Summary of product characteristics (SmPC)—(EMC). Orionintie, Finland: Orion Pharma (UK) Limited; 2019.

22. Du Cheyron D, Debruyne D, Lobbedez T, Richer C, Ryckelynck JP, Hurault de Ligny B. Effect of sulfasalazine on cyclosporin blood concentration. Eur J Clin Pharmacol. 1999;55(3):227–8.
23. Vosevi (sofosbuvir, velpatasvir, voxilaprevir). Summary of product characteristics (SmPC)—(EMC). Carrigtohill, Ireland: Gilead Sciences Ltd.; 2020.
24. Lardieri AB, Crew PE, McCulley L, Kim IE, Waldron P, Diak IL. Cases of Benzocaine-associated methemoglobinemia identified in the FDA adverse event reporting system and the literature. Ann Pharmacother. 2019;53(4):437–8.
25. Olsalazine (olsalazine sodium). Summary of product characteristics (SmPC)—(EMC). Essex, UK: Atnahs Pharma UK Ltd.; 2015.
26. Budenofalk (budesonide). Summary of product characteristics (SmPC)—(EMC). Freiburg, Germany: Dr. Falk Pharma UK Ltd.; 2019.
27. Regueiro M, Loftus EV, Steinhart AH, Cohen RD. Medical management of left-sided ulcerative colitis and ulcerative proctitis: Critical evaluation of therapeutic trials. Inflamm Bowel Dis. 2006;12(10):979–94.
28. Edsbäcker S, Andersson T. Pharmacokinetics of budesonide [Entocort™ EC] capsules for Crohn's disease. Clin Pharmacokinet. 2004;43(12):803–21.
29. Kroger AT, Sumaya CV, Pickering LK, Atkinson WL. General recommendations on immunization: recommendations of the Advisory Committee on Immunization Practices [ACIP]. Morbid Mortal Weekly Rep Centre for Dis Control Prev. 2011;60(2)
30. Johansson C, Adamsson U, Stierner U, Lindsten T. Interaction by cholestyramine on the uptake of hydrocortisone in the gastrointestinal tract. Acta Med Scand. 1978;204(1–6):509–12.
31. Frankel JK, Packer CD. Cushing's syndrome due to antiretroviral-budesonide interaction. Ann Pharmacother. 2011;45(6):823.
32. Jones W, Chastain CA, Wright PW. Iatrogenic Cushing syndrome secondary to a probable interaction between voriconazole and budesonide. Pharmacotherapy. 2014;34(7)
33. Clipper (beclometasone dipropionate). Summary of product characteristics (SmPC)—(EMC). Manchester, United Kingdom: Chiesi Limited; 2019.
34. Van Assche G, Manguso F, Zibellini M, Cabriada Nunõ JL, Goldis A, Tkachenko E, et al. Oral prolonged release beclomethasone dipropionate and prednisone in the treatment of active ulcerative colitis: results from a double-blind, randomized, parallel group study. Am J Gastroenterol. 2015;110(5):708–15.
35. Prantera C, Rizzi M, Cottone M, Casa A, Annese V, Sturniolo GC, et al. Beclomethasone dipropionate in Crohn's ileitis: a randomised, double-blind trial. Dig Liver Dis. 2011;43(6):459–64.
36. Tursi A, Giorgetti GM, Brandimarte G, Elisei W, Aiello F. Beclomethasone dipropionate for the treatment of mild-to-moderate Crohn's disease: an open-label, budesonide-controlled, randomized study. Med Sci Monit. 2006;12(6):PI29–32.
37. Summers RW, Switz DM, Sessions JT, Becktel JM, Best WR, Kern F, et al. National Cooperative Crohn's disease study: results of drug treatment. Gastroenterology. 1979;77(4 Part 2):847–69.
38. Medrone (methyprednisolone). Summary of product characteristics (SmPC)—(EMC). Kent, UK: Pfizer Limited; 2019.
39. Prednisolone (prednisolone). Summary of product characteristics (SmPC)—(EMC). Barnstaple, Devone: Accord-UK Ltd.; 2020.
40. Uribe M, Casian C, Rojas S, Sierra J, Go VLW, Rosa MA, et al. Decreased bioavailability of prednisone due to antacids in patients with chronic active liver disease and in healthy volunteers. Gastroenterology. 1981;80(4):661–5.
41. Lee D, Taylor G, Walker J, James V. The effect of concurrent administration of antacids on prednisolone absorption (letter). Br J Clin Pharmacol. 1979;8(1):92–4.
42. Pecora PG, Kaplan B. Corticosteroids and ulcers: Is there an association? Ann Pharmacother. 1996;30(7–8):870–2.
43. Ellershaw JE, Kelly MJ. Corticosteroids and peptic ulceration. Palliat Med. 1994;8(4):313–9.

44. Harris CL, Raisch DW, Abhyankar U, Marfatia S, Campbell HM, Sather MR. GI risk factors and use of GI protective agents among patients receiving nonsteroidal antiinflammatory drugs. Ann Pharmacother. 2006;40(11):1924–31.
45. Graham GG, Champion GD, Day RO, Paull PD. Patterns of plasma concentrations and urinary excretion of salicylate in rheumatoid arthritis. Clin Pharmacol Ther. 1977;22(4):410–20.
46. Koren G, Roifman C, Gelfand E, Lavi S, Suria D, Stein L. Corticosteroids-salicylate interaction in a case of juvenile rheumatoid arthritis. Ther Drug Monit. 1987;9(2):177–9.
47. Klinenberg JR, Miller F. Effect of corticosteroids on blood salicylate concentration. J Am Med Assoc. 1965;194(6):601–4.
48. Öst L. Impairment of prednisolone metabolism by cyclosporine treatment in renal graft recipients. Transplantation. 1987;44(4):533–5.
49. Langhoff E, Madsen S, Flachs H, Olgaard K, Ladefoged J, Hvidberg EF. Inhibition of prednisolone metabolism by cyclosporine in kidney–transplanted patients. Transplantation. 1985;39(1):107–9.
50. Klintmalm G, Säwe J. High dose methylprednisolone increases plasma cyclosporin levels in renal transplant recipients. Lancet. 1984;323(8379):731.
51. Hricik DE, Moritz C, Mayes JT, Schulak JA. Association of the absence of steroid therapy with increased cyclosporine blood levels in renal transplant recipients. Transplantation. 1990;49(1):221–3.
52. Frey FJ, Schnetzer A, Horber FF, Frey BM. Evidence that cyclosporine does not affect the metabolism of prednisolone after renal transplantation. Transplantation. 1987;43(4):494–8.
53. Rocci ML, Tietze KJ, Lee J, Harris H, Danzeisen J, Burke JF. The effect of cyclosporine on the pharmacokinetics of prednisolone in renal transplant patients. Transplantation. 1988;45(3):656–60.
54. Arnold JC, O'Grady JG, Tredger JM, Williams R. Effects of low-dose prednisolone on cyclosporine pharmacokinetics in liver transplant recipients: radioimmunoassay with specific and non-specific monoclonal antibodies. Eur J Clin Pharmacol. 1990;39(3):257–60.
55. AmBisome (amphotericin b). Summary of product characteristics (SmPC)—(EMC). Abington, Cambridge, UK: Gilead Sciences Ltd.; 2019.
56. Sarma GR, Kailasam S, Nair NG, Narayana AS, Tripathy SP. Effect of prednisolone and rifampin on isoniazid metabolism in slow and rapid inactivators of isoniazid. Antimicrob Agents Chemother. 1980;18(5):661–6.
57. Ciprofloxacin (ciprofloxacin lactate). Summary of product characteristics (SmPC)—(EMC). Terrugem, Portugal: Consilient Health Ltd.; 2020.
58. Van der Linden PD, Sturkenboom MCJM, Herings RMC, Leufkens HMG, Rowlands S, Stricker BHC. Increased risk of Achilles tendon rupture with quinolone antibacterial use, especially in elderly patients taking oral corticosteroids. Arch Intern Med. 2003;163(15):1801–7.
59. Van der Linden PD, Sturkenboom MCJM, Herings RMC, Leufkens HGM, Stricker BHC. Fluoroquinolones and risk of Achilles tendon disorders: case-control study. Br Med J. 2002;324(7349):1306–7.
60. Widmer P, Capaul R, Mueller U, Galeazzi R, Maibach R, Künzi UP, et al. Diuretic-related hypokalaemia: the role of diuretics, potassium supplements, glucocorticoids and β2-adrenoceptor agonists - Results from the comprehensive hospital drug monitoring programme, Berne [CHDM]. Eur J Clin Pharmacol. 1995;49(1–2):31–6.
61. Ruud E, Holmstrøm H, Bergan S, Wesenberg F. Oral anticoagulation with warfarin is significantly influenced by steroids and CYP2C9 polymorphisms in children with cancer. Pediatr Blood Cancer. 2008;50(3):710–3.
62. Hazlewood KA, Fugate SE, Harrison DL. Effect of oral corticosteroids on chronic warfarin therapy. Ann Pharmacother. 2006;40(12):2101–6.
63. Dowd MB, Vavra KA, Witt DM, Delate T, Martinez K. Empiric warfarin dose adjustment with prednisone therapy. A randomized, controlled trial. J Thromb Thrombolysis. 2011;31(4):472–7.

64. Klein RG, Arnaud SB, Gallagher JC, Deluca HF, Riggs BL. Intestinal calcium absorption in exogenous hypercortisonism. Role of 25 hydroxyvitamin D and corticosteroid dose. J Clin Invest. 1977;60(1):253–9.
65. Kimberg DV, Baerg RD, Gershon E, Graudusius RT. Effect of cortisone treatment on the active transport of calcium by the small intestine. J Clin Invest. 1971;50(6):1309–21.
66. Lukert BP, Stanbury SW, Mawer EB. Vitamin D and intestinal transport of calcium: effects of prednisolone. Endocrinology. 1973;93(3):718–22.
67. Murray MJ, Brull SJ, Bolton CF. Brief review: nondepolarizing neuromuscular blocking drugs and critical illness myopathy. Can J Anesth. 2006;53(11):1148–56.
68. Fischer JR, Baer RK. Acute myopathy associated with combined use of corticosteroids and neuromuscular blocking agents. Ann Pharmacother. 1996;30(12):1437–44.
69. Barrons RW. Drug-induced neuromuscular blockade and myasthenia gravis. Pharmacotherapy. 1997;17(6):1220–32.
70. Booker BM, Magee MH, Blum RA, Lates CD, Jusko WJ. Pharmacokinetic and pharmacodynamic interactions between diltiazem and methylprednisolone in healthy volunteers. Clin Pharmacol Ther. 2002;72(4):370–82.
71. Varis T, Backman JT, Kivistö KT, Neuvonen PJ. Diltiazem and mibefradil increase the plasma concentrations and greatly enhance the adrenal-suppressant effect of oral methylprednisolone. Clin Pharmacol Ther. 2000;67(3):215–21.
72. Lichtenstein GR, Loftus EV, Isaacs KL, Regueiro MD, Gerson LB, Sands BE. ACG clinical guideline: management of Crohn's disease in adults. Am J Gastroenterol. 2018;113(4):481–517.
73. McCarthy NE, Hedin CR, Sanders TJ, Amon P, Hoti I, Ayada I, et al. Azathioprine therapy selectively ablates human Vδ2+T cells in Crohn's disease. J Clin Invest. 2015;125(8):3215–25.
74. Tiede I, Fritz G, Strand S, Poppe D, Dvorsky R, Strand D, et al. CD28-dependent Rac1 activation is the molecular target of azathioprine in primary human CD4+ T lymphocytes. J Clin Invest. 2003;111(8):1133–45.
75. A-Rahim YI, Farrell RJ. Overview of azathioprine and mercaptopurine use in inflammatory bowel disease. In: Robson KM, editor. UpToDate; 2019. Retrieved from https://www.uptodate.com/contents/overview-of-azathioprine-and-mercaptopurine-use-in-inflammatory-bowel-disease.
76. Imuran (azathioprine). Summary of product characteristics (SmPC)—(EMC). Dublin, Ireland, UK: Aspen Pharma Trading Limited; 2019.
77. Moreau B, Clement P, Theoret Y, Seidman EG. Allopurinol in combination with thiopurine induces mucosal healing and improves clinical and metabolic outcomes in IBD. Ther Adv Gastroenterol. 2017;10(11):819–27.
78. Xeljanz (tofacitinib citrate). Summary of product characteristics (SmPC)—(EMC). Bruxelles, Belgium: Pfizer Limited; 2020.
79. Lowry PW, Szumlanski CL, Weinshilboum RM, Sandborn WJ. Balsalazide and azathioprine or 6-mercaptopurine: evidence for a potentially serious drug interaction. Gastroenterology. 1999;116(6):1505–6.
80. Kirchgesner J, Lemaitre M, Carrat F, Zureik M, Carbonnel F, Dray-Spira R. Risk of serious and opportunistic infections associated with treatment of inflammatory bowel diseases. Gastroenterology. 2018;155(2):337–346.e10.
81. Kotlyar DS, Osterman MT, Diamond RH, Porter D, Blonski WC, Wasik M, et al. A systematic review of factors that contribute to hepatosplenic T-cell lymphoma in patients with inflammatory bowel disease. Clin Gastroenterol Hepatol. 2011;9(1):36–41.e1.
82. Sultan KS, Berkowitz JC, Khan S. Combination therapy for inflammatory bowel disease. World J Gastrointest Pharmacol Ther. 2017;8(2):103–13.
83. Department of Health. National Health Service Immunisation Against Infectious Disease—"The Green Book". Chapter 6: Contraindications and special considerations. 2017. Available from: https://www.gov.uk/government/publications/contraindications-and-special-considerations-the-green-book-chapter-6.
84. Imvanex Smallpox vaccine (live modified vaccinia virus ankara). Summary of product characteristics (SmPC)—(EMC). Hellerup, Denmark: Bavarian Nordic A/S; 2018.

85. Yokote H, Shinmura Y, Kanehara T, Maruno S, Kuranaga M, Matsui H, et al. Safety of attenuated smallpox vaccine LC16m8 in immunodeficient mice. Clin Vaccine Immunol. 2014;21(9):1261–6.
86. Elijovisch F, Krakoff LR. Captopril-associated granulocytopenia in hypertension after renal transplantation. Lancet; 1980;315(8174):927–928.
87. Gossmann J, Kachel HG, Schoeppe W, Scheuermann EH. Anemia in renal transplant recipients caused by concomitant therapy with azathioprine and angiotensin-converting enzyme inhibitors. Transplantation. 1993;56(3):585–9.
88. Dretchen KL, Morgenroth VH, Standaert FG, Walts LF. Azathioprine: effects on neuromuscular transmission. Anesthesiology. 1976;45(6):604–9.
89. Rivier G, Khamashta MA, Hughes GRV. Warfarin and azathioprine: a drug interaction does exist. Am J Med. 1993;95(3):342.
90. Walker J, Mendelson H, McClure A, Smith MD. Warfarin and azathioprine: clinically significant drug interaction. J Rheumatol. 2002;29(2):398–9.
91. Hulme B, Reeves DS. Leucopenia associated with trimethoprim-sulphamethoxazole after renal transplantation. Br Med J. 1971;3(5775):610–2.
92. Bradley PP, Warden GD, Maxwell JG, Rothstein G. Neutropenia and thrombocytopenia in renal allograft recipients treated with trimethoprim-sulfamethoxazole. Ann Intern Med. 1980;93(4):560–2.
93. Andrès E, Noel E, Maloisel F, Masters PA, O'Bryan TA, Zurlo J, et al. Trimethoprim-sulfamethoxazole-induced life-threatening agranulocytosis (2) [multiple letters]. Arch Intern Med. 2003;163(16):1975–6.
94. Van Der Klauw MM, Goudsmit R, Halie MR, Van't Veer MB, RMC H, JHP W, et al. A population-based case-cohort study of drug-associated agranulocytosis. Arch Intern Med. 1999;159(4):369–74.
95. Van Der Klauw MM, Wilson JH, Stricker BH. Drug-associated agranulocytosis: 20 years of reporting in The Netherlands (1974–1994). Am J Hematol. 1998;57(3):206–11.
96. Myers MW, Jick H. Hospitalization for serious blood and skin disorders following co- trimoxazole. Br J Clin Pharmacol. 1997;43(6):649–51.
97. Feagan BG, Rochon J, Fedorak RN, Irvine EJ, Wild G, Sutherland L, et al. Methotrexate for the treatment of Crohn's disease. N Engl J Med. 1995;332(5):292–7.
98. Wang Y, Macdonald JK, Vandermeer B, Griffiths AM, El-Matary W. Methotrexate for maintenance of remission in ulcerative colitis. Cochrane Database Syst Rev. 2015;2017(12) https://doi.org/10.1002/14651858.CD007560.pub3.
99. Methotrexate (methotrexate). Summary of product characteristics (SmPC)—(EMC). Hurley, UK: Hospira UK Ltd.; 2019.
100. Saag KG, Gim GT, Patkar NM, et al. American College of Rheumatology 2008 recommendations for the use of nonbiologic and biologic disease-modifying antirheumatic drugs in rheumatoid arthritis. Arthritis Care Res. 2008;59(6):762–84.
101. Dupuis LL, Koren G, Shore A, Silverman EDLR. Methotrexate-nonsteroidal antiinflammatory drug interaction in children with arthritis. J Rheumatol. 1990;17(11):1469–73.
102. Takeda M, Khamdang S, Narikawa S, Kimura H, Coceani F. Characterization of methotrexate transport and its drug interactions with human organic anion transporters. J Pharmacol Exp Ther. 2002;302(2):666–71.
103. Nozaki Y, Kusuhara H, Endou H, Sugiyama Y. Quantitative evaluation of the drug-drug interactions between methotrexate and nonsteroidal anti-inflammatory drugs in the renal uptake process based on the contribution of organic anion transporters and reduced folate carrier. J Pharmacol Exp Ther. 2004;309(1):226–34.
104. El-Sheikh AAK, Van Den Heuvel JJMW, Koenderink JB, Russel FGM. Interaction of nonsteroidal anti-inflammatory drugs with multidrug resistance protein [MRP] 2/ABCC2- and MRP4/ABCC4-mediated methotrexate transport. J Pharmacol Exp Ther. 2007;320(1):229–35.
105. Mandel MA. The synergistic effect of salicylates on methotrexate toxicity. Plast Reconstr Surg. 1976;57(6):733–7.

106. Aithal GP. Hepatotoxicity related to antirheumatic drugs. Nat Rev Rheumatol. 2011;7(3):139–50. https://doi.org/10.1038/nrrheum.2010.214.
107. Jobanputra P, Amarasena R, Maggs F, Homer D, Bowman S, Rankin E, et al. Hepatotoxicity associated with sulfasalazine in inflammatory arthritis: a case series from a local surveillance of serious adverse events. BMC Musculoskelet Disord. 2008;9:48.
108. Asacol (mesalazine). Summary of product characteristics (SmPC)—(EMC). Dublin, Ireland: Allergan Ltd.; 2016.
109. Santucci R, Levêque D, Lescoute A, Kemmel V, Herbrecht R. Delayed elimination of methotrexate associated with co-administration of proton pump inhibitors. Anticancer Res. 2010;30(9):3807–10.
110. Reid T, Yuen A, Catolico M, Carlson RW. Impact of omeprazole on the plasma clearance of methotrexate. Cancer Chemother Pharmacol. 1993;33(1):82–4.
111. Beorlegui B, Aldaz A, Ortega A, Aquerreta I, Sierrasesúmega L, Giráldez J. Potential interaction between methotrexate and omeprazole. Ann Pharmacother. 2000;34(9):1024–7.
112. Tröger U, Stötzel B, Martens-Lobenhoffer J, Gollnick H, Meyer FP. Drug points: severe myalgia from an interaction between treatments with pantoprazole and methotrexate. Br Med J. 2002;324(7352):1497.
113. Santucci R, Levêque D, Kemmel V, Lutz P, Gérout AC, N'Guyen A, et al. Severe intoxication with methotrexate possibly associated with concomitant use of proton pump inhibitors. Anticancer Res. 2010;30(3):963–6.
114. McBride A, Antonia SJ, Haura EB, Goetz D. Suspected methotrexate toxicity from omeprazole: a case review of carboxypeptidase G2 use in a methotrexate-experienced patient with methotrexate toxicity and a review of the literature. J Pharm Pract. 2012;25(4):477–85.
115. Breedveld P, Zelcer N, Pluim D, Sönmezer Ö, Tibben MM, Beijnen JH, et al. Mechanism of the pharmacokinetic interaction between methotrexate and benzimidazoles: Potential role for breast cancer resistance protein in clinical drug-drug interactions. Cancer Res. 2004;64(16):5804–11.
116. Suzuki K, Doki K, Homma M, Tamaki H, Hori S, Ohtani H, et al. Co-administration of proton pump inhibitors delays elimination of plasma methotrexate in high-dose methotrexate therapy. Br J Clin Pharmacol. 2009;67(1):44–9.
117. Erttmann R, Landbeck G. Effect of oral cholestyramine on the elimination of high-dose methotrexate. J Cancer Res Clin Oncol. 1985;110(1):48–50.
118. Frusol (furosemide). Summary of product characteristics (SmPC)—(EMC). Leeds, UK: Rosemont Pharmaceuticals Limited; 2017.
119. Glynn-Barnhart AM, Erzurum SC, Leff JA, Martin RJ, Cochran JE, Cott GR, et al. Effect of low-dose methotrexate on the disposition of glucocorticoids and theophylline. J Allergy Clin Immunol. 1991;88(2):180–6.
120. Seifter EJ, Brooks BJ Jr, UW. Possible interactions between warfarin and antineoplastic drugs. Cancer Treat Rep. 1985;69(2):244–5.
121. Bourré-Tessier J, Haraoui B. Methotrexate drug interactions in the treatment of rheumatoid arthritis: a systematic review. J Rheumatol. 2010;37(7):1416–21.
122. Beach BJ, Woods WG, Howell SB. Influence of co-trimoxazole on methotrexate pharmacokinetics in children with acute lymphoblastic leukemia. J Pediatr Hematol Oncol. 1981;3(2):115–20.
123. Liegler DG, Henderson ES, Hahn MA, Oliverio VT. The effect of organic acids on renal clearance of methotrexate in man. Clin Pharmacol Ther. 1969;10(6):849–57.
124. Tortajada-Ituren JJ, Ordovás-Baines JP, Llopis-Salvia P, Victor J-TN. High-dose methotrexate-doxycycline interaction. Ann Pharmacother. 1999;33(7–8):804–8.
125. Bubik RJ, Osmon DR, Oravec CPRC. Two cases of severe neutropenia in patients on low-dose methotrexate and ceftriaxone. Am J Heal Syst Pharm. 2019;76(11):804–9.
126. Ronchera CL, Hernández T, Peris JE, Torres F, Granero L, Jiménez NV, et al. Pharmacokinetic interaction between high-dose methotrexate and amoxycillin. Ther Drug Monit. 1993;15(5):375–9.

127. Dean R, Nachman J, Lorenzana AN. Possible methotrexate-mezlocillin interaction. Am J Pediatr Hematol Oncol. 1992;14(1):88–9.
128. Zarychanski R, Wlodarczyk K, Ariano RBE. Pharmacokinetic interaction between methotrexate and piperacillin/tazobactam resulting in prolonged toxic concentrations of methotrexate. J Antimicrob Chemother. 2006;58(1):228–30.
129. Nierenberg DW, Mamelok RD. Toxic reaction to methotrexate in a patient receiving penicillin and furosemide: a possible interaction. Arch Dermatol. 1983;119(6):449–50.
130. Dalle JH, Auvrignon A, Vassal G, Leverger G. Interaction between methotrexate and ciprofloxacin. J Pediatr Hematol Oncol. 2002;24(4):321–2.
131. Jarfaut A, Santucci R, Levêque D, Herbrecht R. Severe methotrexate toxicity due to a concomitant administration of ciprofloxacin. Med Mal Infect. 2013;43(1):39–41.
132. Tysabri (natalizumab). Summary of product characteristics (SmPC)—(EMC). Badhoevedorp, The Netherlands: Biogen Idec Ltd.; 2020.
133. Mycophenolate Mofetil (mycophenolate mofetil). Summary of product characteristics (SmPC)—(EMC). Hafnarfjordur, Iceland: Accord-UK Ltd; 2016.
134. Lv QK, Liu JX, Li SN, Gao YJ, Lv Y, Xu ZP, et al. Article mycophenolate mofetil modulates differentiation of Th1/Th2 and the secretion of cytokines in an active Crohn's disease mouse model. Int J Mol Sci. 2015;16(11):26654–66.
135. Wenzl HH, Hinterleitner TA, Aichbichler BW, Fickert P, Petritsch W. Mycophenolate mofetil for Crohn's disease: short-term efficacy and long-term outcome. Aliment Pharmacol Ther. 2004;19(4):427–34.
136. Fickert P, Hinterleitner TA, Wenzl HH, Aichbichler BW, Petritsch W. Mycophenolate mofetil in patients with Crohn's disease. Am J Gastroenterol. 1998;93(12):2529–32.
137. Gomollón F, Dignass A, Annese V, Tilg H, Van Assche G, Lindsay JO, et al. 3rd European evidence-based consensus on the diagnosis and management of Crohn's disease 2016: Part 1: Diagnosis and medical management on behalf of ECCO. J Crohns Colitis. 2017:3–25.
138. Gionchetti P, Dignass A, Danese S, José F, Dias M, Rogler G, et al. 3rd European evidence-based consensus on the diagnosis and management of Crohn's disease 2016: Part 2: Surgical management and special situations. J Crohns Colitis. 2017;11(2):135–49.
139. Lichtiger S, Present DH, Kornbluth A, Gelernt I, Bauer J, Galler G, et al. Cyclosporine in severe ulcerative colitis refractory to steroid therapy. N Engl J Med. 1994;330(26):1841–5.
140. D'Haens G, Lemmens L, Geboes K, Vandeputte L, Van Acker F, Mortelmans L, et al. Intravenous cyclosporine versus intravenous corticosteroids as single therapy for severe attacks of ulcerative colitis. Gastroenterology. 2001;120(6):1323–9.
141. Van Assche G, D'Haens G, Noman M, Vermeire S, Hiele M, Asnong K, et al. Randomized, double-blind comparison of 4 mg/kg versus 2 mg/kg intravenous cyclosporine in severe ulcerative colitis. Gastroenterology. 2003;125(4):1025–31.
142. Fernandez-Banares F, Bertran X, Esteve-Comas M, et al. Azathioprine is useful in maintaining long-term remission induced by intravenous cyclosporine in steroid-refractory severe ulcerative colitis. Am J Gastroenterol. 1996;91(12):2498–9.
143. Moskovitz DN, Van Assche G, Maenhout B, et al. Incidence of colectomy during long-term follow-up after cyclosporine-induced remission of severe ulcerative colitis. Clin Gastroenterol Hepatol. 2006;4(6):760–5.
144. Cohen RD, Stein R, Hanauer SB. Intravenous cyclosporin in ulcerative colitis: a five-year experience. Am J Gastroenterol. 1999;94(6):1587–92.
145. Santos JV, Baudet JA, Casellas FJ, Guarner LA, Vilaseca JM, Malagelada JRB. Intravenous cyclosporine for steroid-refractory attacks of Crohn's disease: short- and long-term results. J Clin Gastroenterol. 1995;20(3):207–10.
146. Hermida-Rodriguez C, Cantero Perona J, Garcia-Valriberas R, et al. High-dose intravenous cyclosporine in steroid refractory attacks of inflammatory bowel disease. Hepato-Gastroenterology. 1999;46:2265–8.
147. Egan LJ, Sandborn WJ, Tremaine WJ. Clinical outcome following treatment of refractory inflammatory and fistulizing Crohn's disease with intravenous cyclosporine. Am J Gastroenterol. 1998;93(3):442–8.

148. Nicholls S, Domizio P, Williams CB, et al. Cyclosporin as initial treatment for Crohn's disease. Arch Dis Child. 1994;71(3):243–7.
149. Stange EF, Modigliani R, Peña AS, Wood AJ, Feutren G, Smith PR. European trial of cyclosporine in chronic active Crohn's disease: a 12-month study. Gastroenterology. 1995;109(3):774–82.
150. Feagan BG, Mcdonald JWD, Rochon J, et al. Low-dose cyclosporine for the treatment of Crohn's disease. N Engl J Med. 1994;330(26):1846–51.
151. Sandimmun (ciclosporin). Summary of product characteristics (SmPC)—(EMC). London, UK: Novartis Pharmaceuticals UK LTD; 2020.
152. Hardinger K., Magee CC. Pharmacology of cyclosporine and tacrolimus. in: Lam AQ, editor. UpToDate; 2020. Retrieved from: https://www.uptodate.com/contents/pharmacology-of-cyclosporine-and-tacrolimus?csi=dbc454ce-cbc6-4064-8127-e58820817783&source=contentShare.
153. Peppercorn MA, Farrell RJ. Management of the hospitalized adult patient with severe ulcerative colitis. In: Robson KM, editor. Up to date; 2019. Retrieved from: https://www.uptodate.com/contents/management-of-the-hospitalized-adult-patient-with-severe-ulcerative-colitis?csi=f2b7c01c-5505-46a5-bbd0-24d3760e167e&source=contentShare.
154. Eckardt KU, Kasiske BL, Zeier MG. Special Issue: KDIGO Clinical practice guideline for the care of kidney transplant recipients. Am J Transplant. 2009;9:S1–S155. https://doi.org/10.1111/j.1600-6143.2009.02834.x.
155. Lixiana (edoxaban tosilate). Summary of product characteristics (SmPC)—(EMC). Münich, Germany: Daiichi Sankyo UK Limited; 2020.
156. Chang SH, Chou IJ, Yeh YH, Chiou MJ, Wen MS, Kuo CT, et al. Association between use of non–vitamin K oral anticoagulants with and without concurrent medications and risk of major bleeding in nonvalvular atrial fibrillation. JAMA. 2017;318(13):1250–9.
157. Maltz HC, Balog DL, Cheigh JS. Rhabdomyolysis associated with concomitant use of atorvastatin and cyclosporine. Ann Pharmacother. 1999;33(11):1176–779.
158. Yang WH, Zeng ZS, Ren XW, Li YP, Shang WJ, Feng GW, et al. Simvastatin-induced myopathy with concomitant use of cyclosporine: case report. Int J Clin Pharmacol Ther. 2011;49(12):772–7.
159. Park JW, Siekmeier R, Lattke P, Merz M, Mix C, Schuiler S, et al. Pharmacokinetics and pharmacodynamics of fluvastatin in heart transplant recipients taking cyclosporine A. J Cardiovasc Pharmacol Ther. 2001;6(4):351–61.
160. Simonson SG, Raza A, Martin PD, Mitchell PD, Jarcho JA, Brown CDA, et al. Rosuvastatin pharmacokinetics in heart transplant recipients administered an antirejection regimen including cyclosporine. Clin Pharmacol Ther. 2004;76(2):167–77.
161. Ezetimibe (ezetimibe). Summary of product characteristics (SmPC)—(EMC). North Harrow, UK: Accord Healthcare Limited; 2018.
162. Wadhwa NK, Schroeder TJ, O'Flaherty E, Pesce AJ, Myre SA, First MR. The effect of oral metoclopramide on the absorption of cyclosporine. Transplantation. 1987;43(2):211–3.
163. Zepatier (elbasvir, grazoprevir). Summary of product characteristics (SmPC)—(EMC). Haarlem, The Netherlands: Merck Sharp & Dohme Limited; 2020.
164. Maviret (glecaprevir, pibrentasvir). Summary of product characteristics (SmPC)—(EMC). Ludwigshafen, Germany: AbbVie Ltd.; 2020.
165. Ueda Y, Kaido T, Uemoto S. Fluctuations in the concentration/dose ratio of calcineurin inhibitors after simeprevir administration in patients with recurrent hepatitis C after liver transplantation. Transpl Int. 2015;28(2):251–2.
166. Reichenspurner H, Meiser BM, Muschiol F, et al. The influence of gastrointestinal agents on resorption and metabolism of cyclosporine after heart transplantation: experimental and clinical results. J Hear Lung Transpl. 1993;12(6 Pt 1):987–92.
167. D'Souza MJ, Pollock SH, Solomon HM. Cyclosporine-cimetidine interaction. Drug Metab Dispos. 1988;16:1.
168. Schouler L, Dumas F, Couzigou P, Janvier G, Winnock SSJ. Omeprazole-cyclosporin interaction. Am J Gastroenterol. 1991;86(8):1097.

169. Lorf T, Ramadori G, Ringe B, et al. Pantoprazole does not affect cyclosporin a blood concentration in kidney-transplant patients. Eur J Clin Pharmacol. 2000;55:733–5.
170. Chitwood KK, Abdul-Haqq AJ, Heim-Duthoy KL. Cyclosporine-amiodarone interaction. Ann Pharmacother. 1993;27(5):569–71.
171. Mamprin F, Mullins P, Graham T, et al. Amiodarone-cyclosporine interaction in cardiac transplantation. Am Heart J. 1992;123(6):1725–6.
172. Okamura N, Hirai M, Tanigawara Y, Tanaka K, Yasuhara M, Ueda K, et al. Digoxin-cyclosporin A interaction: modulation of the multidrug transporter P-glycoprotein in the kidney. J Pharmacol Exp Ther. 1993;266(3):1614–9.
173. Dorian P, Strauss M, Cardella C, David T, East SOR. Digoxin-cyclosporine interaction: severe digitalis toxicity after cyclosporine treatment. Clin Invest Med. 1988;11(2):108–12.
174. Dorian P, Cardella C, Strauss M, David T, East S OR. Cyclosporine nephrotoxicity and cyclosporine—digoxin interaction prior to heart transplantation. Transpl Proc 1987;19(1 Pt 2):1825–1827.
175. Noordzij TC, Leunissen KML, Van Hooff JP. Renal handling of urate and the incidence of gouty arthritis during cyclosporine and diuretic use. Transplantation. 1991;52(1):64–7.
176. Christians U, Jacobsen W, Benet LZ, Lampen A. Mechanisms of clinically relevant drug interactions associated with tacrolimus. Clin Pharmacokinet. 2002;41(11):813–51.
177. Kim RB. Drugs as P-glycoprotein substrates, inhibitors, and inducers. Drug Metab Rev. 2002;34(1–2):47–54.
178. Hesselink DA, Van Hest RM, Mathot RAA, Bonthuis F, Weimar W, De Bruin RWF, et al. Cyclosporine interacts with mycophenolic acid by inhibiting the multidrug resistance-associated protein 2. Am J Transplant. 2005;5(5):987–94.
179. Westley IS, Brogan LR, Morris RG, Evans AM, Sallustio BC. Role of MRP2 in the hepatic disposition of mycophenolic acid and its glucuronide metabolites: effect of cyclosporine. Drug Metab Dispos. 2006;34(2):261–6.
180. Humira (adalimumab). Summary of product characteristics (SmPC)—(EMC). Ludwigshafen, Germany: AbbVie Ltd.; 2019.
181. Powles AV, Baker BS, Fry L, Valdimarsson H. Cyclosporin toxicity. Lancet. 1990;335(8689):610.
182. Korstanje MJ, van Breda Vriesman CJP, van de Staak WJBM. Cyclosporine and methotrexate: a dangerous combination. J Am Acad Dermatol. 1990;23(2):320–1.
183. Fox R, Morgan S, Smith H, et al. Treatment of RA patients with methotrexate [MTX] plus cyclosporine A [CSA] leads to elevation of plasma MTX levels and decrease of 7 hydroxy-methotrexate [7-OH] Levels. Arthritis Rheum. 1998;41(Suppl. 9):S138.
184. Stockschlaeder M, Storb R, Pepe M, Longton G, McDonald G, Anasetti C, et al. A pilot study of low-dose cyclosporin for graft-versus-host prophylaxis in marrow transplantation. Br J Haematol. 1992;80(1):49–54.
185. Prograf (tacrolimus monohydrate). Summary of product characteristics (SmPC)—(EMC). Surrey, United Kingdom: Astellas Pharma Ltd.; 2019.
186. Matsuoka K, Saito E, Fujii T, Takenaka K, Kimura M, Nagahori M, et al. Tacrolimus for the treatment of ulcerative colitis. Intest Res. 2015;13(3):219.
187. Mutalib M, Borrelli O, Blackstock S, Kiparissi F, Elawad M, Shah N, et al. The use of sirolimus [rapamycin] in the management of refractory inflammatory bowel disease in children. J Crohn's Colitis. 2014;8(12):1730–4.
188. Farkas S, Hornung M, Sattler C, Guba M, Steinbauer M, Anthuber M, et al. Rapamycin decreases leukocyte migration in vivo and effectively reduces experimentally induced chronic colitis. Int J Color Dis. 2006;21(8):747–53.
189. Thalidomide Celgene (thalidomide). Summary of product characteristics (SmPC)—(EMC). Utrecht, Netherlands: Celgene Ltd.; 2020.
190. Ruemmele FM, Veres G, Kolho KL, Griffiths A, Levine A, Escher JC, et al. Consensus guidelines of ECCO/ESPGHAN on the medical management of pediatric Crohn's disease. J Crohns Colitis. 2014;8(10):1179–207.

191. Akobeng AK, Stokkers PC. Thalidomide and thalidomide analogues for maintenance of remission in Crohn's disease. Cochrane Database Syst Rev. 2009:2. https://doi.org/10.1002/14651858.CD007351.pub2.
192. Srinivasan R, Akobeng AK. Thalidomide and thalidomide analogues for induction of remission in Crohn's disease. Cochrane Database Syst Rev. 2009;(2) https://doi.org/10.1002/14651858.CD007350.pub2.
193. Kammermeier J, Morris MA, Garrick V, Furman M, Rodrigues A, Russell RK. Management of Crohn's disease. Arch Dis Child. 2016;101(5):475–80.
194. Bramuzzo M, Ventura A, Martelossi S, Lazzerini M. Thalidomide for inflammatory bowel disease: systematic review. Med (United States). 2016;95(30):e4239. https://doi.org/10.1097/MD.0000000000004239.
195. Lazzerini M, Martelossi S, Marchetti F, et al. Efficacy and safety of thalidomide in children and young adults with intractable inflammatory bowel disease: long-term results. Aliment Pharmacol Ther. 2007;25(4):419–27.
196. Lazzerini M, Martelossi S, Magazzù G, et al. Effect of thalidomide on clinical remission in children and adolescents with refractory Crohn disease: A randomized clinical trial. J Am Med Assoc. 2013;310(20):2164–73.
197. Felipez LM, Gokhale R, Tierney MP, Kirschner BS. Thalidomide use and outcomes in pediatric patients with crohn disease refractory to infliximab and adalimumab. J Pediatr Gastroenterol Nutr. 2012;54(1):28–33.
198. Hollister L. Interactions of cannabis with other drugs in man. NIDA Res Monogr. 1986;68:110–6.
199. Johnstone RE, Lief PL, Kulp RA, Smith TC. Combination of Δ9 tetrahydrocannabinol with oxymorphone or pentobarbital: effects on ventilatory control and cardiovascular dynamics. Anesthesiology. 1975;42(6):674–84.
200. Entyvio (vedolizumab). Summary of product characteristics (SmPC)—(EMC). Taastrup, Denmark: Takeda UK Ltd.; 2020.

29 Intestinal Inflammation: Biologics and Small Molecules

Marko Banić, Željko Krznarić, Marko Brinar, Marija Urek, and Milenko Bevanda

Abbreviations

CD	Crohn's Disease
CYPs	Cytochromes, a superfamily of enzymes
DMARDs	Disease-modifying anti-rheumatic drugs
EBV	Ebstein Barr Virus
EMA	European Medicine Agency
FDA	Food and Drug Administration (US)

M. Banić (✉)
Division for IBD and Clinical Nutrition, Department of Gastroenterology, Hepatology and Clinical Nutrition, Dubrava University Hospital, Zagreb, Croatia

School of Medicine, University of Zagreb, Zagreb, Croatia

School of Medicine, University of Rijeka, Rijeka, Croatia
e-mail: mbanic@kbd.hr

Ž. Krznarić · M. Brinar
School of Medicine, University of Zagreb, Zagreb, Croatia

Division of Gastroenterology and Hepatology, Department of Internal Medicine, University Hospital Center Zagreb, Zagreb, Croatia
e-mail: zeljko.krznaric1@zg.t-com.hr

M. Urek
Division of Gastroenterology, Hepatology and Clinical Nutrition, Department of Internal Medicine, Dubrava University Hospital, Zagreb, Croatia

School of Medicine, University of Zagreb, Zagreb, Croatia

M. Bevanda
Division of Gastroenterology and Hepatology, Department of Internal Medicine, University Hospital Mostar, Mostar, Bosnia and Herzegovina

School of Medicine, University of Mostar, Mostar, Bosnia and Herzegovina

M. Banić, D. Erceg (eds.), *Drug Interactions in Gastroenterology*, Clinical Gastroenterology, https://doi.org/10.1007/978-3-031-69800-2_29

HSCTL	Hepatosplenic T-cell Lymphoma
IBD	Inflammatory Bowel Disease
JAK	Janus Kinase
JAK-STAT	Janus kinase-signal transducers and activators of transcription family
MAdCAM-1	Mucosal Addressin Cell Adhesion Molecule 1
NHL	Non-Hodgkin Lymphoma
PDE	Phosphodiesterase
TNF	Tumor necrosis factor
UC	Ulcerative colitis
VCAM-1	Vascular Cell Adhesion Protein 1

Introduction

Besides the possible interactions of chemically synthetized molecules, the advent and the present wide clinical use of biologics and small molecules that act on inflammatory mediators, integrins, and hubs of signaling and/or metabolic pathways pave the scenery of the medication decisions and the risk of drug interactions more complicated. The newly designed molecules, either chemically synthesized or produced by methods of biotechnology and used for the treating of intestinal inflammation are no exception.

In the pathogenesis of idiopathic, chronic intestinal inflammation, four components play a major role: the changed intestinal microbiome and genetic/epigenetic background (epi/genome) of each individual, environmental factors (exposome) and altered patterns of immunological reactions (immunome) that initiate, sustain, and perpetuate the inflammation. It has been generally accepted that the crucial events in disease initiation represent the breakdown of tolerance to antigens of self-intestinal microbiota and the breakdown of the intestinal barrier, as well. The methods of systems biology, digital "big data", and efforts of multidisciplinary teams in basic research have broadly expanded our knowledge of multiple interactions of etiopathogenetic components and mechanisms of initiation and perpetuation of inflammation [1].

In parallel, the clinical research teams, collaborating worldwide closely, have strived to identify the precluding factors for the severe and complicated biological course of the disease, along with the development and validation of combined clinical and endoscopic scores that would adequately evaluate the state of disease, during the timeline of cumulative bowel damage. Putting it all together, the networking of translational medicine and "big data" approach has enabled the emerging identification of combined clinical, endoscopic, epi/genetic, metabolomic, immunologic, and microbiomial markers that would recognize different cohorts of patients for targeted therapy and surveillance [2]. At this point, one can differ between preventive/early-stage interventions that are focused on predisposing factors and initiating events of intestinal barrier breakdown and interventions that are focused on treating clinically/endoscopically/histologically established intestinal inflammation.

During the biological course of inflammatory bowel disease (IBD), the established clinical inflammation, in Crohn's disease (CD) going beyond the gut mucosa represents the downstream effects of defective homeostatic modules with altered signaling and metabolic pathways, resulting in overproduction of pro-inflammatory cytokines and accumulation of immune and inflammatory cells in inflamed areas with consequent tissue and organ damage. The therapeutic concept of biologics and newly designed small molecules relies on targeting the specific critical mediators, receptors or processes in key immunologic and inflammatory pathways, presumably providing selective and highly potent regulation [3].

Biologic agents as medicinal products for treating immune-mediated disease are protein-based large molecules, usually monoclonal antibodies or their fragments, produced on living cell lines using recombinant DNA technology [3]. It has been over twenty years, since FDA approval for infliximab, the first anti-TNF biologic drug for the treatment of moderate to severe IBD. The originally designed biological drugs that followed have also targeted different cytokines (IL-12/23) or different adhesion molecules (anti-integrin agents), and are in wide clinical use, today.

These original biologic drugs have been followed by the advent of biosimilar drugs (biosimilars) on the market, after the patent of originally designed biologic drug (reference drug) has expired. The concept of biosimilar drugs evolved due to the possibility of using the shortcuts in the biotechnology process that was originally designed for the production of reference biological drugs. Unlike the chemically synthetized generic active substances that are almost identical to the originally designed reference drug, the biosimilar is not identical but highly similar in regard to physical, chemical, and biological properties to reference biological drug. In regard to the benefits and risks of therapeutic use, by demonstrating biosimilarity, the biosimilar relies on the safety and efficacy experience gained with the reference biologic drug [4].

Medicine agencies in US (FDA) and Europe (EMA) and medicine agencies at the national level in different countries have developed a robust regulatory framework for approval, safety monitoring, traceability in clinical use and pharmacovigilance of biosimilars. One of the key points of the regulatory framework is the extrapolation of the data. If a biosimilar is highly similar to a reference biologic and has comparable safety and efficacy in one therapeutic indication, safety and efficacy data may be extrapolated to other indications approved for the reference biologic [5]. However, the interchangeability, switching, and substitution between biosimilar and reference biologic have been the matter of dispute between medicine agencies and medical societies and patients' associations, as well. In regard to drug interactions, due to complex manufacturing process, the biosimilar product presumably may not mirror the drug interactions profile of the reference biologic, entirely. However, the advent of biosimilars, due to their significantly lower pricing has made biologic therapy to many patients suffering from moderate to severe IBD more accessible.

The therapeutic goals in treating IBD include the achievement of deep and sustained remission with fewer side effects of therapy applied. However, the real-world data have shown that one size does not fit all. The substantial proportion of patients does not elicit the response on given medicine(s) and a substantial proportion experiences a loss of response, over time. In addition, dose escalation in order to optimize therapeutic effect and sustain and/or regain the state of disease remission expose these patients to higher cumulative dose of certain medicine(s), which is of special importance in regard to combination therapy with immunosuppressive drugs and/or corticosteroids. Thus, there is a continuing need for new therapeutic approaches that include the development of substances with targeted anti-inflammatory/immunomodulatory efficacy and new formulations (including the route of application) of already established drugs, as well. A special need for effective and safer medicines that could alter the biological course of disease exists in patients who are refractory to established therapy. The oral preparations, containing small molecules offer possible advantages over parenteral medicines. Oral drugs could be applied with less discomfort, probably less immunogenicity and achieving more stable concentration over time, due to shorter intervals of application. On the other hand, the lesions in the small bowel could affect the absorption of small molecules and there exists the still open question of their efficacy on extraintestinal manifestations of IBD. Nevertheless, the substances designed for oral use could probably offer improved efficacy and a more advantageous safety profile, at least in certain cohorts of patients with IBD [6, 7].

The results of published networking meta-analyses have discussed certain aspects of the efficacy and safety of medicines in the first and second line of therapy for IBD [8]. Still, the answers that should strongly support the concept of evidence-based and personalized medicine should await the results of "head to head" and randomized controlled trials., appropriately designed.

It is almost impossible to predict the potential interactions of different drugs in each and individual patients, with certainty and accuracy. Especially in the clinical situations of polypharmacy and different (epi)genetic backgrounds and comorbidity that could influence the mechanisms of absorption, distribution, metabolism, and excretion that are specific to each drug in use. In clinical decision-making, it is mandatory to be familiar with the most common drug interactions, in order to avoid the major, highly clinically significant interactions, always considering the risks and benefits for the patient. In situations of known and already documented moderate or minor interactions of particular drug combinations, the careful clinical use of these combinations is possible, under special circumstances. The special problem represents the majority of drugs, for which are no data available. However, this nonexistence of data does not mean that these drugs are free from possible interactions in individual patient, taking into account the aforementioned special clinical situations. In spite of the fact that biologics and small molecules are grouped according to the mode of action and targeting certain general or specific inflammatory pathways, there exist significant differences in their biosafety and possible drug interactions, taking into account the differences in selectivity in regard to the inhibition of hub signaling pathways, such as JAK-STAT inhibition.

Table 29.1 Major drug interactions: anti-TNF agents, vedolizumab, ustekinumab, and tofacitinib

Anti-TNF agents	Vedolizumab	Ustekinumab	Tofacitinib
Abatacept	Anti-TNF	Anti-TNF	Abatacept
Anakinra	Etanercept	Ccertolizumab	Anakinra
Azathioprine	Leflunomide	Etanercept	Anti-TNF
BCG	Live vaccines	Leflunomid	Azacitidine
Certolizumab pegol	Natalizumab	Live vaccine	Azathioprine
Corticosteroids	Ozanimod	Natalizumab	Bleomycine
Cyclophosphamide	Tofacitinib	Ozanimod	Cisplatin
Cyclosporine	Upadacitinib	Tocilizumab	Corticosteroids
Cisplatin		Tofacitinib	Cyclosporine
Doxorubicin		Upadacitinib	Etanercept
Etanercept			Everolimus
Everolimus			Fluconazole
Fludarabine			Guselkumab
Ganciclovir			Imatinib
Linezolid			Itraconazole
Live vaccines			Ketoconazole
Methotrexate			Linezolid
Ozanimod			Live vaccine
Risankizumab			lopinavir
Rituximab			Metothrexate
Roflumilast			Natalizumab
Ssecukinumab			Ozanimod
Tacrolimus			Phenobarbital
Tocilizumab			Phenytoin
Tofacitinib			Posaconazole
Upadacitinib			Rifampin
Ustekinumab			Risankizumab
Vedolizumab			Ritonavir
			Rituximab
			Sirolimus
			Tacrolimus
			Tocilizumab
			Upadacitinib
			Vedolizumab
			Voriconazole
			Zidovudine

Tables 29.1 and 29.2, at the end of this chapter, illustrate major and moderate interactions of biologics and JAK inhibitors, widely used in treating intestinal inflammation.

Biologics and Small Molecules in the Treatment of Inflammatory Bowel Disease

During the past 20 years, the general effect of the therapeutic approach to inflammatory bowel disease has been significantly improved, in healing the bowel and improving the patient's quality of life, along with better inclusion into the family

Table 29.2 Moderate drug interactions: anti-TNF agents, vedolizumab, ustekinumab, and tofacitinib

Anti-TNF agents	Vedolizumab	Ustekinumab	Tofacitinib
Alprazolam	Aanakinra	6-MP	Amiodarone
Aminophylline	Azathioprine	Abatacept	Aspirin
Amiodarone	Nonlive vaccines	Albendazole	Atenolol
Amlodipine	Roflumilast	Alprazolam	Bisoprolol
Apixaban	Ustekinumab	Aminophylline	Biprofloxacin
Atorvastatin		Amiodarone	Blonidine
Buprenorphine		Amlodipine	Diltiazem
Cyclosporine		Anakinra	Fentanyl
Inactivated vaccines		Apixaban	Ganciclovir
Isoniazid		Atorvastatin	Nonlive vaccine
Lidocaine		Azathioprine	Ibuprofen
Metronidazole		Bortezomib	Indomethacin
Naltrexone		Buprenorphine	Lansoprazole
Nifedipine		Colchicine	Lidocaine
Nitrofurantoin		Corticosteroids	Methadone
Phenobarbital		Cyclosporine	Omeprazole
Propafenone		Danorubicin	Propafenone
Remdesivir		Diazepam	Roflumilast
Roflumilast		Dverolimus	Tramadol
Rosuvastatin		Fentanyl	Verapamil
Theophylline		Imatinib	
Warfarin		Lidocaine	
		Linezolid	
		Methadone	
		Methotrexate	
		Midazolam	
		Nifedipine	
		Nonlive vaccine	
		Phenobarbital	
		Phenytoin	
		Prošafenone	
		Risankizumab	
		Rituximab	
		Tacrolimus	
		Thalidomide	
		Vedolizumab	
		Warfarin	

and community. The targeted biologic therapy, anti-TNF agents as first have enabled the shorter time in achieving the remission and sustainment of long-lasting remission, along with the change of the biological course of the disease, in a significant number of patients with IBD (see also Chap. 9). However, the certain number of patients on biologic therapy experienced primary nonresponse (20–40% on anti-TNF biologics) during the early stage of therapy and loss of response (20–46% on anti-TNF biologics) during the first years of therapy [9].

In light of those unmet medical needs of IBD patients, the wide variety of biologics and small molecules, already registered for clinical use or continuing/finalizing registration trials and/or in the process of registration feature the strategic approaches (see also Chap. 9). These strategic approaches include inhibition of cytokine pathways, inhibition of JAK (Janus kinases)-STAT (signal transducer and activators of transcription family) signaling, PDE (phosphodiesterase) inhibition, inhibition of immune cells trafficking, lymphocyte trapping by sphingosine-1-phosphate receptor modulators, oligonucleotide therapeutics, and cell-based therapies [10]. However, this chapter on drug interactions in regard to biologics and small molecules is focused on medicines that are already in wide clinical use for treating intestinal inflammation.

Anti-TNF Medicines: Infliximab, Adalimumab, Golimumab, Certolizumab Pegol

Anti-TNF agents inhibit the cytokine TNF-α which plays a central role in the mediation of systemic and mucosal inflammation and this is the first class of biologic agents that has been approved for use in inflammatory bowel diseases (IBD). To date, anti-TNF agents remain most widely used class of biologic medicines, due to relatively rapid onset of action and high anti-inflammatory/immunomodulatory efficacy in both, gastrointestinal and extra-intestinal manifestations of the disease [11–13]. The use of anti-TNF biologics provides immunosuppression and could lead to serious infections, but it has been shown that the risk is lower in real-world settings than predicted, initially. Importantly, the risk of serious infections is lower than the one, associated with steroid use [14]. Furthermore, there have been concerns raised regarding the increased likelihood of malignancy or lymphoma which also appear to be overemphasized, mostly relative to the risk of existing (combo) immunosuppressive therapy with conventional small molecules [15–17]. To date, four different original anti-TNF agents and several biosimilars of infliximab and adalimumab are approved for use in IBD.

Infliximab, the first anti-TNF agent to be in clinical use is a chimeric monoclonal antibody, approved for treating Crohn's disease (CD) and ulcerative colitis (UC), including induction and maintenance therapy, and in treating fistulizing disease [18–21].

More specifically, infliximab is indicated in moderately to severely active CD with inadequate response to conventional therapy (to reduce signs/symptoms and induce and maintain clinical remission) or to reduce the number of draining enterocutaneous and rectovaginal fistulas and maintain fistula closure in adults. In UC, infliximab is indicated in moderately to severely active ulcerative colitis with inadequate response to conventional therapy (to reduce signs/symptoms and induce and maintain clinical remission) or to induce/maintain mucosal healing and eliminate corticosteroid use in adults. Dosing of infliximab in CD and UC is weight-based and is administered 5 mg/kg at 0, 2, and 6 weeks, followed by 5 mg/kg every 8 weeks, with a certain number of patients requiring higher doses (10 mg/kg) or shortened interval (6 or 4 weeks).

Adalimumab is a human IgG1 monoclonal anti-TNF-α antibody approved for use in both CD and UC, in treatment of active moderate to severe disease in patients with an inadequate response to conventional therapy or who have lost response to or are intolerant to infliximab [22–25]. The induction therapy for adalimumab is initiated with a dose of 160 mg subcutaneously on day 1, or split and given over 2 consecutive days, followed by the dose of 80 mg s.c. after two weeks. After the mentioned induction therapy, the maintenance therapy is usually scheduled as 40 mg s.c. every other week. In order to sustain the adequate response/remission, a certain number of patients may require 40 mg every week as maintenance therapy.

Golimumab is a human IgG1 monoclonal antibody directed against TNF-α and is approved for use in UC only in the treatment of moderately to severely active ulcerative colitis in adults with corticosteroid dependence or who have had an inadequate response to conventional therapy (to induce and maintain clinical response, improve mucosal appearance during induction, induce clinical remission, and achieve and sustain remission in induction responders) [26, 27]. The induction therapy with golimumab is started subcutaneously with a dose of 200 mg at week 0, then 100 mg at week two, followed by maintenance therapy at fixed dose of 100 mg every 4 weeks.

Certolizumab pegol is a humanized, pegylated Fab' fragment of an antibody directed against TNF-α, approved for use in CD in treatment of moderately to severely active CD in patients who have inadequate response to conventional therapy [28–31]. Certolizumab pegol is administered subcutaneously, initially 400 mg with repeated doses 2 and 4 weeks after initial dose. Standard dose of maintenance therapy is 400 mg every 4 weeks.

According to the currently available database of drug interactions, there is a total of 395 drugs known to interact with infliximab (230 major, 158 moderate, and 7 minor drug interactions), 381 drugs known to interact with adalimumab (227 major, 147 moderate, and 7 minor), 381 drugs known to interact with golimumab (227 major, 147 moderate, and 7 minor), and 382 known drug interactions with certolizumab (227 major, 148 moderate, and 7 minor) [32–35]. The focus of this chapter is to discuss the clinically most relevant drug interactions of anti-TNF agents.

Anti-Integrin Agent: Vedolizumab

The second class of biologic agents with proven anti-inflammatory and immunomodulatory activity are anti-integrin agents. The main mechanism is interfering with leukocyte migration to sites of inflammation, in contrast to anti-TNF agents which interfere with cytokine molecules, directly. The mechanisms of action of anti-integrins rely on blocking a transmembrane receptor present on a cell surface that mediates cell adhesion, signaling, and migration [36]. The α4 integrins are situated on leukocytes and they interact with cell adhesion molecules on the vascular endothelium VCAM-1 and MAdCAM-1, which is a key point in allowing of cell migration to the site of inflammation and enabling inflammatory cascade. Vedolizumab is a humanized IgG1 monoclonal antibody which specifically binds to

$\alpha 4\beta 7$ that is found primarily on cells localized in the GI tract and biliary system, in that manner blocking the interaction with MAdCAM-1 [37]. In contrast to nonselective anti-integrin molecules, such as natalizumab, and due to its gut selectivity, the major advantage of vedolizumab is a very good safety profile [38]. Vedolizumab is indicated in treatment of UC and CD, administered at a dose of 300 mg at weeks 0, 2, and 6 and then 300 mg every 8 weeks, thereafter. According to the current available database of drug interactions, there is a total 100 drugs known to interact with vedolizumab (30 major, 63 moderate, and 7 minor drug interactions), which is considerably less compared to anti-TNF-a agents [39].

Anti-IL-12/23 Agent: Ustekinumab

Ustekinumab is a human IgG antibody developed to bind to the p40 protein subunit of receptors for cytokines IL-12 and IL-23, the IL-12 being responsible for activation of STAT4 transcription factor with downstream effect of long-term Th1 activation and IL-23 playing a key role in proliferation and stabilization of Th17 cells in gut mucosa. Ustekinumab is indicated for the treatment of moderate to severe or refractory CD and UC. In the induction phase, ustekinumab is administered intravenously, the dose depending on the body weight of an individual patient (≤55 kg: 260 mg as single dose, >55 kg to 85 kg: 390 mg as single dose or > 85 kg: 520 mg as single dose). Maintenance therapy usually starts at week 8, after the induction dose, and continuing with the dose of 90 mg every 12 weeks. However, according to the prescribing information, the dose in maintenance phase could be applied at shorter intervals, such as every 8 weeks [40]. About 360 drug interactions have been described with ustekinumab (33 major, 320 moderate, and 7 minor) [41].

JAK Inhibitor: Tofacitinib

In addition to biologics, there is also an increasing interest in the potential of small molecules, which are specifically designed and have the potential to disrupt intracellular signaling pathways, crucial to IBD pathogenesis. Compared to anti-inflammatory therapy with biologics, the advantages of small molecules would be the targeting of specific intracellular pathways and minimizing the interference, oral administration and relatively stable concentrations in blood and tissue, and the lack of immunogenicity, as well. The Janus kinases (JAKs) represent the family of intracellular tyrosine kinases that enable transmission of signals (via JAK-STAT phosphorylation pathway) from receptors interacting with cytokines, interferons, and hormones to the nucleus, with the downstream effect of synthesis of many biologically active compounds that change the cell metabolism and function. The class I and class II receptors use JAKs as catalytic centers to transmit signals of multiple cytokines and growth factors, including IFN-γ, IL-2, IL-6, IL-12, and IL-23 [42, 43]. Thus, the blockade of JAK-STAT pathway represents deep interference in the immune system with possible suppression of normal immune response and reduction of the organism's self-defense. In that way, the panblockade of JAK-STAT pathway, along with the reduction of inflammation may also induce serious adverse events, toxicity, and represent an increased risk for infections, bone marrow suppression, and increased incidence of cardiovascular events [44]. Tofacitinib is a nonselective JAK inhibitor which preferentially inhibits JAK 3, and to a lesser extent JAK 1 and 2 [44]. Tofacitinib is indicated for the treatment of adult patients with moderately to severely active UC, usually at an induction dose of 10 mg twice daily for 8–16 weeks, based on the obtained therapeutic response [34]. Maintenance dose is usually set at 5–10 mg twice daily, after assessing the benefits and risk of therapy and taking into account the recommendation to use the lowest effective dose to maintain response [45].

A substantial number of significant drug interactions have been noted for tofacitinib, so far. Altogether, 472 drug interactions have been described (266 major, 198 moderate, and 8 minor), according to database [45].

Interactions: Biologics, Conventional, and Newly Designed Small Molecules and Vaccines

Overall, most of the interactions in this group of drugs are due to additive effects, mostly immunosuppressive, and the potential risk of combined immunosuppression and/or immunomodulation should not outweigh the expected clinical benefit in a particular patient. Therefore, the potential clinical situations of significant interactions should be approached carefully. A special issue represents the use of different vaccines in patients on immunosuppressive/immunomodulatory therapy.

Combination of Biological Drugs and/or Small Molecules: Major Interaction

In clinical practice, the concomitant use of more than one biologic should be avoided, whenever possible. The combination of anti-TNF agents (infliximab, adalimumab, golimumab, and certolizumab pegol), vedolizumab, ustekinumab, or tofacitinib in the treatment of IBD is categorized as major interaction and is generally not recommended. However, current therapies for IBD are not effective in all patients and there exists a growing interest in combining biologics with different modes of anti-inflammatory/immunomodulatory action, in order to improve the outcome in each individual patient. On the other hand, in spite of the growing number of different molecules as potential IBD therapies in the pipeline, the therapeutic approach using the combination of registered biologics and small molecules with clinically proven efficacy and already noted adverse effects and interactions of each drug seems to be tempting. Indeed, the results of case reports and case series in both, CD and UC speak in favor of clinical feasibility in using the combination of these drugs. However, the data about this therapeutic paradigm in IBD are limited and the results of randomized controlled trials in other immune-mediated diseases, such as rheumatologic diseases raised concerns in regard to serious adverse reactions [46]. The mechanism of this interaction is hypothesized to be the additive immunosuppressive effect of combined therapy, which brings up the issue of increased risk of infection, simultaneously raising the question of inadequate additive efficacy and increased adverse events, such as in the combination of biologics and disease-modifying antirheumatic drugs (DMARDs). [47–51] In clinical setting of combined therapy with biologics and/or small molecules, it seems that the increased risk of infection is rather the result of the synergistic immunosuppressive/immunomodulatory effect of drug combination than the result of a true drug interaction [52].

Biological Drugs with Corticosteroids: Major Interaction

According to the Drugs interaction database, there is a general rule that applies to the use of biological therapy with both immunosuppressive or myelosuppressive agents in terms of increased risk of infections, serious infections, and sepsis [40]. This is particularly important when using high doses of corticosteroids or adrenocorticotropic agents (greater than 10 mg/day to 1 mg/kg/day, whichever is less, of prednisone or equivalent for more than 2 weeks) [53]. Chronic corticosteroid therapy can lead to an increased risk of adverse events such as Cushing syndrome, acne, infection, increased risk of abdominal and pelvic abscesses in patients with CD, ecchymoses, hypertension, diabetes mellitus, osteoporosis, cataracts, glaucoma, and growth failure in children [54]. It is important to stress that corticosteroids have an effect on the human body's nonspecific defense and entire immune system—innate and adaptive immunity. In addition, the adverse events and drug interactions linked to the combined therapy with corticosteroids and biologics are further complicated by the heterogeneity of IBD phenotypes, across different populations [55].

However, the data from postmarketing surveillance strategies and databases, such as TREAT™ and ENCORE registries offered the tool for estimation and/or calculation of safety outcomes [56]. Therefore, close monitoring for signs and symptoms of developing infections is advised whenever a combination of immunosuppressive therapy is used. In conclusion, anti-TNF-a therapy, vedolizumab, ustekinumab, or tofacitinib should be used with caution in combination with corticosteroids, especially in the cases of higher doses of corticosteroid therapy, and early tapering of corticosteroids during induction therapy with biologics is strongly advised [57].

Live Vaccines and Immunosuppressive Medicines: Major Interaction

Immunosuppressants may enhance adverse or toxic effects of live vaccines or may diminish their therapeutic effect, and therefore should generally be avoided. Overall, the clinical significance of the interaction of immunosuppressive agents and live vaccines may be dose- and duration-dependent. Even though the current data on response to vaccination with live vaccines or on possible secondary transmission of infection by live vaccines in patients receiving anti-TNF therapy are limited, it is considered that such concomitant therapy could result in clinical infection or disseminated infection. Therefore, it is recommended that live vaccines (e.g., BCG vaccine, Measles, Mumps, Rubella, live/trivalent/oral Poliovirus vaccine, Varicella virus vaccine, etc.) should not be given during therapy with anti-TNF therapy (e.g., infliximab, adalimumab, golimumab, certolizumab pegol), neither with other biologic agents/small molecules used in the treatment of IBD (e.g., vedolizumab, ustekinumab, and tofacitinib) [53].

Additionally, live vaccines in infants who have been exposed to infliximab during pregnancy should not be administered within 6 months of age, due to the fact that infliximab is known to cross the placenta and to be present in the serum of infants up to 6 months [48]. Although the current data are scarce, there are some general recommendations. Whenever possible, vaccination should be received prior to initiation of immunosuppressive therapy or after immunosuppressive therapy cessation and after restoring immune function, which may usually take up to 3 months, depending on the elimination half-life [53]. In addition, due to immunosuppressive effects, inadequate immune response to vaccine may also occur. Local immunization guidelines should be consulted for recommendations regarding initiating immunosuppressive therapy after vaccination, especially if there is a relatively short interval between immunization and starting immunosuppressive therapy (e.g., less than 2 weeks).

Inactivated Vaccines: Moderate Interaction

Inactivated vaccines could be used in patients treated with infliximab, adalimumab, golimumab, certolizumab pegol, vedolizumab, ustekinumab, or tofacitinib. The administration of nonalive, inactivated, killed, or otherwise noninfectious vaccines to immunosuppressed patients is generally safe. Another concern is diminished effectiveness, i.e., lower immunologic response. There are some general recommendations of the Advisory Committee on Immunization Practices (ACIP) which state that inactivated vaccines can be safely administered to non-HIV immunosuppressed patients according to the standard procedure. However, such immunization could require higher dosages or more frequent boosters. Immunologic response could be tested using serological testing [58]. Local guidelines should be consulted for more detailed approach, according to the specific type of vaccination. If possible, all age-appropriate vaccinations should be completed at least 2 weeks prior to initiation of an immunosuppressant. If this is not the case, revaccination after the restoration of the immune system (e.g., 3 months after discontinuation of immunosuppressive therapy), could be considered [58]. Some of the inactivated vaccines such as Diphtheria and Tetanus, acellular Pertussis, Hepatitis B (recombinant), Poliovirus (inactivated), Haemophilus influenzae B conjugate (adsorbed) vaccine, Influenza virus vaccine (inactivated), Influenza virus vaccine (recombinant), Pneumococcal conjugate vaccine, etc.

Anti-TNF Agents and Immunosuppressive Therapy

Anti-TNF Agents and Other Targeted Biological Therapy

Concomitant use of anti-TNF agents and biological therapy has been described under section "Anti-TNF Medicines: Infliximab, Adalimumab, Golimumab, Certolizumab Pegol".

Anti-TNF Agents and Thiopurine Analogues: Major Interaction

There are several concerns regarding the concomitant use of azathioprine and anti-TNF agents (infliximab, adalimumab, golimumab, and certolizumab pegol). Firstly, this combination of therapy may increase the risk for T-cell non-Hodgkin's lymphomas (NHL), especially hepatosplenic T-cell lymphoma (HSTCL), which is likely to be a consequence of additive immunosuppression, and secondly, infliximab may lead to increased levels of azathioprine active metabolite with unknown mechanism. Analysis of the FDA Adverse Event Reporting System identified an increased risk of T-cell NHL with the combination of a TNF-alpha inhibitor and a thiopurine and with thiopurine use only, while there was no significant risk observed with the use of TNF-alpha inhibitors only [59]. Furthermore, a pharmacokinetic study on 32 patients with CD reported an increase in the 6-tioguanine levels by 60% 1–3 weeks after treatment with infliximab which returned to baseline values 3 months after treatment [60]. Prescribing information for infliximab states that almost all HSTCL cases were, in addition to anti-TNF agents, treated with azathioprine or 6-mercaptopurine, and that the majority of the affected population were adolescents and young males with CD or UC [48]. Thus, in young males, especially EBV-negative and elderly this concomitant therapy should be generally avoided [61]. This is important to emphasize since the improved efficacy of combination therapy with azathioprine over biologic monotherapy has been proved in a landmark SONIC study in CD and later confirmed in UC SUCCESS study for UC [62, 63].

Patient management should therefore include close monitoring for developing of signs and symptoms suggestive of T-cell NHL, including HSTCL such as splenomegaly, hepatomegaly, abdominal pain, persistent fever, night sweats, and weight loss. Secondly, serious and potentially life-threating infections may occur due to additive immunosuppressive effects. Finally, monitoring for toxic effects of azathioprine such as leukopenia or thrombocytopenia should also be applied.

Methotrexate and Anti-TNF Agents: Major Interaction

Synergistic effect of methotrexate on the efficacy of infliximab has been described, and it has also been shown that, as with azathioprine, methotrexate decreases the formation of infliximab antibodies [64, 65]. According to the prescribing information, no specific drug interaction studies have been conducted with methotrexate and infliximab [48]. Regarding adalimumab, current data do not suggest the need for dose adjustment when combined with methotrexate, even though there have been reports that concomitant use of adalimumab and methotrexate reduces adalimumab clearance, while another study demonstrated no effect of adalimumab on methotrexate pharmacokinetics [66, 67]. Prescribing information on golimumab states that the presence of methotrexate did not influence efficacy or safety in psoriatic arthritis and ankylosing spondylitis [49]. In conclusion, even though there are no strict recommendations, as with other combinations of immunosuppressive drugs, due to their additive immunosuppressive effect, close monitoring for the development of infections should be applied.

Anti-TNF Agents and Cytochrome P450 Substrates: Moderate Interaction

According to the prescribing information, medications that antagonize cytokine activity such as anti-TNF agents, interleukin inhibitors, or interferon inhibitors, could have an influence on drugs that are CYP450 substrates when used in chronic inflammatory diseases [40, 48, 68]. During chronic inflammation increased levels of certain cytokines (e.g., interleukins −1, −6, and − 10, TNF-a) downregulate hepatic CYP450 enzymes. Upon initiation of the treatment with therapy that antagonizes cytokine activity, the lowering of cytokines may allow the normalization or restoration of CYP450 enzyme levels which could result in increased metabolism of the drugs that are cytochrome P450 substrates. In general, when treatments affecting cytokine levels such as anti-TNF-a, interferons, or interleukin are initiated or withdrawn, patients should be closely monitored. This is particularly important with drugs (which represent the cytochrome P450 substrates) that have a narrow therapeutic range (antiarrhythmics, anticonvulsants, immunosuppressants such as cyclosporine, theophylline, and warfarin) or substrates for which the changes in plasma levels may be clinically significant and lead to undesirable effect (oral contraceptives, statins, benzodiazepines, and opioids) [40]. Other medications which interact through cytochrome P450 are alprazolam, aminophylline, amiodarone, amlodipine, apixaban, atorvastatin, etc. (see Table 29.2).

Anti-TNF Agents and Anakinra or Abatacept: Major Interaction

Concomitant use of anti-TNF agents and abatacept or anakinra should be avoided due to an increased risk for serious infection, and if transitioning from one medication to another, patients could be closely monitored for signs of infection. Namely, data on concomitant administration of abatacept with anti-TNF agents report a significantly higher rate of infections (63% vs. 43%) and serious infections (4.4% vs. 0.8%) [69]. Furthermore, substantially more severe infections were reported that were associated with combined anakinra and etanercept than with etanercept alone [70]. Additionally, this combination was also associated with neutropenia which could increase the risk of serious infection [70].

Vedolizumab

Vedolizumab is considered relatively safe due to its gut selectivity. Data regarding interactions are not extensive, but some of them need to be pointed out according to the prescribing information. Overall, for vedolizumab, there have been the least drug interactions reported.

Vedolizumab and Natalizumab: Major Interaction

The comedication with vedolizumab and natalizumab should not be used due to the increased risk of progressive multifocal leukoencephalopathy (PML) and of other infections. Natalizumab is a nonselective integrin inhibitor which has been associated with PML, while this association has not been clearly established for vedolizumab [71, 72].

Vedolizumab and Anti-TNF Agents: Major Interaction

Prescribing information on vedolizumab states that patients who are receiving vedolizumab should not receive anti-TNF agents due to the potential for an increased risk of infection, as already stated before. Vedolizumab as an immunosuppressive agent is associated with an increased risk of infection, most commonly upper respiratory, including some serious infections [72]. However, a recent systematic review with pool analysis that included seven studies with a total of 18 patients, treated with anti-TNF in combination with vedolizumab or ustekinumab noted clinical improvement in 100% of patients, and no serious adverse events were reported [73]. The authors of the mentioned systematic review concluded that the use of dual biological therapy represents an attractive option therapeutic option for patients with refractory IBD.

The therapeutic approach using the combination of biologics and newly designed small molecules for treating intestinal inflammation has also been discussed in section "Anti-TNF Medicines: Infliximab, Adalimumab, Golimumab, Certolizumab Pegol" of this chapter.

Vedolizumab and Live Vaccines: Major Interaction

The interaction of biologics, including vedolizumab has been discussed in section "Anti-IL-12/23 Agent: Ustekinumab" of this chapter.

Ustekinumab

Ustekinumab and Immunomodulators: Moderate Interaction

The use of ustekinumab with immunomodulatory agents, the risk of common infections, serious infections, and sepsis may be increased, due to additive immunosuppressive effects. In addition, caution is advised if ustekinumab is planned to be used in patients with prior immunosuppressive therapy. In this clinical setting, close clinical and laboratory monitoring is advised both, during and after the discontinuation of therapy. According to the data in the prescribing information, the combined use of ustekinumab with immunomodulators (such as 6-MP, azathioprine, or methotrexate) was encountered in approximately 30% of subjects, and the combined use of ustekinumab with corticosteroids was noted in approximately 40% and 50% of Crohn's disease and ulcerative colitis subjects, respectively. According to this data, the use of combined therapy did not influence the overall safety or efficacy of ustekinumab [40].

Ustekinumab and CYP450 Substrates: Moderate Interaction

Medications that antagonize cytokine activity such as anti-TNF agents, other interleukin inhibitors, or interferon inhibitors, could have an influence on drugs that are CYP450 substrates when used in chronic inflammatory diseases [40, 48, 68]. During chronic inflammation, the increased levels of certain pro-inflammatory cytokines downregulate hepatic CYP450 enzymes. Thus, ustekinumab as an antagonist of pro-inflammatory cytokines (IL-12/23) could normalize the formation of CYP450 enzymes, which could result in increased metabolism of these drugs as CYP450 substrates [63] In general, during initiation and/or withdrawal of medicines affecting pro-inflammatory cytokine levels, including TNF-a, interferons, and cytokines, patients should be closely monitored. This is particularly important in regard to the drugs that are CYP450 substrates, having a narrow therapeutic range (antiarrhythmics, anticonvulsants, immunosuppressants such as cyclosporine, theophylline, and warfarin) or substrates where changes or decreases in plasma levels may be clinically significant and lead to undesirable effect (oral contraceptives, statins, benzodiazepines, and opioids) [53]. Other medications which interact through cytochrome P450 include alprazolam, aminophylline, amiodarone, amlodipine, apixaban, atorvastatin, etc.

Ustekinumab and Allergy Immunotherapy: Major Interaction

Ustekinumab has not been evaluated in patients who have undergone allergy immunotherapy. However, there exists the possibility that ustekinumab may decrease the protective effect of immunotherapy which may lead to suboptimal antiallergic effect and increased incidence of allergic episodes. Patients who have received or are currently receiving allergen immunotherapy have to be approached with caution [40].

Ustekinumab and Live Vaccines: Major Interaction

The interactions of ustekinumab with live vaccines have been described in section "Anti-IL-12/23 Agent: Ustekinumab".

Tofacitinib

Tofacitinib in Combination with Biologics: Major Interaction

The detailed description of concomitant use of biological therapy and small molecules can be found in section "Anti-TNF Medicines: Infliximab, Adalimumab, Golimumab, Certolizumab Pegol".

Strong CP3A4 Inhibitors: Major Interaction

A pharmacokinetic study on 12 healthy volunteers showed that the strong CYP3A4 inhibitor ketoconazole increased the plasma concentrations and systemic exposure to tofacitinib. The coadministration of tofacitinib with potent inhibitors of CYP450 3A4, such as ketoconazole, posaconazole, itraconazole, voriconazole, ritonavir, or lopinavir may significantly increase the plasma concentrations of tofacitinib, which is metabolized by the isoenzyme [64]. The therapeutic combinations of tofacotinib with mentioned medicines may lead to clinically significant side effects, such as lymphopenia, neutropenia, anemia, serious infections, and hyperlipidemia. In UC patients, the dose of tofacitinib should be reduced up to 50% when combined with strong CYP3A4 inhibitors. In these clinical situations, in patients taking 10 mg twice daily, it is advised to reduce the dose to 5 mg twice daily, and in patients taking 5 mg twice daily, the dose should be reduced to 5 mg daily [45].

Coadministration of CYP3A4 and CYP2C19 Inhibitors: Major Interaction

The suspected primary mechanism of this interaction is fluconazole-mediated inhibition of CYP3A4 and CYP2C19, enzymes responsible for tofacitinib metabolism. Tofacitinib is metabolized by CYP3A4 and CYP2C19, and coadministration of fluconazole, which is a moderate CYP3A4 inhibitor and a strong CYP2C19 inhibitor, would increase tofacitinib exposure. In these clinical situations, the dose adjustments of tofacitinib are mandatory, in the manner described for the coadministration of tofacitinib with strong CYP3A4 inhibitors [45].

Strong CYP3A4 Inducers

Comedication of strong CYP3A4 inducer rifampin may reduce tofacitinib efficacy and this combination of medicines is not recommended [64]. In addition to rifampin, the list of strong CYP3A4 inducers, among other medicines include phenobarbital and phenytoin. A retrospective analysis of 81 tofacitinib-treated patients showed that patients who were treated with tofacitinib and strong CYP3A4 inducers had significantly higher discontinuation rates of therapy with tofacitinib [74].

Immunosuppressive Drugs: Major Interaction

Tofacitinib should not be used in combination with other JAK inhibitors, DMARDs, or potent immunosuppressants (e.g., azathioprine, cyclosporine, or tacrolimus) [45]. However, the therapeutic use of tofacitinib in combination with antirheumatic doses of methotrexate or even DMARDs is clinically feasible, along with the close monitoring of patients. There is no clear definition of potent immunosuppressives and lower doses of corticosteroids (i.e., equivalent to prednisone 10 mg/day or less), leflunomide and antirheumatic doses of methotrexate have been used in clinical studies [75, 76].

Taking into account the potential risks and cost of anti-inflammatory therapy, reliable risk predictors are needed and the safety profile of biologic medicines and newly designed small molecules needs to be addressed. It is reasonable to assume that the "big data" approach represents the future of IBD research, including the issue of drug interactions in treating intestinal inflammation [77].

Concluding Remarks

The paradigm of chronic, idiopathic intestinal inflammation represents the continuing challenge in regard to therapeutic targets, such as alleviating the symptoms, achieving the clinical and composite (laboratory, endoscopic, and histologic) remission, thus changing the biological course of the disease and improving the patients' quality of life. Current therapies for IBD are not effective in all patients and there exists a growing interest for new molecules in the pipeline, as well as for therapeutic approaches using the combination of medicines that are registered, already. The sequential and combined nature of proposed regimens of anti-inflammatory therapy, along with dose escalation and/or shortening the intervals between the doses and proven immunogenicity of certain biologicals and their biosimilars pave the scenery of medical decisions and possibilities to encounter various drug interactions more complicated. Moreover, in targeting certain general or specific inflammatory pathways, there exist significant differences in anti-inflammatory medicines' biosafety and possible drug interactions, taking into account the differences in selectivity in regard to the inhibition of hub signaling pathways. In clinical decision-making, it is mandatory to be familiar with the most common drug interactions, in order to avoid the major, highly clinically significant interactions, always considering the risks and benefits for the patient. The special problem represents the drugs, for which are no data available. However, this nonexistence of data does not mean that these drugs are free from possible interactions in individual patient and taking into account the special clinical situations. In these situations, the close clinical and laboratory monitoring of the patients is mandatory.

Further Information and Reading

1. Available at: https://www.drugs.com/drug-interactions/infliximab-index.html
2. Available at: https://www.drugs.com/drug-interactions/adalimumab.html
3. Available at: https://www.drugs.com/drug-interactions/golimumab.html
4. Available at: https://www.drugs.com/drug-interactions/certolizumab.html
5. Available at: https://www.drugs.com/drug-interactions/vedolizumab.html
6. Available at: https://www.drugs.com/drug-interactions/ustekinumab.html
7. Available at: https://www.drugs.com/drug-interactions/tofacitinib.html

References

1. Kim DH, Cheon JH. Pathogenesis of inflammatory bowel disease and recent advances in biologic therapies. Immune Netw. 2017;17(1):25–40.
2. Gonczi L, Bessissow T, Lakatos PL. Disease monitoring strategies in inflammatory bowel diseases: what do we mean by tight control? World J Gastroenterol. 2019;23(41):6172–89.
3. Paramsothy S, Rosenstein AK, Mehandru S, Colombel JF. The current state of the art for biological therapies and new small molecules in inflammatory bowel disease. Mucosal Immunol. 2018;11:1558–70.
4. Medicines Agency. Biosimilars in the EU. Information guide for healthprofessionals. https://www.ema.europa.eu/en/documents/leaflet/biosimilars-eu-information-guide-healthcare-professionals_en.pdf. Accessed 12 Dec 2020.
5. Danese S, Fiorino G, Raine T, Ferrante M, Kemp K, Kierkus J, Lakatos PL, Mantzaris G, van der Woude J, Panes J, Peyrin-Biroulet L. ECCO position statement on the use of biosimilars for inflammatory bowel disease-an update. J Crohns Colitis. 2017;11(1):26–34. https://doi.org/10.1093/ecco-jcc/jjw198.
6. Vetter M, Neurath MF. Emerging oral targeted therapies in inflammatory bowel diseases: opportunities and challenges. Ther Adv Gastroenterol. 2017;10(10):773–90.
7. Sabino J, Verstockt B, Vermeire S, Ferrante M. New biologics and small molecules in inflammatory bowel disease: an update. Ther Adv Gastroenterol. 2019;12:1–14.
8. Singh S, Fumery M, Sandborn WJ, Murad MH. Systematic review and network meta-analysis: first- and second-line biologic therapies for moderate-severe Crohn's disease. Aliment Pharmacol Ther. 2018;48:394–409.
9. Ben-Horin S, Kopylov U, Chowers Y. Optimizing anti-TNF treatment in inflammatory bowel disease. Autoimmun Rev. 2014;13(1):24–30.
10. Misselwitz B, Juillerat P, Sulz MC, Siegmund B, Brand S. Emerging treatment options for inflammatory bowel disease: Janus kinases, stem cells, and more. Digestion. 2020;101(Suppl. 1):69–82.
11. Neurath MF, Travis SP. Mucosal healing in inflammatory bowel diseases: a systematic review. Gut. 2012;61:1619–35.

12. Fernandes C, Allocca M, Danese S, Fiorino G. Progress with anti-tumor necrosis factor therapeutics for the treatment of inflammatory bowel disease. Immunotherapy. 2015;7:175–90.
13. Vavricka SR, Scharl M, Gubler M, Rogler G. Biologics for extraintestinal manifestations of IBD. Curr Drug Targets. 2014;15:1064–73.
14. Lichtenstein GR, et al. Serious infection and mortality in patients with Crohn's disease: more than 5 years of follow-up in the TREAT registry. Am J Gastroenterol. 2012;107:1409–22.
15. Nyboe Andersen N, et al. Association between tumor necrosis factor-alpha antagonists and risk of cancer in patients with inflammatory bowel disease. JAMA. 2014;311:2406–13.
16. Lemaitre M, et al. Association between use of thiopurines or tumor necrosis factor antagonists alone or in combination and risk of lymphoma in patients with inflammatory bowel disease. JAMA. 2017;318:1679–86.
17. Hyams JS, et al. Infliximab is not associated with increased risk of malignancy or hemophagocytic lymphohistiocytosis in pediatric patients with inflammatory bowel disease. Gastroenterology. 2017;152:1901–14.
18. Targan SR, et al. A short-term study of chimeric monoclonal antibody cA2 to tumor necrosis factor alpha for Crohn's disease. Crohn's Disease cA2 Study Group. New Engl J Med. 1997;337:1029–35.
19. Hanauer SB, et al. Maintenance infliximab for Crohn's disease: the ACCENT I randomised trial. Lancet. 2002;359:1541–9.
20. Sands BE, et al. Infliximab maintenance therapy for fistulizing Crohn's disease. N Engl J Med. 2004;350:876–85.
21. Rutgeerts P, et al. Infliximab for induction and maintenance therapy for ulcerative colitis. N Engl J Med. 2005;353:2462–76.
22. Hanauer SB, et al. Human anti-tumor necrosis factor monoclonal antibody (adalimumab) in Crohn's disease: the CLASSIC-I trial. Gastroenterology. 2006;130:323–33.
23. Colombel JF, et al. Adalimumab for maintenance of clinical response and remission in patients with Crohn's disease: the CHARM trial. Gastroenterology. 2007;132:52–65.
24. Rutgeerts P, et al. Adalimumab induces and maintains mucosal healing in patients with Crohn's disease: data from the EXTEND trial. Gastroenterology. 2012;142:1102–11.
25. Sandborn WJ, et al. Adalimumab induces and maintains clinical remission in patients with moderate-to-severe ulcerative colitis. Gastroenterology. 2012;142:257–65.
26. Sandborn WJ, et al. Subcutaneous golimumab induces clinical response and remission in patients with moderate-to-severe ulcerative colitis. Gastroenterology. 2014;146:85–95.
27. Sandborn WJ, et al. Subcutaneous golimumab maintains clinical response in patients with moderate-to-severe ulcerative colitis. Gastroenterology. 2014;146:96–109.
28. Sandborn WJ, et al. Certolizumab pegol for the treatment of Crohn's disease. New Engl J Med. 2007;357:228–38.
29. Schreiber S, et al. Maintenance therapy with certolizumab pegol for Crohn's disease. N Engl J Med. 2007;357:239–50.
30. Hebuterne X, et al. Endoscopic improvement of mucosal lesions in patients with moderate to severe ileocolonic Crohn's disease following treatment with certolizumab pegol. Gut. 2013;62:201–8.
31. Schreiber S, et al. Randomised clinical trial: certolizumab pegol for fistulas in Crohn's disease—subgroup results from a placebo-controlled study. Aliment Pharmacol Ther. 2011;33:185–93.
32. Available at: https://www.drugs.com/drug-interactions/infliximab-index.html.
33. Available at: https://www.drugs.com/drug-interactions/adalimumab.html.
34. Available at: https://www.drugs.com/drug-interactions/golimumab.html.
35. Available at: https://www.drugs.com/drug-interactions/certolizumab.html.
36. Akiyama SK. Integrins in cell adhesion and signaling. Hum Cell. 1996;9:181–6.
37. Kempster SL, Kaser A. alpha4beta7 integrin: beyond T cell trafficking. Gut. 2014;63:1377–9.
38. Colombel JF, et al. The safety of vedolizumab for ulcerative colitis and Crohn's disease. Gut. 2017;66:839–51.
39. Internet: https://www.drugs.com/drug-interactions/vedolizumab.html.

40. Food and Drug Administration. Stelara (ustekinumab) [prescribing information]. Horsham, PA: Janssen Biotech; 2020.
41. Available at: https://www.drugs.com/drug-interactions/ustekinumab.html.
42. Yamaoka K, et al. The Janus kinases (Jaks). Genome Biol. 2004;5:253.
43. Danese S, Grisham M, Hodge J, Telliez JB. JAK inhibition using tofacitinib for inflammatory bowel disease treatment: a hub for multiple inflammatory cytokines. Am J Physiol Gastrointest Liver Physiol. 2016;310:G155–62.
44. Kotyla PJ. Are Janus kinase inhibitors superior over classic biologic agents in RA patients. BioMed Research Int. 2018:7492904. https://doi.org/10.1155/2018/7492904.
45. Anon. Xeljanz (tofacitinib) [prescribing information]. New York, NY: Pfizer Inc.; 2016.
46. Hirten RP, Iacucci M, Shah S, Ghosh S, Colombel J-F. Combining biologics in inflammatory bowel disease and other immune mediated inflammatory disorders. Clin Gastroenterol Hepatol. 2018;16:1374–84.
47. Internet: https://www.drugs.com/drug-interactions/tofacitinib.html.
48. Remicade (infliximab) [prescribing information]. Horsham, PA: Janssen Biotech Inc.; 2018.
49. Simponi (golimumab) [prescribing information]. Horsham, PA: Janssen Biotech Inc.; March 2018.
50. FDA Cimzia (certolizumab pegol) [prescribing information]. Smyrna, GA: UCB Inc.; 2019.
51. Saag KG, Teng GG, Patkar NM, et al. American College of Rheumatology 2008 recommendations for the use of nonbiologic and biologic disease-modifying antirheumatic drugs in rheumatoid arthritis. Arthritis Rheum. 2008;59(6):762–84.
52. Armanious M, Vender R. A Review of drug-drug interactions for biologic drugs used in treatment of psoriasis. J Cutan Med Surg. 2020; https://doi.org/10.1177/1203475420952423.
53. Available at: https://www.drugs.com/drug_interactions.html.
54. Torres J, Bonovas S, Doherty G, Kucharzik T, Gisbert JP, Raine T, et al. ECCO guidelines on therapeutics in Crohn's disease: medical treatment. J Crohns Colitis. 2020;14(1):4–22. https://doi.org/10.1093/ecco-jcc/jjz180.
55. Cohn HM, Dave M, Loftus EV Jr. Understanding the cautions and contraindications of immunomodulator and biologic therapies for use in inflammatory bowel disease. Inflamm Bowel Dis. 2017;23(8):1301–15. https://doi.org/10.1097/MIB.0000000000001199.
56. Martínez-Montiel MP, Casis-Herce B, Gómez-Gómez GJ, et al. Pharmacologic therapy for inflammatory bowel disease refractory to steroids. Clin Exp Gastroenterol. 2015;8:257–69. https://doi.org/10.2147/CEG.S58152.
57. Faleck DM, Shmidt E, Huang R, Katta LG, Narula N, Pinotti R, Suarez-Farinas M, Colombel JF. Effect of concomitant therapy with steroids and tumor necrosis factor antagonists for induction of remission in patients with Crohn's disease: a systematic review and pooled meta-analysis. Clin Gastroenterol Hepatol. 2020;S1542-3565(20):30847–8. https://doi.org/10.1016/j.cgh.2020.06.036.
58. National Center for Immunization and Respiratory Diseases. General recommendations on immunization—recommendations of the Advisory Committee on Immunization Practices (ACIP). MMWR Recomm Rep. 2011;60(2):1–64. [published correction appears in MMWR Recomm Rep. 2011;60(29):993]
59. Deepak P, Sifuentes H, Sherid M, Stobaugh D, Sadozai Y, Ehrenpreis ED. T-cell non-Hodgkin's lymphoma reported to the FDA AERS with tumor necrosis factor-alpha inhibitors: results of the REFURBISH study. Am J Gastroenterol. 2013;108(1):99–105.
60. Roblin X, Serre-Debeauvais F, Phelip JM, Bessard G, Bonaz B. Drug interaction between infliximab and azathioprine in patients with Crohn's disease. Aliment Pharmacol Ther. 2003;18(9):917–25.
61. Magro F, et al. Extra-intestinal malignancies in inflammatory bowel disease: results of the 3rd ECCO Pathogenesis Scientific Workshop (III). J Crohn's Colitis. 2014;8:31–44.
62. Colombel JF, et al. Infliximab, azathioprine, or combination therapy for Crohn's disease. N Engl J Med. 2010;362:1383–95.
63. Panaccione R, et al. Combination therapy with infliximab and azathioprine is superior to monotherapy with either agent in ulcerative colitis. Gastroenterology. 2014;146:392–400.

64. Vermeire S, Noman M, Van Assche G, et al. The effectiviness of concomitant immunosuppressive therapy to suppress formation of antibodies to infliximab in Crohn's disease. Gut. 2007;56:1226–31.
65. Maini RN, Breedveld FC, Kalden JR, et al. Therapeutic efficacy of multiple intravenous infusions of anti-tumor necrosis factor alpha monoclonal antibody combined with low-dose weekly methotrexate in rheumatoid arthritis. Arthritis Rheum. 1998;41:1552–63.
66. Humira [package insert]. North Chicago, IL: Abbott Laboratories; 2004.
67. Weisman MH, Moreland LW, Furst DE, et al. Efficacy, pharmacokinetic, and safety assessment of adalimumab, a fully human anti-tumor necrosis factor-alpha monoclonal antibody, in adults with rheumatoid arthritis receiving concomitant methotrexate: a pilot study. Clin Ther. 2003;25(6):1700–21.
68. AbbVie Inc. Humira (adalimumab) [prescribing information]. North Chicago, IL: AbbVie Inc.; 2020.
69. Bristol-Myers Squibb. Orencia (abatacept) [prescribing information]. Princeton, NJ: Bristol-Myers Squibb; 2020.
70. Kineret. Kineret (anakinra) [prescribing information]. Stockholm, Sweden: Swedish Orphan Biovitrum AB (Publ); 2018.
71. Idec B. Tysabri (natalizumab) [prescribing information]. Cambridge, MA: Biogen Idec Inc.; 2013.
72. Entyvio (vedolizumab) [prescribing information]. Deerfield, IL: Takeda Pharmaceuticals America, Inc.; 2014.
73. Ribaldone DG, Pellicano R, Vernero M, Caviglia GP, Saracco GM, Morino M, Astegiano M. Dual biological therapy with anti-TNF, vedolizumab or ustekinumab in inflammatory bowel disease: a systematic review with pool analysis. Scand J Gastroenterol. 2019;54(4):407–13. https://doi.org/10.1080/00365521.2019.1597159.
74. Nam SH, Oh JS, Hong S, et al. Early discontinuation of tofacitinib in patients with rheumatoid arthritis co-treated with rifampin for latent tuberculosis [published online, May 7, 2020]. Joint Bone Spine. 2020;87(5):475–9. https://doi.org/10.1016/j.jbspin.2020.04.010.
75. Charles-Schoeman C, Burmester G, Nash P, et al. Efficacy and safety of tofacitinib following inadequate response to conventional synthetic or biological disease-modifying antirheumatic drugs. Ann Rheum Dis. 2016;75(7):1293–301.
76. Cohen S, Radominski SC, Gomez-Reino JJ, et al. Analysis of infections and all-cause mortality in phase II, phase III, and long-term extension studies of tofacitinib in patients with rheumatoid arthritis. Arthritis Rheumatol. 2014;66(11):2924–37.
77. Olivera P, Danese S, Jay N, Natoli G, Peyrin-Biroulet L. Big data in in IBD: a look into the future. Nat Rev Gastroenterol Hepatol. 2019;16:312–21.

Interactions of Drugs for Liver Diseases

30

Marina Mudrovčić, Lucija Virović Jukić, Doris Ogresta,
and Ivica Grgurević

Introduction

Liver diseases show increasing trends in incidence and prevalence in general, especially referring to the non-alcoholic fatty liver disease (NAFLD), with the overall prevalence of around 25% in general population worldwide [1]. Whereas the fight against chronic viral hepatitis has been increasingly successful due to available vaccine against hepatitis B and very effective direct-acting antiviral (DAA) drugs introduced over the last 10 years, alcohol-related liver disease (ALD) remains the problem. The region with the highest burden of ALD is Europe [2]. It has been estimated that around 60% of the EU28 population is under risk of developing chronic liver disease (based on the prevalence of overweight, obesity, diabetes

M. Mudrovčić
Pharmacies Baričević, Zagreb, Croatia

L. Virović Jukić
Department of Gastroenterology and Hepatology, Sestre Milosrdnice University Hospital Center, Zagreb, Croatia

School of Medicine, University of Zagreb, Zagreb, Croatia

D. Ogresta
Department of Gastroenterology and Hepatology, Sestre Milosrdnice University Hospital Center, Zagreb, Croatia

I. Grgurević (✉)
School of Medicine, University of Zagreb, Zagreb, Croatia

Department of Gastroenterology, Hepatology and Clinical Nutrition, University Hospital Dubrava, Zagreb, Croatia

Faculty of Pharmacy and Biochemistry, University of Zagreb, Zagreb, Croatia
e-mail: ivica.grgurevic@zg.htnet.hr

M. Banić, D. Erceg (eds.), *Drug Interactions in Gastroenterology*, Clinical Gastroenterology, https://doi.org/10.1007/978-3-031-69800-2_30

mellitus, harmful alcohol drinking and the chronic viral hepatitis). Altogether, these data point to the high public health burden of chronic liver disease which is expected to even grow in the time to come. Chronic liver disease finally results with the development of cirrhosis and liver failure, leading to death or the need for liver transplantation. Therefore, it is important to recognize early patients under risk for such a scenario and treat them accordingly including both preventive lifestyle measures and introducing drug treatment when indicated. Interactions of drugs used to treat liver disease may be affected by pharmacokinetic and pharmacodynamic interactions at different levels. Pharmacokinetic interactions may be observed starting from the intestinal absorption, drug uptake by the hepatocytes, biotransformation and the elimination of drugs by the hepatocytes to blood or bile, as well as the influence on renal elimination [3–5]. Some of these steps may be significantly affected by the altered liver function as CLD advances, but also by the inherited genetic variants of the genes involved in these processes. Apart from the well-known interactions of the classical drugs such as diuretics and corticosteroids, newly introduced drugs especially DAA have opened completely new chapter of previously unknown interactions. This chapter will try to analyse clinically most relevant interactions of drugs commonly used to treat liver diseases. Of course, not all clinical situations and drug interactions could have been covered by this volume of the text and the reader is kindly advised to refer to the available databases, some of which have been mentioned in the following text.

Viral Hepatitis

Hepatitis B Virus

Available treatments that are effective in suppressing hepatitis B virus (HBV) replication include interferons and nucleoside/nucleotide analogues (NAs) (see also Chap. 8).

Nucleotide and Nucleoside Analogues

A number of nucleotide/nucleoside analogues have been developed, but the World Health Organization and most current treatment guidelines issued by the International Hepatology Association recommend the use of tenofovir and entecavir as these are the most potent drugs for viral suppression and rarely cause viral resistance to the drug [6–10]. Other nucleoside analogues, such as lamivudine, telbivudine or adefovir dipivoxil, are no longer widely used and will not be elaborated here.

Entecavir

Entecavir is a guanosine nucleoside analogue used in the treatment of chronic HBV infection. Entecavir is activated in vivo to a 5-triphosphate metabolite. Triphosphate forms competes with the natural substrate deoxyguanosine triphosphate (dGTP) for incorporation into viral DNA. The incorporation inhibits the viral RNA-dependent HBV DNA polymerase, and replication of viral DNA [11].

Entecavir is not a CYP450 enzyme substrate. It is predominantly eliminated unchanged by glomerular filtration and tubular excretion [12, 13]. Lactic acidosis and severe hepatomegaly with steatosis have been reported with the use of nucleoside analogues. Since entecavir is a nucleoside analogue, risk of lactic acidosis cannot be excluded [12].

Drug Interactions

Since entecavir is predominantly eliminated by the kidneys, co-administration with medications that reduce renal function or compete for active tubular secretion may increase serum concentrations of either drug. Patients should be monitored closely when entecavir is coadministered with such medications. Entecavir is not a substrate, an inducer or an inhibitor of cytochrome P450 enzyme system. Therefore, CYP450-mediated drug interactions are unlikely to occur with entecavir. Entecavir is observed for positional risk of interactions with tenofovir, adefovir and lamivudine. According to the study, neither drug significantly affected the pharmacokinetics of the other [14, 15].

Antibiotics: **Tazobactam, meropenem, imipenem, cephalexin and gentamicin** should be used with caution since they are renally excreted. Renal function should be closely monitored.

Antivirals: **Acyclovir, oseltamivir, valaciclovir** and **cidofovir** are eliminated by tubular secretion by OAT1 and/or OAT3 transporters. Concentrations of these drugs and entecavir may increase due to competition for renal elimination. If coadministered, monitoring of renal function is necessary.

Acetazolamide: Acetazolamide is predominantly excreted unchanged via active renal tubular secretion and may competitively inhibit the renal transporters OAT1 and OAT3. Entecavir is eliminated primarily in the urine by glomerular filtration and tubular secretion by OAT1. As entecavir can be nephrotoxic, renal function monitoring is recommended.

Furosemide: Furosemide is a substrate and inhibitor of the renal transporters OAT1/OAT3. Entecavir is eliminated primarily in the urine by tubular secretion by OAT1. Entecavir concentrations may increase and renal monitoring may be required.

Cancer Therapy: **Methotrexate** is eliminated by the kidney (OAT1 and OAT3 transporters), and in case of co-administration, entecavir and methotrexate concentrations may alter. **Cisplatin** is eliminated renally via OCT2 and MATE1. Although they are not eliminated through the same pathways, co-administration can increase the risk of nephrotoxicity. Renal function should be closely monitored if entecavir is coadministered with methotrexate or cisplatin [16].

Tenofovir Disoproxil Fumarate

Tenofovir disoproxil fumarate (TDF) is a nucleoside reverse transcriptase inhibitor registered for HBV and HIV treatment. It selectively inhibits viral reverse transcriptase while showing limited inhibition of human enzymes. In vivo TDF is converted to tenofovir. Once incorporated into a growing DNA strand, tenofovir causes premature termination of DNA transcription thus preventing viral replication [16].

Drug Interactions

TDF is not a substrate for the CYP450 enzymes. It is primarily excreted through the kidneys by glomerular filtration and active tubular transport system. Since TDF is excreted by the kidneys, cases of renal impairment, renal failure, hyperphosphatemia and Fanconi syndrome have been reported during TDF treatment. It is recommended that creatinine clearance is calculated prior to initiating therapy and dose of TDF adjusted in case of moderate or severe renal impairment. Co-administration of TDF with other nephrotoxic medications (such as aminoglycosides, amphotericin B, foscarnet, ganciclovir and vancomycin) should be avoided. According to studies, the use of TDF could cause decrease in bone mineral density. Alternative treatment should be considered for patients with osteoporosis and patients who are at high risk for bone fractures [17–19].

Nonsteroidal Anti-inflammatory Drugs: Cases of renal failure have been reported when TDF was coadministered with nonsteroidal anti-inflammatory drugs (NSAIDs). Alternatives to NSAIDs should be considered. If NSAIDs (diclofenac, ketoprofen, ibuprofen, indomethacin, naproxen, COX-2 inhibitors, etc.) are coadministered with TDF, renal function should be adequately monitored. Tramadol, paracetamol, oxycodone, morphine and fentanyl are considered safe.

Amiodarone: Amiodarone is an inhibitor of P-gp. Since TDF is a substrate of P-gp, co-administration of these drugs can increase concentrations of TDF in plasma and cause nephrotoxicity.

Antibiotics: Some groups of antibiotics decrease renal function and can cause increase of TDF concentration in plasma. Special caution is needed if TDF is coadministered with **aminoglycosides** (amikacin, gentamicin, tobramycin and neomycin), **meropenem, clarithromycin, vancomycin** and **tazobactam**. If concomitant use of TDF and nephrotoxic agents is unavoidable, renal function should be closely monitored.

Antiviral Medications: **Acyclovir** is eliminated through kidneys by OAT1 and OAT 3 transporters. TDF and acyclovir compete for the same transporters. Concentrations of both drugs can increase in plasma if they are coadministered. **Valaciclovir, foscarnet** and **cidofovir** also decrease renal function.

Antifungals: **Amphotericin B, ketoconazole** and **itraconazole** are considered nephrotoxic. Amphotericin B is eliminated unchanged by kidneys and biliary excretion. If co-administration of TDF and these medications is necessary, renal function should be monitored.

Pentamidine: If pentamidine is coadministered with TDF, it can cause renal impairment. Combination of these two medications should be avoided.

Cancer Therapies: **Carboplatin, cisplatin** and **methotrexate** are nephrotoxic and can cause serious renal injury if coadministered with TDF. In case of combination of these medications, renal function should be closely monitored.

Hepatitis C Direct-Acting Antivirals (DAAs): If co-administration of TDF with sofosbuvir-based therapies has no alternative, combination should be used with caution and with frequent monitoring of renal function.

Interferons: Patients receiving interferon with ribavirin and NRTIs should be closely monitored. Combination of these drugs is associated with toxicities, especially hepatic decompensation and anaemia.

Hepatitis Nucleoside/Nucleotide Analogues: TDF should not be administered concomitantly with other medicinal products containing **tenofovir disoproxil** or **tenofovir alafenamide**. Co-administration of TDF and **telbivudine** should be done with caution. Lactic acidosis and severe hepatomegaly with steatosis have been reported with the use of telbivudine (alone or in combination with antiretrovirals).

HIV Protease Inhibitors: In patients with renal risk factors, co-administration of tenofovir disoproxil with a boosted protease inhibitor should be carefully evaluated.

Didanosine: Co-administration is not recommended due to increased didanosine concentrations and toxicity. If this combination is strictly necessary, patients should be carefully monitored for efficacy and didanosine-related adverse events [19].

Tenofovir Alafenamide

Tenofovir alafenamide (TAF) is a nucleoside reverse transcriptase inhibitor, phosphonamidate prodrug of tenofovir. It enters hepatocytes by passive diffusion and by organic anion-transporting polypeptide (OATP) 1B1 and OATP1B3 transporters. It is hydrolysed to tenofovir and then phosphorylated to its active metabolite tenofovir diphosphate intracellularly. Tenofovir diphosphate competes with natural 2′-deoxyadenosine triphosphate for incorporation by the viral reverse transcriptase, and when incorporated, results in DNA chain termination. TAF is indicated for the treatment of chronic hepatitis B and in combination with other antivirals for HIV-1 treatment [16, 20].

Drug Interactions

TAF is a substrate of P-glycoprotein (P-gp) and breast cancer resistance protein (BCRP). Drugs that strongly affect P-gp and BCRP activity may cause changes in TAF absorption. Co-administration of TAF with drugs that induce P-gp activity may decrease the absorption of TAF, possibly leading to loss of its therapeutic effect. Drugs that inhibit P-gp and BCRP may increase the absorption and plasma concentration of TAF. TAF is not a substrate for CYP450 enzyme system (CYP1A2, CYP2C8, CYP2C9, CYP2C19 or CYP2D6), with only slow metabolism by CYP3A4. TAF is mainly eliminated following metabolism of tenofovir. Tenofovir is excreted from the body by the kidneys, by glomerular filtration and active tubular secretion.

Amiodarone: Inhibition of P-gp by amiodarone is expected to increase the absorption of TAF and increase its systemic concentration.

Antibiotics: **Clarithromycin** is an inhibitor of P-gp and is expected to increase the absorption of TAF and increase the systemic concentration. If coadministered, monitoring for side effects and renal function is needed. P-gp inducers, such as **rifampicin** and **rifabutin,** are expected to decrease plasma concentrations of TAF, which may lead to loss of the therapeutic effect.

Table 30.1 Established or potentially clinically significant drug interactions of tenofovir alafenamide

Drug class	Drug	Interactions and recommendations
Anticonvulsants	Carbamazepine Oxcarbazepine Phenobarbital Phenytoin	↓ TAF concentration Co-administration is not recommended
Antimycobacterials	Rifabutin Rifampin Rifapentine	↓ TAF concentration Co-administration is not recommended
Herbal products	St. John's wort (*Hypericum perforatum*)	↓ TAF concentration Co-administration is not recommended

Anticonvulsants: **Carbamazepine, phenobarbital, oxcarbazepine and primidone** are P-gp inducers and decrease TAF concentrations in plasma, which can result in loss of therapeutic response. Co-administration of such medications with medications containing TAF is not recommended.

Didanosine: Increased **didanosine** concentrations and toxicity were observed when combined with tenofovir disoproxil fumarate (TDF). There are not enough data about TAF and didanosine co-administration. Since similar effect with TAF cannot be excluded, co-administration of these medications is not recommended [20].

The most important drug interactions with tenofovir alafenamide are shown in Table 30.1.

Pegylated Interferon Alfa

Interferon alfa has been used for more than three decades as antiviral agent active against hepatitis B and hepatitis C virus (HCV). Conventional interferon was later replaced by pegylated interferon alfa (peginterferon alfa), where interferon was linked to a high molecular mass polyethylene glycol (PEG) molecule which improved interferon's pharmacokinetics and enabled more convenient dosing schedule with higher efficacy rates and improved tolerability. Two drug formulations existed and were used in the treatment of chronic viral hepatitis: pegylated interferon alfa-2a and pegylated interferon alfa-2b; however, the discovery of new, direct-acting antiviral agents (DAAs) gradually replaced interferon-based treatments for hepatitis C. Peginterferon alfa, however, still remains as an option for the treatment of chronic hepatitis B infection. Majority of treatment guidelines recommend only pegylated interferons, and conventional interferons are used in a few countries or specific populations. Peginterferon alfa-2a is registered and available in most countries for the treatment of chronic hepatitis B infection, while peginterferon alfa-2b is generally not used for this indication [6–9].

Peginterferon Alfa-2a

Peginterferon alfa-2a is a form of recombinant alfa interferon. It is indicated for the treatment of patients with chronic HBV infection who have compensated liver disease and evidence of viral replication and liver inflammation. It is applied as a subcutaneous injection once a week [16, 21].

Peginterferon Alfa-2b

Peginterferon alfa-2b is a covalent conjugate of recombinant alfa interferon with monomethoxy polyethylene glycol. It was indicated for use alone or in combination with ribavirin for the treatment of chronic hepatitis C. Peginterferon alfa-2b is given as injection subcutaneously once weekly [22].

Drug Interactions with Peginterferons Alfa

Nucleoside analogues: Patients receiving interferon alfa/ribavirin in combination with nucleoside analogues should be closely monitored because they are potentially toxic. In that case, dose reduction or discontinuation of interferon alfa, ribavirin or both, should also be considered. Co-administration of peginterferon alfa, ribavirin and **didanosine** is not recommended. Reports of fatal hepatic failure, as well as peripheral neuropathy, pancreatitis and symptomatic hyperlactatemia/lactic acidosis, have been reported in clinical trials. Patients treated with peginterferon alfa and **zidovudine** (with or without ribavirin) are at increased risk of developing anaemia and severe neutropenia. Co-administration of those medications is not recommended.

Azathioprine: Pancytopenia and bone marrow suppression have been reported to occur within 3–7 weeks after the co-administration of peginterferon and ribavirin with azathioprine. The use of peginterferon alfa and ribavirin concomitantly with azathioprine should be avoided.

Alopurinol: Metabolic pathways for alopurinol are not affected by peginterferon alfa. However, alopurinol can cause leukopenia and thrombocytopenia which should be monitored for when given in combination with interferons.

Cancer therapies: Co-administration has not been studied. The risk of haematological toxicity may be potentially increased as these drugs can cause myelosuppression. Monitoring of haematological parameters is needed.

Theophylline: Co-administration of theophylline and peginterferon alfa can increase theophylline AUC by 25% in healthy subjects. Theophylline serum concentrations should be monitored and appropriate dose adjustments considered if coadministered.

Antipsychotics/neuroleptics: **Chlorpromazine** and **clozapine** are metabolites of CYP1A2. Peginterferon alfa may inhibit CYP1A2 which could potentially lead to a small increase in chlorpromazine concentrations. As chlorpromazine can cause neutropenia, patients should be monitored if treated with combination of interferon and chlorpromazine. Although **haloperidol** and interferon do not have the same metabolic pathways, it has been reported that seizures can be triggered by haloperidol. Interferon can also be associated with increased seizure activity. Caution is needed. Interferon and **sulpiride** can both separately cause neutropenia and leukopenia and this should merit close clinical monitoring.

Warfarin: Caution should be used when administering peginterferon alfa with warfarin as the therapeutic effect of warfarin may be decreased.

Metamizole: Co-administration is not recommended because of increased risk of developing anaemia.

Antifungals: **Amphotericin B** can be associated with anaemia and myelosuppression which may be intensified when coadministered with peginterferon. If coadministration is necessary, monitoring is needed during the therapy [22].

Hepatitis C

Prior to year 2011, the combination of interferon or later pegylated interferon alfa with ribavirin for 24 or 48 weeks represented the standard treatment of chronic HCV infection. Then, new classes of drugs were introduced, which targeted specific HCV enzymes and interfered with the viral life cycle. These molecules are called direct-acting antiviral agents (DAAs) and belong to one of the three classes of drugs: the NS3/4A protease inhibitors, the NS5A protein inhibitors and NS5B RNA polymerase inhibitors. The combinations of drugs with different targets resulted in high efficacy rates without significant side effects. The new, direct-acting antiviral drugs are taken orally, sometimes with ribavirin, for a shorter period of time (8–12 weeks, rarely 16 or 24 weeks). Some of the combinations are genotype-specific (sofosbuvir/ledipasvir, grazoprevir/elbasvir), while others are pangenotypic (glecaprevir/pibrentasvir, sofosbuvir/velpatasvir, sofosbuvir/velpatasvir/voxilaprevir). Since all these drugs are available in fixed combinations, their interactions will be elaborated together, for both (or all three) active compounds of the product.

Some agents like the first- and second-generation protease inhibitors (boceprevir, telaprevir, simeprevir, asunaprevir), and fixed combinations (like ombitasvir/ritonavir-boosted paritaprevir and dasabuvir) have been mostly replaced by new generation drugs with better efficacy and tolerability. Since these drugs, as well as combination of peginterferon and ribavirin, are no longer recommended and are generally not used for the treatment of chronic HCV infection in most countries, they will not be presented in the following text [23–27].

Because of the risk for HBV reactivation during treatment of chronic HCV infection with DAAs, all patients who are candidates for DAA treatment should be tested for evidence of current or prior HBV infection. Monitoring of HCV/HBV coinfected patients for HBV reactivation and hepatitis flare during HCV treatment and post-treatment follow-up is recommended for all DAA treatment regimens.

Successful clearance of HCV with DAA treatment may lead to improved hepatic function, which may impact the effectiveness and safety of concomitant medications. Examples are altered blood glucose control which may result in serious hypoglycaemia in patients taking hypoglycaemic drugs, or changes in international normalized ratio (INR) which may result in loss of therapeutic effect in patients taking warfarin. Frequent monitoring of relevant laboratory parameters, such as INR, blood glucose levels or drug concentrations of medications with a narrow therapeutic index which are substrates of cytochrome P450 enzymes, is recommended, and adequate dose adjustments should be applied when necessary [23, 28].

Sofosbuvir

Sofosbuvir is a pangenotypic inhibitor of the NS5B RNA-dependent RNA polymerase, which is essential for HCV replication. It undergoes extensive first-pass hepatic and intestinal metabolism. In the liver, sofosbuvir is hydrolysed and sequentially phosphorylated to the pharmacologically active uridine nucleoside analogue triphosphate. When incorporated into HCV RNA by the viral polymerase, it acts as a chain terminator. The inactive circulating metabolite GS-331007 is renally excreted. Sofosbuvir has been used for the treatment of chronic HCV infection in combination with peginterferon alfa and ribavirin, ribavirin only or other DAAs like simeprevir or daclatasvir, and is currently used as a component of a fixed combination with ledipasvir, or velpatasvir, or velpatasvir and voxilaprevir [29, 30].

Drug Interactions

Sofosbuvir is a substrate of P-glycoprotein (P-gp) drug transporter and breast cancer resistance protein (BCRP), while pharmacologically inactive metabolite GS-331007 is not. Drugs that are P-gp inducers in the intestine may decrease sofosbuvir plasma concentration and reduce sofosbuvir therapeutic effect. Examples of potent inducers of P-gp are some anticonvulsants (carbamazepine, phenobarbital and phenytoin), antimycobacterials (rifampicin, rifabutin) and St. John's wort (*Hypericum perforatum*); their co-administration is not recommended as it may lead to potential virological failure. Co-administration of sofosbuvir with drugs that inhibit P-gp and BCRP may increase sofosbuvir plasma concentration but without increasing GS-331007 plasma concentration. That means that sofosbuvir may be coadministered with P-gp and BCRP inhibitors. Sofosbuvir and GS-331007 are not inhibitors of P-gp and BCRP and are not expected to increase exposure to drugs that are substrates of these transporters [29, 31].

Sofosbuvir and Ledipasvir

Sofosbuvir/ledipasvir represents a fixed-dose combination of sofosbuvir, a pangenotypic inhibitor of the HCV NS5B RNA polymerase, and ledipasvir, an inhibitor of HCV NS5A, which is essential for RNA replication and the assembly of HCV virions. This drug is indicated for the treatment of patients with HCV genotype 1, 4, 5 and 6 infections [24–27]. It is sometimes used in combination with ribavirin.

Drug Interactions

Sofosbuvir and ledipasvir are both substrates of drug transporters P-gp and BCRP. Drugs that are strong P-gp inducers may therefore significantly decrease sofosbuvir and ledipasvir plasma concentrations and cause reduced therapeutic effect. As this may result in virological failure, co-administration of such drugs with sofosbuvir/ledipasvir is contraindicated. Concomitant use of moderate P-gp inducers is also not recommended. Co-administration of drugs that are inhibitors of P-gp and/or BCRP may increase sofosbuvir and ledipasvir plasma concentrations, without increasing GS-331007 concentration. Clinically significant consequences are not expected, and these drugs can be coadministered. Drug interactions mediated by cytochrome P450 or UGT1A1 enzymes are not expected.

Acid-reducing agents: Since ledipasvir solubility decreases with increased pH, drugs that increase gastric pH are expected to decrease ledipasvir concentration, which may result in loss of therapeutic efficacy. Antacids are recommended to be separated from the administration of sofosbuvir/ledipasvir. H_2-receptor antagonists (**famotidine, cimetidine, ranitidine, nizatidine**) should be administered at a dose not exceeding or equivalent to famotidine 40 mg twice daily, and proton pump inhibitors (**omeprazole, pantoprazole, lansoprazole, rabeprazole, esomeprazole**) should be administered at a dose not exceeding or equivalent to omeprazole 20 mg once daily. They should not be taken before the administration of sofosbuvir/ledipasvir.

Antiarrhythmics: Co-administration of **amiodarone** with a sofosbuvir containing regimen may result in serious symptomatic bradycardia and is not recommended. Concomitant use of **digoxin** may increase the concentration of digoxin so caution is advised. Monitoring of therapeutic concentration of digoxin is recommended.

Anticoagulants: Co-administration of **dabigatran** and sofosbuvir/ledipasvir may increase dabigatran exposure due to inhibition of P-gp. Clinical monitoring is recommended.

Antimycobacterials: **Rifampicin** and **rifabutin** are potent inducers of P-gp and may significantly decrease sofosbuvir and ledipasvir concentrations. This may result in loss of efficacy and potential virological failure. **Rifapentine** is also expected to decrease concentrations of sofosbuvir and ledipasvir; their co-administration is not recommended.

Anticonvulsants: Co-administration of sofosbuvir/ledipasvir with **carbamazepine**, **phenobarbital** and **phenytoin** is contraindicated. These medications may significantly decrease sofosbuvir and ledipasvir concentrations due to P-gp induction. This may lead to reduced therapeutic effect and potential virological failure. Co-administration with **oxcarbazepine** (moderate P-gp inducer) is not recommended.

HIV antiviral medications: Sofosbuvir and ledipasvir can increase **tenofovir** exposure, especially in a regimen containing tenofovir disoproxil fumarate and a pharmacokinetic enhancer (cobicistat or ritonavir). In case of co-administration of such combinations, patients should be carefully monitored for tenofovir-associated adverse reactions. **Ritonavir-boosted tipranavir** is expected to decrease the concentrations of ledipasvir. This may result in reduced therapeutic effect, and co-administration is not recommended.

HMG-CoA reductase inhibitors: Co-administration of statins can significantly increase the concentration of the statin, which increases the risk of myopathy and rhabdomyolysis. **Rosuvastatin** is contraindicated. A reduced dose of other statins should be considered, and careful clinical monitoring for possible statin adverse events is recommended.

St. John's Wort: St. John's wort (*Hypericum perforatum*) is a potent inducer of P-gp. It may significantly decrease concentrations of sofosbuvir and ledipasvir and result in loss of efficacy of sofosbuvir/ledipasvir [31, 32].

Sofosbuvir and Velpatasvir

Sofosbuvir/velpatasvir is a fixed-dose combination of sofosbuvir, an HCV nucleotide analogue NS5B polymerase inhibitor, and velpatasvir, an HCV NS5A inhibitor. This is a pangenotypic combination of DAAs indicated for the treatment of patients with HCV genotype 1, 2, 3, 4, 5 or 6 infection; it is sometimes used in combination with ribavirin [24–27, 33, 34].

Sofosbuvir is dominantly metabolized in the liver into active uridine analogue triphosphate. It is not a metabolite of CYP enzyme system. Velpatasvir is a metabolite of CYP2B6, CYP2C8 and CYP3A4. Renal clearance is the major elimination pathway for sofosbuvir and its pharmacologically inactive metabolite GS-331007, while biliary excretion is a major route of elimination of unchanged velpatasvir [33–35].

Drug Interactions

Sofosbuvir and velpatasvir are both substrates of drug transporters P-gp and BCRP, while velpatasvir is also a substrate of organic anion-transporting polypeptide (OATP) 1B1 and OATP1B3. Drugs, which are strong P-gp inducers and/or strong CYP inducers such as rifampicin, rifabutin, rifapentine, anticonvulsants like carbamazepine, oxcarbazepine, phenobarbital and phenytoin, may decrease concentrations of sofosbuvir and/or velpatasvir leading to reduced therapeutic effect and their use is contraindicated. Since velpatasvir is an inhibitor of drug transporters P-gp and BCRP, co-administration of drugs which are substrates of these transporters such as rosuvastatin, atorvastatin, fluvastatin and lovastatin may result in potential toxicity of lipid-lowering agents and increase risk of myopathy and rhabdomyolysis. Since velpatasvir solubility decreases with increased pH, drugs that increase gastric pH are expected to decrease the concentration of velpatasvir. Use of proton pump inhibitors is therefore not recommended; if required, they should be used at a lower dose and separated from sofosbuvir/velpatasvir. Similar recommendations apply to H_2-receptor antagonists and antacids [31, 33]. Potentially significant drug interactions with sofosbuvir and velpatasvir are shown in Table 30.2.

Sofosbuvir, Velpatasvir and Voxilaprevir

This fixed-dose pangenotypic combination of sofosbuvir, an HCV NS5B polymerase inhibitor, velpatasvir, an HCV NS5A inhibitor, and voxilaprevir, an HCV NS3/4A protease inhibitor, is indicated for the treatment of patients with chronic HCV genotype 1, 2, 3, 4, 5 or 6 infection [25, 27]. Medication is also indicated for the treatment of patients who have previously been treated with an HCV regimen containing sofosbuvir or an NS5A inhibitor [36]. In the liver, sofosbuvir is hydrolysed and sequentially phosphorylated to the pharmacologically active uridine nucleoside analogue triphosphate. It is not a metabolite of CYP enzyme system. Velpatasvir is a metabolite of CYP2B6, CYP2C8 and CYP3A4. Voxilaprevir is metabolized by CYP3A4. Biliary excretion is the major route of elimination of voxilaprevir and velpatasvir, while sofosbuvir is mainly excreted as inactive metabolite by the kidneys [35, 36].

Table 30.2 Potentially significant drug interactions with sofosbuvir/velpatasvir

Drug class	Drug	Interactions and recommendations
Antiarrhythmics	Amiodarone Digoxin	May result in serious symptomatic bradycardia; co-administration not recommended ↑ Digoxin Monitoring of digoxin plasma concentrations is recommended
Antimycobacterials	Rifabutin Rifampicin Rifapentine	↓ Sofosbuvir, ↓ velpatasvir Co-administration not recommended
Anticancer drugs	Topotecan	↑ Topotecan Co-administration not recommended
Anticonvulsants	Carbamazepine Phenobarbital Phenytoin Oxcarbazepine	↓ Sofosbuvir, ↓ velpatasvir Co-administration not recommended
Herbal products	St. John's wort	Induction of P-gp and CYPs ↓ Sofosbuvir, ↓ velpatasvir Co-administration not recommended
HMG-CoA reductase inhibitors	Rosuvastatin Atorvastatin	↑ Rosuvastatin, ↑ atorvastatin Increased risk of myopathy, including rhabdomyolysis; monitoring is required
HIV antiretrovirals	Efavirenz TDF Tipranavir/ritonavir	↓ Velpatasvir Co-administration is not recommended ↑ Tenofovir Monitoring of renal function is recommended ↓ Sofosbuvir, ↓ velpatasvir Co-administration is not recommended
Acid-reducing agents	Antacids H2-receptor antagonists Proton pump inhibitors	Velpatasvir solubility decreases with increased pH Drugs that increase gastric pH are expected to ↓ velpatasvir concentration

Drug Interactions

Sofosbuvir, velpatasvir and voxilaprevir are substrates of drug transporters P-gp and BCRP, while velpatasvir and voxilaprevir are also substrates of OATP1B1 and OATP1B3. Drugs which are strong P-gp inducers and/or strong CYP inducers may decrease concentrations of sofosbuvir, velpatasvir and/or voxilaprevir leading to reduced therapeutic effect and their use is contraindicated. For the same reason, co-administration of sofosbuvir/velpatasvir/voxilaprevir with moderate P-gp inducers and/or CYP inducers is not recommended. Co-administration of sofosbuvir/velpatasvir/voxilaprevir with inhibitors of P-gp or BCRP may increase concentrations of sofosbuvir, velpatasvir and/or voxilaprevir, while inhibitors of OATP, CYP2B6, CYP2C8 and CYP3A4 may increase concentration of velpatasvir and/or voxilaprevir. The use of strong inhibitors of OATP1B (e.g. cyclosporine) is not recommended. Clinically significant interactions of sofosbuvir/velpatasvir/voxilaprevir and P-gp, BCRP or CYP inhibitors are not expected [33].

Velpatasvir and voxilaprevir are inhibitors of P-gp, BCRP, OATP1B1 and OATP1B3, and co-administration of drugs which are substrates of these transporters may increase their exposure and result in potential toxicity. The use of dabigatran etexilate (P-gp substrate) and rosuvastatin (substrate of OATP1B and BCRP) is contraindicated [33].

Since velpatasvir solubility decreases with increased pH, drugs that increase gastric pH are expected to decrease the concentration of velpatasvir. Proton pump inhibitors, H_2-receptor antagonists and antacids may be used, but certain restrictions (separate administration or limited dose) apply.

The most significant drug interactions with sofosbuvir/velpatasvir and voxilaprevir are shown in Table 30.3.

Table 30.3 Potentially significant drug interactions with fixed-dose combination of sofosbuvir/velpatasvir/voxilaprevir

Drug class	Drug	Interactions and recommendations
Antiarrhythmics	Amiodarone Digoxin	May result in serious symptomatic bradycardia; co-administration not recommended ↑ Digoxin Monitoring of digoxin plasma concentrations is recommended
Anticoagulants	Dabigatran Edoxaban	↑ Dabigatran; Clinical monitoring for dabigatran is recommended ↑ Edoxaban; Co-administration is not recommended
Antimycobacterials	Rifampicin Rifabutin Rifapentine	Co-administration with rifampicin or rifabutin is contraindicated; Co-administration with rifapentine is not recommended
Immunosuppressants	Cyclosporine	↑ Voxilaprevir Not recommended
Anticonvulsants	Carbamazepine Phenobarbital Phenytoin Oxcarbazepine	↓ Sofosbuvir, ↓ velpatasvir, ↓voxilaprevir Co-administration is not recommended
Anticancer drugs	Imatinib, methotrexate Irinotecan Vincristine, vinblastine	↑ Imatinib, methotrexate Co-administration is not recommended ↑ Irinotecan, vincristine, vinblastine Clinical monitoring for side effects is required
Oral contraceptives	Ethinyl-oestradiol containing medications	May increase the risk of ALT elevations; Co-administration is contraindicated
Herbal products	St. John's wort	↓ Sofosbuvir, ↓ velpatasvir, ↓ voxilaprevir; Co-administration is not recommended

(continued)

Table 30.3 (continued)

Drug class	Drug	Interactions and recommendations
HMG-CoA reductase inhibitors	Rosuvastatin, pravastatin, atorvastatin, lovastatin etc.	Increased risk of myopathy, including rhabdomyolysis; Monitoring is required
HIV antiretrovirals	Efavirenz Nevirapine TDF Tipranavir/ritonavir Atazanavir, lopinavir, saquinavir, indinavir, fosamprenavir	↓ Velpatasvir, ↓ voxilaprevir Co-administration is not recommended ↓ Sofosbuvir, ↓ velpatasvir, ↓ voxilaprevir; Co-administration is contraindicated ↑ Tenofovir Monitoring of renal function is recommended ↓ Sofosbuvir, ↓ velpatasvir Co-administration is not recommended ↑ Voxilaprevir; risk of ALT elevations Co-administration is not recommended
Acid-reducing agents	Antacids H2-receptor antagonists Proton pump inhibitors	Expected to ↓ concentration of velpatasvir Separate administration May be administered at a dose not exceeding or equivalent to famotidine 40 mg twice daily May be administered at a dose not exceeding or equivalent to omeprazole 20 mg daily

Glecaprevir/Pibrentasvir

Glecaprevir is a pangenotypic inhibitor of HCV NS3/4A protease, which is used in combination with pibrentasvir, a pangenotypic NS5A inhibitor, thus targeting multiple steps in the HCV viral life cycle. This combination therapy is approved for the treatment of patients with chronic HCV infection with genotypes 1–6 [24–27]. Like other DAA regimens containing NS3/4A protease inhibitors, the combination of glecaprevir/pibrentasvir is not recommended or is contraindicated in patients with moderate or severe hepatic impairment (Child Pugh class B or C). The medication is metabolized in the liver by hepatic CYP3A system. Biliary excretion is the major route of elimination [35, 37, 38].

Drug Interactions

Glecaprevir and pibrentasvir are inhibitors of P-gp, BCRP and OATP1B1/3. Co-administration of drugs that are substrates of P-gp (dabigatran etexilate, digoxin), BCRP (rosuvastatin) or OATP1B1/3 (atorvastatin, lovastatin, pravastatin, rosuvastatin, simvastatin) may increase their concentrations.

Glecaprevir and pibrentasvir are weak inhibitors of cytochrome P450 CYP3A and uridine glucuronosyltransferase (UGT) 1A1. Clinically significant increases in exposure were not observed for sensitive substrates of CYP3A or UGT1A1. Significant inhibition of other CYP enzymes and drug transporters is not expected.

Use of glecaprevir/pibrentasvir with strong P-gp and CYP3A inducers (rifampicin, carbamazepine, phenobarbital, phenytoin, primidone or St. John's wort) could significantly decrease glecaprevir or pibrentasvir concentrations and lead to reduced therapeutic effect. Co-administration of such medicinal products is contraindicated. Co-administration of drugs which are moderate inducers of P-gp or CYP3A is not recommended [31, 38].

The most significant drug interactions with sofosbuvir/velpatasvir and voxilaprevir are shown in Table 30.4.

Table 30.4 Potentially significant drug interactions with glecaprevir/pibrentasvir

Therapy group	Drug	Interaction
Antiarrhythmics	Digoxin	↑ Digoxin; Monitoring of digoxin plasma concentrations is recommended
Anticoagulants	Dabigatran	↑ Dabigatran; Clinical monitoring for dabigatran is recommended Co-administration contraindicated (Europe); dose modification of dabigatran dose in patients with renal impairment and co-administration not recommended with severe renal impairment (creatinine clearance <30 mL/min) (United States)
Antimycobacterials	Rifampicin	↓ Glecaprevir ↓ pibrentasvir; co-administration is contraindicated
Immunosuppressants	Cyclosporine	↑ Glecaprevir ↑ pibrentasvir; Co-administration is not recommended
Anticonvulsants	Carbamazepine	↓ Glecaprevir ↓ pibrentasvir; Co-administration is not recommended
Herbal products	St. John's wort	↓ Glecaprevir ↓ pibrentasvir; Co-administration is not recommended
Oral contraceptives	Ethinyl-oestradiol containing medications	May increase the risk of ALT elevations; Co-administration is not recommended
HMG-CoA reductase inhibitors	Rosuvastatin, pravastatin, atorvastatin, lovastatin, etc.	↑ Statin concentrations, increased risk of myopathy, including rhabdomyolysis; Monitoring is required
HIV antiretrovirals	Efavirenz Atazanavir, lopinavir, darunavir	May lead to reduced therapeutic effect of glecaprevir/pibrentasvir; Co-administration is not recommended Co-administration is not recommended

Grazoprevir/Elbasvir

Grazoprevir/elbasvir is a fixed-dose combination product containing grazoprevir, an HCV NS3/4A protease inhibitor and an NS5A inhibitor elbasvir, and is indicated for the treatment of chronic hepatitis C genotype 1 or 4 infection. It can be used with or without ribavirin. Like all regimens containing NS3/4A protease inhibitors, it is contraindicated in patients with moderate or severe hepatic impairment (Child Pugh class B or C). (Zepatier summary, Kiang TKL) Both compounds are partially eliminated by oxidative metabolism, primarily by CYP3A. The primary route of elimination of medication is through faeces [35, 39].

Drug Interactions

Elbasvir and grazoprevir are substrates of CYP3A and P-gp. Co-administration with moderate and strong CYP3A or P-gp inducers is contraindicated because it may decrease elbasvir and grazoprevir plasma concentrations, which may lead to reduced therapeutic effect and loss of virological response. Co-administration of strong CYP3A4 inhibitors may increase elbasvir and grazoprevir plasma concentrations and is not recommended. The role of intestinal P-gp in the absorption of elbasvir and grazoprevir appears to be minimal. Grazoprevir is also a substrate of OATP1B1 and OATP1B3. Co-administration with drugs that inhibit OATP1B1/3 transporters may result in a significant increase in the grazoprevir plasma concentrations. Elbasvir and grazoprevir are inhibitors of the BCRP at the intestinal level and may increase plasma concentrations of coadministered medications which are BCRP substrates. No dose adjustment is required for CYP3A substrates when coadministered with grazoprevir/elbasvir since elbasvir is not a CYP3A inhibitor and grazoprevir is a weak inhibitor. Elbasvir shows minimal intestinal P-gp inhibition, which does not cause clinically relevant increases in concentrations of P-gp substrates [31, 40].

The most significant drug interactions with grazoprevir and elbasvir are shown in Table 30.5.

Other Drugs: When medication is coadministered with **fentanyl**, fentanyl exposure may be increased due to weak CYP3A4 inhibition by grazoprevir, which could prolong fentanyl action or cause adverse effects and potentially fatal respiratory depression. It can be also expected that **midazolam** concentrations may be increased. Co-administration with **ketoconazole** is not recommended. Concomitant use of systemic ketoconazole and elbasvir/grazoprevir increases grazoprevir exposure and may increase the overall risk of hepatotoxicity [31, 40].

Ribavirin

Ribavirin is a synthetic guanosine nucleoside which interferes with the synthesis of viral mRNA and blocks viral mRNA capping. Before the advent of direct-acting antiviral drugs, ribavirin in combination with peginterferons alfa represented the standard treatment for patients with chronic HCV infection. New DAA-based treatment regimens reduced the use of ribavirin, which is often associated with serious adverse effects. Ribavirin should not be used as monotherapy as is not effective in the treatment of chronic hepatitis C.

Table 30.5 Potentially significant drug interactions with grazoprevir/elbasvir

Drug class	Drug	Interactions and recommendations
Anticonvulsants	Phenytoin, phenobarbital Carbamazepine, primidone	↓ Grazoprevir/elbasvir; may lead to loss of virologic response
Antimycobacterials	Rifampicin Rifabutin Rifapentine	May lead to loss of virologic response due to significant decreases in elbasvir and grazoprevir plasma concentrations
Immunosuppressants	Cyclosporine	May increase the risk of ALT elevations due to a significant increase in grazoprevir plasma concentrations
Herbal products	St. John's wort	May lead to loss of virologic response
Antiarrhythmics	Amiodarone	↑ Amiodarone; close monitoring is required
Anticoagulants	Apixaban, rivaroxaban, dabigatran	↑ Apixaban, rivaroxaban and dabigatran; close monitoring for side effects is recommended
HMG-CoA reductase inhibitors	Rosuvastatin, fluvastatin, lovastatin, atorvastatin, simvastatin, pravastatin, pitavastatin, etc.	The dose of rosuvastatin should not exceed a daily dose of 20 mg; the dose of fluvastatin, lovastatin, atorvastatin or simvastatin 10 mg daily, no dose adjustment for pravastatin and pitavastatin; Increased risk of myopathy; monitoring is required
HIV antiretrovirals	Efavirenz, nevirapine, etravirine Atazanavir, darunavir, lopinavir, saquinavir, tipranavir Raltegravir/cobicistat/emtricitabine/TAF Ritonavir, atazanavir, darunavir, fosamprenavir	↓ Grazoprevir, ↓ elbasvir May lead to loss of virologic response; co-administration is contraindicated May increase the risk of ALT elevations due to a significant increase in grazoprevir plasma concentrations; co-administration is contraindicated ↑ Grazoprevir; co-administration is contraindicated ↑ Grazoprevir; co-administration is contraindicated

According to in vitro studies, ribavirin is not a substrate of CYP450 enzymes. The metabolites of ribavirin are renally excreted. The most serious adverse effect of ribavirin is haemolytic anaemia. The anaemia associated with ribavirin therapy may result in worsening of cardiac disease and lead to myocardial ischemia and infarction. Ribavirin is teratogenic and is contraindicated in women who are pregnant and in the male partners of women who are pregnant [41].

Drug Interactions

Ribavirin does not inhibit nor induce liver enzymes. There is a minimal potential for cytochrome P450 enzyme-based interactions with other drugs.

HIV Nucleoside Reverse Transcriptase Inhibitors (NRTIs): Concomitant use of **didanosine, stavudine** or **zidovudine** with ribavirin is not recommended. Exposure to **didanosine** when coadministered with ribavirin is increased in vitro, and it seems it can cause fatal liver failure, as well as peripheral neuropathy, pancreatitis and symptomatic hyperlactatemia/lactic acidosis. According to clinical studies, concomitant use of **stavudine** and ribavirin can cause pancreatitis and lactic acidosis. The concomitant use of ribavirin with **zidovudine** is not recommended due to an increased risk of anaemia. Due to ribavirin's long half-life, potential for interactions may persist for up to 2 months after cessation of ribavirin therapy [31, 41].

HIV protease inhibitors: A certain proportion of patients receiving **atazanavir** have experienced hyperbilirubinemia and jaundice following initiation of ribavirin and peginterferon. Bilirubin clearance by UGT1A1 is inhibited by atazanavir which, in case of ribavirin-related haemolysis, can result in increased production of bilirubin [31].

Immunomodulators: Ribavirin may interfere with **azathioprine** metabolism which has been associated with myelotoxicity. The use of pegylated alfa interferons and ribavirin concomitantly with azathioprine should be avoided [31].

Cancer therapies: Most of the drugs used in cancer treatment can cause myelosuppression. Concomitant use with ribavirin should be done with caution as those drugs are associated with myelosuppression.

Amphotericin B: Amphotericin B can be associated with anaemia and myelosuppression which may be intensified when coadministered with ribavirin. Co-administration is not recommended. If concomitant use is necessary, monitoring is required [31].

Metamizole: Co-administration is not recommended. Patients treated with peginterferon and ribavirin with metamizole are at increased risk of developing anaemia [31].

Alcoholic Liver Disease (ALD)

Pharmacotherapy of alcoholic steatohepatitis (ASH) involves the use of corticosteroids, prednisolone or methylprednisolone, and as another treatment option, pentoxifylline is recommended in patients with sepsis, developed hepatorenal syndrome, and in those with an inadequate response to corticosteroid therapy [42, 43].

Corticosteroids

Prednisolone

Drug-drug interactions of prednisolone are mostly **pharmacokinetic interactions**, associated with the activity of the CYP3A4 enzyme, whose prednisolone is a substrate, and co-administration with potent inducers or inhibitors of CYP3A4 enzymes requires dose adjustment of prednisolone [44]. It also participates in **pharmacodynamic interactions** with drugs with antagonistic (hypoglycaemics and antihypertensives) or additive effect (drugs that lower potassium levels).

Antidiabetics: Assuming that steroid hyperglycaemia is a common side effect of corticosteroid therapy, patients with diabetes may require dose adjustment of oral hypoglycaemics or insulin [45].

Anticonvulsant: *Phenobarbitone, phenytoin, carbamazepine and primidone* are potent inducers of the CYP3A4 enzyme, which co-administration requires an increased dose of prednisolone. According to studies, carbamazepine was increased the total clearance of prednisolone by 42%, which lead to a reduced immunosuppressive effect [46, 47].

NSAID: Corticosteroids co-administered with *acetylsalicylic acid or NSAIDs* significantly increase the risk of **gastrointestinal toxicity**, as a result of the additive ulcerogenic effect of these two drug classes [48–50]. Corticosteroids also increase the renal clearance of salicylates, and their withdrawal from therapy increases the risk of salicylate intoxication. Therefore, caution is required during their co-administration in patients with **hypoprothrombinemia** [51, 52].

Antibiotics: *Rifampicin* as a potent inducer of the CYP3A4 enzyme accelerates the elimination of prednisolone; therefore, concomitant use of these two drugs requires increasing the dose of prednisolone, according to some authors by twofold to threefold [53, 54].

Macrolide antibiotics as CYP3A4 inhibitors can reduce corticosteroid clearance by up to 60%, consequently increasing the risk of their side effects. *Azithromycin* has the weakest potential for this interaction [55].

Tetracyclines should not be used with prednisolone due to the risk of increased intracranial pressure. Rare cases of **intracranial hypertension** have been reported with abrupt discontinuation of corticosteroid therapy from concomitant tetracycline therapy [56].

Antiviral drug *ritonavir* increases the serum concentrations of prednisolone [57].

Antifungal drugs: *Ketoconazole*, as a potent inhibitor of the CYP3A4 enzyme, slows down the elimination of prednisolone. Studies have shown that the impact of the potent inhibitor of the CYP3A4 enzyme, ketoconazole, on decreased prednisolone clearance results in a threefold to sixfold increase in prednisolone exposure and an increased risk of side effects [58]. Corticosteroids increase the risk of *amphotericin*-induced **hypokalaemia**, and it is recommended to avoid their concomitant use. Cases of congestive heart failure have been reported after their co-administration [59].

Anticoagulants: Although there are conflicting reports, co-administration of warfarin with prednisolone had in most cases resulted in a **reduced anticoagulant effect** [52, 60].

Cardiac glycosides: Concomitant use of corticosteroids with cardiac glycosides, such as *digoxin*, may increase the risk of cardiac arrhythmias due to **hypokalaemia** [44].

Cyclosporine: Like prednisolone, cyclosporine is both a substrate and a competitive inhibitor of the CYP3A4 enzyme, so their co-administration can lead to decreased prednisolone clearance [61]. At the same time, an increase in cyclosporine activity, but also toxic effects are possible, and cases of convulsions during their concomitant use have been reported [52].

Methotrexate: Some of the studies demonstrate the possible effect of prednisolone on the reduction of renal clearance of methotrexate, suggesting a possible increased risk of methotrexate toxicity [62].

Vaccines: Patients on corticosteroid therapy should **not** be given **live vaccines,** due to a reduced immune response [44, 61].

If high-dose prednisolone is co-administered with a high dose of a **β2-receptor agonist,** such as *bambuterol, fenoterol, formoterol, ritodrine, salbutamol, salmeterol or terbutaline*, the risk of **hypokalaemia** increases [44, 63].

The use of **drugs with a hypokalaemic** effect with corticosteroids, such as **diuretics** *(acetazolamide, furosemide, torasemide, thiazide diuretics and carbenoxolone)* or ***theophylline*,** increases the risk of **hypokalaemia** due to their additive effect on potassium loss [64].

Antihypertensive agents: Concomitant use of prednisolone and antihypertensives results in a pharmacodynamic interaction, where the expected effect of antihypertensives may be diminished. This effect is dose-dependent, and an increase in cardiovascular risk has been observed with prednisone doses > 7.5 mg/day [65, 66].

Pyridostigmine, neostigmine and ambenonium: Corticosteroids cause an increase in the metabolism of acetylcholinesterase inhibitors (AChE), which leads to a **worsening of myasthenia gravis** [52, 67].

Anticholinergics: Acute myopathies have been reported with high doses of CS and with anticholinergic muscle relaxants *pancuronium* and *vecuronium*, due to their additive action on muscarinic receptors [52, 68].

Methylprednisolone

Methylprednisolone, like prednisolone, is a substrate of the CYP3A4 enzyme, and therefore, all interactions described in the prednisolone section are also implied for methylprednisolone [69–71].

Pentoxifylline

Pentoxifylline undergoes a extensive first-pass through the liver, whereby **active metabolites** are formed, with the main route of **elimination** by urine, while **CYP1A2 enzyme** plays a major role in the hepatic metabolism of pentoxifylline [72].

Hypoglycaemics: Rare cases of increased hypoglycaemic effects of insulin and oral hypoglycaemic agents are reported on high doses of parenterally co-administered pentoxifylline, but no effects have been observed after oral administration of pentoxifylline [72, 73].

Anticoagulants: Cases of bleeding and prothrombin time prolongation have been reported in patients treated with pentoxifylline, therefore is recommended to monitor INR values in case of their concomitant administration with *warfarin*, and also to control prothrombin time in patients on *platelet aggregation inhibitors, ASA and NSAIDs*. This interaction is a result of an additive antiplatelet effect [74, 75].

Theophylline: Theophylline is, like pentoxifylline, a substrate of the CYP1A2 enzyme, so their concomitant use reduces hepatic clearance and increases the serum concentration of theophylline by 30%. Co-administration of these two drugs requires dose adjustment of theophylline, taking into account its narrow therapeutic range [72, 76, 77].

Ciprofloxacin may increase serum concentrations of pentoxifylline when used concomitantly, most likely as a result of inhibition of the CYP1A2 enzyme [78].

Potentially significant drug interactions with drugs used in treatment of alcoholic steatohepatitis are shown in Table 30.6.

Table 30.6 Potentially significant drug interactions with drugs used in treatment of alcoholic steatohepatitis

Drug class	Drug	Interaction
Interactions of prednisolone (methylprednisolone)		
Oral hypoglycaemics Insulin		↑ Risk of hypoglycaemia
Anticonvulsants	Phenobarbital, phenytoin Carbamazepine, primidone	↓ Conc. prednisolone ↓ IMMUNOSUPPRESSIVE effect
NSAIDs Acetylsalicylic acid (ASK)		↑ Risk of GI bleeding ↑ ASK clearance (After discontinuation of KS ↑ risk of salicylate intoxication)
Antibiotics	Rifampicin Macrolide antibiotics Tetracyclines	↓ Conc. prednisolone ↑ Conc. prednisolone ↑ Risk of intracranial hypertension
Antiviral drugs	Ritonavir	↑ Conc. prednisolone
Antifungals	Ketoconazole Amphotericin	↑ Conc. prednisolone ↑ Risk of hypokalaemia
Anticoagulants	Warfarin	↑ Risk of thrombosis
Cardiac glycosides	Digoxin	↑ Risk of hypokalaemia
Immunosuppressants	Cyclosporine	↑ Conc. prednisolone ↑ Conc. cyclosporine
Cytostatics	Methotrexate	↑ Conc. methotrexate
β2-receptor agonists	Bambuterol Fenoterol, formoterol, ritodrine salbutamol, salmeterol, terbutaline	↑ Risk of hypokalaemia
Diuretics	Acetazolamide, furosemide, torasemide, thiazide diuretics, carbenoxolone	↑ Risk of hypokalaemia
Bronchodilators	Theophylline	↑ Risk of hypokalaemia
Antihypertensives		↓ Hypotensive effect
Acetylcholinesterase (AChE) inhibitors	Pyridostigmine, neostigmine, ambenonium	↓ Cholinergic activity
Anticholinergics (muscle relaxants)	Pancuronium, vecuronium	↑ Risk of acute myopathies
Interactions of pentoxifylline		
Anticoagulants	Warfarin	↑ Risk of bleeding
Antiplatelet drugs	Clopidogrel, eptifibatide, tirofiban, epoprostenol, iloprost, abciximab, anagrelide, ticlopidine, dipyridamole	↑ Risk of bleeding
NSAIDs, ASK		↑ Risk of bleeding
Bronchodilators	Theophylline	↑ Conc. teophylline

Non-alcoholic Fatty Liver Disease

Pharmacotherapy of non-alcoholic fatty liver disease (NAFLD) and non-alcoholic steatohepatitis (NASH) involves off-label use of drugs currently available for the treatment of diabetes, metformin, pioglitazone and liraglutide, and the use of statins to treat dyslipidaemia present in patients with NAFLD [79, 80].

Pioglitazone

Pioglitazone is **metabolized** in the liver predominantly by the **CYP2C8** enzyme [81]. When co-administered with strong inhibitors (e.g. gemfibrozil) or inducers (e.g. rifampicin) of the CYP2C8 enzyme, it is necessary to monitor glycemia, and consider pioglitazone dose adjustment, within the recommended dose range, or changing the therapy. In vitro studies have not shown that pioglitazone inhibits or induces any of the cytochrome P450 subtypes, so pioglitazone impact on other drug pharmacokinetics are not expected [82].

Gemfibrozil: According to studies, co-administration of pioglitazone with gemfibrozil resulted in a threefold increase in the AUC of pioglitazone [83, 84]. This interaction may also be further potentiated by CYP2C8 enzyme gene polymorphisms [85].

Rifampicin: Co-administration of pioglitazone with, a potent CYP2C8 inducer, rifampicin has been reported to result in a 54% reduction in pioglitazone AUC. In case of discontinuation of rifampicin from therapy, dose reduction of pioglitazone is mandatory [86].

Metformin

Metformin **does not undergo hepatic metabolism** [87]. Drug-drug interactions of metformin are uncommon and mostly associated with a risk of developing lactic acidosis, either due to their additive effect on serum lactate levels or due to, with other drug-induced, decreased renal clearance of metformin. considering) that risk of lactic acidosis increases with increasing serum concentrations of metformin [88].

Intravenous administration of **iodine contrast agents** in radiological imaging may lead to contrast-induced nephropathy, resulting in metformin accumulation and an increased risk of lactic acidosis. Metformin should be discontinued before and not initiated for at least 48 h after contrast agent, with prior assessment of renal function [89].

The risk of lactic acidosis is increased when metformin is co-administered with drugs that may reduce renal function and thus renal clearance of metformin, such as **NSAIDs** (including **selective COX-II inhibitors), ACE inhibitors, angiotensin II receptor antagonists and loop diuretics.** In case of their concomitant use, it is necessary to monitor renal function. Cases of severe lactic acidosis and hyperkalaemia have been reported with concomitant use of metformin with ibuprofen and enalapril [89–91].

Carboanhydrase Inhibitors (*acetazolamide, dichlorphenamide, topiramate and zonisamide*) can cause hyperchloraemic metabolic acidosis, and concomitant use of these drugs with metformin may increase the risk of lactic acidosis [92].

Drugs with an intrinsic hyperglycaemic effect, such as **glucocorticoids, sympathomimetics** and **β-2 agonists**, may reduce the effect of metformin, so glucose monitoring and dose adjustment of metformin in patients with type 2 diabetes are required. Thiazide diuretics, phenothiazines, thyroid hormones, oestrogens, phenytoin, nicotinic acid, calcium channel blockers and isoniazid have also a similar effect [88].

Liraglutide

According to currently available data, liraglutide does not enter into clinically significant interactions, and its co-administration with other drugs can be considered generally as safe [93].

Warfarin: Since liraglutide slows gastric emptying and may therefore potentially affect the absorption of co-administered oral drugs, the effect on the absorption of a poorly soluble drug with narrow therapeutic range, such as warfarin, cannot be ruled out. Therefore, monitoring of INR values is recommended when used concomitantly [94].

Statins

All statins, except pravastatin, are metabolized by the hepatic CYP450 enzyme system, via the **CYP3A4, CYP2C9 and CYP2C19** isoenzymes. Statin interactions with potent CYP3A4 inhibitors or inducers are of clinical importance. In addition, statin interactions involving competition for **P-gp** and **OATP1B1 transport proteins** have been described [95, 96]. More than 50% of cases of rhabdomyolysis associated with statins are attributed precisely to drug interactions that significantly affected statin metabolism. These most commonly included were mibefradil, fibrates, cyclosporine, macrolide antibiotics, warfarin, digoxin and azole antifungals [97].

Atorvastatin

Atorvastatin is primarily metabolized in the liver by CYP3A4 and is a substrate of hepatic OATP1B1 and OATP1B3 transporters, so co-administration with strong inhibitors of CYP3A4 enzymes or inhibitors of transport proteins poses a potential risk for interaction. A pharmacodynamic interactions are likely with drugs that already carry the risk of rhabdomyolysis in monotherapy, such as fibrates and ezetimibe [98].

Clarithromycin (macrolide antibiotics): Clarithromycin was found to moderately (twofold to fourfold) increase systemic exposure to atorvastatin, while the greatest effect was measured with simvastatin (ten-fold AUC increase). This interaction is largely attributed to inhibition of the CYP3A4 enzyme and is dose-dependent [99]. *Erythromycin* also has significant potential for this interaction, while *azithromycin* has minimal potential to interact with statins [100, 101].

Protease inhibitors (*saquinavir, lopinavir and ritonavir*): Interactions between statins and protease inhibitors (PI) are mainly due to the inhibitory effect of PIs on the CYP3A4 enzyme, among which ***ritonavir*** is the strongest inhibitor, and to a lesser extent on the OATP1B1 transport protein. According to studies, co-administration of atorvastatin with ***tipranavir/ritonavir*** combination resulted in a ninefold increase in atorvastatin AUC, with ***lopinavir/ritonavir*** in a fivefold increase, and with ***saquinavir/ritonavir*** in a fourfold increase [102]. A case of rhabdomyolysis has also been reported in HIV-infected patients treated with ***indinavir*** *f*ollowing with atorvastatin therapy [103]. According to FDA recommendations, concomitant use of atorvastatin with ***tipranavir/ritonavir*** or ***telaprevir*** is not recommended, but with other PI is permitted with caution and the use of the lowest dose of atorvastatin [98, 104].

Itraconazole: A study in healthy subjects showed that itraconazole, as a potent inhibitor of CYP3A4, increased the AUC of atorvastatin by 3.3-fold. In case of co-administration, dose of atorvastatin should not exceed 20 mg/day [105–107].

Cyclosporine: The results of several studies show a ten-fold increase in atorvastatin serum concentrations, while decrease in cyclosporine systemic exposure was clinically insignificant. The mechanism of this interaction is probably due to inhibition of the Pg-p and OATP1B1 transport systems in the liver, rather than CYP3A4 enzyme [108, 109]. If concomitant administration of atorvastatin with cyclosporine is necessary, the dose of atorvastatin should not exceed 10 mg [98].

Rifampicin: According to a study in healthy subjects, rifampicin, as a potent CYP3A4 inducer, reduces the plasma concentrations of atorvastatin and its metabolites by up to 80%. In concomitant use with rifampicin, administration of atorvastatin in the morning may not provide adequate nocturnal drug concentrations for effective cholesterol reduction, and therefore, a higher dose of atorvastatin in the evening is recommended [110].

Gemfibrozil: Although the pharmacokinetic interaction between gemfibrozil and atorvastatin is only moderate, the risk is increased, due to its additive effect, as gemfibrozil monotherapy is associated with an increased risk of rhabdomyolysis [110].

Effect of Atorvastatin on the Pharmacokinetics of Other Drugs

Digoxin. When 80 mg of atorvastatin with digoxin was administered, a 15% increase in digoxin AUC was measured, as a result of the inhibitory effect of atorvastatin on the transport Pg-p protein, of which digoxin is a substrate. Caution is advised when co-administering a statin with digoxin, respecting its narrow therapeutic range [111].

Warfarin: Concomitant use of statins with warfarin results in an increase in INR values. This interaction can largely be attributed to the inhibition of the CYP3A4 system. In clinical practice, atorvastatin appears to have the lowest incidence of reported interactions with warfarin [112–114].

Rosuvastatin

Rosuvastatin undergoes minimal hepatic metabolism, mainly via **CYP2C9**, and to a lesser extent via CYP2C19 enzymes. It is neither an inhibitor nor an inducer of the CYP450 isoenzyme, nor a substrate of the Pg-p transport protein, while it has a high affinity for the **OATP1B2** transport protein. Pharmacokinetic interactions mediated by the CYP enzyme system are unlikely, while interactions with transport protein inhibitors are possible, and may result in increased plasma concentrations of rosuvastatin [115].

Cyclosporine: Co-administration of cyclosporine and rosuvastatin in heart transplant patients was associated with a 7.1-fold increase in rosuvastatin AUC, while rosuvastatin did not affect cyclosporine plasma concentrations. This interaction is considered to be a result of the inhibition of the hepatic intake of rosuvastatin, mediated by the OATP1B2 transport system [115].

Antiviral Drugs: Increased systemic exposure to rosuvastatin has been observed in subjects receiving rosuvastatin concomitantly with various protease inhibitors in combination with *ritonavir*. In a pharmacokinetic study, co-administration of rosuvastatin and the *atazanavir/ritonavir* combination resulted in a triple and *lopinavir/ritonavir* combination in a twofold increase in rosuvastatin AUC. Although the exact mechanism of interaction is unknown, it may be a multiple mechanism involved [116, 117]. Concomitant use of rosuvastatin and some combinations of PIs may be considered with dose adjustment of rosuvastatin [104].

Gemfibrozil: Concomitant administration of rosuvastatin and gemfibrozil resulted in a twofold increase in rosuvastatin AUC, most likely by inhibition of the hepatic OATP2 transport system [118]. No relevant pharmacokinetic interaction with fenofibrate is expected; however, a pharmacodynamic interaction with fibrates may occur due to their additive effect on the risk of developing myopathies [96].

Warfarin: Cases of bleeding have been reported with concomitant administration of rosuvastatin with warfarin. It is possible that the interaction is due to inhibition of the CYP2C9 enzyme, but also due to the displacement of warfarin from the binding site on plasma proteins and an increase in the free fraction of warfarin [119, 120].

Antacids: Co-administration of rosuvastatin with antacids, containing *aluminium or magnesium hydroxide*, resulted in a reduction in systemic exposure to rosuvastatin of approximately 50% [121].

Potentially significant drug interactions with drugs used in treatment of nonalcoholic fatty liver disease are shown in Table 30.7.

Table 30.7 Potentially significant drug interactions with drugs used in treatment of non-alcoholic liver disease

Drug class	Drug	Interaction
Interactions of pioglitazone		
Antibiotic	Rifampicin	↓ Conc. pioglitazone
Lipid-lowering agents	Gemfibrozil	↑ Conc. pioglitazone
Interactions of metformin		
Alcohol		↑ Risk of lactic acidosis
Iodine contrast agents		↑ Risk of lactic acidosis
Analgesics	NSAID, COX-II inhibitors	
Antihypertensives	ACE inhibitors, ARBs	↓ Metformin clearance ↑ Risk of lactic acidosis
Carboanhydrase inhibitors	Acetazolamide Topiramate, Zonisamide	↑ Risk of lactic acidosis
Interactions of atorvastatin		
Antibiotics	Macrolide antibiotics (clarithromycin) Rifampicin	↑ Conc. atorvastatin ↑ Risk of rhabdomyolysis ↓ Conc. atorvastatin
Antifungals	Itraconazole	
Anticoagulants	Warfarin	↑ Risk of bleeding
Antiviral drugs	Boceprevir, lopinavir Saquinavir, darunavir Fosamprenavir Nelfinavir **Tipranavir/ritonavir** **telaprevir**	↑ Conc. atorvastatin ↑ Risk of rhabdomyolysis
Hypolipaemics	Gemfibrozil	↑ Risk of rhabdomyolysis
Immunosuppressants	Cyclosporine	↑ Conc. atorvastatin ↑ Risk of rhabdomyolysis
Cardiac glycosides	Digoxin	↑ Conc. digoxin
Interactions of rosuvastatin		
Anticoagulants	Warfarin	↑ Risk of bleeding
Antiviral drugs	Simeprevir Velpatasvir Atazanavir/ritonavir	↑ Conc. rosuvastatin (~3×)
	Lopinavir/ritonavir Grazoprevir/elbasvir Glecaprevir/pibrentasvir Ombitasvir/paritaprevir Ritonavir/dasabuvir	↑ Conc. rosuvastatin
Hypolipaemics	*Gemfibrozil*	↑ Risk of rhabdomyolysis
Immunosuppressants	*Cyclosporine*	↑ Conc. rosuvastatin **(KI)**

Primary Biliary Cholangitis (PBC) and Primary Sclerosing Cholangitis (PSC)

Ursodeoxycholic acid (UDCA) is recommended as the first-line therapy for all patients with primary biliary cholangitis (PBC), while in patients who do not tolerate UDCA or who have not responded to treatment with UDCA, obeticholic acid (OCA) is considered another pharmacotherapeutic option, as monotherapy or in combination with UDCA [122, 123].

Ursodeoxycholic Acid (UDCA)

UDCA is a weak inducer of CYP3A enzymes, with eightfold smaller effect on CYP3A4 enzyme activity compared to potent CYP3A4 inducers [124]. The clinically significant observed interactions of UDCA with other drugs occur mainly due to decreased absorption, whether the other drug interferes with resorption by binding UDCA or UDCA reduces the absorption of a lipophilic drug [125].

Anionic resins, cholestyramine and colesevelam, bind UDCA and thus interfere with its intestinal absorption. They should be administered with an appropriate delay from UDCA of at least 4 h. **Aluminium hydroxide, sucralfate and antacids** containing aluminium hydroxide and aluminium oxide also form non-absorbable complexes with UDCA and reduce their absorption [125, 126].

Cyclosporine: UDCA may affect the bioavailability of cyclosporine differently in transplant and non-transplant patients. Patients treated with cyclosporin should be closely monitored when using UDCA, as concomitant use in some patients decreased and in some increased the bioavailability of cyclosporin [127].

Ciprofloxacin: Isolated cases of decreased ciprofloxacin absorption have been reported, but the mechanism of this interaction remains unclear [126].

Nitrendipine: In a controlled clinical study, the availability of nitrendipine, a highly lipophilic calcium channel blocker, was found to be significantly reduced during concomitant administration of UDCA, and it is thought to be a metabolic interaction since nitrendipine is a substrate of the CYP3A4 enzyme [125]. A similar interaction, resulting in its reduced efficacy, was observed with **dapsone**, where induction of CYP3A4 by UDCA contributed to enhanced dapsone biotransformation [126, 127].

Rosuvastatin: Co-administration of UDCA with rosuvastatin resulted in a significant increase in rosuvastatin plasma levels of 60%, due to reduced expression of the OAT1B1 transporter by UDCA [128, 129].

Oestrogen hormones, fibrates: A pharmacodynamic interaction is likely with drugs that enhance hepatic cholesterol excretion, such as oestrogen hormones and fibrates, which may thereby promote biliary lithiasis, as opposed to the effect of UDCA on gallstone dissolution [129].

Obeticholic Acid (OCA)

OCA undergoes **hepatic metabolism,** where it is conjugated with glycine or taurine, followed by excretion into the bile, and formed conjugates re-enter the liver by enterohepatic circulation [130].

Weak inhibition of CYP1A2, by OCA, was observed and assessed as clinically insignificant, with the exception of the CYP1A2 substrates with narrow therapeutic range [131]. OCA and its conjugates have an additional effect on certain transport systems (e.g. BSEP, OATP1B), which may affect the pharmacokinetics of other drugs, but also tauro-OCA conjugate is a substrate for the BSEP transport system [132]. Serum concentrations of OCA are mainly affected by drugs that alter its extent of absorption by forming insoluble complexes [133].

Colesevelam, cholestyramine and colestipol: Bile acid sequestrants (colesevelam, cholestyramine, colestipol) bind OCA and its active conjugates (glyco-OCA and tauro-OCA), thus reducing the extent of absorption of OCA. Therefore, in case of their concomitant use, it is recommended to take OCA with an interval of 4–6 h [133].

Warfarin: Concomitant use of OCA may reduce the anticoagulant effect of warfarin, and monitoring of INR values and dose adjustment of warfarin is required. The mechanism of this interaction has not been elucidated [134].

BSEP/ABCB11 inhibitors: Drugs that inhibit bile acid transporters, such as BSEP bile pump, can lead to the accumulation of conjugated bile salts, including tauro-OCA conjugate, in the liver, and result in hepatotoxic side effects. Also, in vitro studies have shown that OCA and its conjugates inhibit BSEP in a dose-dependent manner. If concomitant use with these drugs is required, monitoring of serum transaminases and bilirubin is necessary [134].

CYP1A2 substrates of narrow therapeutic index: Co-administration of **tizanidine** with OCA may increase the risk of potentially dangerous reactions such as hypotension, bradycardia and somnolence [135]. OCA may significantly increase **theophylline** serum concentrations and cause side effects such as restlessness, headache, vomiting or tachycardia. It is recommended to avoid those combinations, and to adjust the dose of theophylline and tizanidine in case of necessary co-administration with OCA. This recommendation also applies to the theophylline derivative aminophylline [134].

Other CYP1A2 Substrates: Although there are not many studies examining OCA interactions, the possibility of OCA interactions with other drugs that are significantly metabolized by CYP1A2 enzymes should not be ruled out, taking into account gene polymorphisms of CYP enzyme activity [131, 136].

Cholestyramine

Cholestyramine is **not absorbed** from the digestive tract, but it reduces the absorption and bioavailability of a number of drugs, and may be a cause of clinically significant interactions with drugs of narrow therapeutic range [137]. This influence is absent in co-administration with an interval of 4 h. Cholestyramine may also affect the effect of drugs administered i.v., which have active metabolites entering the enterohepatic circulation, by reducing their reabsorption from the intestine. Clinically significant is the effect of cholestyramine on the bioavailability of oral anticoagulants, cardiac glycosides and diuretics [138].

Cholestyramine may interfere with the absorption of **mycophenolate mofetil**, but also with its enterohepatic circulation. Reduced AUC measured by an average of 37% is largely attributed to the effect of cholestyramine on reducing enterohepatic reabsorption [139]. This interaction can be almost completely avoided if cholestyramine is administered 6 h before or 2 h after mycophenolate mofetil [140].

Warfarin: Cholestyramine has been shown to significantly affect the absorption of warfarin from the gastrointestinal tract, but also increases the elimination of warfarin by reducing enterohepatic circulation, which ultimately results in a reduced anticoagulant effect of warfarin [141]. A similar effect of cholestyramine was observed on the reduced bioavailability of **digoxin** to, and therefore is recommended to administer oral digoxin at least 1.5–2 h before cholestyramine [142, 143].

Levothyroxine: Cholestyramine reduces absorption of levothyroxine, but also affects its enterohepatic circulation, which further contributes to a decrease in the bioavailability of levothyroxine [144, 145].

Amiodarone: Cholestyramine may interfere with the absorption of amiodarone from the gastrointestinal tract; however, the effect of cholestyramine on increasing the enterohepatic elimination of amiodarone is more significant [146]. This interaction is of the greatest clinical importance in terms of the use of cholestyramine to accelerate the elimination of amiodarone and its active metabolite desethylamiodarone in cases of amiodarone overdose [147].

According to studies, cholestyramine can reduce the absorption of **furosemide** and **hydrochlorothiazide** by almost 95%. This interaction is clinically significant in patients with portal hypertension receiving furosemide therapy [143].

Propranolol: Co-administration of cholestyramine and propranolol resulted in a 43% reduction in serum propranolol concentrations. It is most likely that occurs a decrease in the absorption of propranolol, but also a decrease in the reabsorption of the active metabolite [148].

Cases of severe metabolic acidosis with concomitant use of **spironolactone** and cholestyramine in patients with reduced renal function have been reported. Discontinuation of cholestyramine therapy in these patients is recommended [149].

Cholestyramine binds hydrophilic **ursodeoxycholic acid**, usually prescribed together in the treatment of cholestatic diseases, reducing its absorption from the digestive system, and also binds both **obeticholic acid** and **bezafibrate**, reducing their bioavailability and efficacy. Co-administration of these drugs is recommended with an appropriate interval of 4 h [150].

Potentially significant drug interactions with drugs used in treatment of primary biliary cholangitis are shown in Table 30.8.

Table 30.8 Potentially significant drug interactions with drugs used in treatment of primary biliary cholangitis

Drug class	Drug	Interaction
Interactions with ursodeoxycholic acid (UDCA)		
Anionic resins	Cholestyramine Colesevelam	↓UDCA absorption
Drugs containing aluminium	Al-hydroxide, antacids Sucralfate	↓ UDCA absorption
Immunosuppressants	***Cyclosporine***	↓ Bioavailability of cyclosporine
Antibiotics	Dapsone	↓ Bioavailability of antibiotics
Ca-channel blocker	***Nitrendipine***	↓ Bioavailability of nitrendipine
Hypolipaemics	Rosuvastatin Fibrates	↑ Rosuvastatin conc. ↑ Risk of biliary lithiasis
Hormones	Oestrogens	↑ Risk of biliary lithiasis
Interactions with obeticholic acid (OCA)		
Bile acids sequestrants	Colesevelam Cholestyramine, colestipol	↓ OCA absorption
Anticoagulants	Warfarin	↓ Anticoagulant effect
BSEP/ABCB11 inhibitors	Various drugs	↑ Hepatotoxicity
Ca-channel blocker	Tizanidine	↑ Conc. tizanidine ↑ Risk of bradycardia and hypotension
Bronchodilators	Theophylline	↑ Conc. theophylline ↑ Risk of tachycardia and arrhythmia
Interactions with cholestyramine		
Antiarrhythmics	Amiodarone	↓ Antiarrhythmic effect
Anticoagulants	Warfarin	↓ Anticoagulant effect
Beta-blockers	Propranolol	↓ Conc. propranolol
Diuretics	Furosemide Hydrochlorothiazide Spironolactone	↓ Conc. diuretics ↑ Risk of metabolic acidosis
Hepatoprotectives	UDCA, OCA	↓ Conc. drug
Hormones	Levothyroxine	↓ Conc. levothyroxine
Immunosuppressants	Mofetil-mycophenolate	↓ Conc. immunosuppressive

Autoimmune Hepatitis

Main treatment goals of autoimmune hepatitis are to achieve and maintain complete remission of the disease, in order to prevent further progression of the disease. For induction to disease remission are recommend corticosteroids, primarily prednisolone, or budesonide as a second-line treatment., followed by the immunosuppressant azathioprine. Maintenance therapy is based on azathioprine or mycophenolate mofetil (MMF) monotherapy [151–153].

Corticosteroids

Prednisone/Prednisolone

Prednisone is a prodrug that is converted in the liver into active **drug** prednisolone, and therefore participates in the same interactions as its active metabolite **prednisolone.** The features and drug-drug interactions of prednisolone are described in the section on alcoholic liver disease [154].

Budesonide

Budesonide undergoes **extensive hepatic first-pass clearance.** Budesonide is a **substrate of the CYP3A4 enzyme;** however, its effect on the metabolism of other CYP3A4 enzyme substrate drugs is unlikely. Pharmacokinetic drug-drug **interactions with potent inhibitors of the CYP3A4** enzyme, resulting in multiple increase in budesonide AUC, are much more clinically relevant [155].

Ketoconazole as a potent inhibitor of the CYP3A4 enzyme may decrease the hepatic clearance of budesonide. 6.5-fold increase in budesonide AUC was found during their co-administration, while a significantly lower increase in AUC by 3.8-fold was found with a time lag of 12 h [156]. Cases of severe systemic side effects have been also reported during co-administration of **itraconazole** with budesonide [157].

Other potent inhibitors of CYP3A4, such as **clarithromycin, erythromycin, cyclosporine, indinavir, saquinavir and ritonavir,** are also likely to cause a marked increase of the plasma concentrations of budesonide. Therefore, concomitant intake of budesonide and these drugs should be avoided [158].

Corticosteroids, among them budesonide, lower the serum potassium level, and in combination with other hypokalaemic drugs, resulting in an additive **hypokalaemic** effect. This pharmacodynamic interaction is of clinical significance in co-administration of budesonide with **diuretics** or with drugs with a narrow therapeutic index such as **digoxin** [159].

Thiopurines (Azathioprine)

However, the enzyme hypoxanthine-guanine phosphoribosyl-transferase (HGPRT) and inosine monophosphate dehydrogenase (IMPD) are essential for the conversion of AZA to active metabolites, two other enzymatic pathways, using xanthine oxidase (XO) and thiopurine methyltransferase(TMT) leading to inactive metabolites. Drugs affecting the activity of these enzymes interfere with the metabolism of thiopurines and cause clinically relevant interactions with AZA, with potentially serious toxicities [160].

Severe cases of pancytopenia with bone marrow suppression have been reported, in patients receiving azathioprine, during the concomitant use of the antiviral drug **ribavirin**. Ribavirin co-administration leads to accumulation of an azathioprine metabolite, 6-methylthioionosine monophosphate (6-MTIMP), which is associated with myelotoxicity, through complete blockade of IMPDH activity. Treatment with **IMPDH inhibitors** and purine analogues should be individualized and patients closely monitored. Increased caution is also required considering the narrow therapeutic index of AZA [161].

Potentially very serious interactions, with an increased risk of myelotoxicity, may occur when co-administered azathioprine with **xanthine oxidase (XO) inhibitors,** since inhibition of XO increases the risk of leukopenia [162]. **Allopurinol,** as a XO inhibitor, interferes with the metabolism of azathioprine, and several cases of reversible leukopenia and anaemia are reported in patients given a combination of azathioprine and allopurinol [163]. Patients receiving AZA and allopurinol concomitantly should have a dose reduction of AZA to approximately 25% of the usual dose. Rare cases of AZA interaction with a XO inhibitor **febuxostat** have been reported; therefore, caution is also required, as recommended for allopurinol [164].

Cases of liver necrosis, during co-administration of cyclophosphamide with azathioprine, have been described, possible due to competition for the same elimination pathway. The additive hepatotoxic effect very likely plays a significant role in this interaction [165].

In vitro studies have shown that **aminosalicylates** (mesalazine, sulfasalazine, olsalazine) reversibly inhibit the activity of the enzyme thiopurine methyltransferase (TMT), essential in the metabolism of thiopurines, and increase the concentration of myelotoxic 6-TGN [166]. In vivo study of co-administered azathioprine with **mesalazine** found a clinically significant increase in the incidence of leukopenia of 50% [167].

The administration of **live vaccines** to patients being treated with immunosuppressive drugs, such as azathioprine, is contraindicated. Reduced immune response has been reported with hepatitis B vaccine [168].

Orally administrated **methotrexate** increased 6-mercaptopurine AUC by approximately 31%, and intravenously methotrexate increased 6-MC AUC by 69–93%. Therefore, when azathioprine is administered concomitantly with high-dose methotrexate, the dose should be adjusted to avoid toxic effects [169].

An additive myelotoxic effect is possible during concomitant administration of AZA with **cytostatic drugs**, or **other drugs with myelosuppressive effect**, such as *penicillamine* and *co-trimoxazole,* and it is therefore preferable to avoid their co-administration [168].

Cases of decreased anticoagulant activity of **warfarin** have been reported during co-administration with azathioprine. Azathioprine is a clinically significant inducer of warfarin resistance, but the exact mechanism of the interaction is still unknown. This induction has been shown to be dose-dependent, and is manifested by the administration of AZA at doses >75 mg/daily. Close monitoring of the INR with warfarin dose adjustment is recommended, and in most patients requiring, at least, a 2.5-fold warfarin dose increases [170, 171].

According to a study examining the interaction of azathioprine with **infliximab**, in patients with Crohn's disease, significant decrease in the leucocyte count was found. Possible effect of infliximab is TPMT inhibition, although the full mechanism of this interaction is not known [172].

Mycophenolate Mofetil (MMF)

Mycophenolate mofetil undergoes complete liver metabolism to the active drug, mycophenolic acid (MPA), which is further metabolized to pharmacologically non-active form, the phenolic glucuronide of MPA (MPAG). MPAG is, through entero-hepatic recirculation, then converted back to MPA [173]. Potential mechanisms for interactions with mycophenolate mofetil involve enterohepatic cycling, or renal tubular competition between MPAG and other drugs undergoing transport-mediated renal excretion [139].

According to a study examining the effect of **cholestyramine** on the pharmacokinetics of MMF, there found a 40% reduction in AUC of MPA, which is attributed to the cholestyramine interference in the enterohepatic circulation of MPA. Caution is required in the co-administration of MMF with any drugs that interfere with enterohepatic recirculation to avoid the risk of their reduced efficacy [139].

In several studies, the effect of **cyclosporine** on the decrease in MPA serum concentration, by 30–40%, was confirmed and considered clinically relevant. The mechanism responsible for this interaction is also interference in enterohepatic circulation by inhibition of MRP2 transporter [174].

Antibiotics that alter the gastrointestinal flora and reduce the number of beta-glucuronidase-producing bacteria in the gut (e.g. *aminoglycosides, cephalosporins, fluoroquinolones and penicillin)* can disrupt the enterohepatic recycling of MPA, and cause clinically significant interactions. In vitro studies suggest that direct beta-glucuronidase inhibition by *ciprofloxacin* may also be involved [175]. Co-administration of *co-amoxiclav* in patients taking MMF resulted with median reduction of 46% in MPA trough concentration, which has been shown to be reversible [176]. The combination of *norfloxacin and metronidazole* co-administrated with MMF significantly reduced the AUC of MPA and MPAG, by 33% [177].

Co-administration of *telmisartan* and MMF resulted in an approximately 30% decrease of MPA concentrations. UGT induction by telmisartan may stimulate the metabolism of MPA to MPAG, and lead to MPA underexposure and low clinical efficacy [178].

Calcium-free phosphate-binding agent, ***sevelamer***, interferes with the gastrointestinal uptake of MMF, resulting in decrease of the MPA AUC, and therefore should preferentially be given 2 h after the intake of MMF [179].

Clinically relevant drug interaction has been described with **rifampicin.** Long-term rifampicin therapy caused a marked reduction of about 70% in dose-corrected MPA exposure, when administered simultaneously with MMF. Interaction can be explained by simultaneous induction of renal, hepatic and gastrointestinal transporters, with subsequent functional inhibition of enterohepatic recirculation of MPA [180].

Immunosuppressive agents: Cases of pure red cell aplasia (PRCA) have been reported in patients treated with MMF in combination with other immunosuppressive agents [181].

During treatment with MMF the use of **live attenuated vaccines** should be avoided [181].

Acyclovir pharmacokinetic parameters were modified by co-administration with MMF, with increased AUC of acyclovir by 31%. This interaction should not be ruled out in patients with impaired renal function [182].

Potentially significant drug interactions with drugs used in treatment of autoimmune hepatitis are shown in Table 30.9.

Table 30.9 Potentially significant drug interactions with drugs used in treatment of autoimmune hepatitis

Drug class	Drug	Interaction
Interactions with budesonide		
Antibiotics	Rifampicin Clarithromycin, erythromycin	↓ Conc. budesonide ↑ Conc. budesonide
Antifungal drugs	Ketoconazole	↑ Conc. budesonide
Antiviral drugs	Indinavir, saquinavir ritonavir	↑ Conc. budesonide
Cardiac glycoside	Digoxin	Hypokalaemic effect
Diuretics	Furosemide	Hypokalaemic effect
Interactions with azathioprine		
Aminosalicylates	Mesalazine, sulfasalazine, olsalazine	↑ Risk of myelotoxicity
Antibiotics	Co-trimoxazole	↑ Risk of myelotoxicity
Anticoagulant	Warfarin	↓ Anticoagulant activity
Antigout agents	Allopurinol Febuxostat	↑ Risk of myelotoxicity
Antiviral drugs	Ribavirin	↑ Risk of myelotoxicity
Chelating agent	Penicillamine	↑ Risk of myelotoxicity
Cytostatic drugs	Cyclophosphamide Methotrexate	Hepatotoxicity ↑ Conc. of methotrexate
Immunosuppressive drugs	Infliximab	↑ Risk of myelotoxicity
Interactions with mycophenolate mofetil (MMF)		
Antibiotics	Amoxiclav, ciprofloxacin, norfloxacin, metronidazole, rifampicin	↓ Conc. of MPA
Antihypertensive agent	Telmisartan	↓ Conc. of MPA
Antiviral drug	Acyclovir	Increased AUC of acyclovir by 31% in renal impairment
Ca-free phosphate-binding agent	Sevelamer	↓ Absorption of MMF
Ion exchange resin	Cholestyramine	40% ↓AUC of MPA
Immunosuppressive agents	Cyclosporine	Cases of pure red cell aplasia (PRCA) have been reported 30–40% ↓ conc. of MPA

Wilson's Disease (WD)

The main therapeutic goal in the treatment of Wilson's disease(WD) to maintain normal copper homeostasis is achieved by pharmacotherapy involving the use of chelating agents (penicillamine, trientine or zinc) as a lifelong therapy [183, 184].

Zinc

Zinc is **absorbed** in the small intestine by transport proteins in a dose-dependent manner [185–187]. Observed drug-drug interactions with zinc generally imply a decrease in the intestinal absorption of zinc or co-administered drug, due to the formation of insoluble metal-drug complexes.

Iron: Zinc and iron compete during intestinal absorption, and long-term zinc co-administration can lead to impaired iron status [188].

D-penicillamine: A study on patients with WD, concomitantly receiving zinc and a **chelating agent**, showed a reduced efficacy of both drugs, probably due to the binding of a portion of the zinc dose to the chelating agent. The chelating treatment and zinc acetate should be separated by at least 1 h [189].

Tetracyclines: Absorption of the various cations may be inhibited by the interaction based on formation of tetracycline-metal complexes in the gut. It was found that AUC of tetracycline hydrochloride was reduced by about 30%, while the absorption of doxycycline was not affected [190, 191].

Fluoroquinolones: Drug preparations that contain multivalent cations are known to form chelates with fluoroquinolones (e.g. *ciprofloxacin, norfloxacin, levofloxacin)* in the gastrointestinal tract. This general finding should be applied in their co-administration with zinc, with time interval at least 2 h before or 6 h after preparations containing zinc. The formation of drug-metal chelates is believed to be the primary reason for reduced antimicrobial activity of these drugs [192, 193].

D-penicillamine

D-penicillamine does not appear to be a substrate for the cytochrome P450 system, while small fraction of the drug dose is metabolized in the liver to S-methyl-D-penicillamine. Pharmacokinetic drug-drug interactions of penicillamine with other drugs are, as is the case in other chelating agents, the result of an effect on the absorption, by formation of non-adsorbable complexes, while pharmacodynamic interactions are associated with additive nephrotoxicity and haematological toxicity [194].

Penicillamine should not be used in patients who are receiving concurrently **gold therapy, antimalarial, immunosuppressive, cytotoxic therapy** or any other drugs associated with serious haematologic and renal adverse effects (e.g. clozapine, chloroquine or hydroxychloroquine, oxyphenbutazone or phenylbutazone) [195, 196].

Antacid mixtures containing aluminium and magnesium hydroxides reduce D-penicillamine absorption by 45%. Interaction may be related to reduced stability of penicillamine at higher pH and also further exacerbated by chelation with magnesium or aluminium ions [197].

D- penicillamine may form complexes or chelates with **metals**, including *zinc* or *iron*, and thus reduce their absorption, while after iron discontinuation adverse effects, such as nephropathy, may occur. Co-administration with zinc may result in reduced zinc levels, but also in decreased penicillamine levels. This chelating property underlies also in treatment of some heavy-metal poisonings [197, 198].

It has been observed that oral penicillamine can significantly reduce serum **digoxin**, irrespective of the route of digoxin administration. Mechanism of this interaction is not completely understood. Concomitant digoxin should be administrated within 2 h apart of penicillamine. This effect of penicillamine can be used in the management of digitalis toxicity [199].

Trientine

Trientine is relatively slow and poorly absorbed from the gastrointestinal tract, with a bioavailability of 8–30%. *D*rug–drug interactions with trientine are mainly associated with interference with intestinal absorption [200, 201].

Antacids, Iron and Zinc: *Calcium or magnesium antacids* reduce the absorption of trientine and therefore is recommended to separate their administration [202]. *Iron* and trientine have been found to inhibit absorption of the each other and should be administrated with an interval of 2 h from trientine. Co-administration with iron should be, in generally, avoided since the resulting complex may induce toxicity. The combination of trientine with *zinc* is not recommended as well [201].

Hemochromatosis

The therapeutic approach to hemochromatosis involves phlebotomy as a first choice and a lifelong treatment, while pharmacotherapy with iron chelators (e.g. deferoxamine) can be a treatment option in patients who are intolerant or refractory to phlebotomy or when phlebotomy is contraindicated [203–205].

Deferoxamine

Deferoxamine is mainly metabolized in the plasma, with minimal hepatic metabolism and does not appear to have great potential for entering into clinically significant drug-drug interactions, while observed interactions are mainly pharmacodynamic [206].

Prochlorperazine: It was reported that a combination of standard doses of deferoxamine and the antiemetic D2-receptor blocker prochlorperazine induced a deep coma. Studies demonstrated that the neurological effects were possibly due to fluctuations in intracellular and extracellular iron levels affected the noradrenergic and serotonergic systems. Therefore, it is recommended to avoid concomitant use of deferoxamine and all *phenothiazine derivatives* [207, 208].

Ga-67: It was noticed that Ga-67 scintigraphy imagining results were distorted as a result of the deferoxamine impact on the excretion of Ga-67. It is recommended that deeroxamine to be discontinued for at least 48 h before the use of Ga-67 diagnostic imaging to avoid this impact [209].

Trombotic Conditions Causing Liver Disease

Initial pharmacotherapy of all thrombotic conditions in liver patients involves mandatory anticoagulation using low-molecular-weight heparin (LMWH), in order to achieve rapid anticoagulation, followed with long-term maintenance therapy, with oral vitamin K antagonists (VKAs), to reduce risk of clot extension and to reduce risk of new thrombotic episodes [210].

Heparin

Heparins are, according to their structure, classified as unfractionated heparin (UFH) and low-molecular-weight heparins (LMWH). Today, LMWH is the standard of care instead of UFH, except in certain conditions such as renal failure and acute coronary syndrome, where UFH is preferred because of its easier liver clearance and better reversibility of protamine sulphate. LMWH shows more predictable pharmacokinetic and pharmacodynamic properties and lower risk of non-haemorrhagic side effects, while one limitation of LMWH is their renal clearance; therefore, their use is not preferred in patients with renal failure [211, 212].

Reported heparin drug-drug interactions apply equally to both UFH and LMWH. Of greatest clinical importance are the pharmacodynamic interactions of heparins with drugs that interfere with coagulation, platelet aggregation or with drugs that suppress coagulation, and their concomitant use with heparins may increase the risk of bleeding, due to their additive anticoagulant effect [213]. However, studies examining this risk have shown quite conflicting results.

Warfarin: Oral anticoagulants may prolong prothrombin time (aPTT) in patients receiving heparin, whereas in patients receiving warfarin, heparin may increase INR [214]. However, according to studies, short-term co-administration of heparin with warfarin was not associated with a statistically significant increase in the incidence of severe bleeding events [215].

Platelet Inhibitors: Concomitant use of multiple drugs that interfere with platelet aggregation reactions, such as *dextran, phenylbutazone, ibuprofen, indomethacin, dipyridamole,* implies increased risk of bleeding. Regardless of this, when co-administering heparin with **clopidogrel or ticagrelor** no clinically significant drug-drug interactions were observed [216, 217]. Similar was observed for **acetylsalicylic acid (ASA)** where the rate of major bleeding after administration of the combination of reviparin/ASA) by 2.5% did not differ from that after ASA alone by 2.6% [218].

Co-administration of heparins with drugs that also have hyperkalaemic potential, such as **potassium-sparing diuretics, ACE inhibitors or angiotensin receptor blockers (ARB),** may lead to potentially dangerous hyperkalaemic conditions [219]. The risk of hyperkalaemia increases with longer duration of therapy, but is generally reversible [220].

Vitamin K Antagonists (VKA)

Warfarin

Warfarin is absorbed quickly and completely and is **significantly protein bound**, with a binding rate of 98–99%. It is almost completely eliminated by hepatic metabolism into inactive metabolites, who are excreted in the urine. The more active (S)-warfarin is metabolized by the polymorphic enzyme CYP2C9, while the less active isomer (R)-warfarin is metabolized by CYP1A2, CYP3A4 and carbonyl reductase. Co-administration of the drugs that are **inhibitors or inducers of CYP2C9,** with warfarin leads to clinically significant interactions, in terms of increased risk of bleeding with inhibitors or increased risk of thrombotic events with CYP inducers [221, 222].

The most frequently reported drug-drug interactions with strong CYP2C9 inducers are those involving **carbamazepine** or **rifampicin,** and typically require increasing the dose of warfarin, while special caution is needed after withdrawal of rifampicin from therapy due to the risk of warfarin overdose [223, 224].

Antidepressants of the SNRI class (e.g. *venlafaxine, duloxetine)* and the SSRI class (e.g. *fluoxetine, sertraline*) interfere with warfarin metabolism by inhibiting the CYP2C9 enzyme. SSRIs also contribute to the pharmacodynamic interaction with an additive antiplatelet effect, which significantly increases the risk of major bleeding [225].

Azole Antifungals: *Fluconazole* and *voriconazole* showed a significant effect on the increase in INR, while with itraconazole, this effect was minimal. The interaction is due to inhibition of the CYP2C9 enzyme [226].

Amiodarone inhibits the clearance of both warfarin isomers. Its active metabolite, monodesethylamiodarone (MDEA), is 40–90 times more potent inhibitor of CYP2C9 than the parent drug [227].

Cholestyramine and sucralfate may affect the absorption but also the enterohepatic recirculation of warfarin, **reducing** its bioavailability and the anticoagulant effect of the administered dose [222].

Pharmacodynamic drug interactions with warfarin generally involve some of the following mechanisms: interference with platelet function, injury of gastrointestinal mucosa, reduced synthesis of vitamin K by intestinal flora or interruption of the vitamin K cycle [228].

Antiplatelet Agents: Drugs that affect platelets and primary haemostasis (e.g. *acetylsalicylic acid, NSAIDs, clopidogrel, ticlopidine, dipyridamole, tirofiban, direct-acting oral anticoagulants, UFH and LMWH heparins*) interact with warfarin and may **increase** the risk of severe bleeding. Co-administration of these drugs with warfarin, however, is not contraindicated, but careful monitoring of such therapy is necessary [229].

Antibiotics: *Penicillins* in high doses have a similar effect like antiplatelet agents and may **increase** the risk of bleeding. *Erythromycin* and some *cephalosporins* can directly reduce the synthesis of vitamin K-dependent blood clotting factors and **increase** the effect of warfarin. Antibiotics can also have an indirect effect on warfarin activity, by reducing the intestinal synthesis of vitamin K2 [230, 231].

Orlistat may have a similar effect by reducing the absorption of vitamin K and thus increasing the effect of warfarin [230].

Warfarin may affect the activity of other drugs, with a clinically significant effect on increasing the activity of oral antidiabetics from the class of **sulfonylureas**, leading to increased risk of potentially dangerous **hypoglycaemia** [232].

In terms of frequency and severity of reported interactions, the leading interactions are those with azole antifungals, macrolide and quinolone antibiotics, nonsteroidal anti-inflammatory drugs, including selective COX-2 inhibitors, SSRI antidepressants, omeprazole, hypolipidemic agents, amiodarone and their co-administration with warfarin should be avoided if possible; otherwise, careful monitoring is mandatory [233].

Direct Oral Anticoagulants (DOACs)

Direct oral anticoagulants (DOAC) are a group of five orally administered drugs that act on the coagulation cascade without affecting antithrombin, with more favourable pharmacokinetic profile then warfarin. They were classified into two groups, factor Xa inhibitors (**apixaban, edoxaban and rivaroxaban**) and direct thrombin inhibitors (**argatroban and dabigatran**) [234, 235].

Intestinal absorption of all DOACs is highly dependent on glycoprotein (P-gp). All DOACs undergo some degree of hepatic metabolism, where apixaban most extensively undergoes hepatic elimination (75%), followed by rivaroxaban (65%) and edoxaban (50%), while in dabigatran elimination takes place largely via kidney (80%). None of the DOACs are completely dependent on cytochrome P450 enzymes metabolism; however, apixaban and rivaroxaban are predominantly metabolized by CYP3A4 enzyme, whereas with edoxaban and dabigatran, the metabolism by CYP enzymes is minimal [232].

DOACs have a markedly lower potential for clinically significant interactions with other drugs than warfarin. Pharmacodynamic interactions of DOAC are likely with several drug classes that interfere with blood clotting mechanisms, including other anticoagulants, antiplatelet drugs, nonsteroidal anti-inflammatory drugs (NSAIDs) and selective serotonin and norepinephrine reuptake inhibitors (SSRIs/SNRIs). Since no DOACs are either an inducer or inhibitor of the CYP enzyme, their effect on the metabolism of other drugs is unlikely The potential for pharmacodynamic interactions is equally pronounced in all DOACs, while pharmacokinetic interactions are present in rivaroxaban and apixaban, but in dabigatran, they are lacking due to the absence of hepatic metabolism [236].

Pharmacokinetic Interactions of DOACs

The pharmacokinetic interactions of rivaroxaban and apixaban, respectively, have been shown to be of clinically significance only with those drugs that are both potent inhibitors of the **CYP3A4** enzyme and potent inhibitors of the **P-gp** transport protein.

Interactions with CYP3A4 and P-gp Inhibitors

Azole antifungals showed a significant increase in rivaroxaban exposure during co-administration of *ketoconazole* with more than a twofold increase in rivaroxaban AUC. Ketoconazole resulted in approximately 70% inhibition of rivaroxaban metabolic clearance, but also in 44% inhibition of active renal secretion. Interaction with ketoconazole may be more pronounced in high-risk patients with renal impairment (creatinine clearance <30 ml/min) [237].

Antiviral Protease Inhibitors: *Ritonavir* also significantly decreased total clearance of rivaroxaban by 60% and renal clearance by 82%. A similar interaction is expected with other members of these two drug classes, with the exception of fluconazole [237].

Due to the limited clinical data available with **dronedarone**, concomitant use with rivaroxaban should be avoided [238].

Interactions with Strong CYP3A4 Inductors

Co-administration of rivaroxaban with a strong CYP3A4 inducer **rifampicin** resulted in a reduction in the mean AUC of rivaroxaban of 50%, with a concomitant pharmacodynamic effects. Co-administration of rivaroxaban with other potent CYP3A4 inducers (e.g. **phenytoin, carbamazepine, phenobarbital** or **St. John's wort** (Hypericum perforatum)) may also lead to decreased plasma concentrations of rivaroxaban [238].

Pharmacodynamic Interactions of DOACs

NSAIDs/Platelet Aggregation Inhibitors: A study assessing the potential interactions between rivaroxaban and **clopidogrel** resulted in 3.77-fold increase in bleeding time, in approximately 1/3 of subjects. Caution should be exercised if patients concomitantly treated with **NSAIDs** (including acetylsalicylic acid) or platelet aggregation inhibitors, as these drugs typically increase the risk of bleeding [239, 240].

Warfarin: Although there are no literature reports on pharmacokinetic interaction between warfarin and rivaroxaban, co-administration with warfarin leads to an increased risk of heavy bleeding, as a result of their additive anticoagulant effect [239].

Due to similar pharmacokinetics, all interactions described for rivaroxaban apply equally to apixaban [241].

The pharmacokinetics of dabigatran differ somewhat from apixaban and rivaroxaban pharmacokinetics, which contributes to its lower potential for pharmacokinetic interactions. **Dabigatran** is a substrate for the efflux transporter P-gp, so inhibition of P-gp transporter associated with impaired renal function is a risk factor contributing to increased dabigatran exposure. Dose reduction of dabigatran should be considered when administered concomitantly with a P-gp inhibitor such as **dronedarone** or **ketoconazole,** and in patients with severe renal impairment (CrCl 15–30 mL/min) should be avoided. It is also observed increased dabigatran AUC by 138% when co-administrated with **ketoconazole**. Itraconazole, cyclosporine and glecaprevir/pibrentasvir are also considered contraindicated, while caution is necessary when co-administering tacrolimus [242].

Concomitant use of dabigatran with strong P-gp inducers (e.g. **rifampin**) reduces exposure to dabigatran and should generally be avoided.

Potentially significant drug interactions with drugs used in treatment of thrombotic conditions in liver patients are shown in Table 30.10.

Table 30.10 Potentially significant drug interactions with drugs used in treatment of thrombotic conditions causing liver disease

Drug class	Drug	Interaction
Interactions with UFH or LMWH		
Antihypertensive drugs	ACE inhibitors angiotensin receptor blockers(ARB)	↑ Risk of hyperkalaemia
	Potassium-sparing diuretics	
Oral anticoagulants	Warfarin	↑ Risk of bleeding
Platelet inhibitors	Dipyridamole, clopidogrel, ticagrelor	↑ Risk of bleeding
Interactions with warfarin		
Antibiotics	Rifampicin	↓ Warfarin activity
Antibiotics	Quinolones, macrolides	↑ Risk of bleeding
Analgesics	All NSAIDs, COX-2 inhibitors	↑ Risk of bleeding
Antiarrhythmics	Amiodarone	↑ Risk of bleeding
Anticoagulants Antiplatelet agents	Acetylsalicylic acid, clopidogrel, ticlopidine, dipyridamole, tirofiban, DOACs	↑ Risk of bleeding
Anticonvulsants	Carbamazepine	↓ Warfarin activity
Antidepressants	SSRI (duloxetine, fluoxetine, fluvoxamine, sertraline, venlafaxine)	↑ Risk of bleeding
Antifungals	Fluconazole, itraconazole, ketoconazole, miconazole	↑ Risk of bleeding
Gastrointestinal drugs	Cimetidine, PPIs (e.g. omeprazole)	↑ Risk of bleeding
Hypoglycaemics	Sulfonylureas	Hypoglycaemia
Cholestyramine		↓ Warfarin activity
Interactions with DOACs		
Analgesics	NSAIDs, acetylsalicylic acid	↑ Risk of bleeding
Antiarrhythmic	Dronedarone	↑ Risk of bleeding

(continued)

Table 30.10 (continued)

Drug class	Drug	Interaction
Anticoagulants Antiplatelet agents	Warfarin, enoxaparin Clopidogrel	↑ Risk of bleeding
Antibiotic	Rifampicin	↓ Conc of DOAC
Anticonvulsants	Carbamazepine, phenytoin, phenobarbital	↓ Conc of DOAC
Antiviral drugs	Ritonavir Glecaprevir/pibrentasvir	↑ Risk of bleeding
Azole antifungals	Ketoconazole, itraconazole (KI)	↑ Risk of bleeding
Immunosuppressants	Cyclosporine, tacrolimus	KI

Drug Used for Portal Hypertension and Its Complications

Treatment goal, in patients at an early-stage compensated cirrhosis, is the prevention of developing clinically significant portal hypertension and decompensation. Recommended pharmacotherapy of portal hypertension and ascites in liver cirrhosis is a combination of **diuretics** spironolactone and furosemide. **Non-selective beta-blocker (NSBB)** propranolol is suggested as first-line pharmacological treatment for primary prophylaxis of variceal haemorrhage in cirrhosis, while the standard of care in the treatment of acute varicose haemorrhage is **vasoactive agents**, such as terlipressin or octreotide [243–245].

Pharmacotherapy of hepatic encephalopathy is aimed at reducing the production and increasing elimination of ammonia, and includes use of lactulose, as a first-line treatment, or antibiotic rifaximin, as a second-line, as another therapeutic options may be considered intravenous (IV) L-ornithine L-aspartate (LOLA) [246].

Furosemide

The metabolism of furosemide occurs mainly in the kidneys, who are responsible for about 85% of total furosemide total clearance. About 50% of the furosemide dose is excreted unchanged in urine, while the rest is metabolized into glucuronide in the kidney [247]. Furosemide has the potential for pharmacokinetic drug-drug interactions due to competition for renal excretion, whereas underlying clinically significant pharmacodynamic interactions are additive hypokalaemic or hypotensive effect or additive nephrotoxicity.

Concomitant use of **glucocorticosteroids, carbenoxolone** or **laxatives** may lead to increased potassium loss and the development of **hypokalaemia**. Concomitant use of **corticosteroids** and furosemide may also cause **sodium retention** [248].

Nonsteroidal anti-inflammatory drugs (NSAIDs), such as indomethacin or acetylsalicylic acid, may **reduce** the effect of furosemide. Also, in patients with hypovolaemia or in dehydrated patients, concomitant use of NSAIDs with furosemide may cause acute renal failure [249, 250]. The **toxicity** of **salicylates**, administered at higher doses, may be **increased** when co-administered with furosemide.

Patients receiving high doses of salicylates concomitantly with furosemide, as in rheumatic diseases, may experience a toxic effect of salicylates at lower doses due to a competitive effect on renal excretion sites [251].

A **weaker** effect of furosemide may also occur with concomitant use of **phenytoin, phenobarbitone and cholestyramine.** There is evidence that treatment with phenytoin leads to **decrease** in intestinal furosemide **absorption** [252, 253].

Methotrexate undergoes significant renal tubular secretion and may reduce the effect of furosemide. Conversely, furosemide may **decrease** renal **elimination** of other drugs that undergo tubular secretion. Other **drugs which are mainly excreted by tubular secretion** (e.g. probenecid) may also **reduce** the effect of furosemide. High-dose treatment of both furosemide and these other drugs may result in their elevated serum levels and may potentiate their toxicity as well as the toxicity of furosemide [254, 255].

Cardiac Glycosides and Drugs that can Prolong the QT Interval: Electrolyte disturbances (e.g. hypokalaemia, hypomagnesaemia), caused by furosemide, may increase the toxicity of some other drugs (e.g. digoxin and drugs inducing QT interval prolongation syndrome). Caution is necessary when co-administering furosemide and cardiac glycosides (**digoxin**), due to his narrow therapeutic range. The risk of **arrhythmias** is increased during co-administration furosemide and drugs that may prolong the QT interval (e.g. **terfenadine**, **amiodarone**, disopyramide, flecainide and sotalol) [255–258].

Antihypertensive drugs: Concomitant administration of other diuretics, antihypertensive drugs or other drugs with hypotensive potential may require dose adjustment due his **additive hypotensive effect.** In addition, impaired renal function, including **renal failure,** has been observed in patients with concomitant use of diuretics and ACE inhibitors or diuretics and angiotensin II receptor antagonists [259, 260].

Antibiotics*:* Furosemide may potentiate the ototoxic effect of ***aminoglycosides*** (e.g. *kanamycin, gentamicin, tobramycin*) and other **ototoxic** drugs (*vancomycin, colistin*) and cause irreversible hearing impairment, especially in the presence of impaired renal function, and therefore, the combination of these drugs should be avoided. Concomitant use of furosemide and high doses of ***cephalosporins*** may cause **nephrotoxicity**, reversible **encephalopathy** and acute **renal failure** [261, 262]. Generally, the toxic effects of nephrotoxic drugs (e.g. aminoglycosides, polymyxins) may be increased by concomitant administration of furosemide. There also observed an increased risk of hyponatraemia in co-administration of furosemide with ***trimethoprim*** [263].

There is a risk of ***ototoxicity*** when **cisplatin** is co-administered with furosemide, and furosemide may also increase the ***nephrotoxicity*** of cisplatin, so in case of their concomitant use, furosemide must be given in low doses, only to patients with normal renal function and with normal fluid balance [249, 264].

Antipsychotics*:* In a placebo-controlled clinical trials with ***risperidone*****,** in elderly patients with dementia, a **higher incidence of mortality** was observed in patients treated concomitantly with furosemide and risperidone (7.3%) than in patients treated with risperidone alone (3.1%) or furosemide alone (4.1%).

The exact pathophysiological mechanism of this finding has not been elucidated [265, 266].

Risk of ventricular **arrhythmias** is increased with *amisulpride* or *sertindole*, and it is enhanced hypotensive effect with *phenothiazines*. Furosemide-induced hypokalaemia increases the risk of cardiac toxicity. It is recommended to avoid concurrent use with *pimozide* [249, 257].

Antidepressants*:* Hypotensive effect is enhanced with MAOIs, increased risk of postural hypotension with TCAs (*tricyclic antidepressants*) and increased risk of hypokalaemia with *reboxetine* [249].

Concomitant use of **cyclosporin** and furosemide has been associated with an increased risk of ***uric arthritis*** due to furosemide-induced hyperuricaemia and ciclosporin-induced renal uric acid excretion [267].

In patients at high risk for **contrast**-induced ***nephropathy***, furosemide may that risk further emphasize [268].

Redness with fever, sweating, agitation, nausea, increased blood pressure and tachycardia have been observed in some patients after intravenous administration of furosemide within 24 h of **chloralhydrate** administration. Therefore, concomitant use of chloral hydrate and furosemide is not recommended [249, 269].

Diuretics, including furosemide, may diminish the efficacy of **oral hypoglycaemic** agents of the sulfonylurea class and **insulin** and can cause hyperglycaemia, glucose intolerance, new-onset diabetes mellitus or exacerbation of preexisting diabetes. Dose modification of the hypoglycaemic agent may be required [270].

Furosemide may **potentiate** the effect of **theophylline;** therefore, patients on theophylline treatment should be monitored closely during the addition or discontinuation of furosemide therapy, considering the narrow therapeutic range of theophylline [271].

Spironolactone

Spironolactone is rapidly and **extensively metabolized,** and metabolites are excreted primarily in urine and secondary in bile, but also undergoes **enterohepatic recirculation.** It should be used with caution in patients with impaired hepatic function [272]. The pharmacodynamic drug-drug interactions of spironolactone, resulting from the additive hyperkalaemic effect, are of clinical importance, while clinically significant pharmacokinetic interactions relate mainly to the effect of spironolactone on renal elimination of drugs with a narrow therapeutic range.

ACE inhibitors: During concomitant treatment with spironolactone and ACE inhibitors, there is a risk of significant hypotension and shock, as well as impaired renal function, and in rare cases, to acute renal failure. Therefore, diuretic treatment is recommended to be discontinued 2–3 days before starting ACE inhibitor therapy. *C*o-administration of ACE inhibitors or angiotensin II receptor antagonists (e.g. valsartan, losartan) with potassium-sparing diuretics may also lead to severe ***hyperkalaemia*** [272]. Considering this risk, it is necessary to monitor potassium levels, especially in the initial phase of prescribing spironolactone and when other risk factors are present [273].

Nonsteroidal anti-inflammatory drugs (NSAIDs): Co-administration of NSAIDs, such as indomethacin, with potassium-sparing diuretics has been associated with severe ***hyperkalaemia*** [274]. In case of hyperkalaemia present, spironolactone should be discontinued immediately [272, 275].

Trimethoprim/sulfamethoxazole (co-trimoxazole) has been also observed to increase a risk of severe hyperkalaemia when co-administered with spironolactone [276].

Cyclosporine, **tacrolimus:** Concomitant use of potassium-sparing diuretics with cyclosporine may result in ***hyperkalaemia*** [272, 277].

Corticosteroids: Co-administration of spironolactone with fludrocortisone may result in a paradoxical dose-related increase in urinary potassium excretion and ***hypokalaemia***. If concomitant administration is necessary, closely monitor serum potassium levels [272, 278].

Alcohol, barbiturates, or narcotics: Potentiation of orthostatic ***hypotension*** may occur [272].

Antidiabetics: Cases of hyponatraemia have been reported due to an unusual effect of chlorpropamide on antidiuretic hormone activity [279].

Pressor amines (e.g. norepinephrine): Spironolactone ***reduces*** the ***vascular response*** to norepinephrine; therefore, **caution is needed** in treating patients who have undergone local or general anaesthesia while being treated with spironolactone [272, 280].

Lithium*:* It is generally recommended not to give lithium in combination with any diuretics, as they may ***reduce the renal clearance*** of lithium and increase the risk of ***lithium toxicity*** [272, 281].

Digoxin: Spironolactone inhibits tubular digoxin secretion and leads to an increase in serum digoxin concentration and increases frequency of electrolyte abnormalities and cardiac arrhythmias. This risk is associated with the use of digoxin in combination with any diuretic, although the lowest incidence appears to be with spironolactone. Doses will probably need to be reduced at concomitant administration of digoxin with spironolactone [256, 272].

Coumarins: The interaction of warfarin and spironolactone is the result of increased diuresis with consequent ***reduced anticoagulant effect.*** Monitoring of INR values with warfarin *dose adjustments* is recommended, when initiating or discontinuing spironolactone treatment [272, 282, 283].

Non-selective Beta-blockers (Propranolol)

Propranolol undergoes a rapid **first-pass metabolism** in the liver, with only about 25% of administrated dose reaches the systemic circulation. Considering the metabolism of propranolol, involving multiple pathways in the cytochrome P-450 system (CYP2D6, 1A2, 2C19), concomitant administration of drugs that, either by induction or inhibition, affect the activity of one or more of these enzymes may be the cause of a clinically relevant interaction drugs. By itself, propranolol has no effect on CYP450 enzyme activity and does not interfere with the other drug hepatic metabolism, but possible pharmacokinetic interactions appear to be those at the level of competition for the P-gp transport system [284, 285].

In case of co-administration with **potent CYP2D6, CYP1A2 and CYP2C19 inhibitors,** monitoring patients for ***bradycardia*** and ***hypotension*** is required.

Drugs such as **cholestyramine** and **colestipol** affect the absorption but also the enterohepatic circulation of propranolol, resulting in a **reduced** expected therapeutic effect. Cholestyramine co-administration was associated with a 43% decrease in propranolol AUC [148].

In the literature can be found contradictory case reports on interactions of propranolol with **clonidine,** resulting in enhanced decrease in portal pressure or in paradoxical hypertensive response [286, 287]. Beta-adrenoceptor blocking agents may exacerbate the rebound hypertension which can follow the withdrawal of **clonidine**. It is recommended withdrawal of the beta-blockers few days before discontinuing clonidine. If clonidine is replaced with beta-adrenoceptor therapy, the introduction of the beta-adrenoceptor blocking drug should be delayed for few days after clonidine administration has stopped. The same also applies to **moxonidine** [284, 288].

Hypotensive effect may be enhanced when propranolol is taken with **diuretics**, **methyldopa** or **levodopa** also [284].

It was found that concurrent propranolol with **alpha-blocker prazosin** increased the severity and duration of the postural hypotensive response and has been associated with prolongation of first-dose ***hypotension*** and ***syncope*** [284, 288].

Beta-blockers have a significant **impact** on **dobutamine** stress **testing** with either echocardiography or SPECT imaging. During dobutamine stress testing, beta-blocker therapy attenuates, and in some cases eliminates, evidence of myocardial ischemia [284, 289].

Antidepressants: Concomitant use of *MAO inhibitors* and propranolol is contraindicated, due to the possible occurrence of severe **hypotension**. Rare case of significant inhibition of ***imipramine*** metabolism and near-toxic imipramine levels while receiving both propranolol and imipramine has been reported. ***Fluvoxamine*** inhibits propranolol metabolism which can result in severe **tachycardia** [290, 291].

Neuroleptic drugs: Episodes of **hypotension** have been reported in a patient receiving concomitant **haloperidol** and propranolol therapy [292]. Co-administration of long-acting propranolol at doses greater than or equal to 160 mg/day resulted in ***increased*** **thioridazine** plasma concentrations ranging from 55% to 369% and increased thioridazine metabolite, mesoridazine, concentrations [293]. Co-administration of **chlorpromazine** increases both plasma levels of chlorpromazine (by 70%) and propranolol as well, leading to an **enhanced antipsychotic** effect of chlorpromazine and an **increased antihypertensive** effect of propranolol [294, 295].

Sympathomimetics: Propranolol has an antagonistic effect on beta adrenergic stimulation by sympathomimetics, which is particularly pronounced with ***isoproterenol***. Patients taking propranolol should be given ***adrenaline*** with extreme caution as **severe bradycardia, vasoconstriction** and **hypertension** may occur and may develop grade 1 or 2 **heart block** [296].

Antiarrhythmics: If propranolol is co-administered with antiarrhythmics, such as *amiodarone, disopyramide, flecainide, quinidine or verapamil,* cardiac effects may be stronger, while toxic side effects may be more frequent and severe. In addition, administration of propranolol during *lidocaine* infusion may increase plasma lidocaine concentrations by approximately 30%, so this combination should also be avoided. The metabolism of **propranolol is reduced** by co-administration of *quinidine*, leading to a twofold to threefold increased propranolol serum concentration and more intense beta-blockade [284, 297]. Concomitant use of propranolol with non-dihydropyridine calcium channel blockers, *verapamil* or *diltiazem*, may increase the adverse effects of those drugs on conduction disturbances, especially in patients with impaired ventricular function, and can result in severe **hypotension, bradycardia and heart failure** [298].

Propranolol may reduce glucose tolerance and may prolong the hypoglycaemic response to insulin but also increase the frequency and severity of **hypoglycaemia**. In addition, by inhibiting tachycardia caused by hypoglycaemia, it may mask the symptoms of drug-induced hypoglycaemia. Therefore, caution should be exercised in diabetics when co-administering propranolol and **hypoglycaemic drugs** [299].

Nonsteroidal anti-inflammatory drugs (NSAIDs), e.g. ibuprofen or indomethacin, may **reduce the hypotensive effect** of most antihypertensive drugs, including propranolol, most likely by interfering with prostaglandin synthesis. This impact may be significant in patients with poorly regulated hypertension [300].

Administration of **rizatriptan** during propranolol treatment increased the AUC of rizatriptan by approximately 67% which is presumed to be caused by inhibition of first-passage metabolism of rizatriptan. When prescribing rizatriptan to migraine patients receiving propranolol administration with 2 h apart, dose reduction of rizatriptan is recommended [301].

Co-administration of **theophylline** with propranolol **decreases theophylline** clearance, in a dose-dependent manner, by 30% to 52%. This finding may be clinically significant given the narrow therapeutic range of theophylline [302].

Octreotide

Following **subcutaneous** injection, about 32% of the administered dose is **excreted** unchanged in the urine. In patients with renal impairment, plasma octreotide elimination is prolonged, as well as in patients with liver cirrhosis [303].

Limited published data suggest that octreotide may decrease the metabolic clearance of cytochrome P450 substrate compounds; therefore, drugs that are mainly metabolized by CYP3A4 and have a low therapeutic index (e.g. *quinidine, terfenadine*) should be used with caution [304].

It has been observed that co-administration of octreotide with ***cyclosporine*** may decrease blood levels of cyclosporine and result in transplant rejection. In case of their co-administration, a 50% increase in ciclosporin doses is required [303, 304].

Octreotide characteristic to inhibit the secretion of several peptides, including **insulin,** should be considered in its concomitant use with sulfonylureas or insulin, due to antagonistic effect, and may require dose adjustment of these therapeutic agents [303, 305].

In a study investigating the effect of a long-acting octreotide on the effect of calcium channel blockers, **verapamil**, on gallbladder contraction, was confirmed that the effect of verapamil was completely abolished by the impact of octreotide. When co-administering octreotide with ca-channel blockers, probably dose adjustment will be required [306].

Terlipressin

The primary adverse events associated with terlipressin are decreased cardiac index and decreased heart rate. Although no clinically significant interactions have been reported, extreme caution is required when co-administering terlipressin with drugs that affect cardiac function [307].

Terlipressin may increase the hypotensive effect of **non-selective β-blockers** on the portal vein [308].

Concomitant treatment with drugs known to induce bradycardia (e.g. *propofol, sufentanil*) can cause **severe bradycardia** [308].

Use of terlipressin in patients with a history of QT interval prolongation, electrolytic abnormalities, concomitant **medications that can prolong the QT interval**, such as *class IA and III antiarrhythmics*, *erythromycin*, certain antihistamines and *tricyclic antidepressants* or medications that can cause hypokalaemia or hypomagnesaemia (e.g. some diuretics) can trigger ventricular **arrhythmias** including 'Torsade de pointes' [308].

Lactulose

Because it is not absorbed systemically, lactulose has minimal potential to interact with other drugs [309–311].

However, a study examining the effect of lactulose on the anticoagulant activity of **warfarin** confirmed significantly increased relative risk of overanticoagulation associated with lactulose treatment, probably related to the effect of lactulose on intestinal bacteria and consequently reduced intestinal synthesis of vitamin K. Considering the frequent use of lactulose, also as a laxative, especially in the elderly, awareness of this potential drug interaction is needed [312].

L-Ornithine L-Aspartate (LOLA)

The summary of product characteristics states that no interaction studies have been performed, and so far, no interactions are known, and also, literature reports of suspected LOLA interactions with other drugs are lacking [313].

Rifaximin

Due to its low rate of systemic absorption, rifaximin appears to have a minimal potential for drug-drug interactions, and also has been found to have minimal effects on the normal GI flora [314, 315]. Clinical drug interaction studies, in healthy subjects, demonstrated that rifaximin is a weak inducer of the CYP3A4 and did not significantly affect the pharmacokinetics of CYP3A4 substrates [314].

Co-administration of **cyclosporine**, an inhibitor of P-gp and OATP transport proteins, significantly increased systemic exposure to rifaximin, which can be further increased in patients with hepatic impairment; therefore, caution should be exercised when administering them concomitantly [314].

Intestinal membrane alterations in patients with small intestine bacterial overgrowth (SIBO) lead to increased rifaximin bioavailability enough to induce CYP3A4, causing clinically significant reductions in the bioavailability of CYP3A4 substrates, including **R-warfarin**. Dose adjustment of warfarin may be needed in these patients to maintain target INR range [316].

Potentially significant drug interactions with drug used for treatment of portal hypertension and its complications are shown in Table 30.11.

Table 30.11 Potentially significant drug interactions with drugs used for portal hypertension and its complications

Drug class	Drug	Interaction
Interactions with furosemide		
Antiarrhythmics	Amiodarone, disopyramide, flecainide, sotalol	↑ Risk of arrhythmias
Antibiotics	Cephalosporins	Nephrotoxicity
	Aminoglycosides Vancomycin, colistin	Ototoxicity
	Trimethoprim	Hyponatraemia
Anticonvulsants	Phenytoin, phenobarbitone	↓ Effect of furosemide
Antidepressants	MAO inhibitors Tricyclic antidepressants	↑ Hypotensive effect Hypokalaemia
Antifungal agent	Terfenadine	↑ Risk of arrhythmias
Antihypertensive drugs	ACE inhibitors Angiotensin II receptor antagonists	Additive hypotensive effect ↑ Risk of renal failure
Antipsychotics	Risperidone	Higher incidence of mortality
	Lithium	Cardiotoxicity/neurotoxicity
	Amisulpride Phenothiazines	↑ Risk of arrhythmias ↑ Hypotensive effect
Chloralhydrate		Fever, sweating, agitation, nausea, increased blood pressure, tachycardia
Bronchodilator	Theophylline	↑ Conc. of theophylline
Cardiac glycosides	Digoxin	↑ Digoxin toxicity

(continued)

Table 30.11 (continued)

Drug class	Drug	Interaction
Cytostatics	Cisplatin	Nephrotoxicity
	Methotrexate	↑ Methotrexate toxicity
Hypoglycaemic agents	Sulfonylureas, insulin	Hyperglycaemia
Immunosuppressants	Ciclosporin	↑ Risk of uric arthritis
	Carbenoxolone	Hypokalaemia
	Glucocorticosteroids	Hypokalaemia, sodium retention
NSAIDs	Indomethacin Acetylsalicylic acid	↓ Effect of furosemide ↑ Toxicity of salicylates
Interactions with spironolactone		
Antibiotics	Co-trimoxazole	Hyperkalaemia
Anticoagulants	Warfarin	↓ Anticoagulant effect
Antihypertensive agents	ACE inhibitors	Hyperkalaemia, hypotension ↑ Risk of acute renal failure
Cardiac glycosides	Digoxin	↑ Digitalis toxicity
Immunosuppressants	Corticosteroids (fludrocortisone)	Hypokalaemia
	Cyclosporin, tacrolimus	Hyperkalaemia
Neuroleptics	Lithium	↑ Lithium toxicity
NSAIDs	Indomethacin	Reduced the diuretic effect Hyperkalaemia
Pressor amines	Norepinephrine	Reduced vascular response
Interactions with propranolol		
Alpha-blocker	Prazosin	Hypotension and syncope
Antiarrhythmics	Amiodarone, disopyramide, flecainide, lidocaine, quinidine verapamil	Hypotension, bradycardia, heart failure
Antidepressants	MAOs, TCAs	Hypotension
	SSRIs (fluvoxamine)	Tachycardia
Antihypertensives	All	↑ Hypotensive effect
Bronchodilators	Theophylline	↑ Conc. of theophylline
Hypoglycaemic drugs	Sulfonylureas	↑ Risk of hypoglycaemia
Neuroleptic drugs	Chlorpromazine, haloperidol Thioridazine	↑ Antipsychotic effect Hypotension
NSAIDs	All	↓ Hypotensive effect
Sympathomimetics	Norepinephrine isoproterenol	Severe bradycardia, vasoconstriction, hypertension
Interactions with octreotide		
Antihypertensives	Calcium channel blockers	↓ Effect of calcium channel blockers
Immunosuppressants	Cyclosporine	↓ Conc. of cyclosporine
Oral hypoglycaemic	Sulfonylureas	Antagonistic effect
Interactions with terlipressin		
Drugs inducing bradycardia	Propofol, sufentanil	Bradycardia

(continued)

Table 30.11 (continued)

Drug class	Drug	Interaction
Drugs that prolong the QT interval	Class IA and III antiarrhythmics antihistamines erythromycin tricyclic antidepressants	↑ Risk of arrhythmias including 'Torsade de pointes'
Drugs that cause hypokalaemia or hypomagnesaemia	Diuretics	↑ Risk of arrhythmias
Non-selective β-blockers	Propranolol, carvedilol	↑ Hypotensive effect

References

1. Moon AM, Singal AG, Tapper EB. Contemporary epidemiology of chronic liver disease and cirrhosis. Clin Gastroenterol Hepatol. 2020;18(12):2650–66.
2. Pimpin L, Cortez-Pinto H, Negro F, Corbould E, Lazarus JV, Webber L, Sheron N. EASL HEPAHEALTH Steering Committee. Burden of liver disease in Europe: epidemiology and analysis of risk factors to identify prevention policies. J Hepatol. 2018;69(3):718–35.
3. Egan LJ. Drug interactions in gastroenterology: mechanisms, consequences, and how to avoid. Clin Gastroenterol Hepatol. 2004;2:725–30.
4. Doligalski CT, Logan AT, Silverman A. Drug interactions: a primer for the gastroenterologist. Gastroenterol Hepatol. 2012;8(6):376–83.
5. Palatini P, De Martin S. Pharmacokinetic drug interactions in liver disease: an update. World J Gastroenterol. 2016;22(3):1260–78.
6. World Health Organization. Global hepatitis report, 2017. Available at: https://www.who.int/publications/i/item/global-hepatitis-report-2017 (accessed on August 4, 2020).
7. World Health Organization. Guidelines for the prevention, care and treatment of persons with chronic hepatitis B infection. Geneva, Switzerland: World Health Organization; 2015.
8. Terrault NA, Bzowej NH, Chang KM, Hwang JP, Jonas MM, Murad MH, American Association for the Study of Liver Diseases. AASLD guidelines for treatment of chronic hepatitis B. Hepatology. 2016;63:261–83.
9. European Association for the Study of the Liver. EASL 2017 Clinical Practice Guidelines on the management of hepatitis B virus infection. J Hepatol. 2017;67:370–98.
10. Sarin SK, Kumar M, Lau GK, Abbas Z, Chan HL, Chen CJ, et al. Asian-Pacific clinical practice guidelines on the management of hepatitis B: a 2015 update. Hepatol Int. 2016;10:1–98.
11. PubChem [Internet]. Bethesda (MD): National Library of Medicine (US), National Center for Biotechnology Information; 2004.[cited 2020 Aug. 29]. Available from: https://pubchem.ncbi.nlm.nih.gov.
12. Baraclude (entecavir). Princeton (NJ): Bristol-Myers Squibb Company; 2005.
13. Yan JH, Bifano M, Xie J, Freund J, Rahim S, Zhang D, et al. Effects of renal impairment on single-dose pharmacokinetics of entecavir. Poster presented et: 40th Annual Meeting of the European Association For the Study of the Liver; 2005 April 13–17; Paris, France.
14. Bifano M, Yan JH, Xie J, Rahim S, Elefant E, Zhang D, et al. Lack of a pharmacokinetic interaction when entecavir is co-administered with lamivudine, adefovir, or tenofovir. J Hepatol. 2005;42(Suppl. 2):171.
15. Bifano M, Yan JH, Xie J, Zhang D, Freund J, Rahim S, et al. Hepatic impairment does not alter single-dose pharmacokinetics and safety of entecavir. Hepatology. 2004;40(Suppl. 1):663A.
16. Wishart Research Group. DrugBank online [internet]: Canada: 2018 [update 2020: cited 2020 Nov 25]. Availabe ftom: http://go.drugbank.com/drug/DB14126.

17. Ustiniowski A, Arends JE. Tenofovir: what we have learnt after 7.5 million person-years of use? Infect Dis Ther. 2015;4:145–57.
18. Baranek B, Wang S, Cheung AM, Mishra S, Tan DH. The effect of tenofovir disoproxil fumarate on bone mineral density: a systematic review and meta-analysis. Antivir Ther. 2020;25:21–32.
19. Viread (tenofovir disoproxil fumarate). Foster City (CA): Gilead Sciences Ltd.; 2020.
20. Vemlidy (tenofovir alafenamide). Foster City (CA): Gilead Sciences Ltd.; 2015.
21. Pegasys (peginterferon alpha 2a). San Francisco (CA): Hoffman-La Roche Inc. 2002.
22. Pegintron (peginterferon alpha 2b). Whitehouse Station (NJ): Merc Sharp & Dohme Corp. 2001.
23. World Health Organization. Hepatitis C fact sheet. Available at: https://www.who.int/news-room/fact-sheets/detail/hepatitis-c (27 July 2020, accessed 6 July 2020).
24. European Association for the Study of the Liver. EASL recommendations on treatment of hepatitis C 2018. J Hepatol. 2018;69:461–511.
25. European Association for the Study of the Liver. EASL recommendations on treatment of hepatitis C: final update of the series. J Hepatol. 2020;73:1170–218.
26. AASLD-IDSA HCV Guidance Panel. Hepatitis C Guidance 2018 update: AASLD-IDSA recommendations for testing, managing, and treating hepatitis C virus infection. Clin Infect Dis. 2018;67:1477–92.
27. American Association for the Study of Liver Diseases and Infectious Diseases Society of America. HCV guidance: recommendations for testing, managing, and treating hepatitis C. Available at: https://www.hcvguidelines.org/ (accessed on August 4, 2020).
28. Salam KA, Akimitzu A. Hepatitis C virus NS3 inhibitors: current and future perspectives. BioMed Rese Int 2013: Article ID 467869, 9 pages.
29. Sovaldi (sofosbuvir). Foster City (CA): Gilead Sciences, Inc.; 2013.
30. Kirby BJ, Symonds WT, Kearney BP, Mathias AA. Pharmacokinetic, pharmacodynamic, and drug-interaction profile of the hepatitis C virus NS5B polymerase inhibitor sofosbuvir. Clin Pharmacokinet. 2015;54:677–90.
31. Liverpool Drug Interactions Group. Hep Drug Interactions [internet]. Liverpool (UK): 2010 [updated 2020; cited 2020 Jun 23]. Available from: https://www.hep-druginteractions.org/view_all_interactions/new.
32. Harvoni (ledipasvir and sofobuvir). Foster City (CA): Gilead Science Ltd.; 2014.
33. Epclusa (sofosbuvir and velpatasvir); Foster City (CA): Gilead Sciences, Inc.; 2017.
34. Chahine EB, Sucher AJ, Hemstreet BA. Sofosbuvir/velpatasvir: the first pangenotypic direct-acting antiviral combination for hepatitis C. Ann Pharmacother. 2017;51:44–53.
35. Smolders EJ, Jansen AME, Ter Horst PGJ, Rockstroh J, Back DJ, Burger DM. Viral Hepatitis C Therapy: pharmacokinetic and pharmacodynamic considerations: a 2019 update. Clin Pharmacokinet 2019; 58: 1237–1263.
36. Vosevi (sofosbuvir, velpatasvir, and voxilaprevir). Foster City (CA): Gilead Science Ltd.; 2017.
37. Lin CW, Dutta S, Zhao W, Asatryan A, Campbell A, Liu W. Pharmacokinetic interactions and safety of co-administration of glecaprevir and pibrentasvir in healthy volunteers. Eur J Drug Metab Pharmacokinet. 2018;43:81–90.
38. Mavyret (glecaprevir and pibrentasvir) tablets. North Chicago: AbbVie Inc.; 2019.
39. Kiang TKL. Clinical pharmacokinetics and drug-drug interactions of elbasvir/grazoprevir. Eur J Drug Metab Pharmacokinet. 2018;43:509–31.
40. Zepatier (elbasvir and grazoprevir). U.S.: Merck Sharp & Dohme Corp; 2016.
41. Copegus (ribavirin). San Francisco (CA): Hoffmann-La Roche, Inc. c/o Genentech, Inc; 2002.
42. European Association for the Study of the Liver. EASL clinical practice guidelines: management of alcohol-related liver disease. J Hepatol. 2018;69(1):154–81.
43. Lieber CS. Alcoholic fatty liver: its pathogenesis and mechanism of progression to inflammation and fibrosis. Alcohol. 2004;34(1):9–19.
44. Prednisolone (prednisolone). Devon (UK): Accord-UK Ltd; 2018.

45. Perez A, Jansen-Chaparro S, Saigi I, Bernal-Lopez MR, Miñambres I, Gomez-Huelgas R. Glucocorticoid-induced hyperglycemia. J Diabetes. 2014;6(1):9–20.
46. Olivesi A. Modified elimination of prednisolone in epileptic patients on carbamazepine monotherapy, and in women using low-dose oral contraceptives. Biomed Pharmacother. 1986;40(8):301–8.
47. Frey BM, Frey FJ. Phenytoin modulates the pharmacokinetics of prednisolone and the pharmacodynamics of prednisolone as assessed by the inhibition of the mixed lymphocyte reaction in humans. Eur J Clin Investig. 1984;14(1):1–6.
48. Piper JM, Ray WA, Daugherty JR, Griffin MR. Corticosteroid use and peptic ulcer disease: role of nonsteroidal anti-inflammatory drugs. Ann Intern Med. 1991;114(9):735–40.
49. Masclee GM, Valkhoff VE, Coloma PM, de Ridder M, Romio S, Schuemie MJ, et al. Risk of upper gastrointestinal bleeding from different drug combinations. Gastroenterology. 2014;147(4):784–92.
50. Narum S, Westergren T, Klemp M. Corticosteroids and risk of gastrointestinal bleeding: a systematic review and meta-analysis. BMJ Open. 2014;4(5):e004587.
51. Klinenberg JR, Miller F. Effect of corticosteroids on blood salicylate concentration. JAMA. 1965;194(6):601–4.
52. Orapred OTD (prednisolone sodium phosphate). Eden Prairie (USA): CIMA® LABS INC.; 2010.
53. McAllister WA, Thompson PJ, Al-Habet SM, Rogers HJ. Rifampicin reduces effectiveness and bioavailability of prednisolone. Br Med J (Clin Res Ed). 1983;286(6369):923–5. https://doi.org/10.1136/bmj.286.6369.923.
54. Niemi M, Backman JT, Fromm MF, Neuvonen PJ, Kivistö KT. Pharmacokinetic interactions with rifampicin : clinical relevance. Clin Pharmacokinet. 2003;42(9):819–50.
55. Van Matre ET, Satyanarayana G, Page RL, Levi ME, Lindenfeld J, Mueller SW. Pharmacokinetic drug-drug interactions between immunosuppressant and anti-infective agents: antimetabolites and corticosteroids. Ann Transplant. 2018;23:66–74.
56. Ramana Reddy AM, Prashanth LK, Sharat Kumar GG, Chandana G, Jadav R. Over-the-counter self-medication leading to intracranial hypertension in a young lady. J Neurosci Rural Pract. 2014;5(4):384–6.
57. Penzak SR, Formentini E, Alfaro RM, Long M, Natarajan V, Kovacs J. Prednisolone pharmacokinetics in the presence and absence of ritonavir after oral prednisone administration to healthy volunteers. J Acquir Immune Defic Syndr. 2005;40(5):573–80.
58. Zürcher RM, Frey BM, Frey FJ. Impact of ketoconazole on the metabolism of prednisolone. Clin Pharmacol Ther. 1989;45(4):366–72.
59. Gubbins PO, Heldenbrand S. Clinically relevant drug interactions of current antifungal agents. Mycoses. 2010;53(2):95–113.
60. Hazlewood KA, Fugate SE, Harrison DL. Effect of oral corticosteroids on chronic warfarin therapy. Ann Pharmacother. 2006;40(12):2101–6.
61. Bergmann TK, Barraclough KA, Lee KJ, Staatz CE. Clinical pharmacokinetics and pharmacodynamics of prednisolone and prednisone in solid organ transplantation. Clin Pharmacokinet. 2012;51(11):711–41.
62. Lafforgue P, Monjanel-Mouterde S, Durand A, Catalin J, Acquaviva PC. Is there an interaction between low doses of corticosteroids and methotrexate in patients with rheumatoid arthritis? A pharmacokinetic study in 33 patients. J Rheumatol. 1993;20(2):263–7.
63. Wong CS, Pavord ID, Williams J, Britton JR, Tattersfield AE. Bronchodilator, cardiovascular, and hypokalaemic effects of fenoterol, salbutamol, and terbutaline in asthma. Lancet. 1990;336(8728):1396–9.
64. Widmer P, Maibach R, Künzi UP, Capaul R, Mueller U, Galeazzi R, Hoigné R. Diuretic-related hypokalaemia: the role of diuretics, potassium supplements, glucocorticoids and beta 2-adrenoceptor agonists. Results from the comprehensive hospital drug monitoring programme, berne (CHDM). Eur J Clin Pharmacol. 1995;49(1–2):31–6.
65. Rossi GP, Seccia TM, Maniero C, Pessina AC. Drug-related hypertension and resistance to antihypertensive treatment: a call for action. J Hypertens. 2011;29(12):2295–309.

66. Lovell AR, Ernst ME. Drug-induced hypertension: focus on mechanisms and management. Curr Hypertens Rep. 2017;19(5):39.
67. Aquilonius SM, Hartvig P. Clinical pharmacokinetics of cholinesterase inhibitors. Clin Pharmacokinet. 1986;11(3):236–49.
68. Kindler CH, Verotta D, Gray AT, Gropper MA, Yost CS. Additive inhibition of nicotinic acetylcholine receptors by corticosteroids and the neuromuscular blocking drug vecuronium. Anesthesiology. 2000;92(3):821–32.
69. Rohatagi S, Barth J, Möllmann H, Hochhaus G, Soldner A, Möllmann C, Derendorf H. Pharmacokinetics of methylprednisolone and prednisolone after single and multiple oral administration. J Clin Pharmacol. 1997;37(10):916–25.
70. Zoorob RJ, Cender D. A different look at corticosteroids. Am Fam Physician. 1998;58(2):443–50.
71. Solu-medrol (methylprednisolone sodium succinate). New York (USA): Pharmacia and Upjohn Company LLC; 2019.
72. Trental (pentoxifylline). Bridgewater (USA): Sanofi-Aventis U.S. LLC; 2010.
73. Han SJ, Kim HJ, Kim DJ, Sheen SS, Chung CH, Ahn CW, et al. Effects of pentoxifylline on proteinuria and glucose control in patients with type 2 diabetes: a prospective randomized double-blind multicenter study. Diabetol Metab Syndr. 2015;7:64.
74. Seiffge D, Weithmann KU. Update on the pharmacology of pentoxifylline and its combination with low-dose acetylsalicylic acid (HWA 5112). Semin Thromb Hemost. 1989;15(2):150–8.
75. Vedes EC, Marques LD, Toscano Rico MC. Severe isolated thrombocytopenia after clopidogrel and pentoxifylline therapy: a case report. J Med Case Rep. 2011;5:281.
76. PubChem [Internet]. Bethesda (MD): National Library of Medicine (US), National Center for Biotechnology Information; 2004. PubChem Compound Summary for CID 2153, Theophylline; [cited 2020 Jun.25]. Available from: https://pubchem.ncbi.nlm.nih.gov/compound/Theophylline.
77. Ellison MJ, Horner RD, Willis SE, Cummings DM. Influence of pentoxifylline on steady-state theophylline serum concentrations from sustained-release formulations. Pharmacotherapy. 1990;10(6):383–6.
78. Peterson TC, Peterson MR, Wornell PA, Blanchard MG, Gonzalez FJ. Role of CYP1A2 and CYP2E1 in the pentoxifylline ciprofloxacin drug interaction. Biochem Pharmacol. 2004;68(2):395–402.
79. European Association for the Study of the Liver (EASL), European Association for the Study of Diabetes (EASD), European Association for the Study of Obesity (EASO). EASL-EASD-EASO Clinical Practice Guidelines for the management of non-alcoholic fatty liver disease. J Hepatol. 2016;64(6):1388–402.
80. Chalasani N, Younossi Z, Lavine JE, Charlton M, Cusi K, Rinella M, et al. The diagnosis and management of nonalcoholic fatty liver disease: practice guidance from the American Association for the Study of Liver Diseases. Hepatology. 2018;67(1):328–57.
81. PubChem [Internet]. Bethesda (MD): National Library of Medicine (US), National Center for Biotechnology Information; 2004-. PubChem Compound Summary for CID 4829, Pioglitazone; [cited 2020 Jun. 25]. Available from: https://pubchem.ncbi.nlm.nih.gov/compound/Pioglitazone.
82. Actos (pioglitazone hydrochloride). Deerfield (USA): Takeda Pharmaceuticals America Inc.; 2011.
83. Deng LJ, Wang F, Li HD. Effect of gemfibrozil on the pharmacokinetics of pioglitazone. Eur J Clin Pharmacol. 2005;61(11):831–6.
84. Takagi M, Sakamoto M, Itoh T, Fujiwara R. Underlying mechanism of drug-drug interaction between pioglitazone and gemfibrozil: Gemfibrozil acyl-glucuronide is a mechanism-based inhibitor of CYP2C8. Drug Metab Pharmacokinet. 2015;30(4):288–94.
85. Aquilante CL, Kosmiski LA, Bourne DW, Bushman LR, Daily EB, Hammond KP, et al. Impact of the CYP2C8 *3 polymorphism on the drug-drug interaction between gemfibrozil and pioglitazone. Br J Clin Pharmacol. 2013;75(1):217–26.

86. Jaakkola T, Backman JT, Neuvonen M, Laitila J, Neuvonen PJ. Effect of rifampicin on the pharmacokinetics of pioglitazone. Br J Clin Pharmacol. 2006;61(1):70–8.
87. Pentikäinen PJ, Neuvonen PJ, Penttilä A. Pharmacokinetics of metformin after intravenous and oral administration to man. Eur J Clin Pharmacol. 1979;16(3):195–202.
88. PubChem [Internet]. Bethesda (MD): National Library of Medicine (US), National Center for Biotechnology Information; 2004-. PubChem Compound Summary for CID 4091, Metformin; [cited 2020 Jun. 30]. Available from: https://pubchem.ncbi.nlm.nih.gov/compound/Metformin.
89. Metformin (metformin). Middlesex (UK): Aurobindo Pharma - Milpharm Ltd.; 2019.
90. Chan NN, Fauvel NJ, Feher MD. Non-steroidal anti-inflammatory drugs and metformin: a cause for concern? Lancet. 1998;352(9123):201.
91. Franzetti I, Donnini P, Gaiazzi M, Mazzola E, Zibetti E, Uccella R. Acidosi lattica ed iperpotassiemia grave in un paziente diabetico in terapia con metformina ed enalapril: influenza di patologia renale acuta e farmaci [Lactic acidosis and severe hyperkalemia in a diabetic patient treated with metformin and enalapril: influence of acute renal disease and drugs]. Minerva Med. 1995;86(1–2):49–54. Italianist
92. Zaidi FH, Kinnear PE. Acetazolamide, alternate carbonic anhydrase inhibitors and hypoglycaemic agents: comparing enzymatic with diuresis induced metabolic acidosis following intraocular surgery in diabetes. Br J Ophthalmol. 2004;88(5):714–5.
93. Armstrong MJ, Gaunt P, Aithal GP, Barton D, Hull D, Parker R, et al. Liraglutide safety and efficacy in patients with non-alcoholic steatohepatitis (LEAN): a multicentre, double-blind, randomised, placebo-controlled phase 2 study. Lancet. 2016;387(10019):679–90.
94. Victoza(liraglutide). Bagsvaerd, Denmark: Novo Nordisk A/S; 2017.
95. Schachter M. Chemical, pharmacokinetic and pharmacodynamic properties of statins: an update. Fundam Clin Pharmacol. 2005;19(1):117–25.
96. Bellosta S, Paoletti R, Corsini A. Safety of statins: focus on clinical pharmacokinetics and drug interactions. Circulation. 2004;109(23 Suppl. 1):III50–7.
97. Hu M, Cheung BM, Tomlinson B. Safety of statins: an update. Ther Adv Drug Saf. 2012;3(3):133–44.
98. Lipitor (atorvastatin calcium). Dublin, Ireland: Pfizer Ireland Pharmaceuticals; 2009.
99. Hougaard Christensen MM, Bruun Haastrup M, Øhlenschlaeger T, Esbech P, Arnspang Pedersen S, Bach Dunvald AC, et al. Interaction potential between clarithromycin and individual statins—a systematic review. Basic Clin Pharmacol Toxicol. 2020;126(4):307–17.
100. Siedlik PH, Olson SC, Yang BB, Stern RH. Erythromycin co-administration increases plasma atorvastatin concentrations. J Clin Pharmacol. 1999;39(5):501–4.
101. Amsden GW, Kuye O, Wei GC. A study of the interaction potential of azithromycin and clarithromycin with atorvastatin in healthy volunteers. J Clin Pharmacol. 2002;42(4):444–9.
102. Pham PA, la Porte CJ, Lee LS, van Heeswijk R, Sabo JP, Elgadi MM, et al. Differential effects of tipranavir plus ritonavir on atorvastatin or rosuvastatin pharmacokinetics in healthy volunteers. Antimicrob Agents Chemother. 2009;53(10):4385–92.
103. Chauvin B, Drouot S, Barrail-Tran A, Taburet AM. Drug-drug interactions between HMG-CoA reductase inhibitors (statins) and antiviral protease inhibitors. Clin Pharmacokinet. 2013;52(10):815–31.
104. Food and Drug Administration [Internet]. Interactions between certain HIV or hepatitis C drugs and cholesterol-lowering statin drugs can increase the risk of muscle injury [cited 2020 Jul. 12]. Available from: https://www.fda.gov/drugs/drug-safety-and-availability/fda-drug-safety-communication-interactions-between-certain-hiv-or-hepatitis-c-drugs-and-cholesterol
105. Kantola T, Kivistö KT, Neuvonen PJ. Effect of itraconazole on the pharmacokinetics of atorvastatin. Clin Pharmacol Ther. 1998;64(1):58–65.
106. Mazzu AL, Lasseter KC, Shamblen EC, Agarwal V, Lettieri J, Sundaresen P. Itraconazole alters the pharmacokinetics of atorvastatin to a greater extent than either cerivastatin or pravastatin. Clin Pharmacol Ther. 2000;68(4):391–400.

107. Jacobson TA. Comparative pharmacokinetic interaction profiles of pravastatin, simvastatin, and atorvastatin when coadministered with cytochrome P450 inhibitors. Am J Cardiol. 2004;94(9):1140–6.
108. Asberg A, Hartmann A, Fjeldså E, Bergan S, Holdaas H. Bilateral pharmacokinetic interaction between cyclosporine A and atorvastatin in renal transplant recipients. Am J Transplant. 2001;1(4):382–6.
109. Asberg A. Interactions between cyclosporin and lipid-lowering drugs: implications for organ transplant recipients. Drugs. 2003;63(4):367–78.
110. Backman JT, Luurila H, Neuvonen M, Neuvonen PJ. Rifampin markedly decreases and gemfibrozil increases the plasma concentrations of atorvastatin and its metabolites. Clin Pharmacol Ther. 2005;78(2):154–67.
111. Boyd RA, Stern RH, Stewart BH, Wu X, Reyner EL, Zegarac EA, Randinitis EJ, Whitfield L. Atorvastatin co-administration may increase digoxin concentrations by inhibition of intestinal P-glycoprotein-mediated secretion. J Clin Pharmacol. 2000;40(1):91–8.
112. Shaik AN, Bohnert T, Williams DA, Gan LL, LeDuc BW. Mechanism of drug-drug interactions between warfarin and statins. J Pharm Sci. 2016;105(6):1976–86.
113. Stern R, Abel R, Gibson GL, Besserer J. Atorvastatin does not alter the anticoagulant activity of warfarin. J Clin Pharmacol. 1997;37(11):1062–4.
114. Andrus MR. Oral anticoagulant drug interactions with statins: case report of fluvastatin and review of the literature. Pharmacotherapy. 2004;24(2):285–90.
115. Kostapanos MS, Milionis HJ, Elisaf MS. Rosuvastatin-associated adverse effects and drug-drug interactions in the clinical setting of dyslipidemia. Am J Cardiovasc Drugs. 2010;10(1):11–28.
116. Busti AJ, Bain AM, Hall RG 2nd, Bedimo RG, Leff RD, Meek C, et al. Effects of atazanavir/ritonavir or fosamprenavir/ritonavir on the pharmacokinetics of rosuvastatin. J Cardiovasc Pharmacol. 2008;51(6):605–10.
117. Kiser JJ, Gerber JG, Predhomme JA, Wolfe P, Flynn DM, Hoody DW. Drug/drug interaction between lopinavir/ritonavir and rosuvastatin in healthy volunteers. J Acquir Immune Defic Syndr. 2008;47(5):570–8.
118. Schneck DW, Birmingham BK, Zalikowski JA, Mitchell PD, Wang Y, Martin PD, Lasseter KC, Brown CD, Windass AS, Raza A. The effect of gemfibrozil on the pharmacokinetics of rosuvastatin. Clin Pharmacol Ther. 2004;75(5):455–63.
119. Simonson SG, Martin PD, Mitchell PD, Lasseter K, Gibson G, Schneck DW. Effect of rosuvastatin on warfarin pharmacodynamics and pharmacokinetics. J Clin Pharmacol. 2005;45(8):927–34.
120. Jindal D, Tandon M, Sharma S, Pillai KK. Pharmacodynamic evaluation of warfarin and rosuvastatin co-administration in healthy subjects. Eur J Clin Pharmacol. 2005;61(9):621–5.
121. Martin PD, Schneck DW, Dane AL, Warwick MJ. The effect of a combination antacid preparation containing aluminium hydroxide and magnesium hydroxide on rosuvastatin pharmacokinetics. Curr Med Res Opin. 2008;24(4):1231–5.
122. Lindor KD, Bowlus CL, Boyer J, Levy C, Mayo M. Primary biliary cholangitis: 2018 practice guidance from the american association for the study of liver diseases. Hepatology. 2019;69(1):394–419.
123. Hirschfield GM, Dyson JK, Alexander GJM, et al. The British Society of Gastroenterology/UK-PBC primary biliary cholangitis treatment and management guidelines. Gut. 2018;67:1568–94. https://doi.org/10.1136/gutjnl-2017-315259.
124. Lee S, Yoon S, Chung H, Ji SC, Yoon SH, Yu KS, et al. Pharmacokinetics of ursodeoxycholic acid in elderly volunteers compared with younger adults in a Korean population. J Clin Pharmacol. 2019;59(8):1085–92.
125. Becquemont L, Glaeser H, Drescher S, Hitzl M, Simon N, Murdter TE, et al. Effects of ursodeoxycholic acid on P-glycoprotein and cytochrome P450 3A4-dependent pharmacokinetics in humans. Clin Pharmacol Ther. 2006;79(5):449–60.
126. Hempfling W, Dilger K, Beuers U. Systematic review: ursodeoxycholic acid—adverse effects and drug interactions. Aliment Pharmacol Ther. 2003;18(10):963–72.

127. al-Quaiz MN, O'Grady JG, Tredger JM, Williams R. Variable effect of ursodeoxycholic acid on cyclosporin absorption after orthotopic liver transplantation. Transpl Int. 1994;7(3):190–4.
128. de Vries E, Beuers U. Ursodeoxycholic acid in pregnancy? J Hepatol. 2019;71(6):1237–45.
129. Ursodeoxycholic acid (ursodeoxycholic acid). London (UK): Advanz pharma, 2016.
130. PubChem [Internet]. Bethesda (MD): National Library of Medicine (US), National Center for Biotechnology Information; 2004-. PubChem Compound Summary for CID 447715,Obeticholic acid; [cited 2020 Jul. 25]. Available from: https://pubchem.ncbi.nlm.nih.gov/compound/Obeticholic-acid.
131. Ishida C, Sanoh S, Kotake Y. CYP1A2 downregulation by obeticholic acid: usefulness as a positive control for the in vitro evaluation of drug-drug interactions. J Pharm Sci. 2019;108(12):3903–10.
132. Beuers U, Trauner M, Jansen P, Poupon R. New paradigms in the treatment of hepatic cholestasis: from UDCA to FXR, PXR and beyond. J Hepatol. 2015;62(Suppl. 1):S25–37.
133. Ocaliva (obeticholic acid). Dublin (Ireland): Intercept Pharma International Ltd.; 2019.
134. Edwards JE, Eliot L, Parkinson A, Karan S, MacConell L. Assessment of pharmacokinetic interactions between obeticholic acid and caffeine, midazolam, warfarin, dextromethorphan, omeprazole, rosuvastatin, and digoxin in phase 1 studies in healthy subjects. Adv Ther. 2017;34(9):2120–38.
135. Zanaflex (tizanidine hydrochloride). Athlone (Ireland); Elan Pharmaceuticals Inc.; 2006.
136. Zhou SF, Yang LP, Zhou ZW, Liu YH, Chan E. Insights into the substrate specificity, inhibitors, regulation, and polymorphisms and the clinical impact of human cytochrome P450 1A2. AAPS J. 2009;11(3):481–94.
137. Questran (colestyramine). Greifswald (Germany): Cheplapharm Arzneimittel GmbH; 2019.
138. Muzeeb S, Venkatesh P, Mullangi R, Srinivas NR. Influence of cholestyramine on the pharmacokinetics of rosiglitazone and its metabolite, desmethylrosiglitazone, after oral and intravenous dosing of rosiglitazone: impact on oral bioavailability, absorption, and metabolic disposition in rats. Xenobiotica. 2006;36(9):838–56.
139. Bullingham RE, Nicholls AJ, Kamm BR. Clinical pharmacokinetics of mycophenolate mofetil. Clin Pharmacokinet. 1998;34(6):429–55.
140. Mignat C. Clinically significant drug interactions with new immunosuppressive agents. Drug Saf. 1997;16(4):267–78.
141. Serlin MJ, Breckenridge AM. Drug interactions with warfarin. Drugs. 1983;25(6):610–20.
142. Henderson RP, Solomon CP. Use of cholestyramine in the treatment of digoxin intoxication. Arch Intern Med. 1988 Mar;148(3):745–6.
143. Neuvonen PJ, Kivistö K, Hirvisalo EL. Effects of resins and activated charcoal on the absorption of digoxin, carbamazepine and frusemide. Br J Clin Pharmacol. 1988;25(2):229–33.
144. Skelin M, Lucijanić T, Amidžić Klarić D, Rešić A, Bakula M, et al. Factors affecting gastrointestinal absorption of levothyroxine: a review. Clin Ther. 2017;39(2):378–403.
145. Rosenberg R. Malabsorption of thyroid hormone with cholestyramine administration. Conn Med. 1994;58(2):109.
146. Amiodarone (amiodarone hydrochloride). Galway (Ireland): Mylan Institutional LLC; 2020.
147. Leatham EW, Holt DW, McKenna WJ. Class III antiarrhythmics in overdose. Presenting features and management principles. Drug Saf. 1993;9(6):450–62.
148. Hibbard DM, Peters JR, Hunninghake DB. Effects of cholestyramine and colestipol on the plasma concentrations of propranolol. Br J Clin Pharmacol. 1984;18(3):337–42.
149. Kamar FB, McQuillan RF. Hyperchloremic metabolic acidosis due to cholestyramine: a case report and literature review. Case Rep Nephrol. 2015;2015:309791.
150. Rust C, Sauter GH, Oswald M, Büttner J, Kullak-Ublick GA, Paumgartner G, et al. Effect of cholestyramine on bile acid pattern and synthesis during administration of ursodeoxycholic acid in man. Eur J Clin Investig. 2000;30(2):135–9.
151. Gleeson D. Heneghan MA; British Society of Gastroenterology. British Society of Gastroenterology (BSG) guidelines for management of autoimmune hepatitis. Gut. 2011;60(12):1611–29.

152. European Association for the Study of the Liver. EASL clinical practice guidelines: autoimmune hepatitis. J Hepatol. 2015;63(4):971–1004.
153. Zachou K, Gatselis N, Papadamou G, Rigopoulou EI, Dalekos GN. Mycophenolate for the treatment of autoimmune hepatitis: prospective assessment of its efficacy and safety for induction and maintenance of remission in a large cohort of treatment-naïve patients. J Hepatol. 2011;55(3):636–46.
154. PubChem [Internet]. Bethesda (MD): National Library of Medicine (US), National Center for Biotechnology Information; 2004-. PubChem Compound Summary for CID 5865, Prednisone; [cited 2020 Aug. 2]. Available from: https://pubchem.ncbi.nlm.nih.gov/compound/Prednisone
155. Edsbäcker S, Andersson T. Pharmacokinetics of budesonide (Entocort EC) capsules for Crohn's disease. Clin Pharmacokinet. 2004;43(12):803–21.
156. Seidegård J. Reduction of the inhibitory effect of ketoconazole on budesonide pharmacokinetics by separation of their time of administration. Clin Pharmacol Ther. 2000;68(1):13–7.
157. Bolland MJ, Bagg W, Thomas MG, Lucas JA, Ticehurst R, Black PN. Cushing's syndrome due to interaction between inhaled corticosteroids and itraconazole. Ann Pharmacother. 2004;38(1):46–9.
158. Budenofalk (budesonide). Buckinghamshire (UK): Dr. Falk Pharma UK Ltd.; 2020.
159. Entocort EC (budesonide). Södertälje(Sweden): AstraZeneca AB; 2016.
160. Sahasranaman S, Howard D, Roy S. Clinical pharmacology and pharmacogenetics of thiopurines. Eur J Clin Pharmacol. 2008;64(8):753–67.
161. Peyrin-Biroulet L, Cadranel JF, Nousbaum JB, Oussalah A, Seddik M, Canva V, et al. Interaction of ribavirin with azathioprine metabolism potentially induces myelosuppression. Aliment Pharmacol Ther. 2008;28(8):984–93.
162. Gearry RB, Day AS, Barclay ML, Leong RW, Sparrow MP. Azathioprine and allopurinol: a two-edged interaction. J Gastroenterol Hepatol. 2010;25(4):653–5.
163. Venkat Raman G, Sharman VL, Lee HA. Azathioprine and allopurinol: a potentially dangerous combination. J Intern Med. 1990;228(1):69–71.
164. Kaczmorski S, Doares W, Winfrey S, Al-Geizawi S, Farney A, Rogers J, et al. Gout and transplantation: new treatment option-same old drug interaction. Transplantation. 2011;92(3):e13–4.
165. Shaunak S, Munro JM, Weinbren K, Walport MJ, Cox TM. Cyclophosphamide-induced liver necrosis: a possible interaction with azathioprine. Q J Med. 1988;67(252):309–17.
166. Dewit O, Vanheuverzwyn R, Desager JP, Horsmans Y. Interaction between azathioprine and aminosalicylates: an in vivo study in patients with Crohn's disease. Aliment Pharmacol Ther. 2002;16(1):79–85.
167. Lowry PW, Franklin CL, Weaver AL, Szumlanski CL, Mays DC, Loftus EV, et al. Leucopenia resulting from a drug interaction between azathioprine or 6-mercaptopurine and mesalamine, sulphasalazine, or balsalazide. Gut. 2001;49(5):656–64.
168. Azathioprine (azathioprine). Hafnarfjörður (Iceland): Actavis Group PTC ehf.; 2017.
169. Innocenti F, Danesi R, Di Paolo A, Loru B, Favre C, Nardi M, et al. Clinical and experimental pharmacokinetic interaction between 6-mercaptopurine and methotrexate. Cancer Chemother Pharmacol. 1996;37(5):409–14.
170. Vazquez SR, Rondina MT, Pendleton RC. Azathioprine-induced warfarin resistance. Ann Pharmacother. 2008;42(7):1118–23.
171. Ng HJ, Crowther MA. Azathioprine and inhibition of the anticoagulant effect of warfarin: evidence from a case report and a literature review. Am J Geriatr Pharmacother. 2006;4(1):75–7.
172. Roblin X, Serre-Debeauvais F, Phelip JM, Bessard G, Bonaz B. Drug interaction between infliximab and azathioprine in patients with Crohn's disease. Aliment Pharmacol Ther. 2003;18(9):917–25.
173. PubChem [Internet]. Bethesda (MD): National Library of Medicine (US), National Center for Biotechnology Information; 2004-PubChem Compound Summary for CID 5281078, Mycophenolate mofetil; [cited 2020 Aug. 20]. Available from: https://pubchem.ncbi.nlm.nih.gov/compound/Mycophenolate-mofetil.

174. Hesselink DA, van Hest RM, Mathot RA, Bonthuis F, Weimar W, de Bruin RW, van Gelder T. Cyclosporine interacts with mycophenolic acid by inhibiting the multidrug resistance-associated protein 2. Am J Transplant. 2005;5(5):987–94.
175. Kodawara T, Masuda S, Yano Y, Matsubara K, Nakamura T, Masada M. Inhibitory effect of ciprofloxacin on β-glucuronidase-mediated deconjugation of mycophenolic acid glucuronide. Biopharm Drug Dispos. 2014;35(5):275–83.
176. Ratna P, Mathew BS, Annapandian VM, Saravanakumar K, Basu G, Tamilarasi V, Fleming DH. Pharmacokinetic drug interaction of mycophenolate with co-amoxiclav in renal transplant patients. Transplantation. 2011 Mar 27;91(6):e36–8.
177. Naderer OJ, Dupuis RE, Heinzen EL, Wiwattanawongsa K, Johnson MW, Smith PC. The influence of norfloxacin and metronidazole on the disposition of mycophenolate mofetil. J Clin Pharmacol. 2005;45(2):219–26.
178. Miura M, Satoh S, Kagaya H, Saito M, Inoue T, Ohkubo T, Habuchi T, Suzuki T. Effect of telmisartan, valsartan and candesartan on mycophenolate mofetil pharmacokinetics in Japanese renal transplant recipients. J Clin Pharm Ther. 2009;34(6):683–92.
179. Pieper AK, Buhle F, Bauer S, Mai I, Budde K, Haffner D, et al. The effect of sevelamer on the pharmacokinetics of cyclosporin A and mycophenolate mofetil after renal transplantation. Nephrol Dial Transplant. 2004;19(10):2630–3.
180. Kuypers DR, Verleden G, Naesens M, Vanrenterghem Y. Drug interaction between mycophenolate mofetil and rifampin: possible induction of uridine diphosphate- glucuronosyltransferase. Clin Pharmacol Ther. 2005;78(1):81–8.
181. CellCept (mycophenolatemofetil). Grenzach-Wyhlen (Germany): Roche Pharma AG; 2020.
182. Gimenez F, Foeillet E, Bourdon O, Weller S, Garret C, Bidault R, Singlas E. Evaluation of pharmacokinetic interactions after oral administration of mycophenolate mofetil and valaciclovir or aciclovir to healthy subjects. Clin Pharmacokinet. 2004;43(10):685–92.
183. European Association for Study of Liver. EASL clinical practice guidelines: Wilson's disease. J Hepatol. 2012;56(3):671–85.
184. Roberts EA, Schilsky ML, American Association for Study of Liver Diseases (AASLD). Diagnosis and treatment of Wilson disease: an update. Hepatology. 2008;47(6):2089–111.
185. PubChem [Internet]. Bethesda (MD): National Library of Medicine (US), National Center for Biotechnology Information; 2004-. PubChem Compound Summary for CID 11192, Zinc acetate; [cited 2020 Aug. 25]. Available from: https://pubchem.ncbi.nlm.nih.gov/compound/Zinc-acetate.
186. Galzin (zinc acetate). Parsippany (USA): Teva Pharmaceuticals USA, Inc.; 2020.
187. Krebs NF. Overview of zinc absorption and excretion in the human gastrointestinal tract. J Nutr. 2000;130(Suppl. 5S):1374S–7S.
188. Donangelo CM, Woodhouse LR, King SM, Viteri FE, King JC. Supplemental zinc lowers measures of iron status in young women with low iron reserves. J Nutr. 2002;132(7):1860–4.
189. Brewer GJ, Yuzbasiyan-Gurkan V, Johnson V, Dick RD, Wang Y. Treatment of Wilson's disease with zinc: XI. Interaction with other anticopper agents. J Am Coll Nutr. 1993;12(1):26–30.
190. Penttilä O, Hurme H, Neuvonen PJ. Effect of zinc sulphate on the absorption of tetracycline and doxycycline in man. Eur J Clin Pharmacol. 1975;9(2–3):131–4.
191. Brion M, Lambs L, Berthon G. Metal ion-tetracycline interactions in biological fluids. Part 5. Formation of zinc complexes with tetracycline and some of its derivatives and assessment of their biological significance. Agents Actions. 1985;17(2):229–42.
192. Pitman SK, Hoang UTP, Wi CH, Alsheikh M, Hiner DA, Percival KM. Revisiting oral fluoroquinolone and multivalent cation drug-drug interactions: are they still relevant? Antibiotics (Basel). 2019;8(3):108. https://doi.org/10.3390/antibiotics8030108.
193. Seedher N, Agarwal P. Effect of metal ions on some pharmacologically relevant interactions involving fluoroquinolone antibiotics. Drug Metabol Drug Interact. 2010;25(1–4):17–24.
194. Joyce DA. D-penicillamine. Baillieres Clin Rheumatol. 1990;4(3):553–74.
195. Cuprimine (penicillamine). Laval (CA): Valeant Canada LP; 2014.

196. Pitman SK, Huynh T, Bjarnason TA, An J, Malkhasyan KA. A case report and focused literature review of d-penicillamine and severe neutropenia: a serious toxicity from a seldom-used drug. Clin Case Rep. 2019;7(5):990–4.
197. Osman MA, Patel RB, Schuna A, Sundstrom WR, Welling PG. Reduction in oral penicillamine absorption by food, antacid, and ferrous sulfate. Clin Pharmacol Ther. 1983;33(4):465–70.
198. Netter P, Bannwarth B, Péré P, Nicolas A. Clinical pharmacokinetics of D-penicillamine. Clin Pharmacokinet. 1987;13(5):317–33.
199. Moezzi B, Fatourechi V, Khozain R, Eslami B. The effect of penicillamine on serum digoxin levels. Jpn Heart J. 1978;19(3):366–75.
200. Lu J. Triethylenetetramine pharmacology and its clinical applications. Mol Cancer Ther. 2010;9(9):2458–67.
201. Cuprior (trientine tetrahydrochloride). Paris (FR): Gmp-orphan SA; 2020.
202. Rodriguez-Castro KI, Hevia-Urrutia FJ, Sturniolo GC. Wilson's disease: a review of what we have learned. World J Hepatol. 2015;7(29):2859–70.
203. European Association for the Study of the Liver. EASL clinical practice guidelines for HFE hemochromatosis. J Hepatol. 2010;53(1):3–22.
204. Bacon BR, Adams PC, Kowdley KV, Powell LW, Tavill AS, American Association for the Study of Liver Diseases. Diagnosis and management of hemochromatosis: 2011 practice guideline by the American Association for the Study of Liver Diseases. Hepatology. 2011;54(1):328–43.
205. Bentur Y, McGuigan M, Koren G. Deferoxamine (desferrioxamine). New toxicities for an old drug. Drug Saf. 1991;6(1):37–46.
206. PubChem [Internet]. Bethesda (MD): National Library of Medicine (US), National Center for Biotechnology Information; 2004-. PubChem Compound Summary for CID 2973, Deferoxamine; [cited 2020 Aug. 25]. Available from: https://pubchem.ncbi.nlm.nih.gov/compound/Deferoxamine
207. Blake DR, Winyard P, Lunec J, Williams A, Good PA, Crewes SJ, Gutteridge JM, Rowley D, Halliwell B, Cornish A, et al. Cerebral and ocular toxicity induced by desferrioxamine. Q Med. 1985;56(219):345–55.
208. Smythies J, Edelstein L. The desferrioxamine-prochlorperazine coma-clue to the role of dopamine-iron recycling in the synthesis of hydrogen peroxide in the brain. Front Mol Neurosci. 2014;7:74.
209. Baker DL, Manno CS. Rapid excretion of gallium-67 isotope in an iron-overloaded patient receiving high-dose intravenous deferoxamine. Am J Hematol. 1988;29(4):230–2.
210. DeLeve LD, Valla DC, Garcia-Tsao G, American Association for the Study Liver Diseases. Vascular disorders of the liver. Hepatology. 2009;49(5):1729–64.
211. Garcia DA, Baglin TP, Weitz JI, Samama MM. Parenteral anticoagulants: antithrombotic therapy and prevention of thrombosis, 9th ed.: American College of Chest Physicians Evidence-Based Clinical Practice Guidelines. Chest. 2012;141(2 Suppl):e24S–43S.
212. Oduah EI, Linhardt RJ, Sharfstein ST. Heparin: past, present, and future. Pharmaceuticals (Basel). 2016;9(3):38.
213. Clexane (enoxaparin sodium). Berkshire (UK): Aventis Pharma Limited; 2020.
214. Harder S, Thürmann P. Clinically important drug interactions with anticoagulants. An update. Clin Pharmacokinet. 1996;30(6):416–44.
215. Heit JA, Lahr BD, Petterson TM, Bailey KR, Ashrani AA, Melton LJ 3rd. Heparin and warfarin anticoagulation intensity as predictors of recurrence after deep vein thrombosis or pulmonary embolism: a population-based cohort study. Blood. 2011;118(18):4992–9.
216. Caplain H, D'Honneur G, Cariou R. Prolonged heparin administration during clopidogrel treatment in healthy subjects. Semin Thromb Hemost. 1999;25(Suppl 2):61–4.
217. Teng R, Butler K. Lack of clinically significant pharmacological interactions between ticagrelor and enoxaparin or unfractionated heparin in healthy subjects. J Clin Pharm Ther. 2012;37(6):704–11.
218. Klinkhardt U, Breddin HK, Esslinger HU, Haas S, Kalatzis A, Harder S. Interaction between the LMWH reviparin and aspirin in healthy volunteers. Br J Clin Pharmacol. 2000;49(4):337–41.

219. Oster JR, Singer I, Fishman LM. Heparin-induced aldosterone suppression and hyperkalemia. Am J Med. 1995;98(6):575–86.
220. Heparin sodium (heparin sodium). Wrexham (UK): Wockhardt UK Ltd; 2018.
221. PubChem [Internet]. Bethesda (MD): National Library of Medicine (US), National Center for Biotechnology Information; 2004-. PubChem Compound Summary for CID 54678486, Warfarin; [cited 2020 Aug. 25]. Available from: https://pubchem.ncbi.nlm.nih.gov/compound/Warfarin.
222. Coumadin (warfarin sodium). Princeton (USA): Bristol-Myers Squibb Company; 2020.
223. Krajewski KC. Inability to achieve a therapeutic INR value while on concurrent warfarin and rifampin. J Clin Pharmacol. 2010;50(6):710–3.
224. Parrish RH, Pazdur DE, O'donnell PJ. Effect of carbamazepine initiation and discontinuation on antithrombotic control in a patient receiving warfarin: case report and review of the literature. Pharmacotherapy. 2006;26(11):1650–3.
225. Teles JS, Fukuda EY, Feder D. Warfarin: pharmacological profile and drug interactions with antidepressants. Einstein (Sao Paulo). 2012;10(1):110–5.
226. Yamamoto H, Habu Y, Yano I, Ozaki J, Kimura Y, Sato E, et al. Comparison of the effects of azole antifungal agents on the anticoagulant activity of warfarin. Biol Pharm Bull. 2014;37(12):1990–3.
227. McDonald MG, Au NT, Wittkowsky AK, Rettie AE. Warfarin-amiodarone drug-drug interactions: determination of [I](u)/K(I,u) for amiodarone and its plasma metabolites. Clin Pharmacol Ther 2012;91(4):709–717.
228. Juurlink DN. Drug interactions with warfarin: what clinicians need to know. CMAJ. 2007;177(4):369–71. https://doi.org/10.1503/cmaj.070946.
229. Hermosillo AJ, Spinler SA. Aspirin, clopidogrel, and warfarin: is the combination appropriate and effective or inappropriate and too dangerous? Ann Pharmacother. 2008;42(6):790–805.
230. Warfarin (warfarin sodium). Hoofddorp (NL): Sun Pharmaceutical Industries Europe B.V.; 2017.
231. Baillargeon J, Holmes HM, Lin YL, Raji MA, Sharma G, Kuo YF. Concurrent use of warfarin and antibiotics and the risk of bleeding in older adults. Am J Med. 2012;125(2):183–9.
232. Qamar A, Vaduganathan M, Greenberger NJ, Giugliano RP. Oral anticoagulation in patients with liver disease. J Am Coll Cardiol. 2018;71(19):2162–75.
233. Holbrook AM, Pereira JA, Labiris R, McDonald H, Douketis JD, Crowther M, et al. Systematic overview of warfarin and its drug and food interactions. Arch Intern Med. 2005;165(10):1095–106.
234. Lee SR, Lee HJ, Choi EK, Han KD, Jung JH, Cha MJ, Oh S, Lip GYH. Direct oral anticoagulants in patients with atrial fibrillation and liver disease. J Am Coll Cardiol. 2019;73(25):3295–308.
235. Galgani A, Palleria C, Iannone LF, De Sarro G, Giorgi FS, Maschio M, et al. Pharmacokinetic interactions of clinical interest between direct oral anticoagulants and antiepileptic drugs. Front Neurol. 2018;9:1067.
236. Forbes HL, Polasek TM. Potential drug–drug interactions with direct oral anticoagulants in elderly hospitalized patients. Ther Adv Drug Saf. 2017;8(10):319–28.
237. Mueck W, Kubitza D, Becka M. Co-administration of rivaroxaban with drugs that share its elimination pathways: pharmacokinetic effects in healthy subjects. Br J Clin Pharmacol. 2013;76(3):455–66.
238. Haas S, Bode C, Norrving B, Turpie AG. Practical guidance for using rivaroxaban in patients with atrial fibrillation: balancing benefit and risk. Vasc Health Risk Manag. 2014;10:101–14.
239. Xarelto (rivaroxaban). Leverkusen (DEU): Bayer HealthCare AG; 2011.
240. Kubitza D, Becka M, Mück W, Schwers S. Effect of co-administration of rivaroxaban and clopidogrel on bleeding time, pharmacodynamics and pharmacokinetics: a phase I study. Pharmaceuticals (Basel). 2012;5(3):279–96.
241. Eliquis (apixaban). Princeton (USA): Bristol-Myers Squibb Company; 2012.
242. Pradaxa (dabigatran etexilate mesylate). Ridgefield (USA): Boehringer Ingelheim Pharmaceuticals, Inc.; 2011.

243. European Association for the Study of the Liver. Electronic address: easloffice@easloffice.eu; European Association for the Study of the Liver. EASL Clinical Practice Guidelines for the management of patients with decompensated cirrhosis. J Hepatol. 2018;69(2):406–60.
244. Runyon BA. AASLD. Introduction to the revised American Association for the Study of Liver Diseases Practice Guideline management of adult patients with ascites due to cirrhosis 2012. Hepatology. 2013;57(4):1651–3.
245. Tripathi D, Stanley AJ, Hayes PC, Patch D, Millson C, Mehrzad H, et al. Clinical Services and Standards Committee of the British Society of Gastroenterology. U.K. guidelines on the management of variceal haemorrhage in cirrhotic patients. Gut. 2015;64(11):1680–704.
246. Bass NM. Review article: the current pharmacological therapies for hepatic encephalopathy. Aliment Pharmacol Ther. 2007;25(Suppl. 1):23–31.
247. PubChem [Internet]. Bethesda (MD): National Library of Medicine (US), National Center for Biotechnology Information; 2004-. PubChem Compound Summary for CID 3440, Furosemide; [cited 2020 Aug. 30]. Available from: https://pubchem.ncbi.nlm.nih.gov/compound/Furosemide.
248. Rudolf J, Würker M, Neveling M, Grond M, Haupt WF, Heiss WD. Dyskaliämische Lähmung bei Furosemidtherapie und gleichzeitigem Laxanzienabusus [Hypokalemic paralysis in furosemide therapy and simultaneous laxative abuse]. Med Klin (Munich). 1999;94(7):391–4. Germanica
249. Lasix (furosemide). Bridgewater (USA): Sanofi-aventis U.S. LLC; 2010.
250. Patak RV, Mookerjee BK, Bentzel CJ, Hysert PE, Babej M, Lee JB. Antagonism of the effects of furosemide by indomethacin in normal and hypertensive man. Prostaglandins. 1975;10(4):649–59.
251. Oyekan AO, Laniyonu AA, Ashorobi RB. Interaction between frusemide and aspirin. Gen Pharmacol. 1984;15(2):163–6.
252. Fine A, Henderson IS, Morgan DR, Tilstone WJ. Malabsorption of frusemide caused by phenytoin. Br Med J. 1977;2(6094):1061–2.
253. Palleria C, Di Paolo A, Giofrè C, Caglioti C, Leuzzi G, Siniscalchi A, De Sarro G, Gallelli L. Pharmacokinetic drug-drug interaction and their implication in clinical management. J Res Med Sci. 2013;18(7):601–10.
254. Offerhaus L. Drug interactions at excretory mechanisms. Pharmacol Ther. 1981;15(1):69–78.
255. Nierenberg DW, Mamelok RD. Toxic reaction to methotrexate in a patient receiving penicillin and furosemide: a possible interaction. Arch Dermatol. 1983;119(6):449–50.
256. Wang MT, Su CY, Chan AL, Lian PW, Leu HB, Hsu YJ. Risk of digoxin intoxication in heart failure patients exposed to digoxin-diuretic interactions: a population-based study. Br J Clin Pharmacol. 2010;70(2):258–67.
257. Nachimuthu S, Assar MD, Schussler JM. Drug-induced QT interval prolongation: mechanisms and clinical management. Ther Adv Drug Saf. 2012;3(5):241–53.
258. Neag MA, Muntean DM, Nacu A, Catinean A, Farcas A, Vesa S, Bocsan C, Vlase L, Buzoianu AD. Influence of concomitant medication on plasma concentration of amiodarone in patients with atrial fibrillation—a pilot study. Med Pharm Rep. 2019;92(2):129–33. https://doi.org/10.15386/mpr-1130.
259. Cleland JG, Gillen G, Dargie HJ. The effects of frusemide and angiotensin-converting enzyme inhibitors and their combination on cardiac and renal haemodynamics in heart failure. Eur Heart J. 1988;9(2):132–41.
260. Good JM, Brady AJ, Noormohamed FH, Oakley CM, Cleland JG. Effect of intense angiotensin II suppression on the diuretic response to furosemide during chronic ACE inhibition. Circulation. 1994;90(1):220–4.
261. Norrby R, Stenqvist K, Elgefors B. Interaction between cephaloridine and furosemide in man. Scand J Infect Dis. 1976;8(3):209–12.
262. Smith CR, Lietman PS. Effect of furosemide on aminoglycoside-induced nephrotoxicity and auditory toxicity in humans. Antimicrob Agents Chemother. 1983;23(1):133–7.
263. Stephens K, Miller JL, Lewis TV, Neely S, Johnson PN. Hyponatremia with intravenous sulfamethoxazole/trimethoprim in children. Ann Pharmacother. 2020;54(4):351–8.

264. Li Y, Ding D, Jiang H, Fu Y, Salvi R. Co-administration of cisplatin and furosemide causes rapid and massive loss of cochlear hair cells in mice. Neurotox Res. 2011;20(4):307–19.
265. Whitten JR, Ruehter VL. Risperidone and hyponatremia: a case report. Ann Clin Psychiatry. 1997;9(3):181–3.
266. Spital A. Diuretic-induced hyponatremia. Am J Nephrol. 1999;19(4):447–52.
267. Ben Salem C, Slim R, Fathallah N, Hmouda H. Drug-induced hyperuricaemia and gout. Rheumatology (Oxford). 2017;56(5):679–88.
268. Marenzi G, Ferrari C, Marana I, Assanelli E, De Metrio M, Teruzzi G, Veglia F, Fabbiocchi F, Montorsi P, Bartorelli AL. Prevention of contrast nephropathy by furosemide with matched hydration: the MYTHOS (induced diuresis with matched hydration compared to standard hydration for contrast induced nephropathy prevention) trial. JACC Cardiovasc Interv. 2012;5(1):90–7.
269. Gauillard J, Cheref S, Vacherontrystram MN, Martin JC. L'hydrate de chloral, un hypnotique à oublier? [Chloral hydrate: a hypnotic best forgotten?]. Encephale. 2002;28(3 Pt 1):200–4.
270. Hammad MA, Tangiisuran B, Kharshid AM, Abdul-Aziz N, Hassan Y, Aziz NA, Elsayed TM. Drug-drug Interaction-related uncontrolled glycemia. J Pharm Bioallied Sci. 2017;9(4):221–8.
271. Conlon PF, Grambau GR, Johnson CE, Weg JG. Effect of intravenous furosemide on serum theophylline concentration. Am J Hosp Pharm. 1981;38(9):1345–7.
272. Spironolactone (spironolactone). Devon (UK): Accord-UK Ltd.; 2019.
273. Abbas S, Ihle P, Harder S, Schubert I. Risk of hyperkalemia and combined use of spironolactone and long-term ACE inhibitor/angiotensin receptor blocker therapy in heart failure using real-life data: a population- and insurance-based cohort. Pharmacoepidemiol Drug Saf. 2015;24(4):406–13.
274. Goldszer RC, Coodley EL, Rosner MJ, Simons WM, Schwartz AB. Hyperkalemia associated with indomethacin. Arch Intern Med. 1981;141(6):802–4.
275. Akbarpour F, Afrasiabi A, Vaziri ND. Severe hyperkalemia caused by indomethacin and potassium supplementation. South Med J. 1985;78(6):756–7.
276. Antoniou T, Gomes T, Mamdani MM, Yao Z, Hellings C, Garg AX, Weir MA, Juurlink DN. Trimethoprim-sulfamethoxazole induced hyperkalaemia in elderly patients receiving spironolactone: nested case-control study. BMJ. 2011;343:d5228.
277. Lee CH, Kim GH. Electrolyte and Acid-base disturbances induced by clacineurin inhibitors. Electrolyte Blood Press. 2007;5(2):126–30.
278. Wenzl HH, Fine KD, Santa Ana CA, Porter JL, Fordtran JS. Effect of fludrocortisone and spironolactone on sodium and potassium losses in secretory diarrhea. Dig Dis Sci. 1997;42(1):119–28.
279. Weissman PN, Shenkman L, Gregerman RI. Chlorpropamide hyponatremia: drug-induced inappropriate antidiuretic-hormone activity. N Engl J Med. 1971;284(2):65–71.
280. Buss SJ, Backs J, Kreusser MM, Hardt SE, Maser-Gluth C, Katus HA, Haass M. Spironolactone preserves cardiac norepinephrine reuptake in salt-sensitive Dahl rats. Endocrinology. 2006;147(5):2526–34.
281. Finley PR. Drug interactions with lithium: an update. Clin Pharmacokinet. 2016;55(8):925–41.
282. O'Reilly RA. Spironolactone and warfarin interaction. Clin Pharmacol Ther. 1980;27(2):198–201.
283. Edwards HD, Webb RD, Conway SE. Effect of oral diuretics on chronic warfarin therapy: a retrospective study. Expert Opin Drug Saf. 2012;11(3):375–80.
284. Inderal (propranolol hydrochloride). Philadelphia (USA): Wyeth Pharmaceuticals Inc.; 2010.
285. Routledge PA, Shand DG. Clinical pharmacokinetics of propranolol. Clin Pharmacokinet. 1979;4(2):73–90.
286. Warren SE, Ebert E, Swerdlin AH, Steinberg SM, Stone R. Clonidine and propranolol paradoxical hypertension. Arch Intern Med. 1979;139(2):253.
287. Lin HC, Tsai YT, Yang MC, Hou MC, Lee FY, Chen LS, Lee SD. Haemodynamic effects of a combination of propranolol and clonidine in patients with post-hepatitic cirrhosis. J Gastroenterol Hepatol. 1995;10(3):281–6.

288. Vernon C, Sakula A. Fatal rebound hypertension after abrupt withdrawal of clonidine and propranolol. Br J Clin Pract. 1979;33(4):112. 121
289. Shehata AR, Gillam LD, Mascitelli VA, Herman SD, Ahlberg AW, White MP, Chen C, Waters DD, Heller GV. Impact of acute propranolol administration on dobutamine-induced myocardial ischemia as evaluated by myocardial perfusion imaging and echocardiography. Am J Cardiol. 1997;80(3):268–72.
290. Pacher P, Kecskemeti V. Cardiovascular side effects of new antidepressants and antipsychotics: new drugs, old concerns? Curr Pharm Des. 2004;10(20):2463–75.
291. Gillette DW, Tannery LP. Beta blocker inhibits tricyclic metabolism. J Am Acad Child Adolesc Psychiatry. 1994;33(2):223–4.
292. Burnakis TG. Haloperidol and propranolol in combination. JAMA. 1985;253(11):1557–8.
293. Silver JM, Yudofsky SC, Kogan M, Katz BL. Elevation of thioridazine plasma levels by propranolol. Am J Psychiatry. 1986;143(10):1290–2.
294. Peet M, Middlemiss DN, Yates RA. Pharmacokinetic interaction between propranolol and chlorpromazine in schizophrenic patients. Lancet. 1980;2(8201):978.
295. Miller FA, Rampling D. Adverse effects of combined propranolol and chlorpromazine therapy. Am J Psychiatry. 1982;139(9):1198–9.
296. Foster CA, Aston SJ. Propranolol-epinephrine interaction: a potential disaster. Plast Reconstr Surg. 1983;72(1):74–8.
297. Zhou HH, Anthony LB, Roden DM, Wood AJ. Quinidine reduces clearance of (+)-propranolol more than (−)-propranolol through marked reduction in 4-hydroxylation. Clin Pharmacol Ther. 1990;47(6):686–93.
298. Murdoch DL, Thomson GD, Thompson GG, Murray GD, Brodie MJ, McInnes GT. Evaluation of potential pharmacodynamic and pharmacokinetic interactions between verapamil and propranolol in normal subjects. Br J Clin Pharmacol. 1991;31(3):323–32.
299. Bonifazi E, Acquafredda A, Milano A, Montagna O, Laforgia N. Severe hypoglycemia during successful treatment of diffuse hemangiomatosis with propranolol. Pediatr Dermatol. 2010;27(2):195–6.
300. Polónia J. Interaction of antihypertensive drugs with anti-inflammatory drugs. Cardiology. 1997;88(Suppl. 3):47–51.
301. Goldberg MR, Sciberras D, De Smet M, Lowry R, Tomasko L, Lee Y, Olah TV, Zhao J, Vyas KP, Halpin R, Kari PH, James I. Influence of beta-adrenoceptor antagonists on the pharmacokinetics of rizatriptan, a 5-HT1B/1D agonist: differential effects of propranolol, nadolol and metoprolol. Br J Clin Pharmacol. 2001;52(1):69–76.
302. Miners JO, Wing LM, Lillywhite KJ, Robson RA. Selectivity and dose-dependency of the inhibitory effect of propranolol on theophylline metabolism in man. Br J Clin Pharmacol. 1985;20(3):219–23.
303. Sandostatin (octreotide acetate). Schaftenau (A): Sandoz GmbH; 2010.
304. Landgraf R, Landgraf-Leurs MM, Nusser J, Hillebrand G, Illner WD, Abendroth D, Land W. Effect of somatostatin analogue (SMS201-995) on cyclosporine levels. Transplantation. 1987;44(5):724–5.
305. Lheureux PE, Zahir S, Penaloza A, Gris M. Bench-to-bedside review: Antidotal treatment of sulfonylurea-induced hypoglycaemia with octreotide. Crit Care. 2005;9(6):543–9.
306. Kapîcîoglu S, Sentürk O, Ilgün K, Ovali E. Effect of long-acting somatostatin analogue (octreotide, SMS 201-995) plus calcium channel blocker (verapamil) on gallbladder contraction. Hepato-Gastroenterology. 1998;45(20):420–3.
307. Pesaturo AB, Jennings HR, Voils SA. Terlipressin: vasopressin analog and novel drug for septic shock. Ann Pharmacother. 2006;40(12):2170–7.
308. Terlipressin acetate (terlipressin acetate). Hoofddorp (NL): Sun Pharmaceutical Industries Europe B.V.; 2018.
309. Duphalac (lactulose). Hertfordshire (UK): Mylan; 2018.
310. PubChem [Internet]. Bethesda (MD): National Library of Medicine (US), National Center for Biotechnology Information; 2004-. PubChem Compound Summary for CID 11333, Lactulose; [cited 2020 Sep. 5]. Available from: https://pubchem.ncbi.nlm.nih.gov/compound/Lactulose.

311. Prakash R, Mullen KD. Mechanisms, diagnosis and management of hepatic encephalopathy. Nat Rev Gastroenterol Hepatol. 2010;7(9):515–25.
312. Visser LE, Penning-van Beest FJ, Wilson JH, Vulto AG, Kasbergen AA, De Smet PA, et al. Overanticoagulation associated with combined use of lactulose and acenocoumarol or phenprocoumon. Br J Clin Pharmacol. 2004;57(4):522–4.
313. Hepa-Merz (L-ornithine L-aspartate). Frankfurt/Main (DEU): Merz Pharmaceuticals GmbH; 2020.
314. Xifaxanta (rifaximin). Harefield (UK): Norgine Pharmaceuticals Limited; 2017.
315. Phongsamran PV, Kim JW, Cupo Abbott J, Rosenblatt A. Pharmacotherapy for hepatic encephalopathy. Drugs. 2010;70(9):1131–48.
316. Hoffman JT, Hartig C, Sonbol E, Lang M. Probable interaction between warfarin and rifaximin in a patient treated for small intestine bacterial overgrowth. Ann Pharmacother. 2011;45(5):e25.

Pancreato-Biliary Disorders

31

Tomislav Bokun, Marko Zelenika, and Milan Kujundžić

Pancreato-biliary disorders encompass a variety of conditions related to pancreas and biliary tract, with wide range of therapeutic options, many falling into interventional endoscopy and/or radiology domain, as well as surgery, but also with a number of medications.

Medications can be used for the treatment of conditions by directly interrupting the pathophysiological pathway leading to the conditions, but more often medications are used to treat symptoms and conditions occurring secondary to primary pancreato-biliary disorder such as pain and infection.

Gallstone Diseases and Its Complications

Gallstone disease is very prevalent, with roughly 80% of the patients being asymptomatic (many unaware of the disease), but for the symptomatic ones a lot of health resources is spent for the management of the disease [1]. The most important aspects of the management are surgical and endoscopic, whereas medications have a

T. Bokun (✉) · M. Kujundžić
Department of Gastroenterology, Hepatology and Clinical Nutrition, Dubrava University Hospital, Zagreb, Croatia

Faculty of Pharmacy and Biochemistry, University of Zagreb, Zagreb, Croatia

School of Medicine, University of Zagreb, Zagreb, Croatia
e-mail: milan.kujundzic@kbd.hr

M. Zelenika
Department of Gastroenterology, Hepatology and Clinical Nutrition, Dubrava University Hospital, Zagreb, Croatia

School of Medicine, University of Zagreb, Zagreb, Croatia

M. Banić, D. Erceg (eds.), *Drug Interactions in Gastroenterology*, Clinical Gastroenterology, https://doi.org/10.1007/978-3-031-69800-2_31

small role in the treatment, except for the management of complications such as cholecystitis and cholangitis.

Over 90% of gallstones in the western world are cholesterol stones, containing more than 50% of cholesterol with variable number of other substances such as calcium salts, bile pigments, proteins, and fatty acids, whereas pigment stones are composed of calcium components, and often variable amounts of protein component and small amounts of cholesterol.

Ursodeoxycholic acid (UDCA) [2], also known as ursodiol, is a gallstone solubilizing agent. It is a naturally occurring bile acid present in small quantities in human bile, which suppresses liver synthesis and secretion of cholesterol and inhibits intestinal cholesterol absorption. UDCA is used to dissolve radiolucent gallstones (mostly composed of cholesterol) in selected patients and to prevent gallstones formation in obese patients who are losing weight rapidly (e.g., after bariatric procedures), as well as in recurrent choledocholithiasis. It should not be administrated concomitantly with salt–sequestering agents' cholestyramine and colestipol, nor with antacids containing aluminum hydroxide and/or aluminum oxide, as these preparations bind UDCA in the intestine thereby inhibiting its absorption and efficacy. Adsorption of cyclosporine from the intestine can be affected by UDCA, therefore requiring blood concentration checks and dose adjust if needed. Rarely, the absorption of ciprofloxacin could also be decreased. Calcium antagonist nitrendipine peak plasma concentrations could be reduced if taken concomitantly with UDCA, so either dose adjustment might be needed, or more pragmatically, a replacement antihypertensive therapy could be considered. Therapeutic effect of dapsone could also be reduced. When taken with UDCA, rosuvastatin plasma concentrations raised, but the clinical implications of this interaction for rosuvastatin as well as other statins are not known.

Acute biliary infections—cholecystitis and cholangitis—are frequent complications of gallstone disease. Acute cholecystitis is best managed by surgery—laparoscopic (preferably) or open cholecystectomy [3, 4]. Acute cholangitis is an acute infection of the biliary tree with considerable mortality that is generally managed by biliary drainage, depending of the severity of the disease [5, 6]. Medications used for the treatment of acute biliary infections include broad spectrum antibiotics, and when needed analgesics, antipyretics, and/or antiemetics are given [7].

Many bacteria can cause acute biliary infection, *E. coli*, *Klebsiella* spp., and *Pseudomonas* spp. being the most common among Gram negative, and *Enterococcus* spp. and *Streptococcus* spp. being the most common among Gram-positive microorganisms [7]. Broad spectrum antibiotics are used to cover the most common isolates. They are started empirically and changed upon defining responsible microorganism and obtaining antibiogram. The list of antibiotics that can be used is quite long, and the selection depends on multiple factors such as pharmacokinetics and pharmacodynamics, severity of infection, history of recent antibiotics usage, local epidemiology and resistance to certain antibiotics, possible drug-drug interactions, as well as factors related to the patient such as renal and hepatic function, and history of allergies. Cephalosporins, penicillin derivates, fluoroquinolones, and carbapenems are most commonly used.

Cephalosporines, generally divided into five major groups/generations are in many cases the first choice for empiric therapy. Ceftriaxone [8] has the longest-half life among third-, fourth-, and fifth-generation cephalosporins, being practical for once daily dosage, and because is eliminated by biliary excretion therefore reaching high concentrations in biliary tree. Because of possible precipitation, ceftriaxone should not be diluted with any fluid containing calcium, nor should be applied though the same intravenous administration line together with calcium-containing solutions. If used concomitantly with vitamin K antagonists, international normalized ratio (INR) should be monitored more often, as the effect of this class of oral anticoagulants can be increased therefore increasing the risk of bleeding. This also applies to some other cephalosporines such as cefepime [9]. As with all other medications, special care must be taken for potential allergic reactions. Cephalosporines are contraindicated in case of previous allergic reaction to any of cephalosporines. On the other hand, cross-reactivity between cephalosporins and other β-lactam antibiotics is considerable, and according to Summary of Product Characteristics (SPC) of the drugs, history of severe allergic reaction like anaphylaxis to any β-lactam antibiotic is a contraindication for administration of ceftriaxone or other cephalosporines. There are still controversies around possible cross-reactivity considering the given β-lactam antibiotic that previously caused reaction, as well as the "strength" of hypersensitivity/allergic reaction [10–12]. Lidocaine can be used as solvent (only) for intramuscular application of ceftriaxone and some other cephalosporines, and in that case should also be considered for allergy and drug-drug interaction as well. Ceftazidime [13] and cefotaxime [14] are also third-generation cephalosporines that can be used for the treatment of biliary infections. Both medications and other cephalosporines when used together with nephrotoxic drugs such as aminoglycosides or with potent diuretics such as furosemide could impair renal function, and kidney function should be monitored closely. It is recommended not to combine ceftazidime, cefotaxime, and cefepime—fourth-generation cephalosporine—with medications having bacteriostatic activity (such as tetracyclines, erythromycin, and chloramphenicol), because of potential antagonistic effect.

Penicillin derivate piperacillin combined with tazobactam [15] is very effective for biliary infections. It is contraindicated in the case of history of allergic reaction to other penicillin derivates, as well as severe allergic reaction to any β-lactam antibiotic. While using concomitantly with heparin, oral anticoagulants and other substances that may affect the blood coagulation system and thrombocyte function, appropriate coagulation tests should be performed more frequently. Piperacillin has the potential to reduce the excretion of methotrexate, therefore increasing the risk of clinically significant toxicity, necessitating monitoring of serum levels of methotrexate. The caution is needed for concomitant treatment of piperacillin and vecuronium or other non-depolarizing muscle relaxants, as the prolongation of the neuromuscular blockade is possible.

Meropenem [16] is another wide-spectrum potent antibiotic, from class of carbapenems. It is contraindicated in case of hypersensitivity reaction to other carbapenems, as well as severe allergic reaction to any β-lactam antibiotic. It can be hepatotoxic, especially in patients with liver disease, so close monitoring of liver function is indicated during treatment. Because carbapenems significantly decrease the levels of valproic acid, comedication should be avoided. INR should be monitored closely during and shortly after the treatment with carbapenems in patients receiving vitamin K antagonists, because possible increase in anticoagulant effect.

Fluroquinolones are widely accepted for the treatment of biliary infection, ciprofloxacin [17] and levofloxacin [18] being most commonly prescribed. Fluroquinolones are contraindicated in case of hypersensitivity reaction to other quinolones and should be used with caution in patients receiving drugs known to prolong QT interval. In patients treated with ciprofloxacin and levofloxacin that are receiving vitamin K antagonists, INR should be monitored closely during and shortly after the treatment. Ciprofloxacin must not be used concomitantly with tizanidine-short-acting muscle relaxers. Because of chelation complex formation resulting in reduced absorption, oral ciprofloxacin should not be taken together with multivalent cation-containing drugs and mineral supplements (e.g., calcium, magnesium, aluminum, and iron), polymeric phosphate binders (e.g., sevelamer or lanthanum carbonate), sucralfate or antacids, and highly buffered drugs (e.g., didanosine tablets) containing magnesium, aluminum, or calcium. As with many other medications, probenecid interferes with renal secretion of ciprofloxacin and levofloxacin, therefore increasing its serum concentrations, but this is not known to be clinically relevant. Concomitant use of ciprofloxacin with methotrexate is not recommended. Ciprofloxacin has the potential to significantly increase plasma level of theophylline when taken concomitantly, therefore introducing toxicity. If this comedication is necessary, serum theophylline concentrations should be measured, and dose adjusted if needed. Kidney function should be monitored in case of treatment with ciprofloxacin and cyclosporine. Coadministration with ciprofloxacin may increase blood levels of zolpidem; therefore, concurrent use is not recommended.

Metronidazole has activity against various anaerobic bacteria and is often added to cephalosporines and fluoroquinolones for the treatment of biliary infections. If metronidazole therapy is planned, tapering and discontinuation of lithium therapy is recommended. If this is not convenient close monitoring of plasma concentration of lithium, creatinine, and electrolytes is suggested, while on metronidazole therapy. In patients receiving warfarin, while being treated with metronidazole INR should be monitored and dose reduced if necessary. Psychotic reactions have been reported, while concomitant therapy of disulfiram and metronidazole. Due to risk of ciclosporin serum level elevation, when introduction of metronidazole is needed serum level of ciclosporin, and serum creatinine should be closely monitored. Metronidazole inhibits metabolism of fluorouracil. Therefore, increased toxicity of fluorouracil can result.

To check for possible and/or detailed drug-drug interactions for the above and many other antibiotics, we refer the reader to SPCs of certain antibiotics and/or web-based drug-drug interaction checkers.

Paracetamol [19] can be used as antipyretic and analgetic, and combinations with other analgesics are available. Its hepatotoxicity in high doses (>4 g) is well known, and coadministration with other hepatotoxic substances my increase the risk of toxicity. Patients taking enzyme-inducing drugs such as rifampicin and some antiepileptics (carbamazepine, phenytoin, phenobarbital, and primidone) are at increased risk of hepatotoxicity, as the metabolization of paracetamol is increased resulting in accumulation of a toxic metabolite N-acetyl-p-benzoquinone imine (NAPQI), and the risk is greater if alcohol is consumed during treatment. Therefore, caution is needed is case of such comedication, lower doses of paracetamol considered, and alcohol consumption withhold. Paracetamol dosage should be reduced also while taking probenecid as is causes almost 2-fold reduction in clearance of paracetamol by inhibiting its conjugation with glucuronic acid, therefore, increasing risk of toxicity.

Ketorolac, ketoprofen, and diclofenac are some of non-steroidal anti-inflammatory drugs (NSAIDs) that are used to relieve biliary pain, that also have antipyretic activity. Ketorolac [20] and diclofenac [21] are used for the treatment of short-time moderate to severe acute pain, whereas ketoprofen [22] is used for chronic pain management especially for chronic inflammatory diseases but can also be used for acute pain management in some conditions, including biliary pain. Ketorolac should be used for up to 5 days. It is contraindicated in case of hypersensitivity reaction to other NSAIDs, aspirin, or other prostaglandin synthesis inhibitors and is contraindicated in patients taking ASA and anticoagulants. Ketorolac should not be used in patients on pentoxifylline/oxpentifylline, as well as probenecid or lithium salts. Generally, two different NSAIDs (including cyclo-oxygenase-2 selective inhibitors) should not be used concomitantly because of increased toxicities, especially GI ulceration and bleeding. Caution is needed when coprescribing NSAIDs and corticosteroids also because of increased toxicity. The list of potential interactions of various medications with diclofenac and/or ketoprofen is quite long, including lithium and digoxin, diuretics and antihypertensive drugs, antidiabetics, methotrexate, ciclosporin, tacrolimus, phenytoin, mifepristone, quinolone antibiotics, voriconazole, and zidovudine. So concomitant therapy with these drugs should be avoided if possible, or clinical and appropriate laboratory monitoring should be scheduled, or concentrations of coprescribed drugs should be monitored when applicable. As colestipol and cholestyramine delay or decrease the absorption of diclofenac, it should be administrated at least 1 h before or at least 4 h after administration of colestipol or cholestyramine.

Pethidine (also known as meperidine) [23] is a synthetic opioid medication used to relieve strong pain, that should be used for up to 48 h. Generally opioid analgesics should not be used concomitantly with sedative medicines such as benzodiazepines as comedication can result with respiratory depression, and even coma or death. There is an increased risk of convulsions when taking antipsychotics together with pethidine. Digoxin toxicity is increased when co-prescribed, and pethidine increases anticoagulant effect of coumarins. Carbamazepine reduces the effect of pethidine, and on the other hand pethidine antagonizes the gastro-intestinal activity of domperidone and metoclopramide. Oxycodone [24] is another opioid analgetic that can be used alone or in combination with paracetamol or naloxone for the management of severe pain. Administrated concomitantly with anticholinergics or medicines with anticholinergic activity (e.g., tricyclic antidepressants, antihistamines, antipsychotics, muscle relaxants, and anti-Parkinson drugs) may result in increased anticholinergic adverse effects, and the dosage may need to be adjusted. Monoamine oxidase (MAO) inhibitors can interact with narcotic analgesics causing CNS excitation or depression associated with hypertensive or hypotensive crisis.

To check for possible and detailed drug-drug interactions for the above and many other analgesics, we refer the reader to SPCs of certain analgetic and/or web-based drug-drug interaction checkers.

Among antiemetics of various classes, prochlorperazine and metoclopramide are most used to control nausea and vomiting in acute pancreato-biliary diseases. Due to mutual antagonism, combination of metoclopramide [25] and levodopa or dopaminergic agonists is contraindicated. Alcohol consumption should be avoided while taking metoclopramide because potentiation of sedative effect, the same as comedication with CNS depressants, whereas anticholinergics and morphine derivatives may antagonize the effect of metoclopramide on digestive tract motility. Neuroleptics together with metoclopramide may increase the risk for extrapyramidal disorders, whereas serotonergic drugs such as SSRIs with metoclopramide may increase the risk of serotonin syndrome. When co-prescribed with metoclopramide, monitoring of plasma concentrations of digoxin and cyclosporine is required because of decreased/increased bioavailability. Prochlorperazine [26], among other has anticholinergic activity and its CNS depressant activity may be increased when taken with alcohol or coprescribed with barbiturates and other sedatives, possible leading to respiratory depression. It can reduce antipsychotic effect of neuroleptics, and anticholinergic activity can be raised to cause toxicity manifested with constipation when given together with other anticholinergic drugs. Increased risk of agranulocytosis is possible when used together with drugs that have myelosuppressive potential. It should be used with caution in patients taking QT prolonging drugs as the risk of arrhythmias is increased. Coadministration of desferrioxamine and prochlorperazine has been observed to induce transient metabolic encephalopathy manifested by loss of consciousness for 48–72 h.

Cholestasis and Primary Sclerosing Cholangitis

Cholestasis is caused by various intrahepatic disorders (inflammatory/viral or autoimmune diseases of the liver including cirrhosis, drug-induced, genetic, and hormonal disorders), as well as extrahepatic obstruction of the biliary tree. It can cause jaundice, fatigue, nausea, and abdominal pain, may result with malabsorption and vitamin deficiencies, and the most cumbersome often early symptom is itch or pruritus, with complex pathophysiology and challenging treatment. The management of cholestasis is disease specific and includes the treatment of primary disease; medications are used to relieve symptoms, prevent complications, such as cholangitis, nutritional deficits, and osteoporosis.

Primary sclerosing cholangitis (PSC) is a rare, progressive, debilitating, cholestatic liver disease of unclear etiology, with many drugs being studied, but none showed the ability to stop or slow the progression of the disease. Pruritus is a common symptom in PSC and often is difficult to control.

Couple of drugs is used for the management of cholestasis-associated pruritus including antihistamines, salt–sequestering agents such as cholestyramine and colestipol, rifampin, sertraline, and opiate antagonists such as naltrexone.

In patients with itching due to chronic cholestasis and PSC clinicians might start treatment with antihistamines, which are used off-label in this indication. Generally, these medications cannot be used in patients with severe hepatic impairment, and there are some known interactions with other medications, most without clinical significance, but since this medication class have only limited success, it is not recommended in guidelines.

Most clinicians would start with one of salt–sequestering agents such as cholestyramine and colestipol. Cholestyramine [27] is a basic anion-exchange resin that is potentially effective in case of noncomplete biliary obstruction, which is mostly the case with this disease. It may delay or reduce the absorption of certain drugs, such as tetracycline, chlorothiazide, warfarin, thyroxine, or digitalis. Therefore, patients should take other drugs at least 1 h before or 4–6 h after cholestyramine and closer monitoring is suggested to avoid potential AEs. Like cholestyramine, colestipol [28] may also delay or reduce the absorption of certain concomitant oral drugs such as digitalis and its glycosides, propranolol, hydrochlorothiazide, tetracycline, penicillin G, gemfibrozil, and furosemide, and again taking those drugs 1 h before or at least 4 h after colestipol is considered sufficient to avoid possible interference with their absorption. Even found to be of very low clinical significance in the studies, both cholestyramine and colestipol might interfere with the absorption of fat-soluble vitamins, namely vitamin K, D, and A. Additionally, deficiencies of fat-soluble vitamins are detected in PSC nonrelated to the treatment with these resins. Therefore, the levels of mentioned vitamins should be monitored and supplemented if needed, especially with long-term use of these drugs [27–31].

Rifampin [32] also known as rifampicin is another well-tolerated off-label alternative for the treatment of pruritus. It is an antibiotic used for the treatment of some bacterial infections, including mycobacterium tuberculosis, and is often used in together with other antibiotics. Even though it proved to be effective for pruritus in cholestatic diseases, it has some potential serious side effects including hepatotoxicity, nephrotoxicity, and various others. In patients with hepatic impairment, lower doses are suggested with careful introduction and monitoring of LFTs: before treatment, then weekly for 2 weeks and every 2 weeks for the next 6 weeks. If LFTs deteriorate, withdrawal of the therapy should be considered. On the other hand, there are potential drug-drug interactions concerning this drug. It is contraindicated in patients receiving combination of saquinavir and ritonavir because of increased risk of hepatotoxicity. Concomitant use of halothane or isoniazid also increases the risk of hepatotoxicity, so halothane should be avoided, and with isoniazid closer monitoring is warranted. Rifampicin is a potent inducer of drug metabolizing enzymes and transporters, namely cytochromes P450 (CYP) 1A2, 2B6, 2C8, 2C9, 2C19, and 3A4, UDP- Glucuronosyltransferase (UGT), sulfotransferases, carboxylesterases, and transporters including P-glycoprotein (P-gp) and multidrug resistance-associated protein 2 (MRP2) [32]. Many drugs are metabolized or transported by one or more of these, which increases the risk of potential clinically important drug-drug interactions, calling for safer treatment options [29, 32]. Readers should refer to SPC of rifampicin and/or web-based drug-drug interaction checkers.

Sertraline [33], selective serotonin reuptake inhibitor (SSRI) also demonstrated the effect of relieving pruritus, taken in doses of 75 to 100 mg orally. As sertraline is metabolized by the liver, its use in patients with hepatic disease should be approached with caution. It can be used in lower doses (up to 50% of standard dose) in patients with Child-Turcotte-Pugh (CTP) A cirrhosis but should not be used in CTP B and C cirrhosis. Sertraline therapy should be carefully considered in patients that concomitantly take medications, which prolong QT interval because synergistic effect. Concomitant treatment with irreversible MAObitors is contraindicated, and a combination with reversible and selective MAO inhibitors is also not recommended. Linezolid, which could potentially be considered in patients with cholangitis/sepsis or for other reasons, is a weak reversible, nonselective MAOI, and should not be given to patients treated with sertraline. Sertraline could be started at least 2 weeks after discontinuation of treatment with an irreversible MAOI, and, on the other hand, must be discontinued for at least 1 week before starting treatment with an irreversible MAOI. Sertraline is also contraindicated with pimozide. Caution is needed when administrated together with fentanyl, other serotonergic drugs (including other serotonergic antidepressants, amphetamines, triptans), 5-HT agonists, and with opiate/opioid drugs (e.g., buprenorphine) and opioid antagonists (e.g., naloxone). Due to possible interactions with warfarin, INR should be closely monitored after initiating or stopping sertraline. When coadministrated with drugs modifying platelet function (NSAIDs, acetylsalicylic acid, and ticlopidine), the risk of bleeding may be increased. Concomitant administration of sertraline and various CYP3A4 inhibitors, for example, protease inhibitors, ketoconazole, itraconazole, posaconazole, voriconazole, clarithromycin, telithromycin, nefazodone, aprepitant, erythromycin, fluconazole, verapamil, and diltiazem, would result in sertraline availability, and these drugs should be avoided with sertraline if possible [29, 33].

Opiate antagonist naltrexone [34] has also been shown to be effective in the treatment of pruritus. Although an opioid withdrawal reaction can occur, it is usually self-limited. Naltrexone should not be used with severe liver impairment as has hepatotoxic effect. In patients with PSC, LFTs should be monitored during therapy. It is contraindicated in patients taking opioid derivates (analgesics, antitussives, and substitution treatments), central antihypertensives (alpha-methyldopa), or methadone. Caution is needed when coadministered with barbiturates, benzodiazepines, anxiolytics other than benzodiazepines, hypnotics, sedative antidepressants, sedative antihistamines H1, and neuroleptics [29, 30, 34].

Ursodeoxycholic acid (UDCA), previously studied in various including higher doses showed to modestly improve liver biochemistry but without other benefits, is not recommended for the treatment of PSC as well as chemoprevention of colorectal neoplasia in patients with PSC and ulcerative colitis [29–31].

Broad spectrum antibiotic such as cephalosporin of fluoroquinolone should be administrated after endoscopic or percutaneous biliary intervention or for spontaneously occurring cholangitis, and for the information on drug-drug interactions with antibiotics look at other paragraphs in this chapter.

Acute Pancreatitis

Acute pancreatitis is potentially life-treating inflammatory disease of the pancreas characterized by abdominal pain and elevated levels of pancreatic enzymes. Basic treatment should be initiated immediately, that is, fluid resuscitation started and medications for pain relief applied. Further management of the diseased patient depends on the severity of the disease encompassing organ failure, infections, development of abdominal compartment syndrome, and local complications, as well as etiology (in cases of biliary pancreatitis early ERCP should be considered).

Pain control is effectively provided by opioids such as hydromorphone or fentanyl, as well as pethidine/meperidine (the latter is described in the above sections of this chapter).

Hydromorphone [35], a semi-synthetic derivative of morphine, and fentanyl [36], a powerful synthetic opioid, are both contraindicated in patients taking MAO inhibitors or within 2 weeks of its discontinuation, and alcohol should not be consumed while taking those medications. They should be avoided or used with caution in patients on sedative medicines such as benzodiazepines or other drugs that depress the CNS including anxiolytics, hypnotics, and anesthetics (e.g., barbiturates), neuroleptics, antiemetics, antidepressants, antipsychotics (e.g., phenothiazines), and antihistamines, because the risk of sedation, respiratory depression, or even coma and death; doses of CNS depressants should be reduced. Fentanyl should not be co-administrated with clonidine as fentanyl-induced respiratory depression could be prolonged. Fluconazole or voriconazole (moderate CYP3A4 inhibitors) can increase exposure and/or prolonged exposure to fentanyl when coadministered. Fentanyl should not be combined with non-vagolytic muscle relaxants (e.g., vecuronium) due to possible bradycardia and cardiac arrest. As with MAO inhibitors, fentanyl should also not be administered with serotonergic agent (selective serotonin reuptake inhibitor [SSRI]) or (serotonin norepinephrine reuptake inhibitor [SNRI]) due to increased risk of serotonin syndrome. When coadministered, fentanyl and intravenous midazolam interact resulting in a reduction of plasma clearance of midazolam, requiring dose adjustments. The pharmacological effects of fentanyl citrate can be reversed by naloxone.

NSAIDs such as ketorolac, ketoprofen, and diclofenac can be used for mild-to-moderate pain in acute pancreatitis and are described in the above sections of this chapter. Antiemetics might also be useful (described above).

Antibiotics are generally not indicated for the treatment of acute pancreatitis regardless of type (interstitial or necrotizing) or disease severity (mild, moderate, or severe) [37–39]. Antibiotics are indicated only for infected necrosis, which occurs roughly only in one-third of patients with necrotizing pancreatitis, and the extent of necrosis does not corelate with infection occurrence. Of course, antibiotics should be administrated at the onset of acute pancreatitis or during the disease in case of concomitant cholangitis and/or cholecystitis, or other organ infection (pneumonia, urinary tract infection, etc.). Infected necrosis is best treated with meropenem, as well as the combination of ceftazidime (third-generation) or cefepime (fourth-generation cephalosporine) with anaerobic agent such as metronidazole, interactions of which are well described in the above sections in this chapter.

Chronic Pancreatitis and Pancreatic Exocrine Insufficiency

Chronic pancreatitis is continuous relapsing inflammatory disease of the pancreas, with very challenging treatment requiring multidisciplinary approach. Pain is often the first and the most cumbersome and disabling symptom of chronic pancreatitis, and pain management is very complicated due to its multifactorial etiology. It includes medications, as well as consideration of endoscopic treatment, with surgery reserved for very disabling pain resistant to other less invasive treatment options.

Pain relief medications should be gradually introduced and titrated to effective doses, starting with NSAIDs and moving to long-acting opioids such as morphine or fentanyl, which are often needed. As pancreatic exocrine secretion is suppressed after introducing pancreatic enzyme supplements, this will result in pain relief in some patients.

As other opioids, morphine [40] is contraindicated in patients taking MAO inhibitors or within 2 weeks of its discontinuation, and alcohol should not be consumed while taking morphine (patients should permanently abstinent from alcohol because of disease itself!). It should not be combined with other opioid drugs. Morphine should be avoided if possible or used with caution in patients on sedative medicines such as benzodiazepines or other drugs that depress the CNS including anxiolytics, hypnotics, anesthetics, hypnotics, tricyclic antidepressants and phenothiazines, as well as muscle relaxants and gabapentin, because of the risk of sedation, respiratory depression, or even coma and death. Anti-cholinergic adverse effects may be potentiated by concomitant use of morphine and medicines that block the action of acetylcholine (e.g., antihistamines, anti-parkinsonism, and antiemetics). Comedication and interactions of fentanyl and other medications is well described earlier in this chapter.

Together with pain medications, antidepressants, anticonvulsants, and/or anxiolytics can be used in selected patients. Amitriptyline, nortriptyline, and pregabalin can be used for the treatment of neuropathic pain and in combination with classical pain medications can be effective for the pain management in chronic pancreatitis. Amitriptyline [41] and nortriptyline [42] are tricyclic antidepressants that are contraindicated with MAO inhibitors and are not recommended with many various drugs including sympathomimetic agents, centrally acting antihypertensives, anticholinergic agents, drugs which prolong the QT interval, thioridazine, tramadol, and buprenorphine. Cimetidine, methylphenidate, and calcium-channel blockers (e.g., diltiazem and verapamil) may increase plasma levels of tricyclic antidepressants and therefore potentiate toxicity. Also, antifungals such as fluconazole, terbinafine, ketoconazole, and itraconazole have been observed to increase serum levels of amitriptyline and nortriptyline, and the same is with fluvoxamine. When amitriptyline or nortriptyline are used with valproic acid, their concentration may increase necessitating clinical monitoring. Pregabalin [43] is a safe medication in terms of pharmacokinetic interactions, with rare reports of possible interaction between pregabalin and CNS depressants.

Pancreatic exocrine insufficiency (PEI) is most commonly caused by chronic pancreatitis which among other pathophysiological mechanisms contributes to diarrhea, maldigestion, malabsorption, and weight loss [44]. Clinical evaluation of patient with suspected PEI is hampered by the lack of robust standardized diagnostic test especially for mild-to-moderate PEI, making clinical management of PEI including nonovert forms very challenging. Pancreatic exocrine replacement therapy (PERT) preparations can contain various enzymes such as lipase, amylase, protease, for which no interactions with other medications are described.

References

1. Knab LM, Boller A-M, Mahvi DM. Cholecystitis. Surg Clin North Am. 2014;94(2):455–70.
2. Ursodeoxycholic acid (UDCA), Summary of Product Characteristics (SPC). Available from: https://www.medicines.org.uk/emc/product/7253/smpc.
3. Wakabayashi G, Iwashita Y, Hibi T, Takada T, Strasberg SM, Asbun HJ, et al. Tokyo Guidelines 2018: surgical management of acute cholecystitis: safe steps in laparoscopic cholecystectomy for acute cholecystitis (with videos). J Hepatobiliary Pancreat Sci. 2018;25(1):73–86.
4. Okamoto K, Suzuki K, Takada T, Strasberg SM, Asbun HJ, Endo I, et al. Tokyo Guidelines 2018: flowchart for the management of acute cholecystitis. J Hepatobiliary Pancreat Sci. 2018;25(1):55–72.
5. Miura F, Okamoto K, Takada T, Strasberg SM, Asbun HJ, Pitt HA, et al. Tokyo Guidelines 2018: initial management of acute biliary infection and flowchart for acute cholangitis. J Hepatobiliary Pancreat Sci. 2018;25(1):31–40.
6. Manes G, Paspatis G, Aabakken L, Anderloni A, Arvanitakis M, Ah-Soune P, et al. Endoscopic management of common bile duct stones: European Society of Gastrointestinal Endoscopy (ESGE) guideline. Endoscopy. 2019;51(5):472–91.
7. Gomi H, Solomkin JS, Schlossberg D, Okamoto K, Takada T, Strasberg SM, et al. Tokyo Guidelines 2018: antimicrobial therapy for acute cholangitis and cholecystitis. J Hepatobiliary Pancreat Sci. 2018;25(1):3–16.
8. Ceftriaxone, Summary of Product Characteristics (SPC). Available from: https://www.medicines.org.uk/emc/product/7932/smpc.
9. Cefepime, Summary of Product Characteristics (SPC). Available from: https://www.medicines.org.uk/emc/product/9671/smpc.
10. Shenoy ES, Macy E, Rowe T, Blumenthal KG. Evaluation and management of penicillin allergy: a review. JAMA. 2019;321:188–99.
11. Picard M, Robitaille G, Karam F, Daigle JM, Bédard F, Biron É, et al. Cross-reactivity to cephalosporins and carbapenems in penicillin-allergic patients: two systematic reviews and meta-analyses. J Allergy Clin Immunol Pract. 2019;7(8):2722–2738.e5.
12. Zagursky RJ, Pichichero ME. Cross-reactivity in β-Lactam allergy. J Allergy Clin Immunol Pract. 2018;6(1):72–81.e1.
13. Ceftazidime, Summary of Product Characteristics (SPC). Available from: https://www.medicines.org.uk/emc/product/275/smpc.
14. Cefotaxime, Summary of Product Characteristics (SPC). Available from: https://www.medicines.org.uk/emc/product/8750/smpc.
15. Piperacillin/tazobactam, Summary of Product Characteristics (SPC). Available from: https://www.medicines.org.uk/emc/product/8757.
16. Meronem, Summary of Product Characteristics (SPC). Available from: https://www.medicines.org.uk/emc/product/9834/smpc.
17. Ciprofloxacin, Summary of Product Characteristics (SPC). Available from: https://www.medicines.org.uk/emc/product/885/smpc.

18. Levofloxacin, Summary of Product Characteristics (SPC). Available from: https://www.medicines.org.uk/emc/product/11107/smpc.
19. Paracetamol, Summary of Product Characteristics (SPC). Available from: https://www.medicines.org.uk/emc/product/11948/smpc.
20. Ketorlac, Summary of Product Characteristics (SPC). Available from: https://www.medicines.org.uk/emc/product/11546/smpc.
21. Diclofenac, Summary of Product Characteristics (SPC). Available from: https://www.medicines.org.uk/emc/product/2662/smpc.
22. Ketoprofen, Summary of Product Characteristics (SPC). Available from: https://www.medicines.org.uk/emc/product/2756/smpc.
23. Pethidine/meperidine, Summary of Product Characteristics (SPC). Available from: https://www.medicines.org.uk/emc/product/3402/smpc.
24. Oxycodone, Summary of Product Characteristics (SPC). Available from: https://www.medicines.org.uk/emc/product/5860/smpc.
25. Metoclopramide, Summary of Product Characteristics (SPC). Available from: https://www.medicines.org.uk/emc/product/6213/smpc.
26. Prochlorperazine, Summary of Product Characteristics (SPC). Available from: https://www.medicines.org.uk/emc/product/99/smpc.
27. Colestyramine, Summary of Product Characteristics (SPC). Available from: https://www.medicines.org.uk/emc/product/10588/smpc.
28. Colestipol, Summary of Product Characteristics (SPC). Available from: https://www.medicines.org.uk/emc/product/129/smpc.
29. Lindor KD, Kowdley KV, Harrison ME. ACG clinical guideline: primary sclerosing cholangitis. Am J Gastroenterol. 2015;110(5):646–59.
30. Chapman MH, Thorburn D, Hirschfield GM, Webster GGJ, Rushbrook SM, Alexander G, et al. British Society of Gastroenterology and UK-PSC guidelines for the diagnosis and management of primary sclerosing cholangitis. Gut. 2019;68:356–78.
31. Chapman R, Fevery J, Kalloo A, Nagorney DM, Boberg KM, Shneider B, et al. Diagnosis and management of primary sclerosing cholangitis. Hepatology. 2010;51:660–78.
32. Rifampicin, Summary of Product Characteristics (SPC). Available from: https://www.medicines.org.uk/emc/product/8789/smpc#gref.
33. Sertraline, Summary of Product Characteristics (SPC). Available from: https://www.medicines.org.uk/emc/product/10586/smpc.
34. Naltrexone, Summary of Product Characteristics (SPC). Available from: https://www.medicines.org.uk/emc/product/3559/smpc.
35. Hydromorphone, Summary of Product Characteristics (SPC). Available from: https://www.medicines.org.uk/emc/product/7690/smpc.
36. Fentanyl, Summary of Product Characteristics (SPC). Available from: https://www.medicines.org.uk/emc/product/2852/smpc.
37. Tenner S, Baillie J, DeWitt J, Vege SS, American College of Gastroenterology. American College of Gastroenterology Guideline: management of acute pancreatitis. Am J Gastroenterol. 2013;108(9):1400–15.
38. Working Group IAP/APA Acute Pancreatitis Guidelines. IAP/APA evidence-based guidelines for the management of acute pancreatitis. Pancreatology. 2013;13(4 Suppl. 2):e1–15.
39. Crockett SD, Wani S, Gardner TB, Falck-Ytter Y, Barkun AN, Crockett S, et al. American Gastroenterological Association Institute guideline on initial management of acute pancreatitis. Gastroenterology. 2018;154(4):1096–101.
40. Morphine, Summary of Product Characteristics (SPC). Available from: https://www.medicines.org.uk/emc/product/4689/smpc.
41. Amitriptyline, Summary of Product Characteristics (SPC). Available from: https://www.medicines.org.uk/emc/product/5698/smpc.

42. Nortriptyline, Summary of Product Characteristics (SPC). Available from: https://www.medicines.org.uk/emc/product/11267/smpc.
43. Pregabalin, Summary of Product Characteristics (SPC). Available from: https://www.medicines.org.uk/emc/product/2325/smpc.
44. Löhr JM, Dominguez-Munoz E, Rosendahl J, Besselink M, Mayerle J, Lerch MM, et al. United European Gastroenterology evidence-based guidelines for the diagnosis and therapy of chronic pancreatitis (HaPanEU). United Eur Gastroenterol J. 2017;5(2):153–99.

Comedication and Drug Interactions in Functional Gastrointestinal Disorders

32

Andreea Farcas, Camelia Bucsa, and Dan Dumitrascu

Abbreviations

AEs	Adverse effects
AV	Atrioventricular
CNS	Central nervous system
DDIs	Drug–drug interactions
EMA	European Medicines Agency
EU	European Union
GI	Gastrointestinal
IBS	Irritable bowel syndrome
IBS-D	IBS with diarrhea
IBS-C	IBS with constipation
MAOI	Monoamine oxidase inhibitor
NSAIDs	Non-steroidal anti-inflammatory drugs
OATP1B1	Organic anion transporter peptide
SSRIs	Selective serotonin reuptake inhibitors
TCAs	Tricyclic antidepressants

A. Farcas · C. Bucsa (✉)
Pharmacovigilance Research Center, Iuliu Hatieganu University of Medicine and Pharmacy, Cluj-Napoca, Cluj, Romania
e-mail: afarcas@umfcluj.ro; cfarah@umfcluj.ro

D. Dumitrascu
Department of Internal Medicine, Iuliu Hatieganu University of Medicine and Pharmacy, Cluj-Napoca, Romania
e-mail: ddumitrascu@umfcluj.ro

M. Banić, D. Erceg (eds.), *Drug Interactions in Gastroenterology*, Clinical Gastroenterology, https://doi.org/10.1007/978-3-031-69800-2_32

Irritable bowel syndrome (IBS) is the most common functional gastrointestinal disorder. It is a chronic condition characterized by recurrent abdominal discomfort or pain associated with altered bowel habits (diarrhea [IBS-D], constipation [IBS-C], or both [IBS-M]). The pharmacological treatment of IBS depends on the underlying symptoms and may include prokinetics, antidiarrheals, antispasmodics, probiotics, antidepressants, and newer medications for IBS-D (eluxadoline and rifaximin) and for IBS-C (prucalopride, lubiprostone, and linaclotide). More than one drug is often administered to chronic patients and the concomitant use of drugs raises the awareness of possible drug-drug interactions (DDIs). In this chapter, we offer an overview of the possible DDIs of the drugs used in IBS, with their potential effect, mechanism, and management.

Domperidone

Domperidone is a dopamine antagonist used as an antiemetic for short-term treatment of nausea and vomiting of various etiologies. In the European Union, it is not approved anymore for the management of symptoms such as bloating, discomfort and heartburn [1]. However, due to its prokinetic action, it can be used in functional disorders such as functional dyspepsia and irritable bowel syndrome [2].

The main metabolic pathway of domperidone is by cytochrome P450 isoenzyme CYP3A4; therefore, drugs that are potent inhibitors for this isoenzyme are expected to interact with domperidone [3, 4]. Moreover, domperidone itself has been associated with QT prolongation [5] and coadministration of drugs that prolong the QT interval is expected to have additive effects leading to serious cardiac outcomes [6].

The European Medicines Agency (EMA) has reviewed the existing evidence for the risk of serious cardiac adverse drug reactions related to the use of domperidone in 2013 to 2014. The agency confirmed that the risk of QTc prolongation, torsade de pointes, serious ventricular arrhythmia, and sudden cardiac death is increased with the use of oral domperidone, particularly at doses greater than 30 mg/day, in patients older than 60 years and in those taking QT-prolonging medicines or CYP3A4 inhibitors concomitantly. Following this review, domperidone was contraindicated when coadministered with QT-prolonging medicines or potent CYP3A4 inhibitors [1].

Different manufacturers list in their product label such as summary of product characteristics different drugs interacting with domperidone, being either CYP3A4 inhibitors or drugs prolonging the QT interval. We have summarized the most important ones and the wider used ones below.

Concurrent use of domperidone with potent CYP3A4 inhibitors (regardless of their effects on QT prolongation), such as:

- HIV-protease inhibitors (nelfinavir, ritonavir, and saquinavir)
- macrolides (erythromycin, clarithromycin, and telithromycin)
- systemic azole antifungals (itraconazole and ketoconazole)

may have light-threating or fatal outcome; therefore, concurrent use of domperidone with the above-mentioned drugs are **contraindicated** [1, 7, 8].

Concomitant use with moderate CYP3A4 inhibitors (i.e., diltiazem and verapamil) and some macrolides (azithromycin, roxithromycin) involved in QT-interval prolongation is not recommended [7]. If coadministration is necessary, domperidone should be initiated at the lowest possible dose and titrated with caution. Domperidone should be discontinued if the patient experiences dizziness, palpitations, syncope, or seizure [9].

Concurrent use of domperidone with drugs that prolong the QT interval is also **contraindicated**. A list of drugs that prolong the QT interval for which concomitant use with domperidone is contraindicated/ not recommended due to a potential for additive effects on QT-interval prolongation and an increased risk of serious cardiovascular effects is provided in Table 32.1. Other important drug interactions that should be considered for domperidone are presented in Table 32.2.

Table 32.1 Drugs known to prolong the QT interval for which concomitant use with domperidone is contraindicated [7–9]

Class	Drugs
Antiarrhythmics class IA	Disopyramide, procainamide, hydroquinidine, quinidine
Antiarrhythmics class III	Amiodarone, dofetilide, dronedarone, ibutilide, sotalol
Antipsychotics	Haloperidol, pimozide, sertindole, thioridazine, amisulpride, ziprasidone
Antidepressants	Citalopram, escitalopram, clomipramine
Antibiotics	Erythromycin, levofloxacin, moxifloxacin, gatifloxacin, spiramycin
Antifungal agents	Pentamidine (intravenous use)
Antimalarial	Halofantrine, lumefantrine
Antihistaminics	Mequitazine, mizolastine
Gastrointestinal medicines	Cisapride, ondansetron, dolasetron
Medicines used in cancer	Toremifene, vandetanib
Other medicines	Methadone, metronidazole

Table 32.2 Domperidone main drug–drug interactions and their potential effect, mechanism, and management [7–9]

Domperidone			
Interacting drug/ drug class	Potential effect	Mechanism	Management
Bromocriptine	Decreased bromocriptine efficacy (reduced prolactin lowering effect)	Antagonism at dopamine receptors	Alternatives for domperidone should be considered or close monitoring in order to ensure that bromocriptine effect remain positive
Lithium	Weakness, dyskinesias, increased extrapyramidal symptoms, encephalopathy, and brain damage	Unknown	Monitor patients closely for any signs of toxicity or extrapyramidal symptoms
Apomorphine[a]	Increased risk of QT-interval prolongation	Additive effects on the QT interval	Domperidone should be initiated at the lowest possible dose and titrated with caution. It should be discontinued if the patient experiences dizziness, palpitations, syncope, or seizure

[a]Domperidone is contraindicated with QT-prolonging drugs unless the benefit of the coadministration of apomorphine outweighs the risks. If coadministration is decided, risk factors in each individual patient should be carefully assessed before treatment initiation, and during treatment. Monitoring for an effect on the QTc interval by electrocardiogram is advisable. Important risk factors include serious underlying heart conditions such as congestive cardiac failure, severe hepatic impairment, or significant electrolyte disturbance. Also, medication possibly affecting electrolyte balance, CYP3A4 metabolism, or QT interval should be assessed [10]

Metoclopramide

Metoclopramide has prokinetic and antiemetic properties by stimulating the motility of the upper gastrointestinal tract and increasing gastric peristalsis, leading to accelerated gastric emptying and accelerated intestinal transit time [11]. For the prokinetic action, it can be used in functional disorders such as functional dyspepsia and irritable bowel syndrome [2]. Metoclopramide is known to be associated with extrapyramidal effects, including neuroleptic malignant syndrome [11], its utilization being restricted in the EU, where it is no longer to be used in chronic conditions such as gastroparesis, dyspepsia, and gastroesophageal reflux disease [12]. This recommendation was made within the EMA in order to mainly reduce the risk of neurological side effects.

Concomitant use of metoclopramide for injection with other drugs likely to cause extrapyramidal reactions (i.e., selective serotonin reuptake inhibitors [SSRIs], tricyclic antidepressants [TCAs], and antipsychotics) is contraindicated [9]. Coadministration of oral metoclopramide with serotoninergic antidepressants and neuroleptics was associated with several cases of extrapyramidal symptoms and should be regarded with caution [8, 13].

Levodopa or dopaminergic agonists and metoclopramide have a mutual antagonism [14] and their use should be avoided especially in patients with Parkinson disease, as it may result in exacerbation of Parkinson symptoms due to decreased efficacy of both agents [9]. Table 32.3 lists the most important drug interactions for metoclopramide.

Table 32.3 Metoclopramide main drug-drug interactions and their potential effect, mechanism, and management [8, 9, 13–20]

Metoclopramide			
Interacting drug/drug class	Potential effect	Mechanism	Management
Serotonin norepinephrine reuptake inhibitors Venlafaxine, desvenlafaxine, nefazodone, duloxetine	Increased risk of extrapyramidal reactions and neuroleptic malignant syndrome	Unknown	Patients should be monitored closely for signs of extrapyramidal reactions or neuroleptic malignant syndrome (fever, sweating, confusion, muscle stiffness). If adverse reactions occur, both agents should be discontinued (Micromedex)
SSRIs Fluvoxamine, sertraline citalopram, escitalopram			
Antipsychotics Thioridazine, haloperidol, prochlorperazine, chlorpromazine, trifluoperazine, aripiprazole, clozapine, pimozide, risperidone, olanzapine, sertindole, quetiapine, ziprasidone, amisulpride			
Anticholinergics and opioids	These drugs are commonly used together and the clinical significance of such effects is not clear	Anticholinergics and morphine derivatives may have both a mutual antagonism with metoclopramide on the digestive tract motility Metoclopramide increases the rate of absorption of oral morphine and sedative effects	NA

(continued)

Table 32.3 (continued)

Metoclopramide			
Interacting drug/drug class	Potential effect	Mechanism	Management
Digoxin	Decreased digoxin effectiveness	Metoclopramide may decrease digoxin bioavailability (reduced digoxin absorption)	Careful monitoring of digoxin plasma concentration is required and digoxin dose increase (by approximately 20–40% with oral preparations), if necessary, and continued monitoring
Cyclosporine	The clinical consequence is uncertain.	Metoclopramide increases cyclosporine bioavailability (Cmax by 46% and exposure by 22%)	Careful monitoring of cyclosporine plasma concentration is required and dosage adjustments as needed
Cimetidine	Decreased cimetidine effectiveness	Decreased absorption/ bioavailability	Cimetidine should be administered at least 2 h before the metoclopramide (Micromedex)
Strong CYP2D6 inhibitors: fluoxetine, paroxetine	Increased risk of metoclopramide adverse effects	Inhibition of CYP2D6-mediated metoclopramide metabolism	Decrease the metoclopramide dosage to 5 mg orally four times daily or 10 mg three times daily; maximum dose 20–30 mg/day depending on indication

SSRIs selective serotonin reuptake inhibitors

Loperamide

Loperamide inhibits gut motility and reduces gastrointestinal secretions, being used to treat acute or chronic diarrhea, including diarrhea from irritable bowel syndrome [11, 21]. Loperamide is a substrate for the cytochrome P450 isoenzymes CYP2C8 and CYP3A4 and also for glycoprotein-P. When coadministered with drugs that inhibit glycoprotein-P (quinidine, ritonavir) or CYP2C8 (gemfibrozil) or both CYP3A4 and glycoprotein-P (itraconazole, ketoconazole) exposure to loperamide might be increased up to four- to fivefold [11, 22, 23]. The main loperamide drug interactions are presented in Table 32.4.

Table 32.4 Loperamide main drug–drug interactions and their potential effect, mechanism, and management [8, 9, 11, 22, 24]

Loperamide			
Interacting drug/ drug class	Potential effect	Mechanism	Management
Saquinavir	Reduced antiviral efficacy of saquinavir	Interference of saquinavir absorption and reduction of bioavailability by 50%; reduced metabolic clearance and increased exposure of loperamide, with no clinically significant effect	Concomitant use should be avoided, especially for prolonged therapy
Ritonavir	Clinical relevance not clear, potential for loperamide adverse effects	Inhibition of P-glycoprotein-mediated loperamide metabolism	Monitor patients for adverse effects such as nausea, vomiting, dry mouth, dizziness, or drowsiness
Gemfibrozil	Clinical relevance not clear, potential for loperamide adverse effects	Inhibition of CYP2C8-mediated loperamide metabolism leading to significant increases in loperamide C_{max}, AUC, and the elimination half-life	Monitor patients for adverse effects such as nausea, vomiting, dry mouth, dizziness, or drowsiness
Itraconazole, ketoconazole	Clinical relevance not clear, potential for loperamide adverse effects	Inhibition of CYP3A4 and P-glycoprotein-mediated loperamide metabolism	Monitor patients for adverse effects such as nausea, vomiting, dry mouth, dizziness, or drowsiness
Quinidine	Clinical relevance not clear, potential for loperamide adverse effects	Inhibition of P-glycoprotein-mediated loperamide metabolism	Monitor patients for adverse effects such as nausea, vomiting, dry mouth, dizziness, or drowsiness
Desmopressin	Increased desmopressin plasma concentrations	Slower gastrointestinal motility	Monitor for desmopressin adverse effects

Trimebutine

The antispasmodic agent trimebutine has been effectively used to reduce colonic spasm, abdominal pain and distension, diarrhea, constipation, and flatulence in irritable bowel syndrome in clinical practice and in a few controlled studies [25–27].

The only reported drug interaction is with cisapride, due to pharmacodynamics antagonism, with loss of cisapride efficacy [9].

Table 32.5 Eluxadoline main drug-drug interactions and their potential effect, mechanism, and management [30]

Eluxadoline			
Interacting drug/drug class	Potential effect	Mechanism	Management
Alosetron, anticholinergics, opioids	Enhanced constipation	Additive constipating effect	Avoid combination
Topotecan	May increase the risk for topotecan toxicities	May increase the serum concentration of Topotecan	Avoid combination with oral topotecan; monitor closely for IV topotecan
Rosuvastatin	Increased exposure to rosuvastatin and risk of myopathy or rhabdomyolysis	Unknown	The lowest effective dose of rosuvastatin should be used
OATP1B1 inhibitors cyclosporine, gemfibrozil, antiretrovirals (atazanavir, lopinavir, ritonavir, saquinavir, tipranavir), rifampin	Increased systemic exposure to eluxadoline and risk of adverse effects	Unknown	Concomitant use should be avoided

OATP1B1 organic anion transporter peptide

Eluxadoline

Eluxadoline, a gut targeting μ and κ opioid receptor agonist and a δ opioid receptor antagonist, is used for the treatment of diarrhea predominant irritable bowel syndrome, improving stool consistency, and reducing abdominal pain [28, 29].

Eluxadoline is a substrate for the organic anion transporter peptide OATP1B1. Concomitant use of eluxadoline and OATP1B1 inhibitors can increase eluxadoline exposure with increased risk of adverse effects. The eluxadoline dose should be reduced from 100 mg twice daily to 75 mg twice daily if concurrent use is required, and patients should be monitored for impaired mental or physical abilities [9, 11]. Although not an interaction, chronic use of eluxadoline with loperamide or other medicinal products causing constipation (anticholinergics, opioids) should be avoided due to risk of constipation. Table 32.5 summarizes eluxadoline drug interactions.

Antidepressants

Antidepressants are used in the treatment of IBS for their effects on pain perception, quality of life, and motility. Although they were included in the therapy of IBS, when this was associated with depression and anxiety, antidepressants proved to be also effective against abdominal pain and global IBS symptoms independently of coexistent depression [21]. The antidepressant therapy was showed to improve the

IBS global symptoms by 20% over placebo [28]. There are two classes of antidepressants that are effective in the IBS, tricyclic antidepressants (TCAs), and selective serotonin reuptake inhibitors (SSRIs). Depending on the IBS type and the coexistence of psychological comorbidities, one of these agents may be used for the management of pain and motility [21].

Amitriptyline, imipramine, and desipramine (TCAs) are predominantly used in IBS-D patients for their analgesic and mood-altering effect but also because of their anticholinergic effects. They delay the gastrointestinal transit and by that decrease the frequency of stools and complaints of urgency in IBS-D [28]. The dosages used in IBS are lower than the antidepressant ones in order to avoid the adverse effects.

SSRIs at antidepressive dosages were showed to be effective especially in IBS-C because of their prokinetic effects [21]. Fluoxetine, paroxetine, and citalopram are the SSRIs most studied and used in IBS. Several randomized controlled trials that studied the effect of antidepressants in IBS showed that SSRIs significantly improved IBS symptoms such as pain, severity, bloating, and quality of life compared with placebo [31].

The disadvantage of using antidepressants in IBS is their risk of adverse effects (AEs). Dizziness, dry mouth, and constipation are commonly observed in multiple TCA trials, accounting for high drop-out rates in the treatment groups. In contrast, SSRI use is associated with nausea, vomiting, and diarrhea, making this less desirable in IBS-D [32]. DDIs in patient's therapy increase the risk of AEs. Both TCAs and SSRIs are substrates of several CYP450 enzymes and thus concomitant utilization with other drugs metabolized through the same pathway may lead to DDIs.

TCAs are metabolized mostly via CYP2D6, CYP2C19, CYP3A4, CYP2C9 by demethylation, hydroxylation, and oxidation [9]. When coadministered with other drugs that share the same pathway or drugs that induce or inhibit these enzymes the result might be an AE. Another possible mechanism of drug interaction is the additive toxicity of TCAs and concomitant antimuscarinic drugs or CNS depressants [11]. In addition, TCAs have a potential for QTc prolongation, so the administration of other drugs with effect on QT interval may increase the risk of cardiotoxicity (ventricular arrhythmia, QT prolongation, torsade de pointes, and cardiac arrest). See Table 32.6 for the DDIs that may occur due to the QT prolongation and serotoninergic effect. In Table 32.7 are listed other important DDIs of TCAs together with their potential effect and mechanism.

When TCAs are administered with SSRIs an increased risk of TCA toxicity, QT prolongation and serotonin syndrome may be expected [9].

In addition to being substrates of CYP450 enzymes SSRIs have also inhibitory properties mostly over CYP2D6 but also CYP1A2, CYP2C19, CYP3A4 and thus an increased potential for DDIs when used with drugs metabolized through these enzymes [9]. The serotoninergic properties of SSRIs can lead to an increased risk of serotonin syndrome if these are associated with other drugs that have this potential. Another serious risk for DDIs comes from the SSRIs' potential of QT-interval prolongation (see Table 32.8).

Table 32.6 Drugs that interact with tricyclic antidepressants resulting in QT-interval prolongation and serotoninergic effect [8, 9, 11, 33]

Potential effect Increased risk of cardiotoxicity (QT prolongation, torsade de pointes, and cardiac arrest)
Mechanism Additive effects on the QT interval

Interacting drug/drug class	Management
Antiarrhythmic agents class I (Disopyramide Flecainide, Lorcainide, Moricizine, Propafenone, Quinidine), *class III* (Acecainide, Amiodarone, Azimilide, Bretylium, Dronedarone, Ibutilide, Sematilide, Dofetilide, Sotalol), Bepridil, Ivabradine, *Antipsychotics* (Aripiprazole, Amisulpride, Asenapine, Chlorpromazine, Clozapine, Droperidol, Quetiapine, Iloperidone, Haloperidol, Mesoridazine, Paliperidone, Pimavanserin, Pimozide, Prochlorperazine, Risperidone, Sultopride, Thioridazine, Trifluoperazine, Ziprasidone, Zotepine, Zuclopenthixol), *Antidepressants* (Amoxapine, Clomipramine Venlafaxine, Trazodone), *Antihistaminics* (Astemizole, Terfenadine, Hydroxyzine, Promethazine), *5-HT$_3$ antagonists antiemetics* (Dolasetron, Ondansetron, Palonosetron, Granisetron), *Antineoplastic agents* (Tyrosine kinase inhibitors, Anagrelide, Glasdegib, Panobinostat), *Hormones/analogues and agonists* (Gonadorelin, Leuprolide, Goserelin, Degarelix, Deslorelin, Histrelin, Nafarelin), *Macrolides* (all), *Fluoroquinolones* (all, Grepafloxacin, Sparfloxacin), other *Antimicrobials* (Lefamulin, Pentamidine, Sulfamethoxazole, Metronidazole), *Antimalarials* (Artemether, Halofantrine, Hydroxychloroquine, Lumefantrine, Mefloquine, Piperaquine), *Anesthetics* (Enflurane, Halothane), *Prokinetics* (Cisapride, Domperidone) and Alfuzosin, Delamanid, Donepezil, Efavirenz, Fingolimod, Levomethadyl, Lofexidine, Octreotide, Pasireotide, Pitolisant, Tacrolimus, Vardenafil	Levomethadyl, Dronedarone, Bepridil, Mesoridazine, Pimozide, Thioridazine, Ziprasidone, Terfenadine, Grepafloxacin, Sparfloxacin, Piperaquine, Cisapride, are **contraindicated** in patients being treated with TCAs Major interactions for the rest; association is not recommended. Monitor the patient closely for QT-interval prolongation in case coadministration is necessary

Potential Effect Increased risk of serotonin syndrome (hypertension, hyperthermia, myoclonus, mental status changes)
Mechanism Additive serotonergic effect

Interacting drug/drug class	Management
Antimigraine drugs (*serotonin (5HT$_1$) agonists*, Lasmiditan), Buspirone, Chlorpheniramine, *MAOI* (selective and non-selective), Dextromethorphan, Milnacipran, Linezolid, Lithium, Lorcaserin, Metaxalone, Methylene Blue, *Atypical antidepressives* (Mirtazapine, Nefazodone), Vortioxetine, *HT$_3$ antagonists antiemetics* (Dolasetron, Ondansetron, Palonosetron, Granisetron), Oxycodone, Propoxyphene, Sibutramine, Tryptophan	MAOI, Linezolid and Methylene Blue are **contraindicated** in association with TCA Major interactions for the rest; association is not recommended. Monitoring of patient during treatment and dosage increases is recommended

Contraindicated association is listed if the association was deemed as such in at least one of the consulted references; TCAs, tricyclic antidepressants; MAOI, monoamine oxidase inhibitor

Table 32.7 Drugs that interact with tricyclic antidepressants and their potential effect, mechanism, and management [8, 9, 11, 33]

Interacting drug/drug class	Potential effect	Mechanism	Management
Calcium channel blockers (Diltiazem, Verapamil, piperazine derivates (Lidoflazine, Ranolazine))	Cardiotoxicity	Increased plasma concentration of TCAs	Concomitant use of TCAs and ranolazine is **contraindicated**
HIV-protease inhibitors (Ritonavir, Saquinavir, Lopinavir)	Increased risk of TCA AEs	Increased plasma concentration of TCA	Association with saquinavir is **contraindicated** Monitor patients for signs and symptoms of TCA toxicity
Bromopride, metoclopramide	Increased risk of extrapyramidal reactions	Additive extrapyramidal side effects	Concomitant use is **contraindicated**.
Furazolidone	Neurotoxicity, seizures, or serotonin syndrome	Altered catecholamine uptake and metabolism	**Contraindicated association**
Opioids and derivates (Alfentanil, Benzhydrocodone, Buprenorphine, Codeine, Levorphanol, Pethidine, Methadone, Morphine, Nalbuphine, Pentazocine, Tramadol), Scopolamine	Increased risk of serotonin syndrome and an increased risk of paralytic ileus	Additive serotonergic effects; additive effects on gastric motility	Discontinue opioid if serotonin syndrome is suspected; Monitor patients for signs of urinary retention or reduced gastric motility
NSAIDs	Increased risk of bleeding (intracranial hemorrhage within 30 days of concomitant use was reported)	Unknown	Monitor the patient for signs of increased bleeding
Acenocoumarol, Diflunisal, Phenindione, Phenprocoumon, Warfarin	Increased risk of bleeding	TCAs may increase the half-life and bioavailability of oral anticoagulants	The prothrombin time ratio or INR (international normalized ratio) should be closely monitored
Albuterol (Salbutamol)	Increased risk of cardiovascular system effects (e.g., tachycardia and blood pressure changes)	Potentiation of vascular effects of albuterol	Albuterol should be administered with extreme caution to patients being treated with TCAs, or within 2 weeks of TCA discontinuation

(continued)

Table 32.7 (continued)

Interacting drug/drug class	Potential effect	Mechanism	Management
Simpatomimetics (Adrenaline, Noradrenaline, Ephedrine, Isoprenaline)	Severe prolonged hypertension	Inhibition of vasopressor reuptake	Association should be avoided
Clonidine, Guanetidine, Debrisochine, Betanidine	Decreased antihypertensive effectiveness	Pharmacological antagonism at central alpha-2 receptors	Blood pressure should be monitored for an appropriate clinical response; higher doses of clonidine may be required
Barbiturates	Lowering of convulsive thresholds; increased metabolism of the TCA with decreased serum concentrations	Antagonization of the antiepileptic activity; increased TCA metabolism	Monitor for toxicity when either drug is added to or withdrawn from therapy
Carbamazepine	Decreased TCA effectiveness	Increased amitriptyline metabolism induced by carbamazepine	Monitor for clinical efficacy of the amitriptyline therapy and for any signs of toxicity of carbamazepine
Valproate	Increased risk of TCA AEs (anticholinergic effects, sedation, confusion, cardiac arrhythmias)	Increased plasma concentration of TCAs	Monitor patients for signs and symptoms of TCA toxicity
Phenytoin	Increased risk of phenytoin toxicity (ataxia, hyperreflexia, nystagmus, tremor)	Inhibition of phenytoin metabolism	Monitor serum phenytoin levels
Cimetidine	Amitriptyline toxicity (dry mouth, blurred vision, urinary retention)	Decreased amitriptyline metabolism	If co-administration is required, lower than usual TCA doses may be needed
Fluconazole, Ketoconazole, Posaconazole, Terbinafine, Voriconazole	Increased plasma concentration of TCAs, syncope, torsade de pointes	Additive prolongation of cardiac conduction time	Measure and adjust TCA dosage if necessary
Insulin, *Sulphonylureas*	Decrease insulin requirements	TCA antihyperglycemic activity may decrease insulin requirements	Glycemic monitoring

(continued)

Table 32.7 (continued)

Interacting drug/drug class	Potential effect	Mechanism	Management
Diazepam, Loxapine	Psychomotor deficits (decreased reaction time, decreased vigilance) and an increased risk of respiratory depression, hypotension, profound sedation, and syncope	Additive psychomotor deficits and CNS depression	If co-administration is necessary, consider a dose reduction of the CNS depressant
Estrogens	The pharmacologic effects of tricyclic antidepressants may be increased or decreased by estrogens, with paradoxical loss of antidepressant effect yet tricyclic toxicity being manifested simultaneously	Possible estrogen-enhanced hepatic metabolism of the tricyclic	Dose adjustment downward of either the estrogen or tricyclic component
Diphenhydramine, Glycopyrrolate, Glycopyrronium, Tiotropium	Increased anticholinergic effects (dry mouth, urinary retention)	Additive anticholinergic effects	Lower doses of diphenhydramine should be considered
Peginterferon Alfa-2b	Increased plasma concentrations of TCA metabolized by CYP2D6 and increased risk for toxicities	Inhibition of CYP2D6-mediated metabolism of TCAs by peginterferon alfa-2b	Monitor levels of tricyclic antidepressants when co-administered with a CYP2D6 inhibitor

Contraindicated association is listed if the association was deemed as such in at least one of the consulted references; *TCAs* tricyclic antidepressants, *NSAIDs* non-steroidal anti-inflammatory drugs, *AEs* adverse effects, *CNS* central nervous system

Other new drugs like lubiprostone, linaclotide, and prucalopride may be used in the treatment of IBS with constipation. The evidence for these drug's interactions are either not available yet or the evidence are weak.

Probiotics may have beneficial effects in reducing bloating and flatulence associated with IBS. The probiotics used most frequently in the treatment of IBS include *Lactobacillus* and *Bifidobacterium* strains. As probiotics contain live microorganisms, antibiotics may inactivate them reducing the efficacy of the *Lactobacillus* and *Bifidobacterium* species. It is recommended to separate their administration by at least 2 h. Probiotics should also be used cautiously in patients taking immunosuppressants, such as cyclosporine, tacrolimus, azathioprine, and chemotherapeutic agents, since probiotics could cause an infection or pathogenic colonization in immunocompromised patients [36].

Table 32.8 Selective serotonin reuptake inhibitors main drug-drug interactions and their potential effect, mechanism, and management [8, 9, 11, 34, 35]

Interacting drug/drug class	Potential effect	Mechanism	Management
MAOI, Procarbazine, Linezolid, Furazolidone, Methylene blue, *Anorexigenics* (Lorcaserin, Fenfluramină, Sibutramină), *Antidepressives* (Atomoxetine, Duloxetine, Desvenlafaxine, Trazodone, Milnacipran, Mirtazapine, Venlafaxine), Buspirone, *Ergot derivates*, *Opioids* (Codeine, Dextromethorphan, Fentanyl, Hydrocodone, Morphine, Oxycodone, Pentazocine, Pethidine, Tramadol), *Antiepileptics* (Oxcarbazepine, Carbamazepine, Phenytoin), *Serotonin* ($5HT_1$) *agonists* (triptans), Tryptophan, Lithium, Venlafaxine, Ziprasidone	Increased risk of serotonin syndrome (hypertension, hyperthermia, myoclonus, mental status changes) The analgesic effect of codeine and hydrocodone may be reduced by fluoxetine and paroxetine	Inhibition of metabolization and/or serotonin additive effect	**Contraindicated association** for MAOI, Procarbazine, Linezolid, Furazolidone, Methylene blue, Ziprasidone **Major** DDI for the rest with close patient monitoring
Antipsychotics (Pimozide, *Phenothiazines*, Clozapine, Thioridazine, Ziprasidone), Levomethadyl *Fluoroquinolones* (Sparfloxacin, Gatifloxacin, Moxifloxacin, Gemifloxacin), *Macrolides* (Erythromycin, Clarithromycin, Spiromycin, Azithromycin, Telithromycin), other *Antimicrobials* (Chloramphenicol, Pentamidine), Saquinavir, Piperaquine, *Antiarrhythmic agents Class I* (flecainide, propafenone), *II* (propranolol, metoprolol) and *III* (Amiodarone, Dronedarone, Sotalol), Bepridil, Foscarnet, Cisapride, Domperidone, *Anesthetics* (Enflurane, Halothane), *Antifungals* (Fluconazole, Itraconazole), HT_3 *antagonists antiemetics* (Ondansetron, Dolasetron, Granisetron), Omeprazole, *Antidepressants* (Duloxetine, Trazodone), Eliglustat, Terfenadine	Increased risk of QT-interval prolongation, torsade de pointes, cardiac arrest	Inhibition of metabolization and/or QT-interval prolongation additive effect	**Contraindicated association** for Antipsychotics (Pimozide, *Phenothiazines*, Thioridazine, Ziprasidone), Levomethadyl, Sparfloxacin, Saquinavir, Piperaquine, Dronedarone, Bepridil, Cisapride, Eliglustat, Terfenadine **Major** DDI for the rest with recommendation of close patient monitoring
Tamoxifen	Decreased efficacy of tamoxifen	Paroxetine, Fluoxetine inhibit the CYP2D6 metabolization of tamoxifen to its active metabolite, endoxifen	**Contraindicated association**

Tizanidine	Hypotension, bradycardia, sedation	Marked increase in tizanidine exposure	**Contraindicated association**
Neuromuscular blockers (Mivacurium, Suxamethonium)	Prolongation of neuromuscular blockade	Decreased plasma activity of cholinesterase	NA
Betablockers (Propranolol, Carvedilol, Metoprolol)	Increased risk of bradycardia and AV block	Inhibition of betablocker metabolization through CYP2D6	Clinically more likely to be important for metoprolol + fluoxetine, especially for patients with heart failure, where the combination is contraindicated
NSAIDs, *Anticoagulants* (Acenocumarol, *Heparins*, Warfarină, Apixaban), *Antiplatelets* (Aspirin, Dipyridamole, Ticlopidine, Clopidogrel, Ticagrelor, Ticlopidine)	Increased risk of GI bleeding	Additive effects on bleeding	Caution on the concurrent use of drugs affecting the platelet function; consider adding a PPI, when patient has a high risk of GI bleeding Anticoagulants interact mostly with fluvoxamine, but caution for all SSRIs
Benzodiazepines (Alprazolam, Diazepam), Antidepressives (Atomoxetine, Trazodone)	Increased risk of sedation	Increased plasma concentration of diazepam	Clinically more likely to be important for benzodiazepines + fluoxetine
Phenytoin	Increases risk of phenytoin toxicity (ataxia, hyperreflexia, nystagmus, tremor)	Increased levels of phenytoin	Monitor for early signs of phenytoin toxicity
Bupropione	Psychosis, mania, seizures, serotonin syndrome	Inhibition of CYP2D6 metabolization of bupropione	May need to decrease the dose of SSRI
Metoclopramide, bromopride	Extrapyramidal symptoms		Monitoring for extrapyramidal reactions or neuroleptic malignant syndrome (fever, sweating, confusion, muscle stiffness). If adverse reactions occur, both agents should be discontinued

Contraindicated association is listed if the association was deemed as such in at least one of the consulted references; *NA* information not available, *MAOI* monoamine oxidase inhibitor, *DDI* drug–drug interaction, *AV* atrio-ventricular, *NSAIDs* nonsteroidal anti-inflammatory drugs, *GI* gastrointestinal, *SSRIs* selective serotonin reuptake inhibitors

References

1. European Medicines Agency (EMA): Restrictions on the use of domperidone-containing medicines. European Medicines Agency (EMA). London, United Kingdom. 2014. Available from https://www.ema.europa.eu/en/documents/referral/domperidone-article-31-referral-restrictions-use-domperidone-containing-medicines_en.pdf. Accessed 12 Oct 2019
2. Quigley EMM. Prokinetics in the management of functional gastrointestinal disorders. Curr Gastroenterol Rep. 2017;19(10):53.
3. Templeton I, Ravenstijn P, Sensenhauser C, Snoeys J. A physiologically based pharmacokinetic modeling approach to predict drug-drug interactions between domperidone and inhibitors of CYP3A4. Biopharm Drug Dispos. 2016;37(1):15–27.
4. Boyce MJ, Baisley KJ, Warrington SJ. Pharmacokinetic interaction between domperidone and ketoconazole leads to QT prolongation in healthy volunteers: a randomized, placebo-controlled, double-blind, crossover study. Br J Clin Pharmacol. 2012;73(3):411–21.
5. Straus SM, Sturkenboom MC, Bleumink GS, Dieleman JP, van der Lei J, de Graeff PA, Kingma JH, Stricker BH. Non-cardiac QTc-prolonging drugs and the risk of sudden cardiac death. Eur Heart J. 2005;26(19):2007–12.
6. Buffery PJ, Strother RM. Domperidone safety: a mini-review of the science of QT prolongation and clinical implications of recent global regulatory recommendations. N Z Med J. 2015;128(1416):66–74.
7. National Agency for medicines and medical devices of Romania. Motilium (Terapia) summary of product characteristics. Available from https://www.anm.ro/_/_RCP/rcp_2068_20.10.09.pdf. Accessed 12 Oct 2019.
8. Preston CL, editor. Stockley's drug interactions. Pocket companion. London: Pharmaceutical Press; 2016.
9. Micromedex. IBM Micromedex® Drug Interaction Checking (electronic version). IBM Watson Health, Greenwood Village, Colorado, USA (cited: 12/10/2019).
10. National Agency for Medicines and Medical Devices of Romania. APO-GO 10 mg/ml (STADA Arzneimittel AG) summary of product characteristics. Available from https://www.anm.ro/_/_RCP/rcp_4186_24.01.12.pdf. Accessed 12 Oct 2019.
11. Alison B, editor. Martindale. The complete drug reference. 39th ed. London: Pharmaceutical Press; 2017.
12. European Medicines Agency (EMA): European Medicines Agency recommends changes to the use of metoclopramide. European Medicines Agency (EMA). London, United Kingdom. 2013. Available from https://www.ema.europa.eu/en/medicines/human/referrals/metoclopramide-containing-medicines. Accessed 12 Oct 2019.
13. Baxter K, editor. Stockley's drug interactions. 9th ed. London: Pharmaceutical Press; 2010.
14. National Agency for Medicines and Medical Devices of Romania. Metoclopramid (Terapia) summary of product characteristics. Available from https://www.anm.ro/_/_RCP/RCP_8519_14.01.16.pdf. Accessed 12 Oct 2019.
15. Manara AR, Shelly MP, Quinn K, Park GR. The effect of metoclopramide on the absorption of oral controlled release morphine. Br J Clin Pharmacol. 1988;25:518–21.
16. McNeill MJ, Ho ET, Kenny GNC. Effect of i.v. metoclopramide on gastric emptying after opioid premedication. Br J Anaesth. 1990;64:450–2.
17. Manninen V, Apajalahti A, Melin J, Karesoja M. Altered absorption of digoxin in patients given propantheline and metoclopramide. Lancet. 1973;301:398–400.
18. Wadhwa NK, Schroeder TJ, O'Flaherty E, et al. The effect of oral metoclopramide on the absorption of cyclosporine. Transplant Proc. 1987;19:1730–3.
19. Gugler R, Brand M, Somogyi A. Impaired cimetidine absorption due to antacids and metoclopramide. Eur J Clin Pharmacol. 1981;20:225–8.
20. Barzaghi N, Crema F, Mescoli G, Perucca E. Effects on cimetidine bioavailability of metoclopramide and antacids given two hours apart. Eur J Clin Pharmacol. 1989;37:409–10.

21. Moayyedi P, Mearin F, Azpiroz F, Andresen V, Barbara G, Corsetti M, et al. Irritable bowel syndrome diagnosis and management: a simplified algorithm for clinical practice. United Eur Gastroenterol J. 2017;5(6):773–88.
22. National Agency for Medicines and Medical Devices of Romania. Imodium (MCNEIL HEALTHCARE (IRELAND) LIMITED) summary of product characteristics. Available from https://www.anm.ro/_/_RCP/RCP_11594_29.03.19.pdf. Accessed 12 Oct 2019.
23. Niemi M, Tornio A, Pasanen MK, et al. Itraconazole, gemfibrozil and their combination markedly raise the plasma concentrations of loperamide. Eur J Clin Pharmacol. 2006;62(6):463–72.
24. Mikus G, Schmidt L, Burhenne J, et al. Reduction of saquinavir exposure by coadministration of loperamide: a two-way pharmacokinetic interaction. Clin Pharmacokinet. 2004;43(14):1015–24.
25. Luttecke K. A trial of trimebutine in spastic colon. J Int Med Res. 1978;6:86–8.
26. Moshal MG, Herron M. A clinical trial of trimebutine (Mebutin) in spastic colon. J Int Med Res. 1979;7:231–4.
27. Luttecke K. A three-part controlled study of trimebutine in the treatment of irritable colon syndrome. Curr Med Res Opin. 1980;6:437.
28. Rivkin A, Rybalov S. Update on the Management of Diarrhea-predominant irritable bowel syndrome: focus on rifaximin and eluxadoline. Pharmacotherapy. 2016;36(3):300–16.
29. Weber HC. New treatment options for irritable bowel syndrome with predominant diarrhea. Curr Opin Endocrinol Diabetes Obes. 2017;24(1):25–30.
30. Food and Drug Administration. VIBERZI. Highlights of prescribing information. Available from https://www.accessdata.fda.gov/drugsatfda_docs/label/2016/206940s001lbl.pdf. Accessed 08 Dec 2023.
31. Kułak-Bejda A, Bejda G, Waszkiewicz N. Antidepressants for irritable bowel syndrome—a systematic review. Pharmacol Rep. 2017;69(6):1366–79.
32. Nee J, Zakari M, Lembo AJ. Current and emerging drug options in the treatment of diarrhea predominant irritable bowel syndrome. Expert Opin Pharmacother. 2015;16(18):2781–92.
33. National Agency for Medicines and Medical Devices of Romania. Amitriptilina Arena (ARENA GROUP S.A.—ROMANIA) summary of product characteristics. Available from https://www.anm.ro/_/_RCP/rcp_5704_15.09.05.pdf. Accessed 12 Oct 2019.
34. National Agency for Medicines and Medical Devices of Romania. Seroxat (GLAXOSMITHKLINE (IRELAND) LIMITED—IRLANDA) summary of product characteristics. Available from https://www.anm.ro/_/_RCP/rcp_601_18.03.08.pdf. Accessed 12 Oct 2019.
35. National Agency for Medicines and Medical Devices of Romania. Prozac (ELI LILLY SA—SPANIA) Summary of product characteristics. Available from https://www.anm.ro/_/_RCP/RCP_11794_23.05.19.pdf. Accessed 12 Oct 2019.
36. Williams NT. Probiotics. Am J Health-Syst Pharm. 2010;67(6):449–58.

Index

M. Banić, D. Erceg (eds.), *Drug Interactions in Gastroenterology*, Clinical Gastroenterology, https://doi.org/10.1007/978-3-031-69800-2

MIX
Papier aus verantwortungsvollen Quellen
Paper from responsible sources
FSC® C105338

If you have any concerns about our products,
you can contact us on
ProductSafety@springernature.com

In case Publisher is established outside the EU,
the EU authorized representative is:
Springer Nature Customer Service Center GmbH
Europaplatz 3, 69115 Heidelberg, Germany

Printed by Libri Plureos GmbH
in Hamburg, Germany